Taurine and the Mitochondrion: Applications in the Pharmacotherapy of Human Diseases

Authored By

Reza Heidari
Pharmaceutical Sciences Research Center
Shiraz University of Medical Sciences
Shiraz, Iran

&

M. Mehdi Ommati
Henan Key Laboratory of Environmental
and Animal Product Safety
College of Animal Science and Technology
Henan University of Science and Technology
Luoyang 471000
Henan, China

Taurine and the Mitochondrion:
Applications in the Pharmacotherapy of Human Diseases

Authors: Reza Heidari and M. Mehdi Ommati

ISBN (Online): 978-981-5124-48-4

ISBN (Print): 978-981-5124-49-1

ISBN (Paperback): 978-981-5124-50-7

First published in 2023.

need for a court order if at any point you breach any terms of this License Agreement. In no event will any delay or failure by Bentham Science Publishers in enforcing your compliance with this License Agreement constitute a waiver of any of its rights.

3. You acknowledge that you have read this License Agreement, and agree to be bound by its terms and conditions. To the extent that any other terms and conditions presented on any website of Bentham Science Publishers conflict with, or are inconsistent with, the terms and conditions set out in this License Agreement, you acknowledge that the terms and conditions set out in this License Agreement shall prevail.

Bentham Science Publishers Pte. Ltd.
80 Robinson Road #02-00
Singapore 068898
Singapore
Email: subscriptions@benthamscience.net

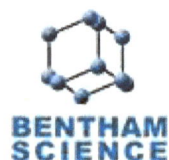

BENTHAM SCIENCE

CONTENTS

PREFACE

The use of safe molecules for treating diseases has always been of special interest in medical sciences. During research on the application of potential drug candidates for the treatment and prevention of human disease, the application of the amino acid taurine received attention from the authors. The use of the amino acid taurine in the treatment of human diseases has also attracted the attention of many researchers in various fields of biomedical sciences. Numerous studies revealed that taurine could treat and prevent a wide range of diseases by affecting the fundamental signaling pathways and cellular function. The effect of taurine on mitochondria is one of this substance's key mechanisms in preventing cell damage. In the present book, the effects of taurine on mitochondria and its relationship with the treatment of various human diseases have been given special attention and widely discussed. Researchers in biomedical sciences could widely use the data provided in this book. We hope that attention to compounds such as the amino acid taurine, a safe molecule that causes no significant side effects even at very high doses, can lead to the development of new and effective strategies in the pharmacotherapy of various human diseases.

CONSENT FOR PUBLICATION

Not applicable.

CONFLICT OF INTEREST

The author declares no conflict of interest, financial or otherwise.

ACKNOWLEDGEMENT

The current study was financially supported by the Vice-Chancellor of Research Affairs, Shiraz University of Medical Sciences, Shiraz, Iran (Grants: 12203/12028/11738/ 12806/12243/23158/23024/16259/13555).

Reza Heidari
Pharmaceutical Sciences Research Center
Shiraz University of Medical Sciences
Shiraz, Iran

&

M. Mehdi Ommati
Henan Key Laboratory of Environmental and Animal Product Safety
College of Animal Science and Technology
Henan University of Science and Technology
Luoyang 471000, Henan, China

The authors contributed equally to this book

DEDICATION

"Everything passes and vanishes; Everything leaves its trace; And often, you see in a footstep What you could not see in a face!" William Allingham

Dedicated to my beloved ones!

Reza Heidari

Mainly thanks to my wife (Samira Sabouri) and my lovely son (Adrian Ommati), who provide a calm and happy environment to create this work. I dedicate it to my parents (Mr. Hossein Ommati and Mrs. Akram Pirouzfar) for all the support and valuable things they have taught me and for their sincere love.

M. Mehdi Ommati

CHAPTER 1

Taurine: Synthesis, Dietary Sources, Homeostasis, and Cellular Compartmentalization

Abstract: Taurine (β-amino acid ethane sulfonic acid; TAU) is a sulfur-containing amino acid abundant in the human body. Although TAU does not corporate in the protein structure, many vital physiological properties have been attributed to this amino acid. TAU could be synthesized endogenously in hepatocytes or come from nutritional sources. It has been found that the source of body TAU varies significantly between different species. For instance, some species, such as foxes and felines, are entirely dependent on the nutritional sources of TAU. On the other hand, TAU is readily synthesized in the liver of animals such as rats and dogs. The TAU synthesis capability of the human liver is negligible, and we receive this amino acid from food sources. The distribution of TAU also greatly varies between various tissues. Skeletal muscle and the heart tissue contain a very high concentration of TAU. At subcellular levels, mitochondria are the primary targets for TAU compartmentalization. It has been found that TUA also entered the nucleus and endoplasmic reticulum. The current chapter discusses the synthetic process and dietary sources of TAU. Then, the transition of TAU to sub-cellular compartments will be addressed. Finally, the importance of TAU homeostasis in the pathogenesis of human disease is mentioned.

Keywords: Amino acid, Food sources, Human disease, Mitochondrion, Mitochondrial cytopathies, Nutraceuticals, Nutrition.

INTRODUCTION

Using endogenous compounds with minimum adverse effects has always been a plausible approach to managing human diseases. In this context, since its discovery in the OX bile in 1827, taurine (TAU) has become the subject of a plethora of investigations in biomedical sciences [1]. Many physiological roles have been detected for TAU. Nowadays, it is well-known that TAU acts as an osmolyte in many biological systems, contributes to many metabolic processes such as bile acids conjugation, and even could be applied as a biomarker on some occasions [2 - 6].

Although TAU is readily synthesized in the liver of many species (*e.g.*, Dogs), some other species, including humans, depend on the dietary sources of this compound [7]. It has been found that some tissues such as the skeletal muscle, heart, brain, and reproductive organs contain a huge amount of TAU in humans. Hence, this amino acid could play a pivotal role in the function of these organs.

Several pharmacological roles have also been identified for TAU, and these effects are growing every year. It has been found that TAU could protect different organs against xenobiotics, provide neuroprotective properties, mitigate skeletal muscle damage and enhance its functionality, improve human reproductive indices, prevent and/or cure cardiovascular disease, provide protection against liver diseases and many other pharmacological properties [8 - 26].

As mentioned, we receive our body TAU from dietary sources. Several TAU-rich foodstuffs have been identified. Seafood is rich in TAU. Hence, in countries that consume the types of foods (*e.g.*, Japan), people benefit from the positive effects of TAU. On the other hand, there is no TAU in herbal products, and herbivores could develop signs of TAU deficiency.

In the current chapter, the dietary sources of TAU are introduced, its absorption from the gastrointestinal tract is discussed, a brief overview of the synthesis of this amino acid in the liver is highlighted, its distribution in different organs is mentioned, and finally, its cellular compartmentalization is described.

TAURINE SYNTHESIS, DIETARY SOURCES, AND CELLULAR COMPARTMENTALIZATION

Taurine (β-amino acid ethane sulfonic acid; TAU) is endogenously synthesized in the liver hepatocytes from the amino acid cysteine and methionine [6, 27, 28] (Fig. **1**). Hence, the liver is the main organ responsible for TAU synthesis. The endogenous synthesis of TAU occurs *via* the cysteine sulfinic acid pathway (Fig. **1**). The enzyme responsible for TAU synthesis is dependent on cysteine bioavailability [28, 29]. Thus, TAU synthesis is dependent on the amount of protein intake and the availability of the precursor amino acids (methionine and cysteine) [6]. On the other hand, the ability of hepatocytes to synthesize TAU is widely variant between different species [30, 31]. Some species, such as foxes and felines, are entirely dependent on the dietary sources of TAU [30, 31]. TAU deficiency in these species could lead to severe anomalies, including retinal degeneration, cardiovascular disturbances, reproduction defects, and even animal death [30 - 34]. This evidence mentions the key physiological roles of TAU in some mammalians. Cysteine sulfonate decarboxylase (CSD) activity as a rate-limiting enzyme involved in TAU synthesis has been measured in the liver of various species (Table **1**). The activity of this enzyme in humans, as well as cats, is negligible (Table **1**). On the other hand, animals such as dogs and rats have a considerable CSD activity in their liver (Table **1**) [1]. Hence, they could readily synthesize TAU from methionine and cysteine (Fig. **1**) and do not need to intake TAU from dietary sources [35].

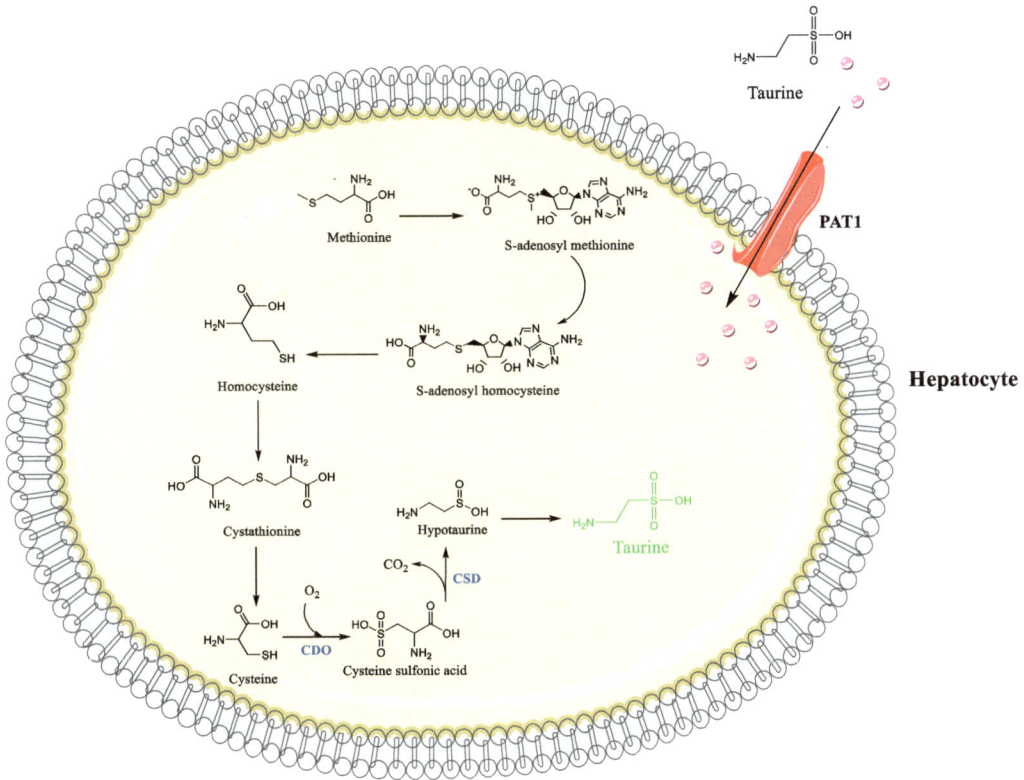

Fig. (1). Specific transporters uptake TAU from the bloodstream to various organs. The TAU uptake capability of different organs is widely varied. Taurine (TAU) is also endogenously synthesized in hepatocytes. TAU synthesis capability of some species such as fox and felines is very low, and these species are entirely dependent on the dietary sources of TAU. TAU could be readily uptaken by cells through transporters (*e.g.*, PAT1). The capacity of our hepatocytes is negligible for TAU synthesis. Thus, humans also greatly rely on the nutritional origins of TAU. CDO: Cysteine deoxygenase; CSD: Cysteinesulfinate decarboxylase; PAT1: Polyamine transporter 1.

It has been found that CSD activity is exceptionally high in oysters (*e.g.*, *Crassostrea gigas*). Therefore, oysters are an excellent food source of TAU in some regions [36] (Fig. **2**). Interestingly, approximately 80% of the total amino-acid content of oysters is TAU [36]. Oysters are widely used in England, Japan, Italy, and Spain [36].

Table 1. The activity of cysteine sulfinic acid decarboxylase (CSD) in the liver of different species.

Species	Liver CSD Enzyme Activity	References
Human	-	[1, 35]
Cat	-	[1, 35]
Fox	-	[1, 35]
Horse	-	[35]
Dog	++++	[35]
Cow	+	[35]
Rabbit	+	[35]
Mouse	++	[35]
Rat	++++	[1, 35]
Guinea pig	++	[35]

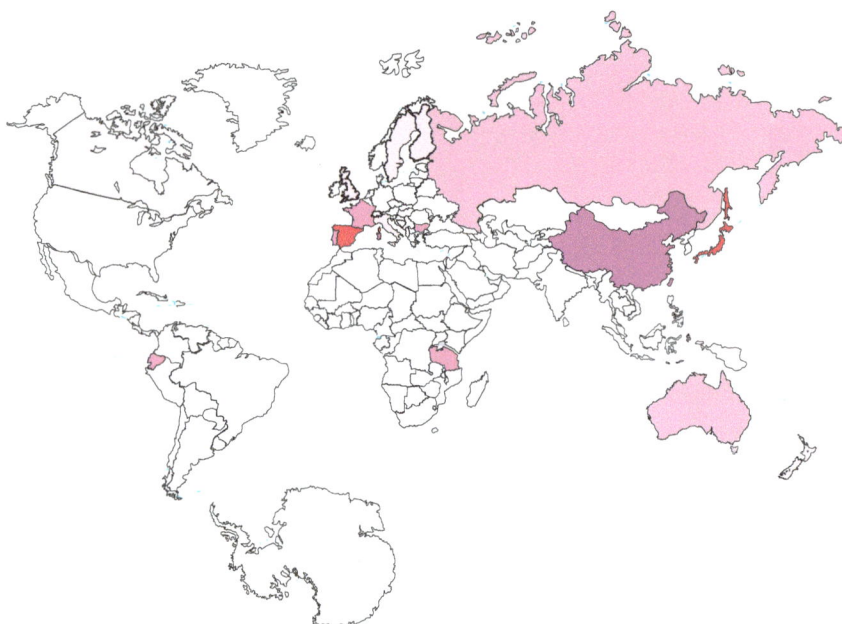

Fig. (2). A schematic representation of the geographic distribution of taurine excretion in urine (and probably most taurine consumption) in different world regions. This figure is re-drawn from the same figure from the manuscript https://doi.org/10.1002/mnfr.201800569. Darker colors indicate the higher consumption of taurine. Japan and Spain are among the most taurine-consuming countries. For countries with no color, no reliable data is available so far.

A schematic presentation of TAU excretion (and probably most TAU-consumed countries) is given in Fig. (**2**). As mentioned, the TAU synthesis capability of the human liver is negligible (Table **1**). Therefore, we also depend on nutritional TAU sources [37 - 39]. While seafood contains the highest taurine concentrations, based on Fig. (**2**), Spain and Japan are the most TAU-consuming countries in the world. Other countries such as France, Russia, China, Australia, Sweden, Finland, Bulgaria, Ecuador, New Zealand, and Tanzania have relatively higher TAU consumption [40] (Fig. **2**). Interestingly, some studies mentioned that higher TAU consumption in countries such as Japan (Fig. **2**) could be related to a lower prevalence of diseases such as cardiovascular complications [41 - 44].

Despite very high concentrations of TAU in tissues such as the lung [45], spleen, and reproductive organs (Fig. **3**), the roles of this amino acid in these systems largely remain unknown. However, some human studies mentioned the osmoregulatory properties of TAU as a physiological role of this amino acid in these organs. Besides, further studies are needed to reveal the exact mechanism of TAU action in biological systems.

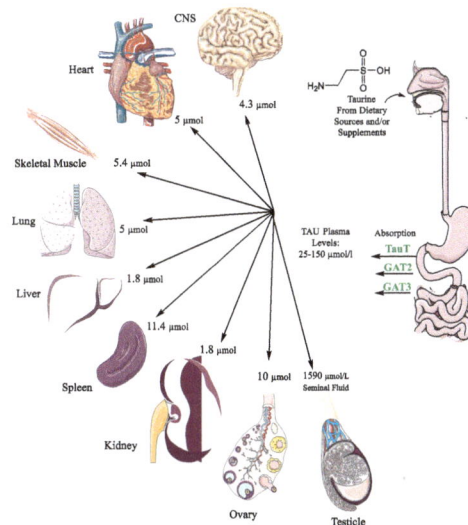

Fig. (3). Tissue distribution of taurine in humans. Concentrations are given as μmol TAU/g tissue wet weight. The ovary TAU level is reported in rats. The written TAU content of human tissues is adapted from "DOI: 10.1152/physrev.1968.48.2.424". TauT: Na$^+$/Cl$^-$-dependent taurine transporter; GAT: γ-aminobutyric acid (GABA) transporter.

It has been found that TAU could readily be absorbed through the small intestinal brush border through specific TAU transporters (TauT, GAT2, and GAT3), resulting in a high plasma concentration of this amino acid [6] (Fig. **3**). It has been found that some factors could influence TAU absorption from the intestine. For instance, some investigations revealed that inflammatory cytokine increases TAU absorption where diseases such as diabetes suppress the intestinal absorption of this amino acid [46 - 49]. When TAU reaches the bloodstream, it is distributed to different organs through TAU transporters (TauT) and polyamine transporters 1 (PAT1) [6] (Fig. **3**).

The γ-aminobutyric acid (GABA) transporter 2 (GAT2) is another crucial transporter identified for TAU uptake by some cell types such as hepatocytes [50]. Because of the active transport of TAU from the bloodstream to the cells, the concentration of this amino acid in plasma is approximately 100 fold lower than its tissue level (Fig. **3**). On the other hand, the effect of the TAU transport system is different between various organs [6]. Therefore, TAU concentration varies widely among tissue types [51] (Fig. **3**). The brain, heart, skeletal muscle, and kidneys contain a high concentration of TAU [6]. It has been well-documented that TAU is localized at higher concentrations in high energy-consuming tissues such as skeletal muscle, heart, and the brain [22, 35, 51 - 55] (Fig. **3**). TAU uptake may not only differ between organs but could also compartmentalize within the various parts of a specific organ. For example, it has been found that there is a zonal distribution of TAU within the liver [56]. Although more studies are needed to clear the zonal distribution of TAU in the liver, investigators such as Miyazaki *et al.* suggested that the variation in TAU level might be involved in the susceptibility to the zonal toxic response of the liver tissue [56]. It has been found that TauT, which is responsible for TAU uptake from the circulation, is predominantly expressed in the pre-central (PC) region of the liver [56]. Moreover, it has also been shown that the enzymes involved in the TAU synthesis process, namely cysteine dehydrogenase, are predominantly localized in the PC region [27, 56]. An exciting finding of TAU excretion from our body is that there is no TAU metabolizing enzyme in human cells, and this amino acid is metabolized by gut bacteria (readers could refer to chapter 9 for more information). The main excretion route for TAU is its conjugation with bile acids or excretion through the kidney.

The uptake of TAU has also been identified at cellular levels, and some transporters involved in this process have been identified. In this context, the cellular uptake of TAU through TauT and the role of factors involved in this process are widely investigated [57] (Fig. **4**). It has been found that factors such as cellular hyper-osmolarity, mammalian target of rapamycin (mTOR) signaling, tonicity-responsive enhancer-binding protein (TonEBP), and several transcription factors such as c-Jun, c-Myb, and WT1 could enhance cellular TAU uptake [57, 58] (Fig. **4**). On the other hand, factors such as ROS formation and oxidative stress, protein kinase C (PKC), and casein kinase 2 (CK2) could inhibit cellular TAU uptake through TauT [57, 59] (Fig. **4**). TAU transport is regulated by the phosphorylation of the intracellular TauT transporter domain [57, 58, 60] (Fig. **4**).

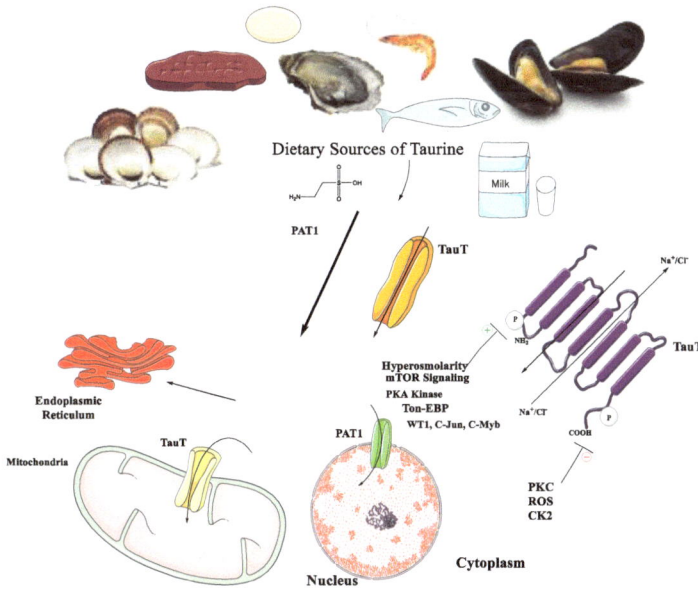

Fig. (4). Taurine transport and cellular compartmentalization. Different transporters are responsible for taurine uptake, transportation to the cytoplasm, and finally to the cellular organelles. At subcellular levels, taurine is accumulated in the endoplasmic reticulum, mitochondria, and nucleus. TauT: Taurine transporter; PAT1: Polyamine transporter 1; mTOR: mammalian target of rapamycin; PKA: protein kinase A; Ton-EBP: tonicity-responsive enhancer-binding protein; PKC: Protein kinase C; CK2: Casein kinase 2. The role of factors involved in the TAU absorption through TauT was inspired by the same figure from reference [57].

As mentioned, several investigations have been conducted to identify the subcellular TAU compartmentalization [61] (Fig. **4**). It has been well-documented that cellular mitochondria are significant reservoirs for TAU storage [62 - 64]. At least one TAU transporter has been identified in cellular mitochondria so far [64] (Figs. **3** and **4**). Interestingly, in addition to TAU transport from the cytoplasm, some studies indicate that TAU synthesis occurs in the mitochondrial matrix [65]. These data could indicate a vital role for TAU in mitochondria. The role of TAU in the mitochondrial function is the subject of various investigations [9 - 11, 16, 21 - 23, 25, 26, 51, 55, 66 - 70]. In the forthcoming chapters of this book, the role of TAU in mitochondrial function and its association with the pathophysiology of human diseases are discussed.

TAU also enters the cellular nucleus through a series of transporters [6] (Fig. **4**). Some studies reported that the nucleus TAU level could change under modifications of cell physiological conditions [6]. These data suggest a putative role for TAU in the nucleus. It has been proposed that TAU could act as an osmolyte in the nucleus [6]. TAU might also contribute to genetic materials stabilization and preventing their damage [6]. It has also been mentioned that the presence of TAU in the nucleus could be related to nuclear shrinking or swelling [61, 71]. Although the significance of such nuclear changes in response to TAU is not fully understood so far, it seems that transporters such as PAT1, which mediate TAU influx to the nucleus, are involved in events such as cell growth [71]. However, the current knowledge regarding TAU mechanisms of action in the cellular nucleus is limited, and more investigations into this topic are warranted.

The endoplasmic reticulum (ER) is another intracellular target for TAU accumulation and function (Fig. **4**). ER plays a pivotal role in cytoplasmic calcium (Ca^{2+}) homeostasis [72, 73]. Dysregulated cytoplasmic Ca^{2+} by xenobiotics or diseases could activate cell death mechanisms and organ injury [15, 20, 72 - 76]. The stabilization of ER and prevention of cytoplasmic Ca^{2+} overload is a critical function of TAU (Fig. **5**). The effects of TAU on ER and Ca^{2+} homeostasis and its relevance in the pathogenesis of human diseases are discussed in the forthcoming chapters.

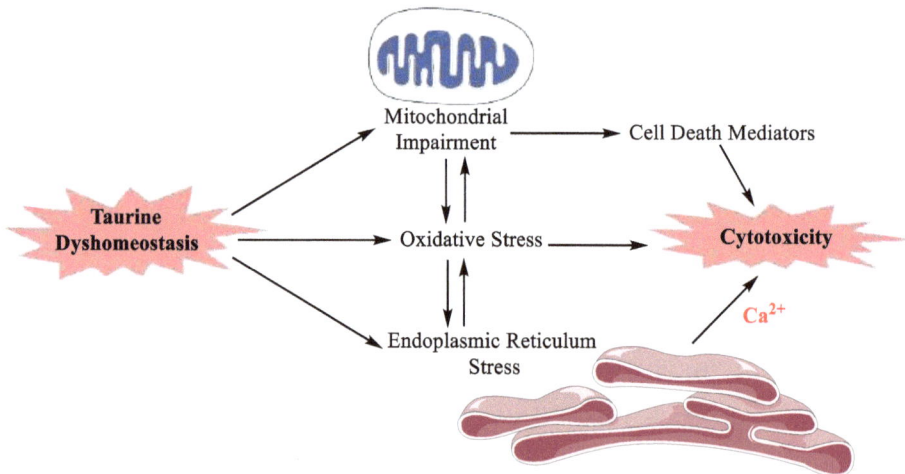

Fig. (5). Taurine dyshomeostasis is related to mitochondrial impairment, oxidative stress, and endoplasmic reticulum stress. These events could finally lead to cell death and organ injury.

Since the human body's ability for TAU synthesis is limited [56, 77 - 79], dietary TUA plays a crucial role in maintaining our body's TAU reservoirs. On the other hand, TAU has not been detected in plants and plant products. Therefore, the lack of this amino acid could occur in vegans [78]. A list of TAU-rich foodstuffs has been represented in Table **2**.

Table 2. The taurine content of common foods. This table is inspired by an identical table in the manuscript [80].

Foodstuff	Taurine Content (mg/100 g weight)	References
Chicken Dark Meat (Broiled)	199	[80]
Turkey Dark Meat (Roasted)	299	[80]
Beef (Broiled)	38	[80]
White Fish (Cooked)	172	[80]
Tuna Fish (Canned)	42	[80]
Cod Fish (Farmed)	106	[81]
Salmon Fish (Farmed)	60	[81]
Shrimp	39	[80]
Oyster	396	[80]
Mussel	655	[80]
Clam	520	[80]
Scallop	827	[80]
Squid	356	[80]
Cow Milk (3.5% fat, Whole)	3.5	[80]
Low-Fat Plain Yogurt	3.3	[80]
Vanilla Ice-cream	1.9	[80]

Most of the TAU-rich materials listed in Table **2** are not found in many parts of the world, or generally, people cannot afford to buy them due to their high cost. It could be suggested that in the comprehensive programs, TAU could be added to the high-consumption diets of the communities to benefit from the positive effects of this compound in human health. On the other hand, vegetarians can also benefit from adding this amino acid to their diet (since the synthetic form of this substance is also available).

It has been found that the destruction in the body TAU homeostasis could seriously compromise the function of several organs such as the heart and skeletal muscle [82 - 84]. TAU concentration in tissues such as skeletal muscle, cardiac tissue, and seminal fluid is very high (Fig. **3**). It has been found that TAU plays a vital role in the physiological activity of tissues such as cardiac and skeletal muscle [40, 44, 85, 86]. In this regard, the role of TAU in regulating mitochondrial function and cellular energy metabolism seems to play a crucial role in its action [44, 84, 86 - 88]. Therefore, it is essential to investigate the effect of TAU deficiency in the pathogenesis of the human disease. It has been well-known that the TAU transporter, TauT, plays a crucial role in regulating tissue TAU homeostasis [57]. TauT also plays a crucial role in transporting this amino acid to the mitochondria [44, 57] (Fig. **4**). Thus, TAU deficiency could play a vital role in the pathogenesis of mitochondrial dysfunction, cellular energy crisis, oxidative stress, and organ injury.

The role of TUA deficiency in the pathogenesis of the human disease is the subject of several studies [89 - 93]. For instance, it has been found that mitochondrial myopathy, encephalopathy, lactic acidosis, and stroke-like episodes (MELAS) syndrome, and TAU deficiency are closely related [89]. TAU deficiency in MELAS leads to a significant decrease in mitochondrial electron transport chain (ETC) synthesis and consequently impaired mitochondrial function [89, 94, 95]. In another study, it has been found that severe muscle weakness and senescence occurred in TAU transporter knock-out animals [84]. All these data indicate the crucial role of TAU in health and disease.

LESSONS LEARNED FROM TAURINE-TRANSPORTER KNOCKOUT EXPERIMENTAL MODELS

A big part of our knowledge about the role of TAU in various organs and the pathological consequences of its deficiency has been obtained from TAU transporter knock-out experimental models [57, 96 - 98]. Physiologically, TAU transporters respond to several stimuli such as changes in the cellular ionic environment, pH, and electrochemical charge [57]. Two major types of TAU transporters have been identified to date. TauT (SLC6A6) is an ion (Na^+ and Cl^-)-sensitive TAU transporter (Fig. **4**). PAT1 (SLC36A1) is another TAU transporter and its activity is pH-dependent [57]. The affinity and capacity of these transporters for TAU are different (The K_m value for TauT is <60 μM where for PAT1 is 4-7 mM) [57, 99]. It has been well-known that TauT is responsible for cellular TAU influx and efflux in various organs [57]. TAU transporters are located on the cell membranes or intracellular organelles (Fig. **4**).

β-alanine, a competitive inhibitor of cellular TAU uptake, has been used for investigating the effect of cellular TAU deficiency in several studies [6, 100 - 103]. However, it has been revealed that β-alanine may not significantly affect the cellular compartmentalization of TAU [104, 105]. For instance, Jong *et al.*

revealed that β-alanine could not significantly influence mitochondrial TAU levels despite inhibiting cellular TAU uptake [104]. In some cases, it has also been found that β-alanine could not affect tissue (*e.g.*, skeletal muscle) TAU content [106]. Therefore, it is crucial to develop a method to investigate the cellular and molecular mechanisms of TAU deficiency in various organs and subcellular compartments. In this context, several studies have been developed to study the role of TAU deficiency in the pathogenesis of organ injury and its cellular and molecular mechanisms. For instance, TAU transporters' knockout experimental models have been widely applied [107 - 112].

It has been found that severe complications occur in TauT knockout models [107 - 110]. Organs with higher TAU levels (*e.g.*, cardiac and skeletal muscle) are the first organs influenced by the TauT knocking-out procedure [84, 109, 111]. Severe muscle weakness, low ATP levels, significant oxidative stress, and muscle wasting are complications reported in TauT knockout models [84, 96, 107, 111]. Moreover, cardiomyopathy and low cardiac output are the dominant pathological changes detected in the TauT knockout animals [82, 83]. Other organs, including the brain, kidney, eye, and liver, are also affected in TauT knockout models [97, 98, 108, 113 - 115].

It is essential to mention that TauT knockout models revealed a crucial role for mitochondrial function and energy metabolism in the mechanism of action of TAU in various organs [83, 116]. These models revealed that the absence of TAU in mitochondria could lead to deleterious consequences such as severe mitochondria-mediated ROS formation, mitochondrial depolarization, impaired ATP synthesis, mitochondrial permeabilization, and the release of cell death mediators from mitochondria [83, 84, 117]. Moreover, it has been found that TAU deficiency is linked with other events such as endoplasmic reticulum (ER) stress, cytoplasmic Ca^{2+} overload, and denaturation of cellular proteins [118] (Fig. **5**). These events could finally lead to cell death and organ injury (Fig. **5**). The role of TauT knockout models and their relevance to cellular TAU concentration and mitochondrial function are discussed in various chapters of this book.

As previously mentioned, TAU deficiency could also lead to severe pathological changes in tissues such as cardiac and skeletal muscles experimental model [82 - 84, 119]. It has been found that mitochondria are among vital targets affected by TAU deficiency [63, 82 - 84, 117, 119 - 121]. All these data indicate an essential role for TAU in the normal function of our body. Hence, TAU deficiency could lead to harmful consequences. Mitochondrial impairment is interconnected with other pivotal intracellular signaling such as ROS formation, endoplasmic reticulum (ER) stress, and finally, cell death and organ injury (Fig. **5**). Therefore, it is crucial to investigate the role of TAU deficiency in the pathogenesis of various human diseases and/or use this safe amino acid as a potential therapeutic strategy against vast pathologic complications.

The essentiality of TAU has not been profoundly highlighted in reference books of human nutrition. Therefore, there is no recommended daily allowance (RDA) for this amino acid by standard dietary references [78]. However, many clinical studies administered TAU at very high doses (*e.g.*, 6 g/day). This could be a beneficial point for the safety of this amino acid. Free TAU is mainly detected in seafood, meat, and at a lower content in dairy products [122 - 126] (Fig. **2**). As mentioned, no significant TAU content is seen in plants and plant products [78]. Therefore, the daily TAU intake of vegetarians is estimated to be zero [78]. The higher dietary intake of TAU or its precursors such as methionine and cysteine might partially compensate for the shortage of TAU in vegans [127, 128]. However, as previously mentioned, the TAU synthesis capability of the human liver is limited. Hence, TAU's fortification of their food is a good choice, and many people could benefit from the positive effects of this amino acid.

CONCLUSION

Based on the data collected in this chapter, TAU plays a vital role in mitochondrial function in various organs. Therefore, changes in the hemostasis of this amino acid could lead to several pathological conditions associated with the energy crisis and mitochondria-mediated cellular and organ injury. In the following chapters, the mechanism involved in the effects of TAU on mitochondria are bolded, and the results of this amino acid on different organs, with a focus on the effects of TAU on mitochondrial function, are highlighted. The data collected in this book could lead to a better understanding of the mechanisms of action of TAU in the body and, finally, its application as a therapeutic option against a wide range of human diseases.

REFERENCES

[1]   Ripps H, Shen W. Review: taurine: a "very essential" amino acid. Mol Vis 2012; 18: 2673-86.
[PMID: 23170060]

[2]   Lambert IH. Regulation of the cellular content of the organic osmolyte taurine in mammalian cells. Neurochem Res 2004; 29(1): 27-63.
[http://dx.doi.org/10.1023/B:NERE.0000010433.08577.96] [PMID: 14992263]

[3]   Burg MB, Ferraris JD. Intracellular organic osmolytes: function and regulation. J Biol Chem 2008; 283(12): 7309-13.
[http://dx.doi.org/10.1074/jbc.R700042200] [PMID: 18256030]

[4]   Pasantes-Morales H, Quesada O, Morán J. Taurine: An osmolyte in mammalian tissues.Taurine 3: Cellular and Regulatory Mechanisms Advances in Experimental Medicine and Biology. Boston, MA: Springer US 1998; pp. 209-17.
[http://dx.doi.org/10.1007/978-1-4899-0117-0_27]

[5]   Schuller-Levis G, Park E. Is taurine a biomarker? Adv Clin Chem 2006; 41: 1-21.

[http://dx.doi.org/10.1016/S0065-2423(05)41001-X] [PMID: 28682746]

[6]   Lambert IH, Kristensen DM, Holm JB, Mortensen OH. Physiological role of taurine - from organism to organelle. Acta Physiol (Oxf) 2015; 213(1): 191-212.
[http://dx.doi.org/10.1111/apha.12365] [PMID: 25142161]

[7]   Bouckenooghe T, Remacle C, Reusens B. Is taurine a functional nutrient? Curr Opin Clin Nutr Metab Care 2006; 9(6): 728-33.
[http://dx.doi.org/10.1097/01.mco.0000247469.26414.55] [PMID: 17053427]

[8]   Heidari R, Ommati MM, Alahyari S, Azarpira N, Niknahad H. Amino acid-containing Krebs-Henseleit buffer protects rat liver in a long-term organ perfusion model. Ulum-i Daruyi 2018; 24(3): 168-79.
[http://dx.doi.org/10.15171/PS.2018.25]

[9]   Niknahad H, Jamshidzadeh A, Heidari R, Zarei M, Ommati MM. Ammonia-induced mitochondrial dysfunction and energy metabolism disturbances in isolated brain and liver mitochondria, and the effect of taurine administration: relevance to hepatic encephalopathy treatment. Clin Exp Hepatol 2017; 3(3): 141-51.
[http://dx.doi.org/10.5114/ceh.2017.68833] [PMID: 29062904]

[10]   Heidari R, Babaei H, Eghbal MA. Amodiaquine-induced toxicity in isolated rat hepatocytes and the cytoprotective effects of taurine and/or N-acetyl cysteine. Res Pharm Sci 2014; 9(2): 97-105.
[PMID: 25657778]

[11]   Heidari R, Babaei H, Eghbal MA. Cytoprotective effects of taurine against toxicity induced by isoniazid and hydrazine in isolated rat hepatocytes. Arh Hig Rada Toksikol 2013; 64(2): 201-10.
[http://dx.doi.org/10.2478/10004-1254-64-2013-2297] [PMID: 23819928]

[12]   Heidari R, Jamshidzadeh A, Niknahad H, *et al.* Effect of taurine on chronic and acute liver injury: Focus on blood and brain ammonia. Toxicol Rep 2016; 3: 870-9.
[http://dx.doi.org/10.1016/j.toxrep.2016.04.002] [PMID: 28959615]

[13]   Heidari R, Jamshidzadeh A, Niknahad H, Safari F, Azizi H, Abdoli N, *et al.* The hepatoprotection provided by taurine and glycine against antineoplastic drugs induced liver injury in an ex vivo model of normothermic recirculating isolated perfused rat liver. Trends Pharmacol Sci 2016; 2(1): 59-76.

[14]   Heidari R, Jamshidzadeh A, Keshavarz N, Azarpira N. Mitigation of methimazole-induced hepatic injury by taurine in mice. Sci Pharm 2015; 83(1): 143-58.
[http://dx.doi.org/10.3797/scipharm.1408-04] [PMID: 26839807]

[15]   Heidari R, Abdoli N, Ommati MM, Jamshidzadeh A, Niknahad H. Mitochondrial impairment induced by chenodeoxycholic acid: The protective effect of taurine and carnosine supplementation. Trends in Pharmaceutical Sciences 2018; 4: 2.

[16]   Heidari R, Behnamrad S, Khodami Z, Ommati MM, Azarpira N, Vazin A. The nephroprotective properties of taurine in colistin-treated mice is mediated through the regulation of mitochondrial function and mitigation of oxidative stress. Biomed Pharmacother 2019; 109: 103-11.
[http://dx.doi.org/10.1016/j.biopha.2018.10.093] [PMID: 30396066]

[17]   Karamikhah R, Jamshidzadeh A, Azarpira N, Saeidi A, Heidari R. Propylthiouracil-induced liver injury in mice and the protective role of taurine. Pharm Sci 2015; 21(2): 94-101.
[http://dx.doi.org/10.15171/PS.2015.23]

[18]   Heidari R, Sadeghi N, Azarpira N, Niknahad H. Sulfasalazine-induced hepatic injury in an *ex vivo* model of isolated perfused rat liver and the protective role of taurine. Pharm Sci 2015; 21(4): 211-9.
[http://dx.doi.org/10.15171/PS.2015.39]

[19]   Heidari R, Rasti M, Shirazi Yeganeh B, Niknahad H, Saeedi A, Najibi A. Sulfasalazine-induced renal and hepatic injury in rats and the protective role of taurine. Bioimpacts 2016; 6(1): 3-8.
[http://dx.doi.org/10.15171/bi.2016.01] [PMID: 27340618]

[20]   Jamshidzadeh A, Abdoli N, Niknahad H, Azarpira N, Mardani E, Mousavi S, *et al.* Taurine alleviates

brain tissue markers of oxidative stress in a rat model of hepatic encephalopathy. Trends Pharmacol Sci 2017; 3(3): 181-92.

[21]   Mohammadi H, Ommati MM, Farshad O, Jamshidzadeh A, Nikbakht MR, Niknahad H, *et al.* Taurine and isolated mitochondria: A concentration-response study. Trends Pharmacol Sci 2019; 5(4): 197-206.

[22]   Ommati MM, Farshad O, Jamshidzadeh A, Heidari R. Taurine enhances skeletal muscle mitochondrial function in a rat model of resistance training. PharmaNutrition 2019; 9: 100161.
[http://dx.doi.org/10.1016/j.phanu.2019.100161]

[23]   Ahmadi N, Ghanbarinejad V, Ommati MM, Jamshidzadeh A, Heidari R. Taurine prevents mitochondrial membrane permeabilization and swelling upon interaction with manganese: Implication in the treatment of cirrhosis-associated central nervous system complications. J Biochem Mol Toxicol 2018; 32(11): e22216.
[http://dx.doi.org/10.1002/jbt.22216] [PMID: 30152904]

[24]   Heidari R, Jamshidzadeh A, Ghanbarinejad V, Ommati MM, Niknahad H. Taurine supplementation abates cirrhosis-associated locomotor dysfunction. Clin Exp Hepatol 2018; 4(2): 72-82.
[http://dx.doi.org/10.5114/ceh.2018.75956] [PMID: 29904723]

[25]   Jamshidzadeh A, Heidari R, Abasvali M, *et al.* Taurine treatment preserves brain and liver mitochondrial function in a rat model of fulminant hepatic failure and hyperammonemia. Biomed Pharmacother 2017; 86: 514-20.
[http://dx.doi.org/10.1016/j.biopha.2016.11.095] [PMID: 28024286]

[26]   Ommati MM, Heidari R, Ghanbarinejad V, Abdoli N, Niknahad H. Taurine treatment provides neuroprotection in a mouse model of manganism. Biol Trace Elem Res 2019; 190(2): 384-95.
[http://dx.doi.org/10.1007/s12011-018-1552-2] [PMID: 30357569]

[27]   Bella DL, Hirschberger LL, Kwon YH, Stipanuk MH. Cysteine metabolism in periportal and perivenous hepatocytes: perivenous cells have greater capacity for glutathione production and taurine synthesis but not for cysteine catabolism. Amino Acids 2002; 23(4): 453-8.
[http://dx.doi.org/10.1007/s00726-002-0213-z] [PMID: 12436215]

[28]   Stipanuk MH. Role of the liver in regulation of body cysteine and taurine levels: a brief review. Neurochem Res 2004; 29(1): 105-10.
[http://dx.doi.org/10.1023/B:NERE.0000010438.40376.c9] [PMID: 14992268]

[29]   de la Rosa J, Stipanuk MH. Evidence for a rate-limiting role of cysteinesulfinate decarboxylase activity in taurine biosynthesis in vivo. Comp Biochem Physiol B 1985; 81(3): 565-71.
[http://dx.doi.org/10.1016/0305-0491(85)90367-0] [PMID: 4028681]

[30]   Moise NS, Pacioretty LM, Kallfelz FA, Stipanuk MH, King JM, Gilmour RF Jr. Dietary taurine deficiency and dilated cardiomyopathy in the fox. Am Heart J 1991; 121(2): 541-7.
[http://dx.doi.org/10.1016/0002-8703(91)90724-V] [PMID: 1990761]

[31]   Pion PD, Kittleson MD, Skiles ML, Rogers QR, Morris JG. Dilated cardiomyopathy associated with taurine deficiency in the domestic cat: relationship to diet and myocardial taurine content Taurine. Springer 1992; pp. 63-73.

[32]   Hayes KC, Trautwein EA. Taurine deficiency syndrome in cats. Vet Clin North Am Small Anim Pract 1989; 19(3): 403-13.
[http://dx.doi.org/10.1016/S0195-5616(89)50052-4] [PMID: 2658282]

[33]   Pion PD, Kittleson MD, Thomas WP, Skiles ML, Rogers QR. Clinical findings in cats with dilated cardiomyopathy and relationship of findings to taurine deficiency. J Am Vet Med Assoc 1992; 201(2): 267-74.
[PMID: 1500323]

[34]   Dow SW, Fettman MJ, Smith KR, Ching SV, Hamar DW, Rogers QR. Taurine depletion and cardiovascular disease in adult cats fed a potassium-depleted acidified diet. Am J Vet Res 1992; 53(3):

402-5.
[PMID: 1534475]

[35]   Jacobsen JG, Smith LH. Biochemistry and physiology of taurine and taurine derivatives. Physiol Rev 1968; 48(2): 424-511.
[http://dx.doi.org/10.1152/physrev.1968.48.2.424] [PMID: 4297098]

[36]   Zhao X, Li Q, Meng Q, Yue C, Xu C. Identification and expression of cysteine sulfinate decarboxylase, possible regulation of taurine biosynthesis in Crassostrea gigas in response to low salinity. Sci Rep 2017; 7(1): 5505.
[http://dx.doi.org/10.1038/s41598-017-05852-6] [PMID: 28710376]

[37]   Hansen SH, Grunnet N. Taurine, Glutathione and Bioenergetics.Taurine 8 Advances in Experimental Medicine and Biology: Springer New York. 2013; pp. 3-12.

[38]   Huxtable RJ. Taurine in nutrition and neurology: Springer Science & Business Media; 2013.

[39]   Xu Y-J, Arneja AS, Tappia PS, Dhalla NS. The potential health benefits of taurine in cardiovascular disease. Exp Clin Cardiol 2008; 13(2): 57-65.
[PMID: 19343117]

[40]   Seidel U, Huebbe P, Rimbach G. Taurine: A regulator of cellular redox homeostasis and skeletal muscle function. Mol Nutr Food Res 2019; 63(16): 1800569.
[http://dx.doi.org/10.1002/mnfr.201800569] [PMID: 30211983]

[41]   Ishikawa M, Arai S, Takano M, Hamada A, Kunimasa K, Mori M. Taurine's health influence on Japanese high school girls. J Biomed Sci 2010; 17(S1) (Suppl. 1): S47.
[http://dx.doi.org/10.1186/1423-0127-17-S1-S47] [PMID: 20804624]

[42]   Yamori Y, Liu L, Mori M, *et al.* Taurine as the nutritional factor for the longevity of the Japanese revealed by a world-wide epidemiological survey. Adv Exp Med Biol 2009; 643: 13-25.
[http://dx.doi.org/10.1007/978-0-387-75681-3_2] [PMID: 19239132]

[43]   Qaradakhi T, Gadanec LK, McSweeney KR, Abraham JR, Apostolopoulos V, Zulli A. The anti-inflammatory effect of taurine on cardiovascular disease. Nutrients 2020; 12(9): 2847.
[http://dx.doi.org/10.3390/nu12092847] [PMID: 32957558]

[44]   Schaffer S, Kim HW. Effects and mechanisms of taurine as a therapeutic agent. Biomol Ther (Seoul) 2018; 26(3): 225-41.
[http://dx.doi.org/10.4062/biomolther.2017.251] [PMID: 29631391]

[45]   Zachmann M, Tocci P, Nyhan WL. The occurrence of gamma-aminobutyric acid in human tissues other than brain. J Biol Chem 1966; 241(6): 1355-8.
[http://dx.doi.org/10.1016/S0021-9258(18)96782-7] [PMID: 4222879]

[46]   Mochizuki T, Satsu H, Nakano T, Shimizu M. Regulation of the human taurine transporter by TNF-α and an anti-inflammatory function of taurine in human intestinal Caco-2 ⁻ cells. Biofactors 2004; 21(1-4): 141-4.
[http://dx.doi.org/10.1002/biof.552210128] [PMID: 15630186]

[47]   Ishizuka K, Miyamoto Y, Satsu H, Sato R, Shimizu M. Characteristics of lysophosphatidylcholine in its inhibition of taurine uptake by human intestinal Caco-2 cells. Biosci Biotechnol Biochem 2002; 66(4): 730-6.
[http://dx.doi.org/10.1271/bbb.66.730] [PMID: 12036043]

[48]   Mochizuki T, Satsu H, Shimizu M. Signaling pathways involved in tumor necrosis factor α-induced upregulation of the taurine transporter in Caco-2 cells. FEBS Lett 2005; 579(14): 3069-74.
[http://dx.doi.org/10.1016/j.febslet.2005.04.063] [PMID: 15907840]

[49]   Merheb M, Daher RT, Nasrallah M, Sabra R, Ziyadeh FN, Barada K. Taurine intestinal absorption and renal excretion test in diabetic patients: a pilot study. Diabetes Care 2007; 30(10): 2652-4.
[http://dx.doi.org/10.2337/dc07-0872] [PMID: 17666467]

[50] Ikeda S, Tachikawa M, Akanuma S, Fujinawa J, Hosoya K. Involvement of γ-aminobutyric acid transporter 2 in the hepatic uptake of taurine in rats. Am J Physiol Gastrointest Liver Physiol 2012; 303(3): G291-7.
[http://dx.doi.org/10.1152/ajpgi.00388.2011] [PMID: 22678999]

[51] Hansen SH, Andersen ML, Birkedal H, Cornett C, Wibrand F. The important role of taurine in oxidative metabolism. Adv Exp Med Biol 2006; 583: 129-35.
[http://dx.doi.org/10.1007/978-0-387-33504-9_13] [PMID: 17153596]

[52] Goodman CA, Horvath D, Stathis C, Mori T, Croft K, Murphy RM, *et al.* Taurine supplementation increases skeletal muscle force production and protects muscle function during and after high-frequency *in vitro* stimulation. Journal of Applied Physiology (Bethesda, Md: 1985) 2009; 107(1): 144-54.
[http://dx.doi.org/10.1152/japplphysiol.00040.2009]

[53] De Carvalho FG, Galan BSM, Santos PC, *et al.* Taurine: A potential ergogenic aid for preventing muscle damage and protein catabolism and decreasing oxidative stress produced by endurance exercise. Front Physiol 2017; 8: 710.
[http://dx.doi.org/10.3389/fphys.2017.00710] [PMID: 28979213]

[54] Takahashi Y, Hatta H. Effects of taurine administration on exercise-induced fatigue and recovery. J Phys Fit Sports Med 2017; 6(1): 33-9.
[http://dx.doi.org/10.7600/jpfsm.6.33]

[55] Mousavi K, Niknahad H, Ghalamfarsa A, *et al.* Taurine mitigates cirrhosis-associated heart injury through mitochondrial-dependent and antioxidative mechanisms. Clin Exp Hepatol 2020; 6(3): 207-19.
[http://dx.doi.org/10.5114/ceh.2020.99513] [PMID: 33145427]

[56] Miyazaki T, Matsuzaki Y. Taurine and liver diseases: a focus on the heterogeneous protective properties of taurine. Amino Acids 2014; 46(1): 101-10.
[http://dx.doi.org/10.1007/s00726-012-1381-0] [PMID: 22918604]

[57] Baliou S, Kyriakopoulos A, Goulielmaki M, Panayiotidis M, Spandidos D, Zoumpourlis V. Significance of taurine transporter (TauT) in homeostasis and its layers of regulation (Review). Mol Med Rep 2020; 22(3): 2163-73.
[http://dx.doi.org/10.3892/mmr.2020.11321] [PMID: 32705197]

[58] Hansen DB, Friis MB, Hoffmann EK, Lambert IH. Downregulation of the taurine transporter TauT during hypo-osmotic stress in NIH3T3 mouse fibroblasts. J Membr Biol 2012; 245(2): 77-87.
[http://dx.doi.org/10.1007/s00232-012-9416-8] [PMID: 22383044]

[59] Jacobsen JH, Clement CA, Friis MB, Lambert IH. Casein kinase 2 regulates the active uptake of the organic osmolyte taurine in NIH3T3 mouse fibroblasts. Pflugers Arch 2008; 457(2): 327-37.
[http://dx.doi.org/10.1007/s00424-008-0517-2] [PMID: 18542993]

[60] Hoffmann EK, Lambert IH. Amino acid transport and cell volume regulation in Ehrlich ascites tumour cells. J Physiol 1983; 338(1): 613-25.
[http://dx.doi.org/10.1113/jphysiol.1983.sp014692] [PMID: 6875973]

[61] Voss JW, Pedersen SF, Christensen ST, Lambert IH. Regulation of the expression and subcellular localization of the taurine transporter TauT in mouse NIH3T3 fibroblasts. Eur J Biochem 2004; 271(23-24): 4646-58.
[http://dx.doi.org/10.1111/j.1432-1033.2004.04420.x] [PMID: 15606752]

[62] Hansen S, Andersen M, Cornett C, Gradinaru R, Grunnet N. A role for taurine in mitochondrial function. J Biomed Sci 2010; 17(Suppl 1): S23.
[http://dx.doi.org/10.1186/1423-0127-17-S1-S23] [PMID: 20804598]

[63] Jong CJ, Azuma J, Schaffer S. Mechanism underlying the antioxidant activity of taurine: prevention of mitochondrial oxidant production. Amino Acids 2012; 42(6): 2223-32.

[http://dx.doi.org/10.1007/s00726-011-0962-7] [PMID: 21691752]

[64]   Suzuki T, Suzuki T, Wada T, Saigo K, Watanabe K. Taurine as a constituent of mitochondrial tRNAs: new insights into the functions of taurine and human mitochondrial diseases. EMBO J 2002; 21(23): 6581-9.
[http://dx.doi.org/10.1093/emboj/cdf656] [PMID: 12456664]

[65]   Ubuka T, Okada A, Nakamura H. Production of hypotaurine from l-cysteinesulfinate by rat liver mitochondria. Amino Acids 2008; 35(1): 53-8.
[http://dx.doi.org/10.1007/s00726-007-0633-x] [PMID: 18219548]

[66]   Abdoli N, Sadeghian I, Azarpira N, Ommati MM, Heidari R. Taurine mitigates bile duct obstruction-associated cholemic nephropathy: effect on oxidative stress and mitochondrial parameters. Clin Exp Hepatol 2021; 7(1): 30-40.
[http://dx.doi.org/10.5114/ceh.2021.104675] [PMID: 34027113]

[67]   Heidari R, Ghanbarinejad V, Ommati MM, Jamshidzadeh A, Niknahad H. Mitochondria protecting amino acids: Application against a wide range of mitochondria-linked complications. PharmaNutrition 2018; 6(4): 180-90.
[http://dx.doi.org/10.1016/j.phanu.2018.09.001]

[68]   Eftekhari A, Ahmadian E, Azarmi Y, Parvizpur A, Fard JK, Eghbal MA. The effects of cimetidine, N-acetylcysteine, and taurine on thioridazine metabolic activation and induction of oxidative stress in isolated rat hepatocytes. Pharm Chem J 2018; 51(11): 965-9.
[http://dx.doi.org/10.1007/s11094-018-1724-6]

[69]   Shimada K, Jong CJ, Takahashi K, Schaffer SW. Role of ROS production and turnover in the antioxidant activity of taurine. Adv Exp Med Biol 2015; 803: 581-96.

[70]   Heidari R, Babaei H, Eghbal MA. Ameliorative effects of taurine against methimazole-induced cytotoxicity in isolated rat hepatocytes. Sci Pharm 2012; 80(4): 987-99.
[http://dx.doi.org/10.3797/scipharm.1205-16] [PMID: 23264945]

[71]   Jensen A, Figueiredo-Larsen M, Holm R, Broberg ML, Brodin B, Nielsen CU. PAT1 (SLC36A1) shows nuclear localization and affects growth of smooth muscle cells from rats. Am J Physiol Endocrinol Metab 2014; 306(1): E65-74.
[http://dx.doi.org/10.1152/ajpendo.00322.2013] [PMID: 24222668]

[72]   Zhao L, Ackerman SL. Endoplasmic reticulum stress in health and disease. Curr Opin Cell Biol 2006; 18(4): 444-52.
[http://dx.doi.org/10.1016/j.ceb.2006.06.005] [PMID: 16781856]

[73]   Carreras-Sureda A, Pihán P, Hetz C. Calcium signaling at the endoplasmic reticulum: fine-tuning stress responses. Cell Calcium 2018; 70: 24-31.
[http://dx.doi.org/10.1016/j.ceca.2017.08.004] [PMID: 29054537]

[74]   Pinton P, Giorgi C, Siviero R, Zecchini E, Rizzuto R. Calcium and apoptosis: ER-mitochondria Ca^{2+} transfer in the control of apoptosis. Oncogene 2008; 27(50): 6407-18.
[http://dx.doi.org/10.1038/onc.2008.308] [PMID: 18955969]

[75]   Nedergaard M, Verkhratsky A. Calcium dyshomeostasis and pathological calcium signalling in neurological diseases. Cell Calcium 2010; 47(2): 101-2.
[http://dx.doi.org/10.1016/j.ceca.2009.12.011] [PMID: 20079921]

[76]   Ommati MM, Mobasheri A, Ma Y, *et al.* Taurine mitigates the development of pulmonary inflammation, oxidative stress, and histopathological alterations in a rat model of bile duct ligation. Naunyn Schmiedebergs Arch Pharmacol 2022; 395(12): 1557-72.
[http://dx.doi.org/10.1007/s00210-022-02291-7] [PMID: 36097067]

[77]   Lourenço R, Camilo ME. Taurine: a conditionally essential amino acid in humans? An overview in health and disease. Nutr Hosp 2002; 17(6): 262-70.
[PMID: 12514918]

[78]   Stapleton PP, Charles RP, Redmond HP, Bouchier-Hayes DJ. Taurine and human nutrition. Clin Nutr 1997; 16(3): 103-8.
[http://dx.doi.org/10.1016/S0261-5614(97)80234-8] [PMID: 16844580]

[79]   Yamori Y, Taguchi T, Hamada A, Kunimasa K, Mori H, Mori M. Taurine in health and diseases: consistent evidence from experimental and epidemiological studies. J Biomed Sci 2010; 17(Suppl 1) (Suppl. 1): S6.
[http://dx.doi.org/10.1186/1423-0127-17-S1-S6] [PMID: 20804626]

[80]   Laidlaw SA, Grosvenor M, Kopple JD. The taurine content of common foodstuffs. JPEN J Parenter Enteral Nutr 1990; 14(2): 183-8.
[http://dx.doi.org/10.1177/0148607190014002183] [PMID: 2352336]

[81]   Gormley TR, Neumann T, Fagan JD, Brunton NP. Taurine content of raw and processed fish fillets/portions. Eur Food Res Technol 2007; 225(5-6): 837-42.
[http://dx.doi.org/10.1007/s00217-006-0489-4]

[82]   Ito T, Hanahata Y, Kine K, Murakami S, Schaffer SW. Tissue taurine depletion induces profibrotic pattern of gene expression and causes aging-related cardiac fibrosis in heart in mice. Biol Pharm Bull 2018; 41(10): 1561-6.
[http://dx.doi.org/10.1248/bpb.b18-00217] [PMID: 30270325]

[83]   Ito T, Kimura Y, Uozumi Y, *et al.* Taurine depletion caused by knocking out the taurine transporter gene leads to cardiomyopathy with cardiac atrophy. J Mol Cell Cardiol 2008; 44(5): 927-37.
[http://dx.doi.org/10.1016/j.yjmcc.2008.03.001] [PMID: 18407290]

[84]   Ito T, Yoshikawa N, Inui T, Miyazaki N, Schaffer SW, Azuma J. Tissue depletion of taurine accelerates skeletal muscle senescence and leads to early death in mice. PLoS One 2014; 9(9): e107409.
[http://dx.doi.org/10.1371/journal.pone.0107409] [PMID: 25229346]

[85]   Thirupathi A, Pinho RA, Baker JS, István B, Gu Y. Taurine reverses oxidative damages and restores the muscle function in overuse of exercised muscle. Front Physiol 2020; 11: 582449.
[http://dx.doi.org/10.3389/fphys.2020.582449] [PMID: 33192592]

[86]   Schaffer SW, Ju Jong C, Kc R, Azuma J. Physiological roles of taurine in heart and muscle. J Biomed Sci 2010; 17(Suppl 1): S2.
[http://dx.doi.org/10.1186/1423-0127-17-S1-S2] [PMID: 20804594]

[87]   Yang Y, Zhang Y, Liu X, *et al.* Exogenous taurine attenuates mitochondrial oxidative stress and endoplasmic reticulum stress in rat cardiomyocytes. Acta Biochim Biophys Sin (Shanghai) 2013; 45(5): 359-67.
[http://dx.doi.org/10.1093/abbs/gmt034] [PMID: 23619568]

[88]   Oudit GY, Trivieri MG, Khaper N, *et al.* Taurine supplementation reduces oxidative stress and improves cardiovascular function in an iron-overload murine model. Circulation 2004; 109(15): 1877-85.
[http://dx.doi.org/10.1161/01.CIR.0000124229.40424.80] [PMID: 15037530]

[89]   Schaffer SW, Jong CJ, Warner D, Ito T, Azuma J. Taurine deficiency and MELAS are closely related syndromes. Adv Exp Med Biol 2013; 776: 153-65.
[http://dx.doi.org/10.1007/978-1-4614-6093-0_16] [PMID: 23392880]

[90]   Schaffer SW, Jong CJ, Ito T, Azuma J. Role of taurine in the pathologies of MELAS and MERRF. Amino Acids 2014; 46(1): 47-56.
[http://dx.doi.org/10.1007/s00726-012-1414-8] [PMID: 23179085]

[91]   Asano K, Suzuki T, Saito A, *et al.* Metabolic and chemical regulation of tRNA modification associated with taurine deficiency and human disease. Nucleic Acids Res 2018; 46(4): 1565-83.
[http://dx.doi.org/10.1093/nar/gky068] [PMID: 29390138]

[92]   Kirino Y, Yasukawa T, Ohta S, *et al.* Codon-specific translational defect caused by a wobble

modification deficiency in mutant tRNA from a human mitochondrial disease. Proc Natl Acad Sci USA 2004; 101(42): 15070-5.
[http://dx.doi.org/10.1073/pnas.0405173101] [PMID: 15477592]

[93]   Tsutomu S, Asuteka N, Takeo S. Human mitochondrial diseases caused by lack of taurine modification in mitochondrial tRNAs. Wiley Interdiscip Rev RNA 2011; 2(3): 376-86.
[http://dx.doi.org/10.1002/wrna.65] [PMID: 21957023]

[94]   Rikimaru M, Ohsawa Y, Wolf AM, *et al.* Taurine ameliorates impaired the mitochondrial function and prevents stroke-like episodes in patients with MELAS. Intern Med 2012; 51(24): 3351-7.
[http://dx.doi.org/10.2169/internalmedicine.51.7529] [PMID: 23257519]

[95]   Ohsawa Y, Hagiwara H, Nishimatsu S, *et al.* Taurine supplementation for prevention of stroke-like episodes in MELAS: a multicentre, open-label, 52-week phase III trial. J Neurol Neurosurg Psychiatry 2019; 90(5): 529-36.
[http://dx.doi.org/10.1136/jnnp-2018-317964] [PMID: 29666206]

[96]   Warskulat U, Flögel U, Jacoby C, *et al.* Taurine transporter knockout depletes muscle taurine levels and results in severe skeletal muscle impairment but leaves cardiac function uncompromised. FASEB J 2004; 18(3): 577-9.
[http://dx.doi.org/10.1096/fj.03-0496fje] [PMID: 14734644]

[97]   Qvartskhava N, Jin CJ, Buschmann T, *et al.* Taurine transporter (TauT) deficiency impairs ammonia detoxification in mouse liver. Proc Natl Acad Sci USA 2019; 116(13): 6313-8.
[http://dx.doi.org/10.1073/pnas.1813100116] [PMID: 30862735]

[98]   Kubo Y, Akanuma S, Hosoya K. Impact of SLC6A transporters in physiological taurine transport at the blood–retinal barrier and in the liver. Biol Pharm Bull 2016; 39(12): 1903-11.
[http://dx.doi.org/10.1248/bpb.b16-00597] [PMID: 27904033]

[99]   Anderson CMH, Howard A, Walters JRF, Ganapathy V, Thwaites DT. Taurine uptake across the human intestinal brush-border membrane is via two transporters: H^+-coupled PAT1 (SLC36A1) and Na^+- and Cl^--dependent TauT (SLC6A6). J Physiol 2009; 587(4): 731-44.
[http://dx.doi.org/10.1113/jphysiol.2008.164228] [PMID: 19074966]

[100] Schaffer S, Ito T, Azuma J, Jong C, Kramer J. Mechanisms underlying development of taurine-deficient cardiomyopathy. Hearts 2020; 1(2): 86-98.
[http://dx.doi.org/10.3390/hearts1020010]

[101] Shetewy A, Shimada-Takaura K, Warner D, *et al.* Mitochondrial defects associated with β-alanine toxicity: relevance to hyper-beta-alaninemia. Mol Cell Biochem 2016; 416(1-2): 11-22.
[http://dx.doi.org/10.1007/s11010-016-2688-z] [PMID: 27023909]

[102] Schaffer SW, Solodushko V, Kakhniashvili D. Beneficial effect of taurine depletion on osmotic sodium and calcium loading during chemical hypoxia. Am J Physiol Cell Physiol 2002; 282(5): C1113-20.
[http://dx.doi.org/10.1152/ajpcell.00485.2001] [PMID: 11940527]

[103] Sturman JA, Lu P, Messing JM, Imaki H. Depletion of Feline Taurine Levels by β-Alanine and Dietary Taurine Restriction.Taurine 2: Basic and Clinical Aspects Advances in Experimental Medicine and Biology. Boston, MA: Springer US 1996; pp. 19-36.
[http://dx.doi.org/10.1007/978-1-4899-0182-8_3]

[104] Jong C, Ito T, Mozaffari M, Azuma J, Schaffer S. Effect of β-alanine treatment on mitochondrial taurine level and 5-taurinomethyluridine content. J Biomed Sci 2010; 17(Suppl 1): S25.
[http://dx.doi.org/10.1186/1423-0127-17-S1-S25] [PMID: 20804600]

[105] García-Ayuso D, Di Pierdomenico J, Valiente-Soriano FJ, *et al.* β-alanine supplementation induces taurine depletion and causes alterations of the retinal nerve fiber layer and axonal transport by retinal ganglion cells. Exp Eye Res 2019; 188: 107781.
[http://dx.doi.org/10.1016/j.exer.2019.107781] [PMID: 31473259]

[106] Saunders B, Franchi M, de Oliveira LF, *et al.* 24-Week β-alanine ingestion does not affect muscle taurine or clinical blood parameters in healthy males. Eur J Nutr 2020; 59(1): 57-65.
[http://dx.doi.org/10.1007/s00394-018-1881-0] [PMID: 30552505]

[107] Warskulat U, Heller-Stilb B, Oermann E, *et al.* Phenotype of the taurine transporter knockout mouse. Methods Enzymol 2007; 428: 439-58.
[http://dx.doi.org/10.1016/S0076-6879(07)28025-5] [PMID: 17875433]

[108] Warskulat U, Borsch E, Reinehr R, *et al.* Chronic liver disease is triggered by taurine transporter knockout in the mouse. FASEB J 2006; 20(3): 574-6.
[http://dx.doi.org/10.1096/fj.05-5016fje] [PMID: 16421246]

[109] Warskulat U, Borsch E, Reinehr R, *et al.* Taurine deficiency and apoptosis: Findings from the taurine transporter knockout mouse. Arch Biochem Biophys 2007; 462(2): 202-9.
[http://dx.doi.org/10.1016/j.abb.2007.03.022] [PMID: 17459327]

[110] Rascher K, Servos G, Berthold G, *et al.* Light deprivation slows but does not prevent the loss of photoreceptors in taurine transporter knockout mice. Vision Res 2004; 44(17): 2091-100.
[http://dx.doi.org/10.1016/j.visres.2004.03.027] [PMID: 15149840]

[111] Ito T, Nakanishi Y, Yamaji N, Murakami S, Schaffer SW. Induction of growth differentiation factor 15 in skeletal muscle of old taurine transporter knockout mouse. Biol Pharm Bull 2018; 41(3): 435-9.
[http://dx.doi.org/10.1248/bpb.b17-00969] [PMID: 29491220]

[112] Oermann E, Warskulat U, Heller-Stilb B, Häussinger D, Zilles K. Taurine-transporter gene knockout-induced changes in GABAA, kainate and AMPA but not NMDA receptor binding in mouse brain. Anat Embryol (Berl) 2005; 210(5-6): 363-72.
[http://dx.doi.org/10.1007/s00429-005-0024-6] [PMID: 16222546]

[113] Sergeeva OA, Chepkova AN, Doreulee N, *et al.* Taurine-induced long-lasting enhancement of synaptic transmission in mice: role of transporters. J Physiol 2003; 550(3): 911-9.
[http://dx.doi.org/10.1113/jphysiol.2003.045864] [PMID: 12824447]

[114] Heller-Stilb B, Roeyen C, Rascher K, *et al.* Disruption of the taurine transporter gene (*taut*) leads to retinal degeneration in mice. FASEB J 2002; 16(2): 1-18.
[http://dx.doi.org/10.1096/fj.01-0691fje] [PMID: 11772953]

[115] Han X, Patters AB, Ito T, Azuma J, Schaffer SW, Chesney RW. Knockout of the TauT gene predisposes C57BL/6 mice to streptozotocin-induced diabetic nephropathy. PLoS One 2015; 10(1): e0117718.
[http://dx.doi.org/10.1371/journal.pone.0117718] [PMID: 25629817]

[116] De Luca A, Pierno S, Camerino DC. Taurine: the appeal of a safe amino acid for skeletal muscle disorders. J Transl Med 2015; 13(1): 243.
[http://dx.doi.org/10.1186/s12967-015-0610-1] [PMID: 26208967]

[117] Jong CJ, Azuma J, Schaffer SW. Role of mitochondrial permeability transition in taurine deficiency-induced apoptosis. Exp Clin Cardiol 2011; 16(4): 125-8.
[PMID: 22131855]

[118] Bhat MA, Ahmad K, Khan MSA, *et al.* Expedition into taurine biology: structural insights and therapeutic perspective of taurine in neurodegenerative diseases. Biomolecules 2020; 10(6): 863.
[http://dx.doi.org/10.3390/biom10060863] [PMID: 32516961]

[119] Ito T, Oishi S, Takai M, *et al.* Cardiac and skeletal muscle abnormality in taurine transporter-knockout mice. J Biomed Sci 2010; 17(Suppl 1): S20.
[http://dx.doi.org/10.1186/1423-0127-17-S1-S20] [PMID: 20804595]

[120] Jong C, Ito T, Prentice H, Wu JY, Schaffer S. Role of mitochondria and endoplasmic reticulum in taurine-deficiency-mediated apoptosis. Nutrients 2017; 9(8): 795.
[http://dx.doi.org/10.3390/nu9080795] [PMID: 28757580]

[121] Schaffer SW, Shimada-Takaura K, Jong CJ, Ito T, Takahashi K. Impaired energy metabolism of the taurine-deficient heart. Amino Acids 2016; 48(2): 549-58.
[http://dx.doi.org/10.1007/s00726-015-2110-2] [PMID: 26475290]

[122] Dragnes BT, Larsen R, Ernstsen MH, Mæhre H, Elvevoll EO. Impact of processing on the taurine content in processed seafood and their corresponding unprocessed raw materials. Int J Food Sci Nutr 2009; 60(2): 143-52.
[http://dx.doi.org/10.1080/09637480701621654] [PMID: 18608559]

[123] Pasantes-Morales H, Quesada O, Alcocer L, Olea RS. Taurine content in foods. Nutr Rep Int 1989; 40: 793-801.

[124] Larsen R, Eilertsen K-E, Mæhre H, Jensen I-J, Elvevoll EO. Taurine content in marine foods: Beneficial health effects. Bioactive compounds from marine foods: Plant and animal sources. 2013; 249-68.

[125] Jeong J-S, Choi M-J. The intake of taurine and major food source of taurine in elementary school children in Korea Taurine 11. Springer 2019; pp. 349-58.

[126] Han SH, Park SH, Chang KJ. Dietary taurine intake and its food sources in Korean young adults using 2015 Korea national health and nutrition examination survey data. Adv Exp Med Biol 2019; 1155: 223-30.
[http://dx.doi.org/10.1007/978-981-13-8023-5_21] [PMID: 31468401]

[127] Stipanuk MH, Coloso RM, Garcia RAG, Banks MF. Cysteine concentration regulates cysteine metabolism to glutathione, sulfate and taurine in rat hepatocytes. J Nutr 1992; 122(3): 420-7.
[http://dx.doi.org/10.1093/jn/122.3.420] [PMID: 1542000]

[128] Terriente-Palacios C, Castellari M. Levels of taurine, hypotaurine and homotaurine, and amino acids profiles in selected commercial seaweeds, microalgae, and algae-enriched food products. Food Chem 2022; 368: : 130770..
[http://dx.doi.org/10.1016/j.foodchem.2021.130770] [PMID: 34399181]

CHAPTER 2

Taurine and the Mitochondrion

Abstract: Several studies have evaluated the subcellular compartmentalization of taurine (TAU) and its cellular and molecular mechanisms of action. Meanwhile, it has been found that TAU is largely uptaken by mitochondria. TAU could improve mitochondrial function by incorporating it into the basic mitochondrial structures and protein synthesis (*e.g.*, mainly mitochondrial electron transport chain components). Several other mechanisms, including the enhancement of mitochondrial calcium sequestration, regulation of mitochondria-mediated reactive oxygen species (ROS) formation, prevention of mitochondria-mediated cell death, and mitochondrial pH buffering, are also involved in the mitochondrial function regulatory properties of TAU. Therefore, TAU has been used against a wide range of pathologies, including mitochondrial injury. In the current chapter, a review of the approved molecular mechanism for the effects of TAU on mitochondria is provided. Then, the applications of TAU on a wide range of complications linked with mitochondrial impairment are discussed. The data collected here could give a better insight into the application of TAU as a therapeutic agent against a wide range of human diseases.

Keywords: Amino acid, Bioenergetics, Energy metabolism, Mitochondrial cytopathies, Mitochondrial disease, Mitochondrial impairment.

INTRODUCTION

The mechanisms of cytoprotection provided by taurine (TAU) have been widely investigated. Earlier, it was proposed that TAU could act as a direct radical scavenger [1 - 4]. However, later it became clear that TAU is a weak scavenger of reactive species [1 - 4]. Further studies revealed that mitochondria are the major place where TAU provides its cytoprotective properties by regulating this organelle [3, 5 - 11]. Nowadays, it is clear that TAU accumulates in mitochondria in high quantities [7, 12 - 14].

Several essential roles have been attributed to TAU in cellular mitochondria [7, 12, 13]. First, it is well-known that TAU contributes to basic mitochondrial structures such as tRNA [4, 13]. It has been found that mitochondria lacking TAU-modified tRNA couldn't synthesize their proteins (*e.g.*, mitochondrial respiratory chain complexes), and their function is impaired [13, 15]. On the other hand, it has been found that TAU regulates mitochondrial calcium homeostasis,

Reza Heidari and M. Mehdi Ommati

prevents the release of cell death mediators from forming this organelle, and finally boosts energy (ATP metabolism) [10, 13, 16 - 22].

Many examples of human diseases are connected to mitochondrial impairment and disturbed energy metabolism. Skeletal muscle disease, neurodegenerative disorders, cardiovascular complications, liver disease, and reproductive anomalies have been identified with mitochondrial disturbances [23 - 37]. Therefore, it seems that targeting mitochondria in these complications could serve as a viable therapeutic option.

A plethora of investigations revealed the positive effects of TAU supplementation on human diseases. Interestingly, TAU provides its protective properties mainly by affecting cellular power plants. In the current chapter, the basic concepts of the effects of TAU on mitochondrial function are highlighted. Then, the potential application of this amino acid for a wide range of human diseases focusing on the effects of TAU on mitochondria and its related complications are highlighted.

TAURINE IN THE BASIC MITOCHONDRIAL STRUCTURES

The positive effects of TAU on mitochondria have been repeatedly documented [5, 18, 38 - 40]. Many studies have also mentioned that TAU significantly suppresses mitochondria-mediated cell death [18, 41 - 43]. Several mechanisms have been noted regarding the effects of TAU on mitochondrial function and its association with cellular energy metabolism and cytoprotective mechanisms [17, 20]. Recently, an exciting finding revealed the incorporation of TAU in the synthesis and regulation of basic mitochondrial structures [15, 44, 45]. These results mention that TAU is not just a supplement agent but is essential for proper mitochondrial function. The pivotal role of TAU in mitochondrial function and structure is discussed herein.

Recent studies revealed that TAU incorporates the structure of transfer RNA (tRNA) in mitochondria [4, 13] (Fig. **1**). tRNA is a molecule that serves as a link between messenger RNA (mRNA) and protein synthesis. tRNA carries amino acids to ribosomes (Fig. **1**). Hence, tRNA is necessary for mRNA translation and protein synthesis [4, 13]. Mitochondrial DNA (mtDNA) encodes several proteins (*e.g.,* electron transport chain components) independently from the nuclear DNA. Hence, any defect in the mitochondrial tRNA structure could influence protein synthesis and, finally, mitochondrial function (Fig. **1**). Mechanistically, it has been found that TAU forms a conjugate with a uridine base in mitochondrial tRNA [13, 15]. This TAU conjugation leads to structural changes in mitochondrial tRNA, making it functional for amino acid transportation to ribosomes and, finally, appropriate mitochondrial protein synthesis [13, 15] (Fig. **1**). On the other hand, recent data revealed that defective mitochondrial tRNA

TAU modification activates several protease enzymes, leading to cell death [45]. Therefore, it is crucial to manage tRNA taurine deficiency in patients.

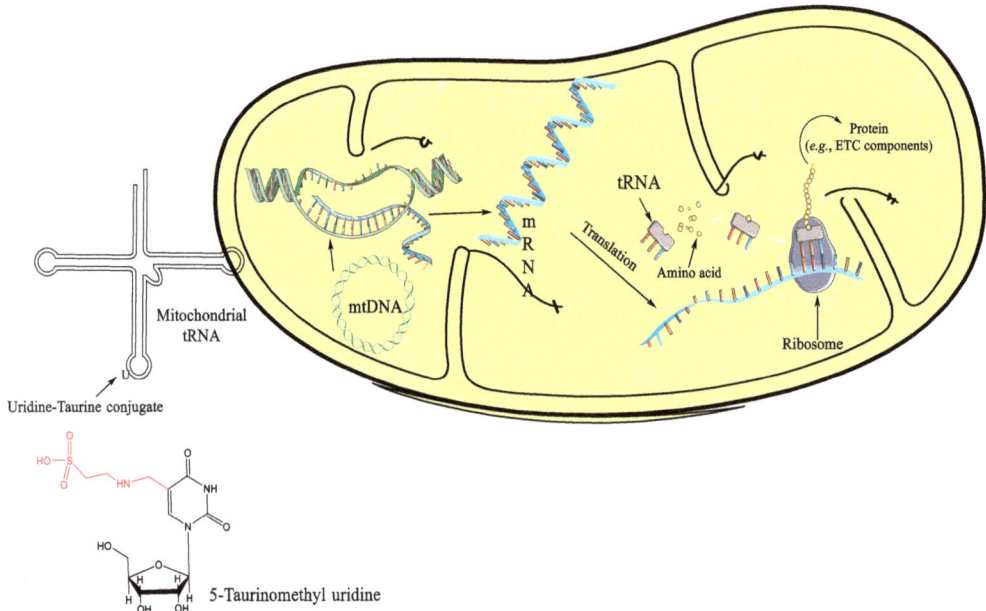

Fig. (1). Functional mitochondrial transfer RNA (tRNA) forms a conjugate with taurine. Mitochondrial tRNA lacking taurine modification cannot efficiently transport amino acids to ribosomes. Consequently, the synthesis of many proteins, including the mitochondrial respiratory chain components, could be disturbed. ETC: Electron transport chain. Taurine could find an application to alleviate mitochondrial tRNA defects in clinical settings.

Interestingly, it has been revealed that the formation of TAU-tRNA conjugate is hampered in several mitochondria-linked diseases [13, 46 - 48]. Mitochondrial tRNA lacking TAU modification is unstable and could not synthesize proteins correctly [65]. Consequently, the expression of several mitochondria-encoded proteins (*e.g.*, respiratory chain complexes) is suppressed [13, 46 - 48]. Excitingly, when mitochondrial oxidative phosphorylation is diminished (*e.g.*, lack of tRNA in TAU deficiency), an elevation in the glycolysis process and lactate production will occur, leading to metabolic acidosis. It has been found that TAU supplementation could significantly improve symptoms of patients with mitochondrial disorders related to impaired tRNA TAU modification [49, 50]. These findings provide clues for TAU application as a therapeutic option in clinical settings.

Several pathogenic mutations in human mtDNA have been identified that are suspected to be linked with impaired mitochondrial tRNA function [51]. These mutations could be associated with specific clinical manifestations [51]. A mutation in mtDNA has been recognized, related to deficient TAU modification of mitochondrial tRNA [48]. Mitochondrial myopathy, encephalopathy, lactic acidosis, stroke-like syndrome (MELAS), myoclonic epilepsy, and ragged red fiber syndrome (MERRF) are two severe mitochondrial diseases in humans that are linked with the lack of TAU modification in mitochondrial tRNA [49, 50, 52] (Fig. **1**). It is well-identified that the synthesis and assembly of mitochondrial respiratory chain complexes are hampered in MELAS and MERRF [49, 50] (Fig. **1**). As we receive all our mitochondria from our mother, MELAS and MERRF are maternally-inherited genetic disorders. These data mention the importance of genetic defects in mitochondria-related to the amino acid TAU.

Excitingly, a phase III clinical trial confirmed the beneficial role of TAU in MELAS patients [49]. It was found that TAU significantly decreased the recurrence of stroke-like syndrome episodes as the most acute symptom of MELAS [49]. Another interesting finding of TAU supplementation in MELAS patients is the increase in TAU-modified mitochondrial tRNA [49].

As mitochondrial oxidative phosphorylation is diminished in TAU deficiency, an elevation in glycolysis and lactate production will occur [49]. In phase III clinical trial, Ohsawa *et al.* found that "taurine supplementation was effective and safe for the prevention of stroke-like episodes in patients with MELAS by ameliorating the modification defect in the first anticodon nucleotide of mitochondrial tRNA$^{Leu(UUR)}$" [49]. These data are an example of a case that TAU supplementation could change the future of a genetic disorder.

Based on the abovementioned data, it could be concluded that TAU is not only a supplementary amino acid. TAU contributes to basic mitochondrial structures (*e.g.*, tRNA) and is involved in vital pathways such as protein synthesis in cellular mitochondria. Moreover, TAU supplementation might also benefit other mitochondrial diseases where TAU modification of mitochondrial tRNA is impaired. Besides, the effects of TAU on mitochondrial tRNA and mtDNA mutations in healthy subjects have not been evaluated so far.

TAURINE REGULATES MITOCHONDRIA-FACILITATED OXIDANTS PRODUCTION

In the current section, we focus on the primary mechanisms involved in the antioxidant properties of TAU. Previously, it was mainly thought TAU is a direct radical scavenger and provides its antioxidant capacity through removing reactive species. However, it is now known that TAU is a weak radical scavenger and is practically unable to scavenge many ROS forms [53]. More studies on the antioxidative properties of TAU revealed that this amino acid directly affects mitochondria-originated ROS formation [10, 13, 16 - 22]. It has been demonstrated that TAU deficiency dramatically decreased the synthesis of mitochondria-encoded proteins and enhanced the mitochondria-facilitated ROS formation [7]. The mitochondrial electron transport chain (ETC) is the primary source of intracellular ROS, especially the superoxide anion ($O_2^{\cdot-}$) [54]. Enhanced mitochondrial-mediated ROS formation could lead to dangerous events such as mitochondria permeabilization and swelling [54, 55]. Finally, cell death and organ injury could occur [54, 55]. Besides, as mitochondria have a less potent antioxidant system than the cytosol, many intra-mitochondrial components could be damaged by ROS. Mitochondria impairment and oxidative stress are the primary mechanisms of cytotoxicity induced by a wide range of xenobiotics [56 - 60]. Besides, the enhancement of mitochondria-mediated ROS formation could further damage intracellular targets, including mtDNA, proteins, and lipids.

It has been found that TAU significantly decreased superoxide generation by the mitochondria respiratory chain [10, 23, 61, 62]. On the other hand, some studies mentioned that the potentiation of cellular antioxidant mechanisms upon TAU supplementation could also be involved in its antioxidant mechanism [18, 63 - 68]. It has been found that the brain, heart, liver, and kidney antioxidant capacity was significantly increased with TAU treatment [69 - 76]. The increase in the activity of glutathione peroxidase, catalase, superoxide dismutase, and glutathione-s-transferase has been documented in association with TAU treatment [69 - 71].

As previously mentioned, some other investigations questioned the role of TAU in boosting the activity of cellular antioxidant enzymes [6, 17, 77, 78]. These discrepancies in results might be due to the dose of TAU administered, the duration of treatment, and the sensitivity of methods used to assess cellular antioxidant capacity. Based on these data, the regulatory properties of mitochondria of TAU could be the dominant mechanism that contributes to the antioxidant effects of this amino acid [39, 69, 79 - 83]. It has been found that TAU deficiency significantly decreases the expression of specific mitochondrial proteins [10]. TAU could prevent the diversion of electrons from the ETC to the cytosol, which in turn substantially reduces the formation of reactive species (Fig. **2**).

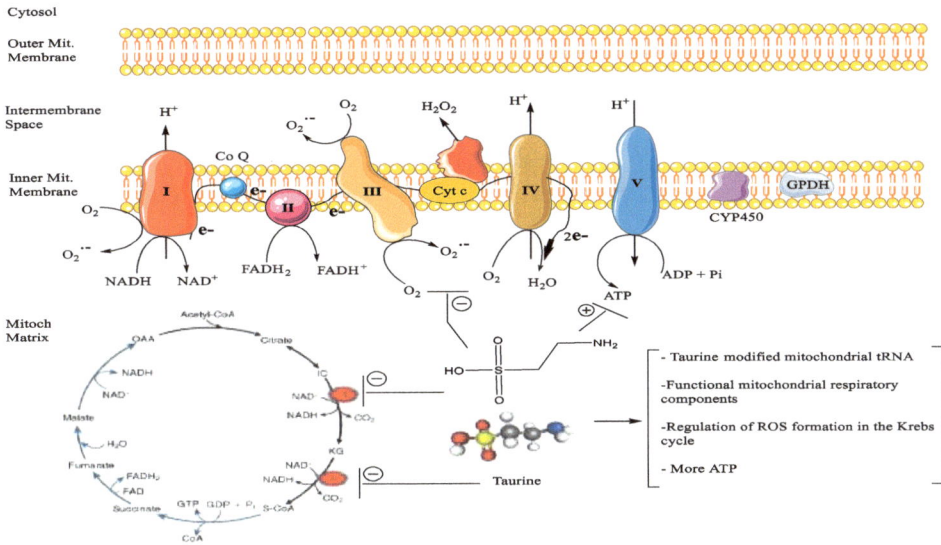

Fig. (2). Taurine significantly decreases mitochondria-facilitated reactive oxygen species (ROS) formation during oxidative phosphorylation. The effects of taurine on the appropriate synthesis of mitochondrial respiratory chain complexes could profoundly affect mitochondria-mediated ROS formation. Unfortunately, there is a lack of experimental evidence on the role of taurine in the synthesis or regulation of ROS formation by mitochondrial matrix-embedded enzymes. GPDH: Glycerol-3-phosphate dehydrogenase. AC: Aconitase; KG: Ketoglutarate; S-CoA: Succinyl Co-A; Co-A: Co-enzyme A; OAA: Oxaloacetate.

As mitochondria-mediated oxidative stress plays a fundamental role in the pathogenesis of several diseases, TAU treatment could be considered a preventive/therapeutic option against these complications. ROS could also be formed by P450 or glycerol-3-phosphate dehydrogenase (GPDH) located in the mitochondria's inner membrane (Fig. **2**). Moreover, many mitochondrial matrix-located enzymes, such as α-KGD, aconitase, and pyruvate dehydrogenase, can generate superoxide anions (Fig. **2**). Unfortunately, there is little data on the effects of TAU on mitochondrial matrix-embedded enzymes and their contribution to this amino acid antioxidant property.

The effects of TAU on mitochondria-dependent cell death and apoptosis are another interesting mechanism involved in the cytoprotective properties of this amino acid [43, 84 - 88]. It has been found that TAU significantly prevents the release of cell death mediators (*e.g.*, cytochrome *c*) from mitochondria [43, 84 - 88]. It has been found that TAU significantly regulates signaling pathways related to mitochondria-mediated apoptosis [88]. For example, it has been revealed that TAU significantly down-regulated the expression of apoptosis-inducing factors such as Bax, Fas ligand (FasL), Fas, caspase 3, and caspase 9 [86, 88]. On the other hand, TAU significantly enhanced the expression of anti-apoptotic factors such as Bcl-2 [88]. The effects of TAU on mitochondrial permeabilization as well as mitochondrial membrane potential play a crucial role in its antiapoptotic properties [86, 89]. All these data indicate that TAU significantly regulates mitochondria-mediated apoptosis and cell death.

It has been found that TAU supplementation could improve mitochondrial function by restoring mitochondrial protein synthesis (*e.g.,* respiratory chain complexes) [6, 17, 77]. As previously mentioned, in some pathological conditions, the lack of TAU in mitochondrial tRNA could lead to various diseases [23, 46 - 50, 90 - 92]. However, it has been found that TAU supplementation to healthy subjects could also enhance the capability of this organelle for ATP metabolism [17, 93]. All these data confirm that the effect of TAU on ETC components and mitochondrial matrix-embedded enzymes could play a primary role in its impact on regulating mitochondria-originated oxidant production (Fig. **2**).

TAURINE AND CELLULAR ENERGY METABOLISM

As mentioned in the previous section, TAU efficiently improves mitochondrial protein synthesis (*e.g.*, electron transport chain complexes). Therefore, this amino acid could significantly preserve mitochondrial energy (ATP) metabolism (Fig. **2**). Many investigations documented that TAU depletion caused severe complications, including energy crises and cell death [31]. The effects of TAU on mitochondrial energy metabolism could be mediated through several ways. The most important pathway for the effects of TAU on mitochondrial ATP production was described in the previous sections about the incorporation of this amino acid in the biosynthesis of mitochondrial respiratory chain complexes. In the forthcoming section, another important mechanism involved in the TAU-induced enhancement of mitochondrial function and ATP metabolism is discussed.

Some studies described the buffering properties of TAU and mentioned this feature as an essential factor for proper mitochondrial function (Fig. **3**). TAU is a well-known physiological buffering agent [94]. This means that TAU could prevent fluctuations in the pH of physiological fluids and maintain it in a constant range [94]. It has been found that TAU could tightly regulate mitochondrial matrix pH [94] (Fig. **3**). Preserving the pH gradient between mitochondrial matrix and cytosol is a critical mechanism for the effects of TAU in mitochondrial function [94]. Hence, the presence of TAU is critical for mitochondrial matrix pH buffering [94]. TAU (PK_a = 8.6 at 37°C) is a well-known physiological pH regulator. Because of the H^+ gradient, the pH of the mitochondrial matrix is slightly alkaline in normal conditions (pH = 7.9-8.1). Hansen *et al.* reported that TAU acts as a mitochondrial buffer regulatory agent and preserves mitochondrial pH at the range of 7.7-8.1 [6] (Fig. **3**). On the other hand, the activity of some mitochondria-embedded enzymes seems to be pH-dependent [94]. Interestingly it has been established that the activity of some mitochondrial matrix enzymes, especially those involved in energy metabolism, are increased in the presence of higher mitochondrial TAU concentrations [94] (Fig. **3**). Hansen *et al.* found that enzymes such as isocitrate dehydrogenase (involved in the citric acid cycle) have maximum capacity in alkaline pH (7.7-8.1) [94]. It has also been documented that TAU promotes fatty acids beta-oxidation by enhancing the uptake of fatty acids into the cellular mitochondria [10]. Acyl-CoA dehydrogenases (ACDDs) are other essential enzymes involved in the fatty acid β-oxidation. It has been found that ACDDs have maximum activity at mildly alkaline pH (pH = 8-8.5) [94] (Fig. **3**). The effect of TAU on ACADs activity might play a fundamental role in the effects of this amino acid in lipid metabolism disorders (*e.g.,* fatty liver, obesity) or drug-induced steatohepatitis (*e.g.,* valproic acid-induced liver injury). Based on the data provided in this section, the effects of TAU on oxidative phosphorylation (OXOPHOS) and ATP production could be mediated through several mechanisms. All these data highlight the importance of TAU in mitochondrial ATP synthesis and its vital role in managing human diseases associated with impaired energy metabolism. Future studies on experimental animals or clinical trials could reveal the beneficial effects of TAU in human diseases linked with mitochondrial impairment.

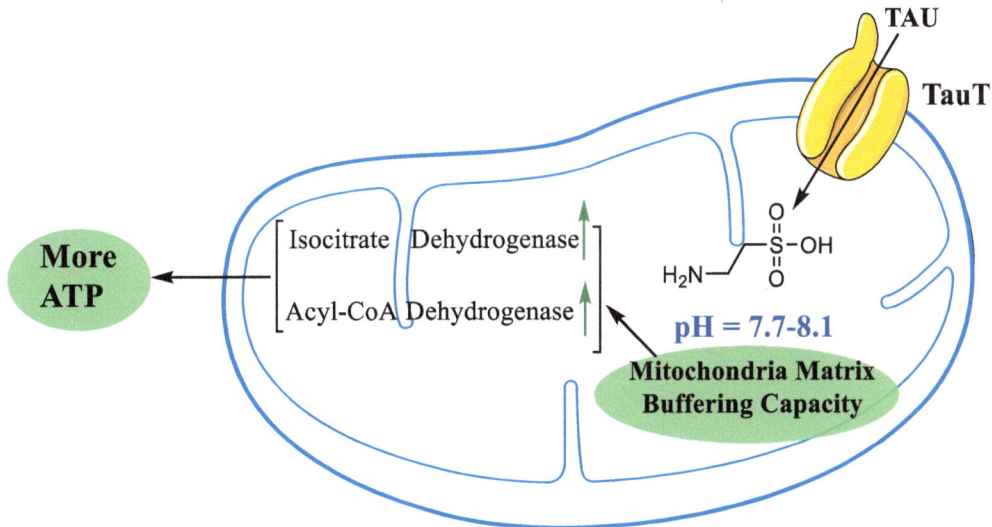

Fig. (3). Mitochondrial buffering capacity play an essential role in the positive effects of this amino acid in cellular mitochondria. Regulating mitochondrial matrix pH is a critical parameter regulated by compounds such as taurine. Several mitochondria matrix-embedded enzymes, especially those involved in the energy (ATP) metabolism, have maximum activity at alkaline pH (pH = 7.7-8.1).

TAURINE AND CELLULAR CALCIUM HOMEOSTASIS

Disturbance in cellular Ca^{2+} homeostasis is linked to a cascade of deleterious events, which finally lead to cytotoxicity [95] (Fig. **4**). High intracellular Ca^{2+} activates several proteolytic enzymes involved in cell death [95, 96]. Interestingly, modulation of cellular Ca^{2+} levels is an essential feature of TAU [97, 98]. In response to moderately high Ca^{2+} levels, it has been found that TAU increases the Ca^{2+} sequestration capability of mitochondria [97, 98] (Fig. **4**). Actually, mitochondria act as safety valves to prevent cytoplasmic Ca^{2+} overload and cell death [97, 98]. The smooth endoplasmic reticulum is the primary storage of Ca^{2+} in the cytoplasm. The mechanisms of the cytotoxicity induced by many xenobiotics rely on ER stress and cytoplasmic Ca^{2+} overload [99] (Fig. **4**). ER stress and cellular Ca^{2+} disturbances are also well-known mechanisms involved in the pathogenesis of several human diseases [100, 101]. As the ER is the primary site for the folding and modification of proteins, ER stress could lead to unfolded protein response (UPR) [100, 101]. UPR could lead to a series of events that finally lead to cellular and organ malfunction [102, 103]. An intricate set of signaling pathways could be involved in the ER and UPR [100, 101]. Therefore, the effects of TAU on ER stress could play a big role in its cytoprotective mechanisms (Fig. **4**).

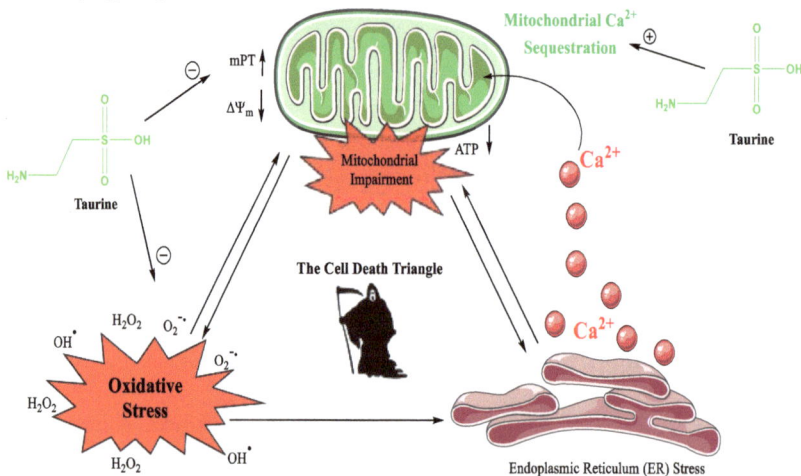

Fig. (4). Mitochondrial impairment, oxidative stress, and cytoplasmic calcium disturbances are firmly interrelated events. Disturbances in each factor could lead to severe complications, including cell death and organ injury. The amino acid taurine could prevent these deleterious events. It has also been well-established that taurine enhanced mitochondrial Ca^{2+} sequestration. Moreover, taurine significantly diminished mitochondria-mediated ROS formation and oxidative stress. Finally, it should be mentioned that taurine can enhance mitochondrial ATP metabolism. mPT: Mitochondrial permeability transition; ROS: Reactive oxygen species; RNS: Reactive nitrogen species; $\Delta\Psi$: Mitochondrial membrane potential; ATP: Adenosine triphosphate.

It has been well-documented that TAU effectively prevents ER stress, cellular Ca^{2+} overload, and oxidative stress in different experimental models [38, 104, 105]. Therefore, controlling the release of Ca^{2+} from intracellular stores (*e.g.*, ER) plays a fundamental role in the cytoprotective properties of TAU (Fig. **4**). TAU affects different transporters involved in regulating cytoplasmic and mitochondrial Ca^{2+} homeostasis (Fig. **5**). It has been found that TAU inhibits Na^+/Ca^{2+} exchangers in different subcellular compartments, including the endoplasmic reticulum and mitochondria [21]. TAU also promotes Ca^{2+} efflux from the cytoplasm through Na^+/Ca^{2+} exchanger [21]. Cellular mitochondria also play a fundamental role in cytoplasmic Ca^{2+} homeostasis [106, 107] (Fig. **5**). Several lines of evidence indicate that TAU facilitates the Ca^{2+} buffering capacity of mitochondria [106, 107]. TAU could positively affect the mitochondrial ability for Ca^{2+} sequestration in moderate cases of Ca^{2+} overload and enhance cell survival during toxic insults [106, 107]. Interestingly, it has been found that when cytoplasmic pH is declined (*e.g.*, in ischemia-reperfusion injury), the Na^+/H^+ exchanger is activated and promotes the exchange between extracellular Na^+ and intracellular H^+ (Fig. **5**). The effects of TAU on mitochondrial calcium uniporter (CUP) have been reported as a mechanism for enhancing the mitochondrial buffering capacity of this amino acid [108] (Fig. **5**). Consequently, intracellular Na^+ is increased and leads to the export of Ca^{2+} through the Na^+/Ca^{2+} exchanger (Fig. **5**). Based on the data provided in this section, TAU restrictedly regulates cytoplasmic Ca^{2+} and inhibits ER stress signaling, which could finally lead to cell death [109] (Fig. **4**). ER stress and cytoplasmic Ca^{2+} overload play a pivotal role in the pathogenesis of various diseases [100]. Hence, the effects of TAU on mitochondrial Ca^{2+} sequestration could act as a cytoprotective mechanism and play a role in its protective properties in several human diseases.

TAURINE THERAPY IN MITOCHONDRIA-LINKED PATHOLOGIES

In many old references, TAU is considered a semi-conditional amino acid. On the other hand, increasing evidence indicates that this chemical could play a crucial role in the human body. Besides the physiological roles of TAU as a bile acid conjugator and cellular osmoregulator, many pharmacological roles, including the antioxidant, anti-inflammatory, and anti-apoptotic properties, have also been attributed to this amino acid [44]. The pivotal role of TAU in modulating proper mitochondrial function makes this amino acid an inseparable component of cellular energy metabolism. Many experimental and clinical studies indicate that TAU could enhance mitochondrial function and cellular energy in a wide range of diseases [23, 110 - 112]. On the other hand, several human diseases are connected to impaired mitochondrial function [113 - 117]. Hence, manipulating mitochondrial function and energy metabolism could be a potential point of intervention in these complications. In the forthcoming section, the therapeutic capability of TAU in two specific mitochondrial disorders in humans is discussed. Obviously, many other disorders associated with mitochondrial injury could benefit from TAU administration. The diseases discussed in the next section are selected because they are directly linked to the lack of TAU, and the administration of this amino acid could readily blunt their signs and symptoms.

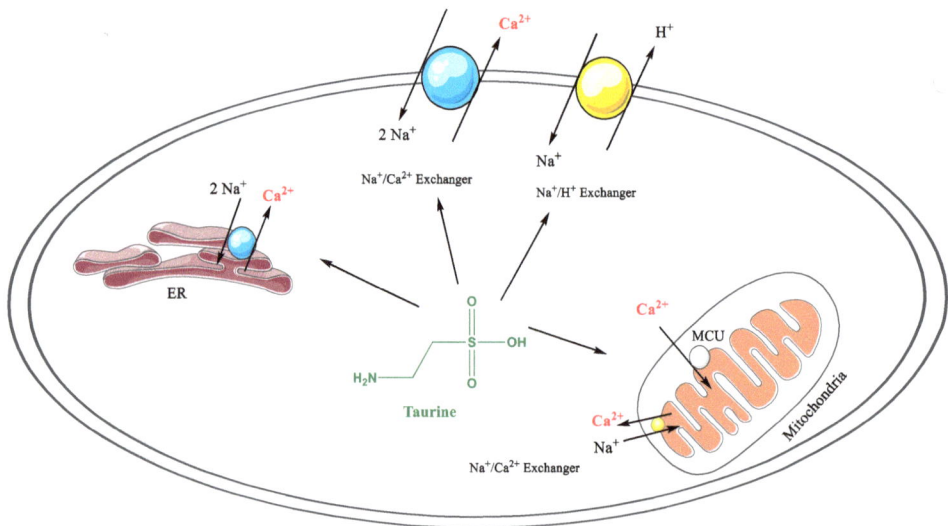

Fig. (5). Taurine sensitive calcium (Ca^{2+}) transporters. The regulation of cytoplasmic calcium (Ca^{2+}) homeostasis plays a critical role in the cytoprotective properties of taurine. MCU: mitochondrial calcium uniporter.

TAURINE AND HUMAN MITOCHONDRIAL CYTOPATHIES

Human mitochondrial cytopathies (MCs) are heterogeneous disorders characterized by diminished biosynthesis and assembly of mitochondrial respiratory chain proteins [15, 118]. Different types of MCs have been identified [13]. MCs could be associated with the mutation in the nuclear or mtDNA [119]. Interrupted cellular energy metabolism is the common endpoint of MCs [119]. MCs are usually associated with a cluster of clinical symptoms [119]. Muscle weakness, severe disability, neurological disorders, metabolic derangements, and premature death are related to different types of MCs [119, 120].

Although genetic engineering could serve as a therapeutic intervention in the different forms of MCs [119, 121], this option may not be available worldwide or could not be economically beneficial (*e.g.*, due to the rare nature of some types of MCs). Hence, finding pharmacological options that could improve MCs' symptoms and enhance patients' quality of life has great value. Lactic acidosis, and stroke-like syndrome (MELAS) and myoclonic epilepsy, and ragged red fiber syndrome (MERRF) are two well-known MCs that significantly debilitate patients [122, 123] (Fig. **6**).

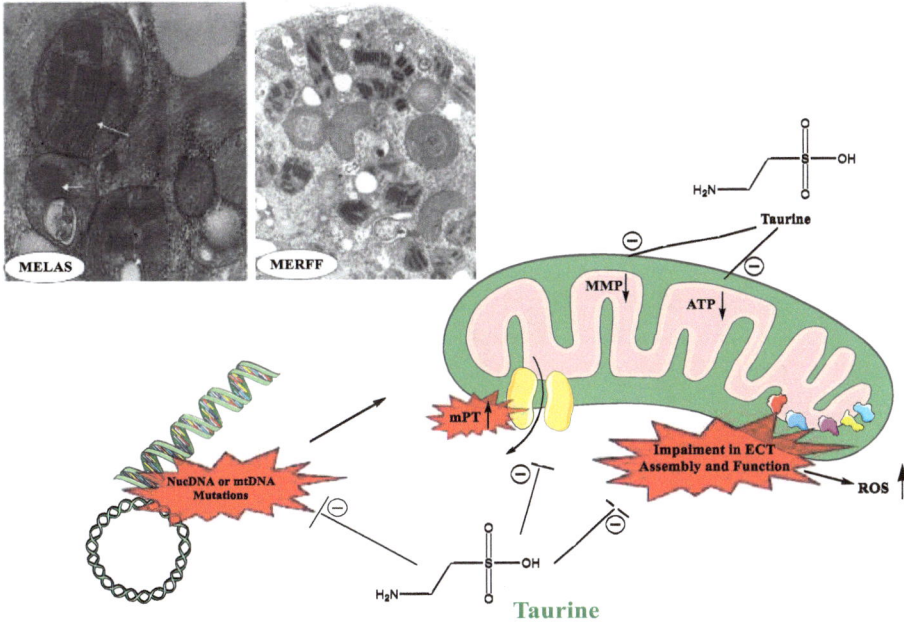

Fig. (6). Taurine could enhance mitochondrial function and improve the condition of patients with mitochondrial cytopathies. mPT: Mitochondrial permeability transition; ROS: Reactive oxygen species; MMP: Mitochondrial membrane potential; ATP: Adenosine triphosphate. Electron microscopic analysis of cellular mitochondria in patients with MELAS (Adapted from Abu-Amero *et al.* [124]; CC-BY 2.0) revealed the abnormal collection of mitochondria with paracrystalline inclusions (arrowhead), osmiophilic inclusions (large arrowhead), and mitochondrial vacuoles (small arrowhead). Abnormal and abundant mitochondria with crystal inclusions also have been detected in MERRF patients (Electron microscope image for MERRF has been adapted from http://neuropathology-web.org/chapter10/chapter10dMitochondria.html). MELAS and MRRF are directly related to impaired taurine-associated tRNA modification.

Interestingly, it has been detected that MELAS and MERRF are directly related to impaired mitochondrial tRNA modification by TAU [23, 123]. This point suggests TAU as a potential therapeutic option against these disorders. Excitingly, several clinical studies revealed that TAU could significantly improve the symptoms of MELAS and MERRF [23, 50, 91]. Finally, it should be noted that high doses of TAU are needed (up to 12 g/day) to subside mitochondrial dysfunction and clinical manifestation of mitochondrial diseases such as MELAS [49, 92]. Hence, designing mitochondria-targeted formulations of this amino acid might significantly enhance its therapeutic value.

CONCLUSION

TAU is a non-protein amino acid with a wide range of physiological and pharmacological properties. TAU could be synthesized from amino acid cysteine *in vivo*. However, the ability of endogenous TAU biosynthesis is highly variable between different species [125 - 127]. In this context, liver TAU synthesis capacity is low in humans [20, 128]. Hence, this amino acid is primarily provided by dietary sources. TAU containing supplements, meat, and kinds of seafood provide a tremendous daily demand for body TAU [129]. Several epidemiological studies revealed that TAU intake is reversely correlated with the mortality associated with many diseases (*e.g.*, cardiovascular and liver disease) [130 - 132].

TAU provides a wide range of protective properties *in vivo* and *in vitro*. Hence, understanding the cellular and molecular mechanisms underlying these protective effects allows us to use this amino acid in various human diseases. It seems that the positive impact of TAU on mitochondria could be critical for the maintenance of cellular homeostasis. Many investigations mentioned that TAU could enhance mitochondrial membrane potential ($\Delta\Psi_m$), improve ATP synthesis, decrease mitochondria-facilitated ROS formation, and prevent mitochondria-mediated cell death [4, 11, 17, 61, 69, 133 - 139]. Based on these data, TAU could be administered for many human diseases (Fig. **7**).

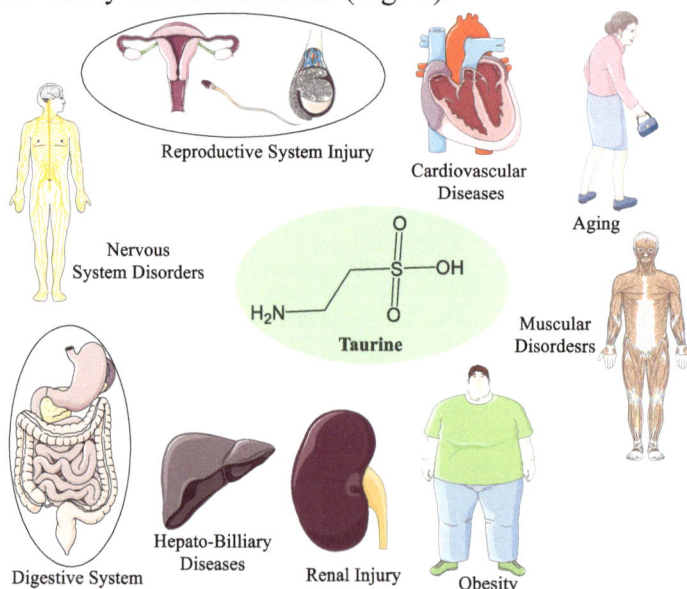

Fig. (7). The pleiotropic effects of taurine on cellular function make this amino acid a mind-provoking compound for managing a battery of human diseases. The enhancement of mitochondrial function and cellular energy metabolism seems to play a fundamental role in the mechanisms of cytoprotection provided by taurine.

Considering the pivotal role of TAU in cellular energy metabolism, this amino acid could be applied against several mitochondria-linked complications. TAU is a safe, naturally occurring nutraceutical with a wide range of beneficial effects against several diseases. On the other hand, this amino acid exhibits few and negligible adverse effects in humans [140, 141]. Therefore, TAU might be applicable as a supplemental/therapeutic agent in clinical settings (Fig. **7**).

In various chapters of the current book, we will discuss the therapeutic role of TAU in various human diseases and highlight the positive effects of this amino acid on cellular mitochondria and energy metabolism as a fundamental mechanism that contributed to its cytoprotective properties. These data could lead to the clinical applications of TAU against mitochondria-linked disorders and finally improve the health condition of many patients (Fig. **7**).

REFERENCES

[1]   Oliveira MWS, Minotto JB, de Oliveira MR, Zanotto-Filho A, Behr GA, Rocha RF, *et al.* Scavenging and antioxidant potential of physiological taurine concentrations against different reactive oxygen/nitrogen species. Pharmacological reports: PR. 2010; 62(1): 185-93.

[2]   Kim JH, Jang HJ, Cho WY, Yeon SJ, Lee CH. *In vitro* antioxidant actions of sulfur-containing amino acids. Arab J Chem 2020; 13(1): 1678-84.
        [http://dx.doi.org/10.1016/j.arabjc.2017.12.036]

[3]   Jong CJ, Schaffer S. Mechanism underlying the antioxidant activity of taurine. The FASEB Journal 2013; 27(S1): 1086.1-1.
        [http://dx.doi.org/10.1096/fasebj.27.1_supplement.1086.1]

[4]   Schaffer SW, Azuma J, Mozaffari M. Role of antioxidant activity of taurine in diabetesThis article is one of a selection of papers from the NATO Advanced Research Workshop on Translational Knowledge for Heart Health (published in part 1 of a 2-part Special Issue). Can J Physiol Pharmacol 2009; 87(2): 91-9.
        [http://dx.doi.org/10.1139/Y08-110] [PMID: 19234572]

[5]   Heidari R, Babaei H, Eghbal MA. Amodiaquine-induced toxicity in isolated rat hepatocytes and the cytoprotective effects of taurine and/or N-acetyl cysteine. Res Pharm Sci 2014; 9(2): 97-105.
        [PMID: 25657778]

[6]   Hansen SH, Andersen ML, Birkedal H, Cornett C, Wibrand F. The important role of taurine in oxidative metabolism. Taurine 6 Advances in Experimental Medicine and Biology. Springer US 2006; pp. 129-35.
        [http://dx.doi.org/10.1007/978-0-387-33504-9_13]

[7]   Jong CJ, Azuma J, Schaffer S. Mechanism underlying the antioxidant activity of taurine: prevention of mitochondrial oxidant production. Amino Acids 2012; 42(6): 2223-32.
        [http://dx.doi.org/10.1007/s00726-011-0962-7] [PMID: 21691752]

[8]   Jong C, Ito T, Prentice H, Wu JY, Schaffer S. Role of mitochondria and endoplasmic reticulum in taurine-deficiency-mediated apoptosis. Nutrients 2017; 9(8): 795.
        [http://dx.doi.org/10.3390/nu9080795] [PMID: 28757580]

[9]   Jong CJ, Sandal P, Schaffer SW. The role of taurine in mitochondria health: More than just an antioxidant. Molecules 2021; 26(16): 4913.
        [http://dx.doi.org/10.3390/molecules26164913] [PMID: 34443494]

[10]   Seidel U, Huebbe P, Rimbach G. Taurine: A regulator of cellular redox homeostasis and skeletal

muscle function. Mol Nutr Food Res 2019; 63(16): 1800569.
[http://dx.doi.org/10.1002/mnfr.201800569] [PMID: 30211983]

[11] Ahmadian E, Babaei H, Mohajjel Nayebi A, Eftekhari A, Eghbal MA. Venlafaxine-induced cytotoxicity towards isolated rat hepatocytes involves oxidative stress and mitochondrial/lysosomal dysfunction. Adv Pharm Bull 2016; 6(4): 521-30.
[http://dx.doi.org/10.15171/apb.2016.066] [PMID: 28101459]

[12] Jong C, Ito T, Mozaffari M, Azuma J, Schaffer S. Effect of β-alanine treatment on mitochondrial taurine level and 5-taurinomethyluridine content. J Biomed Sci 2010; 17(Suppl 1): S25.
[http://dx.doi.org/10.1186/1423-0127-17-S1-S25] [PMID: 20804600]

[13] Suzuki T, Suzuki T, Wada T, Saigo K, Watanabe K. Taurine as a constituent of mitochondrial tRNAs: new insights into the functions of taurine and human mitochondrial diseases. EMBO J 2002; 21(23): 6581-9.
[http://dx.doi.org/10.1093/emboj/cdf656] [PMID: 12456664]

[14] Voss JW, Pedersen SF, Christensen ST, Lambert IH. Regulation of the expression and subcellular localization of the taurine transporter TauT in mouse NIH3T3 fibroblasts. Eur J Biochem 2004; 271(23-24): 4646-58.
[http://dx.doi.org/10.1111/j.1432-1033.2004.04420.x] [PMID: 15606752]

[15] Tsutomu S, Asuteka N, Takeo S. Human mitochondrial diseases caused by lack of taurine modification in mitochondrial tRNAs. Wiley Interdiscip Rev RNA 2011; 2(3): 376-86.
[http://dx.doi.org/10.1002/wrna.65] [PMID: 21957023]

[16] Shimada K, Jong CJ, Takahashi K, Schaffer SW, Eds. Role of ROS production and turnover in the antioxidant activity of taurine 2015. Cham: Springer International Publishing 2015.

[17] Hansen SH, Grunnet N. Taurine, glutathione and bioenergetics.Taurine 8 Advances in Experimental Medicine and Biology: Springer New York. 2013; pp. 3-12.

[18] Das J, Ghosh J, Manna P, Sinha M, Sil PC. Taurine protects rat testes against NaAsO$_2$-induced oxidative stress and apoptosis via mitochondrial dependent and independent pathways. Toxicol Lett 2009; 187(3): 201-10.
[http://dx.doi.org/10.1016/j.toxlet.2009.03.001] [PMID: 19429265]

[19] Chang L, Xu J, Yu F, Zhao J, Tang X, Tang C. Taurine protected myocardial mitochondria injury induced by hyperhomocysteinemia in rats. Amino Acids 2004; 27(1): 37-48.
[http://dx.doi.org/10.1007/s00726-004-0096-2] [PMID: 15309570]

[20] Schuller-Levis GB, Park E. Taurine: new implications for an old amino acid. FEMS Microbiol Lett 2003; 226(2): 195-202.
[http://dx.doi.org/10.1016/S0378-1097(03)00611-6] [PMID: 14553911]

[21] Schaffer S, Azuma J, Takahashi K, Mozaffari M. Why is taurine cytoprotective? Taurine 5: Beginning the 21st Century. Advances in Experimental Medicine and Biology.. Boston, MA: Springer US 2003; pp. 307-21.
[http://dx.doi.org/10.1007/978-1-4615-0077-3_39]

[22] Palmi M, Youmbi GT, Sgaragli G, Meini A, Benocci A, Fusi F, et al. The mitochondrial permeability transition and taurine Taurine 4. Springer 2002; pp. 87-96.

[23] Schaffer S, Kim HW. Effects and mechanisms of taurine as a therapeutic agent. Biomol Ther (Seoul) 2018; 26(3): 225-41.
[http://dx.doi.org/10.4062/biomolther.2017.251] [PMID: 29631391]

[24] Zulli A. Taurine in cardiovascular disease. Curr Opin Clin Nutr Metab Care 2011; 14(1): 57-60.
[http://dx.doi.org/10.1097/MCO.0b013e328340d863] [PMID: 21076292]

[25] Bouckenooghe T, Remacle C, Reusens B. Is taurine a functional nutrient? Curr Opin Clin Nutr Metab Care 2006; 9(6): 728-33.
[http://dx.doi.org/10.1097/01.mco.0000247469.26414.55] [PMID: 17053427]

[26]   Menzie J, Pan C, Prentice H, Wu JY. Taurine and central nervous system disorders. Amino Acids 2014; 46(1): 31-46.
[http://dx.doi.org/10.1007/s00726-012-1382-z] [PMID: 22903433]

[27]   Prentice H, Gharibani PM, Ma Z, Alexandrescu A, Genova R, Chen P-C, *et al.* Neuroprotective functions through inhibition of ER stress by taurine or taurine combination treatments in a rat stroke model Taurine 10 Advances in Experimental Medicine and Biology. Springer 2017; pp. 193-205.

[28]   Jakaria M, Azam S, Haque ME, *et al.* Taurine and its analogs in neurological disorders: Focus on therapeutic potential and molecular mechanisms. Redox Biol 2019; 24: 101223.
[http://dx.doi.org/10.1016/j.redox.2019.101223] [PMID: 31141786]

[29]   Bhat MA, Ahmad K, Khan MSA, *et al.* Expedition into taurine biology: Structural insights and therapeutic perspective of taurine in neurodegenerative diseases. Biomolecules 2020; 10(6): 863.
[http://dx.doi.org/10.3390/biom10060863] [PMID: 32516961]

[30]   Warskulat U, Heller-Stilb B, Oermann E, *et al.* Phenotype of the taurine transporter knockout mouse. Methods Enzymol 2007; 428: 439-58.
[http://dx.doi.org/10.1016/S0076-6879(07)28025-5] [PMID: 17875433]

[31]   Ito T, Yoshikawa N, Inui T, Miyazaki N, Schaffer SW, Azuma J. Tissue depletion of taurine accelerates skeletal muscle senescence and leads to early death in mice. PLoS One 2014; 9(9): e107409.
[http://dx.doi.org/10.1371/journal.pone.0107409] [PMID: 25229346]

[32]   De Luca A, Pierno S, Camerino DC. Taurine: the appeal of a safe amino acid for skeletal muscle disorders. J Transl Med 2015; 13(1): 243.
[http://dx.doi.org/10.1186/s12967-015-0610-1] [PMID: 26208967]

[33]   Heidari R, Jamshidzadeh A, Niknahad H, *et al.* Effect of taurine on chronic and acute liver injury: Focus on blood and brain ammonia. Toxicol Rep 2016; 3(3): 870-9.
[http://dx.doi.org/10.1016/j.toxrep.2016.04.002] [PMID: 28959615]

[34]   Heidari R, Jamshidzadeh A, Keshavarz N, Azarpira N. Mitigation of methimazole-induced hepatic injury by taurine in mice. Sci Pharm 2015; 83(1): 143-58.
[http://dx.doi.org/10.3797/scipharm.1408-04] [PMID: 26839807]

[35]   Abdoli N, Sadeghian I, Azarpira N, Ommati MM, Heidari R. Taurine mitigates bile duct obstruction-associated cholemic nephropathy: effect on oxidative stress and mitochondrial parameters. Clin Exp Hepatol 2021; 7(1): 30-40.
[http://dx.doi.org/10.5114/ceh.2021.104675] [PMID: 34027113]

[36]   Heidari R, Babaei H, Eghbal MA. Ameliorative effects of taurine against methimazole-induced cytotoxicity in isolated rat hepatocytes. Sci Pharm 2012; 80(4): 987-99.
[http://dx.doi.org/10.3797/scipharm.1205-16] [PMID: 23264945]

[37]   Mousavi K, Niknahad H, Ghalamfarsa A, *et al.* Taurine mitigates cirrhosis-associated heart injury through mitochondrial-dependent and antioxidative mechanisms. Clin Exp Hepatol 2020; 6(3): 207-19.
[http://dx.doi.org/10.5114/ceh.2020.99513] [PMID: 33145427]

[38]   Yang Y, Zhang Y, Liu X, *et al.* Exogenous taurine attenuates mitochondrial oxidative stress and endoplasmic reticulum stress in rat cardiomyocytes. Acta Biochim Biophys Sin (Shanghai) 2013; 45(5): 359-67.
[http://dx.doi.org/10.1093/abbs/gmt034] [PMID: 23619568]

[39]   Jamshidzadeh A, Heidari R, Latifpour Z, *et al.* Carnosine ameliorates liver fibrosis and hyperammonemia in cirrhotic rats. Clin Res Hepatol Gastroenterol 2017; 41(4): 424-34.
[http://dx.doi.org/10.1016/j.clinre.2016.12.010] [PMID: 28283328]

[40]   Das J, Ghosh J, Manna P, Sil PC. Taurine protects acetaminophen-induced oxidative damage in mice kidney through APAP urinary excretion and CYP2E1 inactivation. Toxicology 2010; 269(1): 24-34.

[http://dx.doi.org/10.1016/j.tox.2010.01.003] [PMID: 20067817]

[41] Chen K, Zhang Q, Wang J, *et al.* Taurine protects transformed rat retinal ganglion cells from hypoxia-induced apoptosis by preventing mitochondrial dysfunction. Brain Res 2009; 1279: 131-8.
[http://dx.doi.org/10.1016/j.brainres.2009.04.054] [PMID: 19427840]

[42] Lakshmi Devi S, Anuradha CV. Mitochondrial damage, cytotoxicity and apoptosis in iron-potentiated alcoholic liver fibrosis: amelioration by taurine. Amino Acids 2010; 38(3): 869-79.
[http://dx.doi.org/10.1007/s00726-009-0293-0] [PMID: 19381777]

[43] Roy A, Manna P, Sil PC. Prophylactic role of taurine on arsenic mediated oxidative renal dysfunction via MAPKs/ NF- κ B and mitochondria dependent pathways. Free Radic Res 2009; 43(10): 995-1007.
[http://dx.doi.org/10.1080/10715760903164998] [PMID: 19672740]

[44] Lambert IH, Kristensen DM, Holm JB, Mortensen OH. Physiological role of taurine - from organism to organelle. Acta Physiol (Oxf) 2015; 213(1): 191-212.
[http://dx.doi.org/10.1111/apha.12365] [PMID: 25142161]

[45] Fakruddin M, Wei FY, Suzuki T, *et al.* Defective Mitochondrial tRNA Taurine Modification Activates Global Proteostress and Leads to Mitochondrial Disease. Cell Rep 2018; 22(2): 482-96.
[http://dx.doi.org/10.1016/j.celrep.2017.12.051] [PMID: 29320742]

[46] Kirino Y, Yasukawa T, Ohta S, *et al.* Codon-specific translational defect caused by a wobble modification deficiency in mutant tRNA from a human mitochondrial disease. Proc Natl Acad Sci USA 2004; 101(42): 15070-5.
[http://dx.doi.org/10.1073/pnas.0405173101] [PMID: 15477592]

[47] Kirino Y, Goto Y, Campos Y, Arenas J, Suzuki T. Specific correlation between the wobble modification deficiency in mutant tRNAs and the clinical features of a human mitochondrial disease. Proc Natl Acad Sci USA 2005; 102(20): 7127-32.
[http://dx.doi.org/10.1073/pnas.0500563102] [PMID: 15870203]

[48] Yasukawa T, Kirino Y, Ishii N, *et al.* Wobble modification deficiency in mutant tRNAs in patients with mitochondrial diseases. FEBS Lett 2005; 579(13): 2948-52.
[http://dx.doi.org/10.1016/j.febslet.2005.04.038] [PMID: 15893315]

[49] Ohsawa Y, Hagiwara H, Nishimatsu S, *et al.* Taurine supplementation for prevention of stroke-like episodes in MELAS: a multicentre, open-label, 52-week phase III trial. J Neurol Neurosurg Psychiatry 2019; 90(5): 529-36.
[http://dx.doi.org/10.1136/jnnp-2018-317964] [PMID: 29666206]

[50] Schaffer SW, Jong CJ, Ito T, Azuma J. Role of taurine in the pathologies of MELAS and MERRF. Amino Acids 2014; 46(1): 47-56.
[http://dx.doi.org/10.1007/s00726-012-1414-8] [PMID: 23179085]

[51] Taylor RW, Turnbull DM. Mitochondrial DNA mutations in human disease. Nat Rev Genet 2005; 6(5): 389-402.
[http://dx.doi.org/10.1038/nrg1606] [PMID: 15861210]

[52] Ji K, Lin Y, Xu X, *et al.* MELAS-associated m.5541C>T mutation caused instability of mitochondrial tRNA ^{Trp} and remarkable mitochondrial dysfunction. J Med Genet 2022; 59(1): 79-87.
[http://dx.doi.org/10.1136/jmedgenet-2020-107323] [PMID: 33208382]

[53] Mehta TR, Dawson R Jr. Taurine is a weak scavenger of peroxynitrite and does not attenuate sodium nitroprusside toxicity to cells in culture. Amino Acids 2001; 20(4): 419-33.
[http://dx.doi.org/10.1007/s007260170038] [PMID: 11452985]

[54] Venditti P, Di Stefano L, Di Meo S. Mitochondrial metabolism of reactive oxygen species. Mitochondrion 2013; 13(2): 71-82.
[http://dx.doi.org/10.1016/j.mito.2013.01.008] [PMID: 23376030]

[55] Ott M, Gogvadze V, Orrenius S, Zhivotovsky B. Mitochondria, oxidative stress and cell death. Apoptosis 2007; 12(5): 913-22.

[http://dx.doi.org/10.1007/s10495-007-0756-2] [PMID: 17453160]

[56] Heidari R. The footprints of mitochondrial impairment and cellular energy crisis in the pathogenesis of xenobiotics-induced nephrotoxicity, serum electrolytes imbalance, and Fanconi's syndrome: A comprehensive review. Toxicology 2019; 423: 1-31.
[http://dx.doi.org/10.1016/j.tox.2019.05.002] [PMID: 31095988]

[57] Ommati MM, Heidari R, Ghanbarinejad V, Abdoli N, Niknahad H. Taurine treatment provides neuroprotection in a mouse model of manganism. Biol Trace Elem Res 2019; 190(2): 384-95.
[http://dx.doi.org/10.1007/s12011-018-1552-2] [PMID: 30357569]

[58] Ahmadi N, Ghanbarinejad V, Ommati MM, Jamshidzadeh A, Heidari R. Taurine prevents mitochondrial membrane permeabilization and swelling upon interaction with manganese: Implication in the treatment of cirrhosis-associated central nervous system complications. J Biochem Mol Toxicol 2018; 32(11): e22216.
[http://dx.doi.org/10.1002/jbt.22216] [PMID: 30152904]

[59] Ommati MM, Farshad O, Niknahad H, *et al.* Cholestasis-associated reproductive toxicity in male and female rats: The fundamental role of mitochondrial impairment and oxidative stress. Toxicol Lett 2019; 316: 60-72.
[http://dx.doi.org/10.1016/j.toxlet.2019.09.009] [PMID: 31520699]

[60] Heidari R. Brain mitochondria as potential therapeutic targets for managing hepatic encephalopathy. Life Sci 2019; 218: 65-80.
[http://dx.doi.org/10.1016/j.lfs.2018.12.030] [PMID: 30578865]

[61] Chang L, Zhao J, Xu J, Jiang W, Tang CS, Qi YF. Effects of taurine and homocysteine on calcium homeostasis and hydrogen peroxide and superoxide anions in rat myocardial mitochondria. Clin Exp Pharmacol Physiol 2004; 31(4): 237-43.
[http://dx.doi.org/10.1111/j.1440-1681.2004.03983.x] [PMID: 15053820]

[62] Li CY, Deng YL, Sun BH. Taurine protected kidney from oxidative injury through mitochondrial-linked pathway in a rat model of nephrolithiasis. Urol Res 2009; 37(4): 211-20.
[http://dx.doi.org/10.1007/s00240-009-0197-1] [PMID: 19513707]

[63] Fang YZ, Yang S, Wu G. Free radicals, antioxidants, and nutrition. Nutrition 2002; 18(10): 872-9.
[http://dx.doi.org/10.1016/S0899-9007(02)00916-4] [PMID: 12361782]

[64] Tabassum H, Rehman H, Banerjee BD, Raisuddin S, Parvez S. Attenuation of tamoxifen-induced hepatotoxicity by taurine in mice. Clin Chim Acta 2006; 370(1-2): 129-36.
[http://dx.doi.org/10.1016/j.cca.2006.02.006] [PMID: 16556438]

[65] Sinha M, Manna P, Sil PC. Taurine, a conditionally essential amino acid, ameliorates arsenic-induced cytotoxicity in murine hepatocytes. Toxicol. *In Vitro.* 2007; 21(8): 1419-28.
[http://dx.doi.org/10.1016/j.tiv.2007.05.010] [PMID: 17624716]

[66] Manna P, Sinha M, Sil PC. Taurine plays a beneficial role against cadmium-induced oxidative renal dysfunction. Amino Acids 2009; 36(3): 417-28.
[http://dx.doi.org/10.1007/s00726-008-0094-x] [PMID: 18414974]

[67] Sevgiler Y, Karaytug S, Karayakar F. Antioxidative effects of N-acetylcysteine, lipoic acid, taurine, and curcumin in the muscle of Cyprinus carpio L. exposed to cadmium. Arh Hig Rada Toksikol 2011; 62(1): 1-9.
[http://dx.doi.org/10.2478/10004-1254-62-2011-2082] [PMID: 21421527]

[68] Acharya M, Lau-Cam CA. Comparative evaluation of the effects of taurine and thiotaurine on alterations of the cellular redox status and activities of antioxidant and glutathione-related enzymes by acetaminophen in the rat.Taurine 8 Advances in Experimental Medicine and Biology: Springer New York. 2013; pp. 199-215.
[http://dx.doi.org/10.1007/978-1-4614-6093-0_20]

[69] Heidari R, Behnamrad S, Khodami Z, Ommati MM, Azarpira N, Vazin A. The nephroprotective

properties of taurine in colistin-treated mice is mediated through the regulation of mitochondrial function and mitigation of oxidative stress. Biomed Pharmacother 2019; 109: 103-11.
[http://dx.doi.org/10.1016/j.biopha.2018.10.093] [PMID: 30396066]

[70]   Sochor J, Nejdl L, Ruttkay-Nedecky B, *et al.* Investigating the influence of taurine on thiol antioxidant status in Wistar rats with a multi-analytical approach. J Appl Biomed 2014; 12(2): 97-110.
[http://dx.doi.org/10.1016/j.jab.2013.01.002]

[71]   Mas MR, Isik AT, Yamanel L, *et al.* Antioxidant treatment with taurine ameliorates chronic pancreatitis in an experimental rat model. Pancreas 2006; 33(1): 77-81.
[http://dx.doi.org/10.1097/01.mpa.0000222316.74607.07] [PMID: 16804416]

[72]   Heidari R, Rasti M, Shirazi Yeganeh B, Niknahad H, Saeedi A, Najibi A. Sulfasalazine-induced renal and hepatic injury in rats and the protective role of taurine. Bioimpacts 2016; 6(1): 3-8.
[http://dx.doi.org/10.15171/bi.2016.01] [PMID: 27340618]

[73]   Heidari R, Jamshidzadeh A, Ghanbarinejad V, Ommati MM, Niknahad H. Taurine supplementation abates cirrhosis-associated locomotor dysfunction. Clin Exp Hepatol 2018; 4(2): 72-82.
[http://dx.doi.org/10.5114/ceh.2018.75956] [PMID: 29904723]

[74]   Jamshidzadeh A, Abdoli N, Niknahad H, Azarpira N, Mardani E, Mousavi S, *et al.* Taurine alleviates brain tissue markers of oxidative stress in a rat model of hepatic encephalopathy. Trends Pharmacol Sci 2017; 3(3): 181-92.

[75]   Karamikhah R, Jamshidzadeh A, Azarpira N, Saeidi A, Heidari R. Propylthiouracil-induced liver injury in mice and the protective role of taurine. Pharm Sci 2015; 21(2): 94-101.
[http://dx.doi.org/10.15171/PS.2015.23]

[76]   Heidari R, Sadeghi N, Azarpira N, Niknahad H. Sulfasalazine-induced hepatic injury in an ex vivo model of isolated perfused rat liver and the protective role of taurine. Pharm Sci 2015; 21(4): 211-9.
[http://dx.doi.org/10.15171/PS.2015.39]

[77]   Hansen SH, Birkedal H, Wibrand F, Grunnet N. Taurine and regulation of mitochondrial metabolism Taurine 9. Springer 2015; pp. 397-405.

[78]   Hansen S, Andersen M, Cornett C, Gradinaru R, Grunnet N. A role for taurine in mitochondrial function. J Biomed Sci 2010; 17(Suppl 1): S23.
[http://dx.doi.org/10.1186/1423-0127-17-S1-S23] [PMID: 20804598]

[79]   Niknahad H, Jamshidzadeh A, Heidari R, Zarei M, Ommati MM. Ammonia-induced mitochondrial dysfunction and energy metabolism disturbances in isolated brain and liver mitochondria, and the effect of taurine administration: relevance to hepatic encephalopathy treatment. Clin Exp Hepatol 2017; 3(3): 141-51.
[http://dx.doi.org/10.5114/ceh.2017.68833] [PMID: 29062904]

[80]   Heidari R, Babaei H, Eghbal MA. Cytoprotective effects of taurine against toxicity induced by isoniazid and hydrazine in isolated rat hepatocytes. Arh Hig Rada Toksikol 2013; 64(2): 201-10.
[http://dx.doi.org/10.2478/10004-1254-64-2013-2297] [PMID: 23819928]

[81]   Heidari R, Abdoli N, Ommati MM, Jamshidzadeh A, Niknahad H. Mitochondrial impairment induced by chenodeoxycholic acid: The protective effect of taurine and carnosine supplementation. Trends in Pharmaceutical Sciences 2018; 4: 2.

[82]   Homma K, Toda E, Osada H, *et al.* Taurine rescues mitochondria-related metabolic impairments in the patient-derived induced pluripotent stem cells and epithelial-mesenchymal transition in the retinal pigment epithelium. Redox Biol 2021; 41: 101921.
[http://dx.doi.org/10.1016/j.redox.2021.101921] [PMID: 33706170]

[83]   Ommati MM, Farshad O, Jamshidzadeh A, Heidari R. Taurine enhances skeletal muscle mitochondrial function in a rat model of resistance training. PharmaNutrition 2019; 9: 100161.
[http://dx.doi.org/10.1016/j.phanu.2019.100161]

[84]   Wu G, San J, Pang H, *et al.* Taurine attenuates AFB1-induced liver injury by alleviating oxidative

stress and regulating mitochondria-mediated apoptosis. Toxicon 2022; 215: 17-27.
[http://dx.doi.org/10.1016/j.toxicon.2022.06.003] [PMID: 35688267]

[85]   Das J, Ghosh J, Manna P, Sil PC. Protective role of taurine against arsenic-induced mitochondria-dependent hepatic apoptosis via the inhibition of PKCdelta-JNK pathway. PLoS One 2010; 5(9): e12602.
[http://dx.doi.org/10.1371/journal.pone.0012602] [PMID: 20830294]

[86]   Takatani T, Takahashi K, Uozumi Y, *et al.* Taurine inhibits apoptosis by preventing formation of the Apaf-1/caspase-9 apoptosome. Am J Physiol Cell Physiol 2004; 287(4): C949-53.
[http://dx.doi.org/10.1152/ajpcell.00042.2004] [PMID: 15253891]

[87]   Li S, Guan H, Qian Z, *et al.* Taurine inhibits 2,5-hexanedione-induced oxidative stress and mitochondria-dependent apoptosis in PC12 cells. Ind Health 2017; 55(2): 108-18.
[http://dx.doi.org/10.2486/indhealth.2016-0044] [PMID: 27840369]

[88]   Wu G, Yang J, Lv H, *et al.* Taurine prevents ethanol-induced apoptosis mediated by mitochondrial or death receptor pathways in liver cells. Amino Acids 2018; 50(7): 863-75.
[http://dx.doi.org/10.1007/s00726-018-2561-3] [PMID: 29626300]

[89]   Aly HAA, Khafagy RM. Taurine reverses endosulfan-induced oxidative stress and apoptosis in adult rat testis. Food Chem Toxicol 2014; 64: 1-9.
[http://dx.doi.org/10.1016/j.fct.2013.11.007] [PMID: 24262488]

[90]   Meseguer S, Martínez-Zamora A, García-Arumí E, Andreu AL, Armengod ME. The ROS-sensitive microRNA-9/9* controls the expression of mitochondrial tRNA-modifying enzymes and is involved in the molecular mechanism of MELAS syndrome. Hum Mol Genet 2015; 24(1): 167-84.
[http://dx.doi.org/10.1093/hmg/ddu427] [PMID: 25149473]

[91]   Schaffer SW, Jong CJ, Warner D, Ito T, Azuma J. Taurine deficiency and MELAS are closely related syndromes. Adv Exp Med Biol 2013; 776: 153-65.
[http://dx.doi.org/10.1007/978-1-4614-6093-0_16] [PMID: 23392880]

[92]   Rikimaru M, Ohsawa Y, Wolf AM, *et al.* Taurine ameliorates impaired the mitochondrial function and prevents stroke-like episodes in patients with MELAS. Intern Med 2012; 51(24): 3351-7.
[http://dx.doi.org/10.2169/internalmedicine.51.7529] [PMID: 23257519]

[93]   Papet I, Rémond D, Dardevet D, Mosoni L, Polakof S, Peyron M-A, *et al.* Sulfur amino acids and skeletal muscle.Nutrition and Skeletal Muscle. Academic Press 2019; pp. 335-63.
[http://dx.doi.org/10.1016/B978-0-12-810422-4.00020-8]

[94]   Hansen SH, Andersen ML, Birkedal H, Cornett C, Wibrand F. The important role of taurine in oxidative metabolism Taurine 6. Springer 2006; pp. 129-35.

[95]   Brookes PS, Yoon Y, Robotham JL, Anders MW, Sheu SS. Calcium, ATP, and ROS: a mitochondrial love-hate triangle. Am J Physiol Cell Physiol 2004; 287(4): C817-33.
[http://dx.doi.org/10.1152/ajpcell.00139.2004] [PMID: 15355853]

[96]   Pinton P, Giorgi C, Siviero R, Zecchini E, Rizzuto R. Calcium and apoptosis: ER-mitochondria Ca2+ transfer in the control of apoptosis. Oncogene 2008; 27(50): 6407-18.
[http://dx.doi.org/10.1038/onc.2008.308] [PMID: 18955969]

[97]   El Idrissi A. Taurine increases mitochondrial buffering of calcium: role in neuroprotection. Amino Acids 2008; 34(2): 321-8.
[http://dx.doi.org/10.1007/s00726-006-0396-9] [PMID: 16955229]

[98]   Leon R, Wu H, Jin Y, *et al.* Protective function of taurine in glutamate-induced apoptosis in cultured neurons. J Neurosci Res 2009; 87(5): 1185-94.
[http://dx.doi.org/10.1002/jnr.21926] [PMID: 18951478]

[99]   Cribb AE, Peyrou M, Muruganandan S, Schneider L. The endoplasmic reticulum in xenobiotic toxicity. Drug Metab Rev 2005; 37(3): 405-42.
[http://dx.doi.org/10.1080/03602530500205135] [PMID: 16257829]

[100] Lin JH, Walter P, Yen TSB. Endoplasmic reticulum stress in disease pathogenesis. Annu Rev Pathol 2008; 3(1): 399-425.
[http://dx.doi.org/10.1146/annurev.pathmechdis.3.121806.151434] [PMID: 18039139]

[101] Oakes SA, Papa FR. The role of endoplasmic reticulum stress in human pathology. Annu Rev Pathol 2015; 10(1): 173-94.
[http://dx.doi.org/10.1146/annurev-pathol-012513-104649] [PMID: 25387057]

[102] Wang S, Kaufman RJ. The impact of the unfolded protein response on human disease. J Cell Biol 2012; 197(7): 857-67.
[http://dx.doi.org/10.1083/jcb.201110131] [PMID: 22733998]

[103] Hiramatsu N, Chiang WC, Kurt TD, Sigurdson CJ, Lin JH. Multiple mechanisms of unfolded protein response-induced cell death. Am J Pathol 2015; 185(7): 1800-8.
[http://dx.doi.org/10.1016/j.ajpath.2015.03.009] [PMID: 25956028]

[104] Nonaka H, Tsujino T, Watari Y, Emoto N, Yokoyama M. Taurine prevents the decrease in expression and secretion of extracellular superoxide dismutase induced by homocysteine: amelioration of homocysteine-induced endoplasmic reticulum stress by taurine. Circulation 2001; 104(10): 1165-70.
[http://dx.doi.org/10.1161/hc3601.093976] [PMID: 11535574]

[105] Pan C, Giraldo GS, Prentice H, Wu JY. Taurine protection of PC12 cells against endoplasmic reticulum stress induced by oxidative stress. J Biomed Sci 2010; 17(Suppl 1): S17.
[http://dx.doi.org/10.1186/1423-0127-17-S1-S17] [PMID: 20804591]

[106] Orrenius S, McCabe MJ Jr, Nicotera P. Ca^{2+}-dependent mechanisms of cytotoxicity and programmed cell death. Toxicol Lett 1992; 64-65(Spec No): 357-64.
[http://dx.doi.org/10.1016/0378-4274(92)90208-2] [PMID: 1335178]

[107] Nicotera P, Bellomo G, Orrenius S. The role of calcium in cell killing. Chem Res Toxicol 1990; 3(6): 484-94.
[http://dx.doi.org/10.1021/tx00018a001] [PMID: 2103319]

[108] Schaffer SW, Lombardini JB, Huxtable RJ. Taurine 3: Cellular and Regulatory Mechanisms: Springer Science & Business Media; 2013.

[109] Pan C, Prentice H, Price AL, Wu JY. Beneficial effect of taurine on hypoxia- and glutamate-induced endoplasmic reticulum stress pathways in primary neuronal culture. Amino Acids 2012; 43(2): 845-55.
[http://dx.doi.org/10.1007/s00726-011-1141-6] [PMID: 22080215]

[110] Wu G. Important roles of dietary taurine, creatine, carnosine, anserine and 4-hydroxyproline in human nutrition and health. Amino Acids 2020; 52(3): 329-60.
[http://dx.doi.org/10.1007/s00726-020-02823-6] [PMID: 32072297]

[111] Huxtable RJ. Physiological actions of taurine. Physiol Rev 1992; 72(1): 101-63.
[http://dx.doi.org/10.1152/physrev.1992.72.1.101] [PMID: 1731369]

[112] Bkaily G, Jazzar A, Normand A, Simon Y, Al-Khoury J, Jacques D. Taurine and cardiac disease: state of the art and perspectives. Can J Physiol Pharmacol 2020; 98(2): 67-73.
[http://dx.doi.org/10.1139/cjpp-2019-0313] [PMID: 31560859]

[113] Gerbitz KD, Gempel K, Brdiczka D. Mitochondria and diabetes. Genetic, biochemical, and clinical implications of the cellular energy circuit. Diabetes 1996; 45(2): 113-26.
[http://dx.doi.org/10.2337/diab.45.2.113] [PMID: 8549853]

[114] Ramalho-Santos J, Amaral S, Oliveira P. Diabetes and the impairment of reproductive function: possible role of mitochondria and reactive oxygen species. Curr Diabetes Rev 2008; 4(1): 46-54.
[http://dx.doi.org/10.2174/157339908783502398] [PMID: 18220695]

[115] Finsterer J. Mitochondrial disorders, cognitive impairment and dementia. J Neurol Sci 2009; 283(1-2): 143-8.
[http://dx.doi.org/10.1016/j.jns.2009.02.347] [PMID: 19268975]

[116] Jemmerson R, Dubinsky JM, Brustovetsky N. Cytochrome C release from CNS mitochondria and potential for clinical intervention in apoptosis-mediated CNS diseases. Antioxid Redox Signal 2005; 7(9-10): 1158-72.
[http://dx.doi.org/10.1089/ars.2005.7.1158] [PMID: 16115019]

[117] Johannsen DL, Ravussin E. The role of mitochondria in health and disease. Curr Opin Pharmacol 2009; 9(6): 780-6.
[http://dx.doi.org/10.1016/j.coph.2009.09.002] [PMID: 19796990]

[118] Duchen MR. Mitochondria in health and disease: perspectives on a new mitochondrial biology. Mol Aspects Med 2004; 25(4): 365-451.
[http://dx.doi.org/10.1016/j.mam.2004.03.001] [PMID: 15302203]

[119] Teplova VV, Deryabina YI, Isakova EP. Mitochondrial cytopathies: their causes and correction pathways. Biochemistry (Moscow). Supplement Series A: Membrane and Cell Biology 2017; 11(2): 87-102.

[120] El-Hattab AW, Scaglia F. Mitochondrial cytopathies. Cell Calcium 2016; 60(3): 199-206.
[http://dx.doi.org/10.1016/j.ceca.2016.03.003] [PMID: 26996063]

[121] Thangaraj K, Khan NA, Govindaraj P, Meena AK. Mitochondrial disorders: Challenges in diagnosis & treatment. Indian J Med Res 2015; 141(1): 13-26.
[http://dx.doi.org/10.4103/0971-5916.154489] [PMID: 25857492]

[122] Agresti CA, Halkiadakis PN, Tolias P. MERRF and MELAS: current gene therapy trends and approaches. Journal of Translational Genetics and Genomics 2018; 2(7): 9.
[http://dx.doi.org/10.20517/jtgg.2018.05]

[123] Chinnery P, Howell N, Lightowlers RN, Turnbull DM. Molecular pathology of MELAS and MERRF. The relationship between mutation load and clinical phenotypes. Brain 1997; 120(10): 1713-21.
[http://dx.doi.org/10.1093/brain/120.10.1713] [PMID: 9365365]

[124] Abu-Amero KK, Al-Dhalaan H, Bohlega S, Hellani A, Taylor RW. A patient with typical clinical features of mitochondrial encephalopathy, lactic acidosis and stroke-like episodes (MELAS) but without an obvious genetic cause: a case report. J Med Case Reports 2009; 3(1): 77.
[http://dx.doi.org/10.1186/1752-1947-3-77] [PMID: 19946553]

[125] Stipanuk MH. Role of the liver in regulation of body cysteine and taurine levels: a brief review. Neurochem Res 2004; 29(1): 105-10.
[http://dx.doi.org/10.1023/B:NERE.0000010438.40376.c9] [PMID: 14992268]

[126] Saxena R, Zucker SD, Crawford JM. Anatomy and physiology of the liver. Hepatology: A Textbook of Liver Disease. 2003; 3-30.

[127] Huxtable RJ, Michalk D. Taurine in health and disease: Springer Science & Business Media; 2013. 447 p.

[128] Miyazaki T, Matsuzaki Y. Taurine and liver diseases: a focus on the heterogeneous protective properties of taurine. Amino Acids 2014; 46(1): 101-10.
[http://dx.doi.org/10.1007/s00726-012-1381-0] [PMID: 22918604]

[129] Redmond HP, Stapleton PP, Neary P, Bouchier-Hayes D. Immunonutrition: the role of taurine. Nutrition 1998; 14(7-8): 599-604.
[http://dx.doi.org/10.1016/S0899-9007(98)00097-5] [PMID: 9684263]

[130] Yamori Y, Taguchi T, Hamada A, Kunimasa K, Mori H, Mori M. Taurine in health and diseases: consistent evidence from experimental and epidemiological studies. J Biomed Sci 2010; 17(Suppl 1): S6.
[http://dx.doi.org/10.1186/1423-0127-17-S1-S6] [PMID: 20804626]

[131] Murakami S, Yamori Y. Taurine and longevity–preventive effect of taurine on metabolic syndrome Bioactive Food as Dietary Interventions for the Aging Population. Elsevier 2013; pp. 159-71.

[http://dx.doi.org/10.1016/B978-0-12-397155-5.00027-1]

[132]   Hsieh YL, Yeh YH, Lee YT, Huang CY. Effect of taurine in chronic alcoholic patients. Food Funct 2014; 5(7): 1529-35.
[http://dx.doi.org/10.1039/C3FO60597C] [PMID: 24841875]

[133]   Schaffer S, Ito T, Azuma J, Jong C, Kramer J. Mechanisms underlying development of taurine-deficient cardiomyopathy. Hearts 2020; 1(2): 86-98.
[http://dx.doi.org/10.3390/hearts1020010]

[134]   Mohammadi H, Ommati MM, Farshad O, Jamshidzadeh A, Nikbakht MR, Niknahad H, *et al.* Taurine and isolated mitochondria: A concentration-response study. Trends Pharmacol Sci 2019; 5(4): 197-206.

[135]   Heidari R, Ghanbarinejad V, Ommati MM, Jamshidzadeh A, Niknahad H. Mitochondria protecting amino acids: Application against a wide range of mitochondria-linked complications. PharmaNutrition 2018; 6(4): 180-90.
[http://dx.doi.org/10.1016/j.phanu.2018.09.001]

[136]   Jamshidzadeh A, Heidari R, Abasvali M, *et al.* Taurine treatment preserves brain and liver mitochondrial function in a rat model of fulminant hepatic failure and hyperammonemia. Biomed Pharmacother 2017; 86: 514-20.
[http://dx.doi.org/10.1016/j.biopha.2016.11.095] [PMID: 28024286]

[137]   Schaffer SW, Shimada-Takaura K, Jong CJ, Ito T, Takahashi K. Impaired energy metabolism of the taurine-deficient heart. Amino Acids 2016; 48(2): 549-58.
[http://dx.doi.org/10.1007/s00726-015-2110-2] [PMID: 26475290]

[138]   Xu S, He M, Zhong M, *et al.* The neuroprotective effects of taurine against nickel by reducing oxidative stress and maintaining mitochondrial function in cortical neurons. Neurosci Lett 2015; 590 (Suppl. C): 52-7.
[http://dx.doi.org/10.1016/j.neulet.2015.01.065] [PMID: 25637701]

[139]   Sun M, Gu Y, Zhao Y, Xu C. Protective functions of taurine against experimental stroke through depressing mitochondria-mediated cell death in rats. Amino Acids 2011; 40(5): 1419-29.
[http://dx.doi.org/10.1007/s00726-010-0751-8] [PMID: 20862501]

[140]   Schwarzer R, Kivaranovic D, Mandorfer M, *et al.* Randomised clinical study: the effects of oral taurine 6g/day vs placebo on portal hypertension. Aliment Pharmacol Ther 2018; 47(1): 86-94.
[http://dx.doi.org/10.1111/apt.14377] [PMID: 29105115]

[141]   Shao A, Hathcock JN. Risk assessment for the amino acids taurine, l-glutamine and l-arginine. Regul Toxicol Pharmacol 2008; 50(3): 376-99.
[http://dx.doi.org/10.1016/j.yrtph.2008.01.004] [PMID: 18325648]

CHAPTER 3

Applications of Taurine in the Central Nervous System Disorders Linked with Mitochondrial Impairment

Abstract: Taurine (TAU) reaches a high concentration in the central nervous system (CNS). The physiological role of TAU in the CNS is the subject of many investigations. It has been suggested that this amino acid could act as a membrane stabilizer, a modulator of calcium signaling, a trophic factor for neuronal development, and even be proposed as a neurotransmitter in the CNS. Besides, several investigations revealed the neuroprotective properties of TAU in various experimental models. Multiple mechanisms, including the inhibition of the excitotoxic response, the blockade of cytoplasmic calcium overload, regulation of oxidative stress, and the positive effects of TAU on mitochondrial parameters, have been proposed for the neuroprotective properties of this amino acid. Today, it is well-known that mitochondrial function and energy metabolism play a pivotal role in the pathogenesis of various neurodegenerative disorders and xenobiotics-induced neurotoxicity. Hence, targeting mitochondria with safe and clinically applicable agents is a viable therapeutic option in various neurodegenerative disorders. In the current chapter, the effects of TAU on the CNS will be highlighted, focusing on the positive effects of this amino acid on mitochondrial parameters. The data could help the development of safe therapeutic agents against CNS complications.

Keywords: Brain injury, Energy crisis, Mitochondrial dysfunction, Neurodegenerative disease, Neurotoxicity, Oxidative stress.

INTRODUCTION

Neurological complications debilitate a large population worldwide annually. Stroke and brain ischemia, various types of head trauma, seizures, and hepatic encephalopathy are among the neurological complications that need urgent medical interventions [1 - 5]. On the other hand, neurodegenerative diseases refer to a wide range of complications that have become a crucial issue in the recent century [6, 7]. Neurodegenerative diseases are among the leading cause of disability worldwide [6, 7]. Alzheimer's disease, Parkinsonism, and Huntington's disease are debilitating neurodegenerative complications. Based on these data, it

Reza Heidari and M. Mehdi Ommati

is crucial to identify the mechanism of brain injury in these complications and find safe and clinically applicable options against these disorders.

Although the mechanisms involved in CNS complications and neurodegenerative disease could be pleiotropic and multifactorial. Several interconnected mechanisms have been identified in these complications [8 - 18]. These mechanisms could serve as a therapeutic point of intervention to manage serious neurological complications as well as neurodegenerative diseases.

Based on a plethora of investigations over activation of n-methyl-D-aspartate (NMDA) receptors, named excitotoxicity, cytoplasmic calcium overload, oxidative stress, and mitochondrial impairment are the point of convergence for the mechanism of neuronal injury in central nervous system disorders [8 - 18]. All these events finally influence mitochondrial function and mitochondria-mediated cell death. On the other hand, brain tissue is a high energy (ATP) consuming organ [17, 18]. Therefore, it seems reasonable that targeting mitochondria could be a viable therapeutic approach against a wide range of neurological disorders. In this regard, several antioxidants and mitochondria-targeted compounds have been tested, and had more and less therapeutic properties against these complications.

Taurine (TAU) is abundantly found in the brain tissue [19 - 22]. On the other hand, it has been found that this amino acid and its derivatives could significantly alleviated neurological disorders associated with mitochondrial complications [17, 23 - 28]. More interestingly, TAU revealed tremendous protective effects against neurodegenerative disorders in clinical trials [18, 29 - 32]. All these data make TAU an excellent candidate for the management of neurological disorders in humans.

The neuroprotective properties of TAU seem to be mediated through the positive effects of this amino acid on mitochondrial function [17, 23 - 27]. It has been found that TAU prevents mitochondria-mediated cell death, suppresses excitotoxicity-mediated neuronal damage, decreases oxidative stress in CNS, and enhances ATP metabolism [17, 23 - 27].

In the current chapter, the effects of TAU on a wide range of human neurological disorders is discussed focusing on the positive effects of this amino acid on mitochondrial indices. These data could provide clues for future drug development against many neurological disorders.

THE PLEIOTROPIC ROLES OF TAURINE IN THE CENTRAL NERVOUS SYSTEM (CNS)

Brain tissue contains a high concentration of taurine (TAU) [33]. The transfer of

TAU to the CNS and neural cells is a transporter-mediated process [34, 35]. Some physiological roles, including the osmoregulatory properties, have been attributed to TAU in the CNS [36]. However, it has been repeatedly mentioned that several neurological disorders benefit from exogenous TAU supplementation [32, 37 - 39]. The effects of TAU on seizure and epilepsy, Alzheimer's disease (AD), brain trauma, Huntington's disease (HD), stroke, and Parkinson's disease (PD) have experimentally or clinically been investigated [32, 38, 39]. Some investigations even mentioned that TAU plays a role in neuromodulation and neurotransmission [40 - 42]. Nevertheless, the mechanism of action of this amino acid in the CNS is not fully cleared so far.

Some investigations mentioned that TAU could act as an osmolyte to regulate cell volume in astrocytes and neurons during stressful conditions [43, 44]. Although many studies have approved the osmoregulatory properties of TAU, today, we know that other and more important mechanisms could also be involved in the positive effects of TAU in the CNS. The positive impact of TAU on mitochondrial function and energy metabolism in the brain is one of the most elusive mechanisms of action of this amino acid in the CNS. The current chapter will discuss the effects of TAU on stroke and stroke-like episodes, AD, HD, hepatic encephalopathy, PD, trauma, and seizure, which are connected to mitochondrial impairment and energy crisis.

Before discussing the role of mitochondrial impairment in CNS disorders, we should explain a term named "excitotoxicity", which is believed to be involved in the pathogenesis of numerous CNS disorders. Excitotoxicity is also directly connected to mitochondrial impairment and oxidative stress. Glutamate (Glu) is the primary excitatory neurotransmitter in the CNS. It has been found that Glu levels are increased in several neurodegenerative diseases such as HD, AD, stroke, seizure, and brain trauma [8 - 16]. Increased Glu activates the N-Methyl-D-aspartate (NMDA) receptors. The hyper-activation of NMDA receptors is known as the excitotoxic response [45 - 47] (Fig. **1**). Excitotoxicity has several consequences in the CNS [45 - 47]. Detrimental events such as dramatically increased ROS levels, high nitric oxide (NO) levels, and peroxynitrite (NOO⁻) formation could occur upon excitotoxicity [10, 48]. Hence, the excitotoxic response is connected to oxidative/nitrosative stress. The disturbances in cellular Ca^{2+} homeostasis are another deleterious event that ensues NMDA receptors' hyper-activation and excitotoxicity [10, 48] (Fig. **1**). There are several clues that neural mitochondria are also severely damaged during excitotoxicity. It has long been known that oxidative/nitrosative stress is firmly linked to mitochondrial impairment [49]. On the other hand, high cytoplasmic Ca^{2+} levels disturbed mitochondrial function and dissipated mitochondrial membrane potential ($\Delta\Psi_m$). Hence, Ca^{2+} overload and excitotoxicity could impair mitochondrial function in some CNS disorders discussed in this chapter. Interestingly, many studies revealed that TAU is an effective inhibitor of the excitotoxicity response linked with different CNS disorders [35, 50]. The anti-excitotoxic response properties of TAU will be discussed in various neurological disorders mentioned in the current chapter.

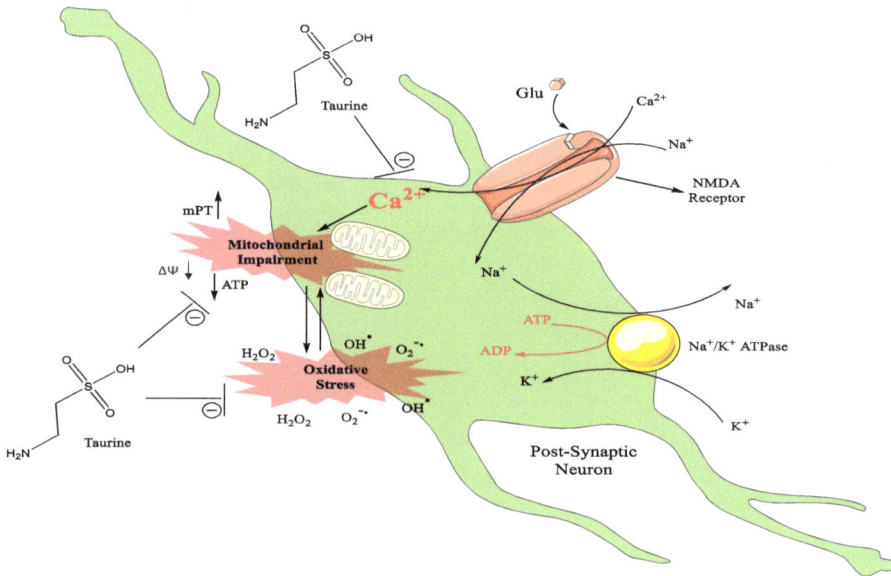

Fig. (1). Mechanisms of excitotoxicity-induced neuronal injury and the protective effects of taurine. Excitotoxicity is directly associated with mitochondrial impairment and oxidative stress in neurons. This complication could entail neurotoxicity. The pathogenic role of excitotoxic response has been repeatedly investigated in human neurodegenerative disorders. Glu: Glutamate; Ca^{2+}: Calcium ion; mPT: mitochondrial permeability transition; NMDA: N-methyl-D-aspartate.

Another critical issue that should be discussed here is the connection between mitochondrial Ca^{2+} sequestration and its relationship with the neuroprotective properties of TAU. It is well-established that the mitochondrial Ca^{2+} sequestering capability of neurons could play a pivotal role in attenuating excitotoxicity [51]. It has been found that TAU could significantly enhance Ca^{2+} sequestration by mitochondria in various models of excitotoxicity [51, 52]. It is well-known that cytoplasmic Ca^{2+} overload could activate a plethora of cell death mechanisms by activating various protease enzymes [53, 54]. Eventually, these events could lead to neural cell death [53, 54]. Therefore, the role of TAU in regulating mitochondrial Ca^{2+} homeostasis could act as a mechanism for the anti-excitotoxicity properties of this compound.

In the forthcoming sections of this chapter, the involvement of mitochondrial injury in the pathogenesis of a wide range of CNS disorders is discussed. Then, the protective effects of TAU against these diseases are highlighted, focusing on the effects of this amino acid on cellular mitochondria.

EFFECTS OF TAURINE ON STROKE AND BRAIN ISCHEMIA

Stroke is a serious clinical complication with different etiologies that could lead to permanent disabilities and death. Brain tissue suffers from local or general ischemia in stroke. Stroke and brain ischemia could occur in response to a wide range of etiologies (*e.g.*, brain vessels occlusion) [55, 56]. Previous studies have well identified the importance of the brain energy level and oxidative stress in stroke and brain ischemia [57, 58]. Besides, several investigations revealed the neuroprotective effects of TAU against stroke and stroke-like disorders (readers could refer to mitochondrial cytopathies section; chapter 2) [59].

The brain is one of the most energy-demanding organs, which contains numerous mitochondria. The importance of mitochondrial dysfunction and cellular energy crisis has also been repeatedly mentioned in critical conditions such as stroke [58, 60]. Cerebral ischemia occurs during the stroke. The ischemia might be global or partial based on the etiology of stroke. Insufficient oxygen in the ischemic brain could lead to a severe decrease in oxidative phosphorylation, cellular energy crisis, and cell death. Therefore, preserving cellular ATP at a high level (*e.g.*, by enhancing mitochondrial function) might be a vital step in preventing stroke-induced brain damage.

As mentioned, several cellular mechanisms are involved in the pathogenesis of stroke. Rather than a severe decrease in mitochondrial oxidative phosphorylation because of oxygen deprivation, other mechanisms, including excitotoxicity, and cellular Ca^{2+}, imbalance (ER stress), could occur during the stroke [61 - 63] (Fig. **2**). Interestingly, it has been found that TAU could provide neuroprotection in stroke models by mechanisms such as the inhibition of ER stress [64]. All these events further deteriorate mitochondrial function and ATP synthesis. Interestingly, it has been found that TAU is a compound that could alleviate all these adverse effects in experimental and/or clinical models of brain ischemia and stroke [18, 31, 32].

In an exciting *in vitro* study, it was found that TAU could robustly protect human neuroblastoma cell lines against hypoxia and oxygen/glucose deprivation [65]. These data mention that TAU as a potential candidate against stroke and brain ischemia in humans. In this context, the protective effects of TAU have been investigated in animal models of brain ischemia . Menzie *et al.* revealed that TAU supplementation significantly improved signs of ischemic stroke [18]. It has been found that TAU could effectively ameliorate stroke-associated brain injury through a mitochondria-dependent mechanism [17, 18]. These mechanisms included preventing cytoplasmic Ca^{2+} overload, inhibiting mitochondrial permeability, enhancing mitochondrial ATP production, and preventing mitochondria-mediated cell death [17, 18]. TAU administration also significantly ameliorated stroke-induced oxidative stress and its linked complications in the brain tissue [17, 18, 66].

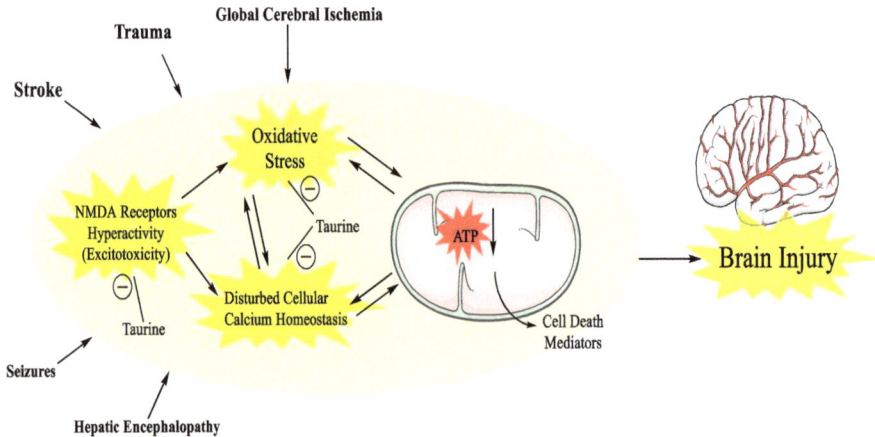

Fig. (2). The effects of taurine in preventing oxidative stress, mitochondrial impairment, and cellular energy (ATP) crisis could play a fundamental role in the protective role of this amino acid in nervous system disorders. NMDA: N-methyl-D-aspartate; ATP: Adenosine triphosphate.

Disturbances in cellular Ca^{2+} homeostasis also play a role in stroke-associated brain injury [18, 31] (Fig. **2**). It has been demonstrated that TAU could effectively mitigate Ca^{2+}-dependent oxidative stress and cell death in experimental stroke models [18, 31, 32]. It has been detected that the release of cell death mediators (*e.g.*, cytochrome *c*) from mitochondria was significantly mitigated by TAU treatment [17]. TAU treatment decreased brain infarct size and improved neurological scores in these studies [17, 31]. Moreover, TAU administration improved brain tissue ATP level [17]. Therefore, TAU treatment could be a therapeutic option against stroke complications in human cases.

Interestingly, several clinical trials revealed the neuroprotective effects of TAU in stroke-like episodes [18, 30]. TAU improved the number and annual relapse of stroke-associated focal neurological deficits [67, 68]. The study by Rikimaru *et al.* emphasized that the positive effects of TAU on cellular mitochondria is due to improvement in TAU-modified mitochondrial tRNA (readers could refer to mitochondrial cytopathies section for more information; chapter 2) [30]. However, as Menzie *et al.* suggested, "more credible extrapolation from experimental studies to patients" is needed for using TAU in human stroke cases [18]. On the other hand, the studies by Ohsawa *et al.* mentioned the small number of participants as a limitation for clinical studies on the effects of TAU on stroke and brain ischemia. Finally, it should be emphasized that TAU is a very hydrophilic compound. Therefore, the transition of this amino acid through the blood-brain barrier (BBB) is limited. Thus, proper formulations of TAU and its efficient delivery to CNS might be a novel approach in treating different types of stroke and brain ischemia in the future.

Taurine and Traumatic Brain Injury

The brain is one of the main organs continuously dependent on energy (ATP) to maintain cellular integrity and organ functionality. Traumatic brain injury (TBI) is an urgent health problem. TBI is accompanying with a high mortality rate [69, 70]. Several therapeutic strategies have been suggested to treat TBI [71 - 74]. However, none of these options have promising effects in clinical settings. Therefore, understanding the mechanisms of TBI could lead to the development of therapeutic strategies against this clinical complication.

Pathophysiological mechanisms of TBI are heterogeneous [72, 75]. At the cellular level, disturbances in cytoplasmic Ca^{2+} ion, excitotoxicity, oxidative/nitrosative stress, and different modes of cell death, including necrosis and apoptosis, are involved in the mechanisms of neurons injury during TBI [75 - 78] (Fig. **2**). Some investigations suggested the administration of antioxidants such as melatonin, resveratrol, curcumin, lipoic acid, selenium, vitamins E and C, beta-carotene, and the iron chelator deferoxamine in TBI [73, 79]. These studies found that these therapeutic options could significantly prevent TBI sequela, such as oxidative stress-linked lipid peroxidation [73, 80]. These studies highlight the importance of oxidative stress-associated complications in TBI.

Impaired cerebral blood flow and ischemia are the primary events in TBI [72]. Consequently, oxygen deprivation will impair the mitochondrial oxidative phosphorylation process and energy metabolism. Compelling evidence indicates a role for mitochondrial impairment and cellular energy crisis during head trauma [81 - 83]. There are also reports on the connections between perturbation of cellular Ca^{2+} levels, mitochondrial dysfunction, and brain damage in TBI [84]. Cheng *et al.* reported a synergistic effect between oxidative stress, ER stress, excitotoxicity, and mitochondrial impairment in the TBI [69] (Fig. **2**). The mitochondrial release of apoptotic factors and a decrease in anti-apoptotic agents could also play a critical role in the fate of neural cells in TBI [77, 85 - 87]. Mitochondrial dysfunction and the failure of ATP production are severe issues in the CNS as the brain consumes a considerable amount of ATP.

The effects of TAU on TBI have been explored in several studies [88 - 93]. Investigators revealed that TAU had a favorable impact on improving the survival rate and prognosis of patients with TBI [88]. Interestingly, the neuroprotection provided by TAU in TBI seems to be mediated through a mitochondria-dependent mechanism [88]. Effects of TAU on mitochondria respiratory chain components and ATP metabolism play a pivotal role in its positive impact on TBI [88]. As mentioned, post-traumatic excitotoxicity is another fundamental mechanism involved in the pathogenesis of TBI [17, 18, 31]. On the other hand, excitotoxicity is associated with mitochondrial dysfunction and cellular energy crisis [94]. Hence, a part of mitochondria-protecting effects of TAU in TBI might be related to its effects on the excitotoxicity process.

Another interesting finding of the protective role of TAU in TBI is the effects of this amino acid on cerebral blood flow (CBF) [88, 90]. Although CBF regulation is a complex process, some mechanisms for the effects of TAU on TBI-induced decrease of CBF have been suggested [88]. Several investigations suggested that the effects of TAU on the coagulation process seem to play a crucial role in its effects on CBF [88, 95, 96]. Wang *et al.* reported that TAU improved the hypercoagulable state as same as the anticoagulant drugs [88]. Therefore, the improvement in CBF could deliver higher oxygen to the brain and lead to enhanced mitochondrial oxidative phosphorylation and energy metabolism in TBI patients.

Lamade *et al.* mentioned mitochondria target therapy as a new strategy for managing TBI complications [97]. They suggested unique strategies for the localization of anti-TBI pharmaceuticals in the mitochondria [97]. Based on these investigations, agents such as TAU that provide significant protective effects in TBI could be directly delivered to mitochondria. All the data collected in this section suggest TAU as a promising therapeutic tool for alleviating TBI and its linked complications. Unfortunately, BBB might be a barrier to effective TAU therapy, like other neurological disorders discussed before, even though BBB integrity is partially disrupted in TBI. Hence, delivering sufficient concentrations of TAU to the CNS in TBI might need appropriate formulations of this amino acid and could be the subject of future studies in this field.

Taurine and Hepatic Encephalopathy

Hepatic encephalopathy (HE) is a severe clinical complication that affects the nervous system. HE could lead to cognitive and motor dysfunction, coma, permanent brain injury, or death [98 - 100]. Ammonium ion (NH_4^+) is suspected as the primary contributor to neurotoxicity in HE [98 - 100]. Several mechanisms, including excitotoxicity, oxidative/nitrosative stress, ER stress, as well as mitochondrial impairment, could be involved in HE [94, 100] (Fig. **2**).

NH_4^+ could affect mitochondrial function by several mechanisms [94]. It has been found that NH_4^+ is an inducer of mPT, inhibits mitochondrial respiratory chain complexes, enhances mitochondria-mediated ROS formation, and finally decreases cellular energy stores [94]. Excitotoxicity also has been identified as one of the basic mechanisms for NH_4^+ neurotoxicity [94, 101] (Fig. **2**). As repeatedly mentioned in the current chapter, excitotoxicity is firmly associated with other deleterious events such as disturbances in cellular Ca^{2+} homeostasis, oxidative/nitrosative stress, and mitochondrial dysfunction. A plethora of studies indicate a central role for mitochondrial dysfunction in the pathogenesis of brain injury during HE [94, 102 - 104].

Despite the etiology of mitochondrial impairment in HE, enhancing the function of this organelle seems to be an elusive therapeutic option [94, 102]. Several investigations mentioned brain mitochondria and energy crisis in the brain tissue as a pathological condition in HE [94, 105 - 109]. In this regard, some studies suggested the importance of antioxidants and mitochondria protecting agents in HE management [110 - 113].

Brain edema and increased intracranial pressure are severe HE complications [114 - 116]. Although there is no precise mechanism for brain edema during HE, some studies mentioned the importance of astrocytes mitochondrial impairment and brain edema [108, 117 - 122]. Induction of mPT in astrocytes could lead to astrocyte swelling. Astrocytes swelling seems to be a key component of brain edema in HE [108, 117 - 122]. Astrocytes are neural cells with unique morphological and functional characteristics. Several functions, including controlling the BBB permeability, synaptogenesis, and conducting some neuronal activities, are attributed to astrocytes [123]. In the context of HE, it has been found that the blockade of mPT could prevent astrocyte swelling and, consequently, brain edema [94, 120, 124, 125]. All these data mentioned the importance of mitochondrial impairment and disturbances in brain energy metabolism in the pathogenesis of HE.

Some investigations mentioned the positive effects of TAU in HE and its associated complications [126 - 128]. Several mechanisms, including the osmoregulatory properties of TAU, the effects of this amino acid on the excitotoxicity response, and mitochondria protecting properties of TAU, have been proposed for the positive impacts of TAU in HE [126 - 128]. It has been found that TAU treatment improved brain edema and intracranial pressure and decreased locomotor and cognitive dysfunction in different models of HE [127]. These studies suggested that mechanisms, including the osmoregulatory, antioxidative, NMDA inhibitory effects, and improving mitochondrial function, are involved in the neuroprotective effects of TAU in HE [126, 127, 129, 130].

An exciting finding of the neuroprotective effects of TAU in preventing brain damage in HE is associated with the effects of this amino acid on astrocytes and probably neurons mitochondria [131]. The osmoregulatory effect of TAU in astrocytes is an essential mechanism of neuroprotection during HE [132, 133]. As mentioned, astrocyte swelling is believed as a fundamental mechanism involved in brain edema as a harmful consequence of HE. Brain edema could lead to a dramatic increase in intracranial pressure and even brain herniation in severe cases.

Although the positive effects of TAU have been mentioned in various experimental models, unfortunately, there is no clinical investigation on the effects of TAU on CNS function in HE patients to date. However, some clinical trials reported the positive effects of this amino acid on liver cirrhosis-linked adverse effects such as portal hypertension [29]. A clinical trial also revealed the positive effects of TAU supplementation on chronic liver disease-associated complications (*e.g.*, muscle cramps) [134]. Finally, like the other neurological disorders discussed in the current chapter, brain-targeted formulations of TAU, which could easily pass the BBB, might be more effective against complications such as HE and could be considered in future investigations.

THE LONG STORY OF USING TAURINE IN SEIZURE AND EPILEPSY

Epilepsy is one of the most frequent neurological complications worldwide [135]. As a medical term, the seizure is a single and occasional event linked to a wide range of pathologies, where epilepsy is the condition that attacks frequently. A large group of neurons' synchronized discharge interrupts brain function in epilepsy. Several factors, such as brain trauma, inflammation, tumors, and gene mutations, could lead to different forms of epilepsy [135]. Besides, the role of mitochondrial disease in the pathogenesis of epilepsy has been widely investigated [136, 137].

As previously mentioned, mitochondria are vital organelles in the CNS and provide ATP for this high energy-demand organ. Moreover, like other cells, neuronal mitochondria regulate Ca^{2+} homeostasis, redox signaling, and cell survival and death [138, 139]. It is also well-known that sufficient ATP is essential for normal synaptic transmission. Therefore, changes in synaptic mitochondrial function could significantly impair neurotransmitters' discharge and/or uptake. Impaired neurotransmitter balance (discharge and synaptic uptake) is a well-known phenomenon in the etiology of different forms of epilepsy [140]. Several forms of epilepsies have been identified connected to the mutation in mitochondrial DNA (mtDNA) [141 - 143]. These mutations subsequently deteriorate mitochondrial oxidative phosphorylation and enhance ROS formation in neurons mitochondria [144 - 146]. These data mention the importance of mitochondria in different types of epilepsy.

It has long been known that mitochondria-facilitated ROS formation and oxidative stress play a significant role in neuronal cell death during epilepsy [147]. The decrease in the mitochondrial complex I activity seems to be the most frequent mitochondrial impairment form noted in the acute phase of seizure in different experimental models of epilepsy [148 - 150]. Impairment in mitochondrial complex I activity is accompanied by severe ROS formation, oxidative stress, and damage of several targets in mitochondria [148, 149]. Interestingly, it has been found that TAU plays a crucial role in the proper activity of mitochondria complex I [151]. The decrease in mitochondrial TAU levels is directly associated with diminished complex I activity [151]. Jong *et al.* revealed that mitochondrial TAU depletion caused a significant elevation in superoxide anion ($O_2^{\cdot-}$) levels in the mitochondria [151]. They revealed that TAU is involved in mitochondrial ND6 (MT-ND6) gene expression [151]. The MT-ND6 protein is a subunit of mitochondrial respiratory complex I [150]. Although there is no experimental evidence in this field so far, based on the mentioned data, TAU might improve complex I activity and decrease mitochondrial impairment and ROS formation in some types of epilepsy associated with complex I activity impairment. The decrease in mitochondrial complex I might also be involved in other conditions such as aging (refer to taurine and aging section), where TAU could act as a mitochondrion protecting agent. Other mitochondria-connected parameters, such as cytoplasmic Ca^{2+} disturbances, ER stress, excitotoxicity, and oxidative stress, are involved in the pathogenesis of epilepsy [152] (Fig. **2**). In this context, TAU might act as a protective agent in epilepsy by modulating all these parameters (Fig. **2**).

TAU is also known as an agonist of $GABA_A$ receptors [153]. Hence, several studies mentioned that the effects of TAU on GABA receptors could also play a role in the neuroprotective effects of this amino acid in epilepsy [153]. However, $GABA_A$ receptors have different subtypes (ρ, γ, β, α) and it has been found that the affinity of these subunits of $GABA_A$ receptor for TAU is widely variable (EC_{50} from 5 µM to 10 mM) [153]. It has been reported that TAU acts as a potent agonist for the $\beta2$ subunit of $GABA_A$ receptors, which are frequently found in the substantia nigra, dentate gyrus, cerebrum, hippocampal CA3 field, and medial thalamic nuclei [154, 155]. Therefore, the inhibitory neuromodulation of TAU is widely discussed in previous studies [156]. Several studies searched for specific TAU receptors or interference of this amino acid on other neurotransmission pathways in the CNS [156]. The interference of TAU with GABA and glycine receptors is one of the most interesting features of this amino acid [157, 158]. It has been found that TAU could bind to the benzodiazepine sites on GABA receptors [159, 160]. It has been revealed that high TAU concentration increased chloride (Cl⁻) flux into the synaptic membrane through the GABA receptors [156, 159]. It has also been found that TAU and glycine act on the same receptors to induce Cl⁻ ion current and neuro-inhibitory mechanisms [161]. As previously mentioned, although some studies declared the potential pharmacological value of TAU on GABA receptors, the exact interaction between TAU and GABA is not fully determined and is also variable in different experimental models. Moreover, designing TAU-based chemicals with a high affinity for GABA subunits for the treatment of epilepsy warranted further investigations.

Several clinical trials were also designed to evaluate the antiepileptic effects of TAU [154]. However, the impact of TAU in patients was partial and controversial [154]. The controversies between these studies could be related to several factors, including small numbers of patients, almost always missing adequate control groups, selecting different types of epilepsies, variations in taurine doses and routes of administration, and the continuation of other anticonvulsant medications during clinical trials on the antiepileptic effects of TAU [154].

As mentioned, several studies suggested that mitochondrial energy metabolism and oxidative stress could readily serve as potential therapeutic targets in managing epilepsy and its consequences [162, 163]. In this case, TAU might act as a good contender. Some studies mentioned "the inability to enhance the antioxidant levels within mitochondria" [138] as a big challenge for antioxidant therapy in epilepsy. Fortunately, TAU is accumulated in the mitochondrial matrix in a transporter-dependent manner [164]. This makes TAU a good candidate against epilepsy complications associated with mitochondrial disorders. Obviously, as previously mentioned, brain mitochondria-targeted formulations of TAU might significantly enhance its beneficial effects in epilepsy. Based on these data, further studies on the targeted delivery of TAU to mitochondria might suggest a viable and safe therapeutic approach against different forms of epilepsy.

ROLE OF TAURINE IN NEURODEGENERATIVE DISORDERS

The role of mitochondrial impairment in several neurodegenerative diseases has been widely reviewed [165 - 167]. Alzheimer's disease (AD), Parkinson's disease (PD), and Huntington's disease (HD) are all neurodegenerative disorders in which mitochondrial dysfunction could play a vital role in their pathogenesis [165 - 167]. The following sections discuss the potential application of TAU in neurodegenerative diseases, focusing on the decisive role of this amino acid on cellular powerhouses.

Taurine in Alzheimer's Disease (AD)

AD is mainly associated with decreased levels of acetylcholine and impaired balance of other neurotransmitters in the brain [168, 169]. Other mechanisms, such as the appearance of extracellular amyloid-β (Aβ) plaques, hyperphosphorylation of the microtubule-binding protein tau, and intracellular neurofibrillary tangles (NFTs) are also involved in the molecular mechanism of AD [47, 170]. However, the major mechanisms related to mitochondrial impairment in AD are associated with neural Ca^{2+} dis-homeostasis and NMDA receptors hyperactivity (excitotoxicity) as two interrelated events [47, 171, 172] (Fig. 1). Excitotoxicity and its associated disturbances in cellular Ca^{2+} could severely affect mitochondrial function in AD.

As repeatedly mentioned in the current chapter, it has been found that TAU could protect neurons in a mitochondria-related mechanism [24]. It is well-known that TAU could effectively prevent cellular Ca^{2+} disturbances and excitotoxicity [24]. On the other hand, it has been found that apoptosis is a significant mechanism of neural cell death linked with the excitotoxicity response [24]. It has been shown that TAU effectively prevented the release of cell death mediators from mitochondria, probably by inhibiting mPT (mostly induced by Ca^{2+} overload) [173] (Fig. 1). These events finally prevent neural cell death in AD [24]. Based on these data, the effects of TAU on cellular mitochondria could play a role in treating or preventing AD complications.

Although several experiments revealed the positive effects of TAU in experimental AD models [26, 174 - 176], unfortunately, there is no clinical examination on TAU in AD patients to date. As previously mentioned, TAU is a lipophobic amino acid, and TAU transport through BB is difficult (Refer to the perspectives section). Interestingly, the integrity of BBB is impaired in AD because of amyloidogenesis that disrupts the tight junction [177]. Hence, TAU might reach higher concentrations in AD patients. However, this cannot keep us from designing an appropriate formulation for TAU delivery, aiming to prevent or ameliorate the signs of neurodegenerative diseases such as AD.

Another interesting finding of TAU on AD that may not be related to its effects on cellular mitochondria is the effects of this amino acid on Aβ plaques formation. It has been found that TAU could significantly prevent Aβ aggregation in AD [175, 178]. This effect is assumed to be associated with the role of TAU in preventing protein misfolding [179, 180]. Collectively, TAU might be an appropriate preventive/therapeutic approach against AD. Indeed, the proper formulation and target delivery of this amino acid to the brain would play a crucial role in this process.

Taurine and Parkinson's Disease

Parkinson's disease (PD) is a motor development dysfunction associated with damaging some brain regions [181, 182]. Substantia nigra (SN) and dopaminergic systems of CNS are corrupted in PD. A wide range of movement disorders occurs in PD. Interestingly, it has been proved that the mechanism of dopaminergic cell death in PD is directly associated with mitochondrial impairment [183 - 185]. The 1-methyl-4-phenyl-1,2,3,6-tetrahydropyridine (MPTP) is a chemical that accidentally leads scientists to discover the mechanism of dopaminergic neural cell death [186, 187]. MPTP is oxidized to MPP^+ in the CNS. It has been found that MPP^+ is a potent mitochondria toxin [187]. These findings lead to extensive investigations on the role of mitochondrial impairment in PD [187 - 189]. Today, it is clear that the mutation in some mitochondrial respiratory complexes (*e.g.*, Complex I) or overexpression of some proteins such as α-synuclein, which adversely affects mitochondrial function, is involved in the pathogenesis of PD [190 - 192]. Moreover, oxidative stress, Ca^{2+} dyshomeostasis, and ER stress play critical roles in dopaminergic cell injury and PD [193, 194]. These events could lead to the energy crisis and cell death in dopaminergic neurons.

Based on the pathogenic role of mitochondrial impairment in PD, several investigations revealed that protecting this organelle could significantly improve signs and symptoms of PD [195 - 198]. Excitingly, it has been found that TAU is present at high concentrations in SN [19, 199]. The age-related decrease in TAU levels in different parts of the brain tissue has also been reported [22, 200]. These data could emphasize a role for TAU in the proper function of mitochondria and its relevance as a protective agent in PD. Herein, the protective effects of TAU in different PD models focusing on the role of this amino acid on mitochondrial function are discussed.

Several investigations revealed that TAU and its derivatives play a protective role in different PD models [201, 202]. Stabilizing mitochondrial function and preventing oxidative stress seem to play a significant role in the neuroprotective effects of TAU in PD. In this context, it has been mentioned that TAU protects the dopaminergic system against excitotoxicity and Ca^{2+} overload [203]. On the other hand, several studies revealed that mitochondrial respiratory complexes are defected in PD [197, 204]. The defect in mitochondrial function could initiate the cell death cascade in the dopaminergic neurons [197, 204]. As previously mentioned, TAU-modified mitochondrial tRNA plays an essential role in synthesizing different proteins (*e.g.*, mitochondrial electron transport chain proteins). The role of TAU in mitochondrial respiratory complexes synthesis might compensate for the defect in complex I activity in PD and finally improve the mitochondrial function in the dopaminergic system, counteract mitochondria-facilitated ROS formation, and prevent cell death. However, this direct effect of TAU on the mitochondria of dopaminergic neurons has not been investigated so far and deserves future investigations to become clear.

Like the case of AD, the effective cross of exogenous TAU from BBB could be a challenge for pharmacological intervention against PD using this amino acid. Again, preparing a suitable brain-targeted formulation of TAU could also be valuable in this case (refer to chapter 13 for more information).

Huntington's Disease: The Therapeutic Potential of Taurine

Huntington's disease (HD) is another locomotor disorder characterized by involuntary movements in patients [205]. Psychiatric disturbances and cognitive dysfunction could also develop in HD [205]. HD is a progressive neurodegenerative disease that severely affects patients' quality of life. Hence, it is essential to develop therapeutic options against this disorder.

Although the pathophysiology of HD is complicated and multifactorial, compelling evidence suggests that mitochondrial impairment plays a crucial role in the pathogenesis of HD [206 - 208]. Disturbed Ca^{2+} homeostasis is a critical factor linked with mitochondrial dysfunction in HD [206 - 208]. Mitochondrial-facilitated ROS formation and oxidative stress, as well as mitochondria-mediated cell death, have also been mentioned to be implicated in the pathogenesis of HD [206 - 208]. Hence, mitochondria could be a viable target for the management of HD.

The brain striatum shows HD's earliest and most prominent neuropathological changes [205]. On the other hand, the atrophy and degeneration of the hypothalamus and, finally, whole-brain injury occur at the final stages of HD [205, 209]. Several models of HD have been developed to date [210, 211]. Interestingly, different types of mitochondrial defects have been observed in the HD experimental models [206, 212, 213]. The dissipation of mitochondrial membrane potential ($\Delta\Psi_m$), disturbances in Ca^{2+} buffering capacity of mitochondria, the high sensitivity of mPT to Ca^{2+} ion, and a significant decrease in the expression and activity of mitochondrial respiratory chain complexes have been evident in HD models [208, 214, 215]. Moreover, a substantial defect in the vesicle trafficking of the neurotransmitters (as an ATP-dependent process) has been developed in HD [216]. All these data mention the importance of cellular mitochondria as well as their interrelated events in the pathogenesis of HD (Fig. 1). Like other previously mentioned CNS complications in this chapter (*e.g.*, stroke, AD, PD, and trauma), the hyperactivation of NMDA receptors also plays a critical role in HD [217 - 219]. As repeatedly mentioned, excitotoxicity is associated with Ca^{2+} disturbances, mitochondrial impairment and cell death.

Fortunately, all the mitochondria-related parameters involved in the pathogenesis of HD are processes that TAU could have a significant effect on them. As mentioned in different parts of this chapter, TAU enhances Ca^{2+} buffering capacity of mitochondria, prevents deleterious effects of excitotoxicity by inhibiting NMDA receptors, enhances the mitochondrial synthesis of respiratory chain complexes, boosts mitochondrial membrane potential, prevents mitochondrial permeabilization and mitochondria-mediated cell death, and finally improves cellular energy metabolism and ATP levels. These findings raised the idea of using this amino acid in HD. In this context, animal models reported the positive effects of TAU against motor deficits, cognitive dysfunction, and the brain histopathological changes in HD [220]. The inhibitory effects of TAU on ER stress, oxidative stress, neural cell apoptosis, and defects in mitochondria respiration have all been documented in the experimental models of HD [220, 221]. Another indirect effect of TAU on cellular mitochondria in HD patients could be associated with its role in increasing the γ-aminobutyric acid (GABA) level in the brain [222]. Higher GABA levels in HD patients could significantly decrease the excitatory output (induced by Glu) from the basal ganglia to the thalamus [39, 222]. Therefore, the effects of TAU on GABA receptors could also play a role in its positive effects in HD.

Unfortunately, there is no clinical study on the effects of TAU in HD patients to date. On the other hand, similar to the previously mentioned neurological disorders, BBB could act as a barrier for target TAU delivery in HD. Hence, designing the appropriate formulations of this amino acid to overcome BBB as an obstacle warranted further research in this field.

CONCLUSION

Conclusively, the data provided in the current chapter indicate a potential role for TAU supplementation in the treatment/prevention of neurological disorders [38]. Hence, this safe amino acid may play a role in treating neurological diseases in clinical settings. On the other hand, several other neurological disorders are known that are associated with mitochondrial impairment (*e.g.*, autism, hypotonia, and amyotrophic lateral sclerosis) [28, 223, 224]. Hence, the effect of TAU on mitochondrial function in other neurological disorders warranted further investigations to be cleared.

REFERENCES

[1]   Iqubal A, Iqubal MK, Khan A, Ali J, Baboota S, Haque SE. Gene therapy, a novel therapeutic tool for neurological disorders: Current progress, challenges and future prospective. Curr Gene Ther 2020; 20(3): 184-94.
[http://dx.doi.org/10.2174/1566523220999200716111502] [PMID: 32674730]

[2]   Angdisen J, Moore VDG, Cline JM, Payne RM, Ibdah JA. Mitochondrial trifunctional protein defects: molecular basis and novel therapeutic approaches. Curr Drug Targets Immune Endocr Metabol Disord 2005; 5(1): 27-40.
        [http://dx.doi.org/10.2174/1568008053174796] [PMID: 15777202]

[3]   Vaquero J, Butterworth RF. Mechanisms of brain edema in acute liver failure and impact of novel therapeutic interventions. Neurol Res 2007; 29(7): 683-90.
        [http://dx.doi.org/10.1179/016164107X240099] [PMID: 18173908]

[4]   Farshad O, Keshavarz P, Heidari R, Farahmandnejad M, Azhdari S, Jamshidzadeh A. The potential neuroprotective role of citicoline in hepatic encephalopathy. J Exp Pharmacol 2020; 12: 517-27.
        [http://dx.doi.org/10.2147/JEP.S261986] [PMID: 33235522]

[5]   Mohammadi H, Heidari R, Niknezhad SV, Jamshidzadeh A, Farjadian F. *In vitro* and *in vivo* evaluation of succinic acid-substituted mesoporous silica for ammonia adsorption: potential application in the management of hepatic encephalopathy. Int J Nanomedicine 2020; 15: 10085-98.
        [http://dx.doi.org/10.2147/IJN.S271883] [PMID: 33363368]

[6]   Zahra W, Rai SN, Birla H, Singh SS, Dilnashin H, Rathore AS, *et al.* The global economic impact of neurodegenerative diseases: Opportunities and challenges. Bioeconomy for Sustainable Development. Singapore: Springer 2020; pp. 333-45.
        [http://dx.doi.org/10.1007/978-981-13-9431-7_17]

[7]   Fereshtehnejad SM, Vosoughi K, Heydarpour P, *et al.* Burden of neurodegenerative diseases in the Eastern Mediterranean Region, 1990–2016: findings from the Global Burden of Disease Study 2016. Eur J Neurol 2019; 26(10): 1252-65.
        [http://dx.doi.org/10.1111/ene.13972] [PMID: 31006162]

[8]   Mehta A, Prabhakar M, Kumar P, Deshmukh R, Sharma PL. Excitotoxicity: Bridge to various triggers in neurodegenerative disorders. Eur J Pharmacol 2013; 698(1-3): 6-18.
        [http://dx.doi.org/10.1016/j.ejphar.2012.10.032] [PMID: 23123057]

[9]   Schulz JB, Henshaw DR, Siwek D, *et al.* Involvement of free radicals in excitotoxicity *in vivo*. J Neurochem 1995; 64(5): 2239-47.
        [http://dx.doi.org/10.1046/j.1471-4159.1995.64052239.x] [PMID: 7536809]

[10]   Mattson MP. Excitotoxicity Stress: Physiology, Biochemistry, and Pathology. Elsevier 2019; pp. 125-34.

[11]   Tehse J, Taghibiglou C. The overlooked aspect of excitotoxicity: Glutamate-independent excitotoxicity in traumatic brain injuries. Eur J Neurosci 2019; 49(9): 1157-70.
        [PMID: 30554430]

[12]   Ng SY, Lee AYW. Traumatic brain injuries: Pathophysiology and potential therapeutic targets. Front Cell Neurosci 2019; 13: 528.
        [http://dx.doi.org/10.3389/fncel.2019.00528] [PMID: 31827423]

[13]   Hynd M, Scott HL, Dodd PR. Glutamate-mediated excitotoxicity and neurodegeneration in Alzheimer's disease. Neurochem Int 2004; 45(5): 583-95.
        [http://dx.doi.org/10.1016/j.neuint.2004.03.007] [PMID: 15234100]

[14]   Esposito Z, Belli L, Toniolo S, Sancesario G, Bianconi C, Martorana A. Amyloid β, glutamate, excitotoxicity in Alzheimer's disease: are we on the right track? CNS Neurosci Ther 2013; 19(8): 549-55.
        [http://dx.doi.org/10.1111/cns.12095] [PMID: 23593992]

[15]   Estrada Sánchez AM, Mejía-Toiber J, Massieu L. Excitotoxic neuronal death and the pathogenesis of Huntington's disease. Arch Med Res 2008; 39(3): 265-76.
        [http://dx.doi.org/10.1016/j.arcmed.2007.11.011] [PMID: 18279698]

[16]   Iovino L, Tremblay ME, Civiero L. Glutamate-induced excitotoxicity in Parkinson's disease: The role of glial cells. J Pharmacol Sci 2020; 144(3): 151-64.

[http://dx.doi.org/10.1016/j.jphs.2020.07.011] [PMID: 32807662]

[17]   Sun M, Gu Y, Zhao Y, Xu C. Protective functions of taurine against experimental stroke through depressing mitochondria-mediated cell death in rats. Amino Acids 2011; 40(5): 1419-29.
[http://dx.doi.org/10.1007/s00726-010-0751-8] [PMID: 20862501]

[18]   Menzie J, Prentice H, Wu JY. Neuroprotective mechanisms of taurine against ischemic stroke. Brain Sci 2013; 3(4): 877-907.
[http://dx.doi.org/10.3390/brainsci3020877] [PMID: 24961429]

[19]   Palkovits M, Elekes I, Láng T, Patthy A. Taurine levels in discrete brain nuclei of rats. J Neurochem 1986; 47(5): 1333-5.
[http://dx.doi.org/10.1111/j.1471-4159.1986.tb00761.x] [PMID: 3760864]

[20]   Wade JV, Olson JP, Samson FE, Nelson SR, Pazdernik TL. A possible role for taurine in osmoregulation within the brain. J Neurochem 1988; 51(3): 740-5.
[http://dx.doi.org/10.1111/j.1471-4159.1988.tb01807.x] [PMID: 3411323]

[21]   Lallemand F, De Witte P. Taurine concentration in the brain and in the plasma following intraperitoneal injections. Amino Acids 2004; 26(2): 111-6.
[http://dx.doi.org/10.1007/s00726-003-0058-0] [PMID: 15042438]

[22]   Suárez LM, Muñoz MD, Martín del Río R, Solís JM. Taurine content in different brain structures during ageing: effect on hippocampal synaptic plasticity. Amino Acids 2016; 48(5): 1199-208.
[http://dx.doi.org/10.1007/s00726-015-2155-2] [PMID: 26803657]

[23]   Bhat MA, Ahmad K, Khan MSA, et al. Expedition into taurinebiology: Structural insights and therapeutic perspective of taurine in neurodegenerative diseases. Biomolecules 2020; 10(6): 863.
[http://dx.doi.org/10.3390/biom10060863] [PMID: 32516961]

[24]   Leon R, Wu H, Jin Y, et al. Protective function of taurine in glutamate-induced apoptosis in cultured neurons. J Neurosci Res 2009; 87(5): 1185-94.
[http://dx.doi.org/10.1002/jnr.21926] [PMID: 18951478]

[25]   Ye HB, Shi HB, Yin SK. Mechanisms underlying taurine protection against glutamate-induced neurotoxicity. Can J Neurol Sci 2013; 40(5): 628-34.
[http://dx.doi.org/10.1017/S0317167100014840] [PMID: 23968934]

[26]   Sun Q, Hu H, Wang W, Jin H, Feng G, Jia N. Taurine attenuates amyloid β 1–42-induced mitochondrial dysfunction by activating of SIRT1 in SK-N-SH cells. Biochem Biophys Res Commun 2014; 447(3): 485-9.
[http://dx.doi.org/10.1016/j.bbrc.2014.04.019] [PMID: 24735533]

[27]   Xu S, He M, Zhong M, et al. The neuroprotective effects of taurine against nickel by reducing oxidative stress and maintaining mitochondrial function in cortical neurons. Neurosci Lett 2015; 590: 52-7.
[http://dx.doi.org/10.1016/j.neulet.2015.01.065] [PMID: 25637701]

[28]   Khalaf K, Tornese P, Cocco A, Albanese A. Tauroursodeoxycholic acid: a potential therapeutic tool in neurodegenerative diseases. Transl Neurodegener 2022; 11(1): 33.
[http://dx.doi.org/10.1186/s40035-022-00307-z] [PMID: 35659112]

[29]   Schwarzer R, Kivaranovic D, Mandorfer M, et al. Randomised clinical study: the effects of oral taurine 6g/day vs placebo on portal hypertension. Aliment Pharmacol Ther 2018; 47(1): 86-94.
[http://dx.doi.org/10.1111/apt.14377] [PMID: 29105115]

[30]   Rikimaru M, Ohsawa Y, Wolf AM, et al. Taurine ameliorates impaired the mitochondrial function and prevents stroke-like episodes in patients with MELAS. Intern Med 2012; 51(24): 3351-7.
[http://dx.doi.org/10.2169/internalmedicine.51.7529] [PMID: 23257519]

[31]   Gharibani PM, Modi J, Pan C, Menzie J, Ma Z, Chen P-C, et al. The mechanism of taurine protection against endoplasmic reticulum stress in an animal stroke model of cerebral artery occlusion and stroke-related conditions in primary neuronal cell culture Taurine 8. Springer 2013; pp. 241-58.

[http://dx.doi.org/10.1007/978-1-4614-6093-0_23]

[32]   Jakaria M, Azam S, Haque ME, *et al.* Taurine and its analogs in neurological disorders: Focus on therapeutic potential and molecular mechanisms. Redox Biol 2019; 24: 101223.
[http://dx.doi.org/10.1016/j.redox.2019.101223] [PMID: 31141786]

[33]   Lambert IH, Kristensen DM, Holm JB, Mortensen OH. Physiological role of taurine - from organism to organelle. Acta Physiol (Oxf) 2015; 213(1): 191-212.
[http://dx.doi.org/10.1111/apha.12365] [PMID: 25142161]

[34]   Benrabh H, Bourre JM, Lefauconnier JM. Taurine transport at the blood-brain barrier: an *in vivo* brain perfusion study. Brain Res 1995; 692(1-2): 57-65.
[http://dx.doi.org/10.1016/0006-8993(95)00648-A] [PMID: 8548320]

[35]   Wu JY, Prentice H. Role of taurine in the central nervous system. J Biomed Sci 2010; 17(Suppl 1) (Suppl. 1): S1.
[http://dx.doi.org/10.1186/1423-0127-17-S1-S1] [PMID: 20804583]

[36]   Solís J, Herranz AS, Herreras O, Lerma J, del Río RM. Does taurine act as an osmoregulatory substance in the rat brain? Neurosci Lett 1988; 91(1): 53-8.
[http://dx.doi.org/10.1016/0304-3940(88)90248-0] [PMID: 3173785]

[37]   Barbeau A, Huxtable RJ. Taurine and neurological disorders. J Neuropathol Exp Neurol 1978; 37(5): 558.
[http://dx.doi.org/10.1097/00005072-197809000-00010]

[38]   Kumari N, Prentice H, Wu JY. Taurine and its neuroprotective role. Adv Exp Med Biol 2013; 775: 19-27.
[http://dx.doi.org/10.1007/978-1-4614-6130-2_2] [PMID: 23392921]

[39]   Menzie J, Pan C, Prentice H, Wu JY. Taurine and central nervous system disorders. Amino Acids 2014; 46(1): 31-46.
[http://dx.doi.org/10.1007/s00726-012-1382-z] [PMID: 22903433]

[40]   Kilb W, Fukuda A. Taurine as an essential neuromodulator during perinatal cortical development. Front Cell Neurosci 2017; 11: 328.
[http://dx.doi.org/10.3389/fncel.2017.00328] [PMID: 29123472]

[41]   Oja SS. Saransaari PJMbd. Taurine as osmoregulator and neuromodulator in the brain. 1996;11(2):153-64.

[42]   Kilb W. Putative role of taurine as neurotransmitter during perinatal cortical development Taurine 10. Springer 2017; pp. 281-92.

[43]   Pasantes-Morales H, Schousboe A. Role of taurine in osmoregulation in brain cells: Mechanisms and functional implications. Amino Acids 1997; 12(3-4): 281-92.
[http://dx.doi.org/10.1007/BF01373008]

[44]   Hussy N, Deleuze C, Desarménien MG, Moos FC. Osmotic regulation of neuronal activity: a new role for taurine and glial cells in a hypothalamic neuroendocrine structure. Prog Neurobiol 2000; 62(2): 113-34.
[http://dx.doi.org/10.1016/S0301-0082(99)00071-4] [PMID: 10828380]

[45]   Dong X, Wang Y, Qin Z. Molecular mechanisms of excitotoxicity and their relevance to pathogenesis of neurodegenerative diseases. Acta Pharmacol Sin 2009; 30(4): 379-87.
[http://dx.doi.org/10.1038/aps.2009.24] [PMID: 19343058]

[46]   Armada-Moreira A, Gomes JI, Pina CC, *et al.* Going the extra (synaptic) mile: Excitotoxicity as the road toward neurodegenerative diseases. Front Cell Neurosci 2020; 14: 90.
[http://dx.doi.org/10.3389/fncel.2020.00090] [PMID: 32390802]

[47]   Olloquequi J, Cornejo-Córdova E, Verdaguer E, *et al.* Excitotoxicity in the pathogenesis of neurological and psychiatric disorders: Therapeutic implications. J Psychopharmacol 2018; 32(3):

265-75.
[http://dx.doi.org/10.1177/0269881118754680] [PMID: 29444621]

[48] Nguyen D, Alavi MV, Kim K-Y, *et al.* A new vicious cycle involving glutamate excitotoxicity, oxidative stress and mitochondrial dynamics. Cell Death Dis 2011; 2(12): e240.
[http://dx.doi.org/10.1038/cddis.2011.117] [PMID: 22158479]

[49] Brookes PS, Yoon Y, Robotham JL, Anders MW, Sheu SS. Calcium, ATP, and ROS: a mitochondrial love-hate triangle. Am J Physiol Cell Physiol 2004; 287(4): C817-33.
[http://dx.doi.org/10.1152/ajpcell.00139.2004] [PMID: 15355853]

[50] Prentice H, Modi JP, Wu J-Y. Mechanisms of neuronal protection against excitotoxicity, endoplasmic reticulum stress, and mitochondrial dysfunction in stroke and neurodegenerative diseases. Oxid Med Cell Longev 2015.

[51] El Idrissi A, Trenkner E. Taurine regulates mitochondrial calcium homeostasis. Adv Exp Med Biol 2003; 526: 527-36.
[http://dx.doi.org/10.1007/978-1-4615-0077-3_63] [PMID: 12908639]

[52] Chen WQ, Jin H, Nguyen M, *et al.* Role of taurine in regulation of intracellular calcium level and neuroprotective function in cultured neurons. J Neurosci Res 2001; 66(4): 612-9.
[http://dx.doi.org/10.1002/jnr.10027] [PMID: 11746381]

[53] Artal-Sanz M, Tavernarakis N. Proteolytic mechanisms in necrotic cell death and neurodegeneration. FEBS Lett 2005; 579(15): 3287-96.
[http://dx.doi.org/10.1016/j.febslet.2005.03.052] [PMID: 15943973]

[54] Leist M, Volbracht C, Kühnle S, Fava E, Ferrando-May E, Nicotera P. Caspase-mediated apoptosis in neuronal excitotoxicity triggered by nitric oxide. Mol Med 1997; 3(11): 750-64.
[http://dx.doi.org/10.1007/BF03401713] [PMID: 9407551]

[55] Smith WS, Lev MH, English JD, *et al.* Significance of large vessel intracranial occlusion causing acute ischemic stroke and TIA. Stroke 2009; 40(12): 3834-40.
[http://dx.doi.org/10.1161/STROKEAHA.109.561787] [PMID: 19834014]

[56] Regenhardt RW, Das AS, Stapleton CJ, *et al.* Blood pressure and penumbral sustenance in stroke from large vessel occlusion. Front Neurol 2017; 8: 317.
[http://dx.doi.org/10.3389/fneur.2017.00317] [PMID: 28717354]

[57] Chen H, Yoshioka H, Kim GS, *et al.* Oxidative stress in ischemic brain damage: mechanisms of cell death and potential molecular targets for neuroprotection. Antioxid Redox Signal 2011; 14(8): 1505-17.
[http://dx.doi.org/10.1089/ars.2010.3576] [PMID: 20812869]

[58] Sims NR, Muyderman H. Mitochondria, oxidative metabolism and cell death in stroke. Biochim Biophys Acta Mol Basis Dis 2010; 1802(1): 80-91.
[http://dx.doi.org/10.1016/j.bbadis.2009.09.003]

[59] Pan C, Prentice H, Price AL, Wu JY. Beneficial effect of taurine on hypoxia- and glutamate-induced endoplasmic reticulum stress pathways in primary neuronal culture. Amino Acids 2012; 43(2): 845-55.
[http://dx.doi.org/10.1007/s00726-011-1141-6] [PMID: 22080215]

[60] Yang JL, Mukda S, Chen SD. Diverse roles of mitochondria in ischemic stroke. Redox Biol 2018; 16: 263-75.
[http://dx.doi.org/10.1016/j.redox.2018.03.002] [PMID: 29549824]

[61] Lai TW, Zhang S, Wang YT. Excitotoxicity and stroke: Identifying novel targets for neuroprotection. Prog Neurobiol 2014; 115: 157-88.
[http://dx.doi.org/10.1016/j.pneurobio.2013.11.006] [PMID: 24361499]

[62] Han Y, Yuan M, Guo YS, Shen XY, Gao ZK, Bi X. Mechanism of endoplasmic reticulum stress in cerebral ischemia. Front Cell Neurosci 2021; 15: 704334.
[http://dx.doi.org/10.3389/fncel.2021.704334] [PMID: 34408630]

[63]   Hazell A. Excitotoxic mechanisms in stroke: An update of concepts and treatment strategies. Neurochem Int 2007; 50(7-8): 941-53.
[http://dx.doi.org/10.1016/j.neuint.2007.04.026] [PMID: 17576023]

[64]   Prentice H, Gharibani PM, Ma Z, Alexandrescu A, Genova R, Chen P-C, *et al.* Neuroprotective functions through inhibition of ER stress by taurine or taurine combination treatments in a rat stroke model Taurine 10 Advances in Experimental Medicine and Biology. Springer 2017; pp. 193-205.

[65]   Chen PC, Pan C, Gharibani PM, Prentice H, Wu JY. Taurine exerts robust protection against hypoxia and oxygen/glucose deprivation in human neuroblastoma cell culture. Adv Exp Med Biol 2013; 775: 167-75.
[http://dx.doi.org/10.1007/978-1-4614-6130-2_14] [PMID: 23392933]

[66]   Schaffer SW, Jong CJ, Ito T, Azuma J. Effect of taurine on ischemia–reperfusion injury. Amino Acids 2014; 46(1): 21-30.
[http://dx.doi.org/10.1007/s00726-012-1378-8] [PMID: 22936072]

[67]   Ohsawa Y, Hagiwara H, Nishimatsu S-i, Hirakawa A, Kamimura N, Ohtsubo H, *et al.* Taurine supplementation for prevention of stroke-like episodes in MELAS: a multicentre, open-label, 52-week phase III trial. J Neurol Neurosurg Psychiatry 2019; 90(5): 529-536.

[68]   Schaffer SW, Jong CJ, Ito T, Azuma J. Role of taurine in the pathologies of MELAS and MERRF. Amino Acids 2014; 46(1): 47-56.
[http://dx.doi.org/10.1007/s00726-012-1414-8] [PMID: 23179085]

[69]   Cheng G, Kong R, Zhang L, Zhang J. Mitochondria in traumatic brain injury and mitochondrial-targeted multipotential therapeutic strategies. Br J Pharmacol 2012; 167(4): 699-719.
[http://dx.doi.org/10.1111/j.1476-5381.2012.02025.x] [PMID: 23003569]

[70]   Bruns J Jr, Hauser WA. The epidemiology of traumatic brain injury: a review. Epilepsia 2003; 44(s10): 2-10.
[http://dx.doi.org/10.1046/j.1528-1157.44.s10.3.x] [PMID: 14511388]

[71]   Lucke-Wold BP, Logsdon AF, Nguyen L, *et al.* Supplements, nutrition, and alternative therapies for the treatment of traumatic brain injury. Nutr Neurosci 2018; 21(2): 79-91.
[http://dx.doi.org/10.1080/1028415X.2016.1236174] [PMID: 27705610]

[72]   Werner C, Engelhard K. Pathophysiology of traumatic brain injury. Br J Anaesth 2007; 99(1): 4-9.
[http://dx.doi.org/10.1093/bja/aem131] [PMID: 17573392]

[73]   Hall ED, Vaishnav RA, Mustafa AG. Antioxidant therapies for traumatic brain injury. Neurotherapeutics 2010; 7(1): 51-61.
[http://dx.doi.org/10.1016/j.nurt.2009.10.021] [PMID: 20129497]

[74]   Curtis L, Epstein P. Nutritional treatment for acute and chronic traumatic brain injury patients. J Neurosurg Sci 2014; 58(3): 151-60.
[PMID: 24844176]

[75]   Raghupathi R. Cell death mechanisms following traumatic brain injury. Brain Pathol 2004; 14(2): 215-22.
[http://dx.doi.org/10.1111/j.1750-3639.2004.tb00056.x] [PMID: 15193035]

[76]   Weber JT. Altered calcium signaling following traumatic brain injury. Front Pharmacol 2012; 3: 60.
[http://dx.doi.org/10.3389/fphar.2012.00060] [PMID: 22518104]

[77]   Stoica BA, Faden AI. Cell death mechanisms and modulation in traumatic brain injury. Neurotherapeutics 2010; 7(1): 3-12.
[http://dx.doi.org/10.1016/j.nurt.2009.10.023] [PMID: 20129492]

[78]   O'Connell KM, Littleton-Kearney MT. The role of free radicals in traumatic brain injury. Biol Res Nurs 2013; 15(3): 253-63.
[http://dx.doi.org/10.1177/1099800411431823] [PMID: 22345426]

[79] Institute of Medicine Committee on Nutrition T, the B Nutrition and traumatic brain injury: Improving acute and subacute health outcomes in military personnel Washington (DC). US: National Academies Press 2011.

[80] Cornelius C, Crupi R, Calabrese V, *et al.* Traumatic brain injury: oxidative stress and neuroprotection. Antioxid Redox Signal 2013; 19(8): 836-53.
[http://dx.doi.org/10.1089/ars.2012.4981] [PMID: 23547621]

[81] Mustafa AG, Singh IN, Wang J, Carrico KM, Hall ED. Mitochondrial protection after traumatic brain injury by scavenging lipid peroxyl radicals. J Neurochem 2010; 114(1): 271-80.
[http://dx.doi.org/10.1111/j.1471-4159.2010.06749.x] [PMID: 20403083]

[82] Hill RL, Kulbe JR, Singh IN, Wang JA, Hall ED. Synaptic mitochondria are more susceptible to traumatic brain injury-induced oxidative damage and respiratory dysfunction than non-synaptic mitochondria. Neuroscience 2018; 386: 265-83.
[http://dx.doi.org/10.1016/j.neuroscience.2018.06.028] [PMID: 29960045]

[83] Hubbard WB, Davis LM, Sullivan PG. Mitochondrial damage in traumatic CNS injury Acute Neuronal Injury. Springer 2018; pp. 63-81.

[84] Xiong Y, Gu Q, Peterson PL, Muizelaar JP, Lee CP. Mitochondrial dysfunction and calcium perturbation induced by traumatic brain injury. J Neurotrauma 1997; 14(1): 23-34.
[http://dx.doi.org/10.1089/neu.1997.14.23] [PMID: 9048308]

[85] Clark RSB, Chen J, Watkins SC, *et al.* Apoptosis-suppressor gene bcl-2 expression after traumatic brain injury in rats. J Neurosci 1997; 17(23): 9172-82.
[http://dx.doi.org/10.1523/JNEUROSCI.17-23-09172.1997] [PMID: 9364064]

[86] Luo CL, Chen XP, Yang R, *et al.* Cathepsin B contributes to traumatic brain injury-induced cell death through a mitochondria-mediated apoptotic pathway. J Neurosci Res 2010; 88(13): 2847-58.
[http://dx.doi.org/10.1002/jnr.22453] [PMID: 20653046]

[87] Lifshitz J, Sullivan PG, Hovda DA, Wieloch T, McIntosh TK. Mitochondrial damage and dysfunction in traumatic brain injury. Mitochondrion 2004; 4(5-6): 705-13.
[http://dx.doi.org/10.1016/j.mito.2004.07.021] [PMID: 16120426]

[88] Wang Q, Fan W, Cai Y, *et al.* Protective effects of taurine in traumatic brain injury *via* mitochondria and cerebral blood flow. Amino Acids 2016; 48(9): 2169-77.
[http://dx.doi.org/10.1007/s00726-016-2244-x] [PMID: 27156064]

[89] Gupte R, Christian S, Keselman P, Habiger J, Brooks WM, Harris JL. Evaluation of taurine neuroprotection in aged rats with traumatic brain injury. Brain Imaging Behav 2018; 1-11.
[PMID: 29656312]

[90] Su Y, Fan W, Ma Z, *et al.* Taurine improves functional and histological outcomes and reduces inflammation in traumatic brain injury. Neuroscience 2014; 266: 56-65.
[http://dx.doi.org/10.1016/j.neuroscience.2014.02.006] [PMID: 24530657]

[91] Sun M, Zhao Y, Gu Y, Zhang Y. Protective effects of taurine against closed head injury in rats. J Neurotrauma 2015; 32(1): 66-74.
[http://dx.doi.org/10.1089/neu.2012.2432] [PMID: 23327111]

[92] Vahdat M, Hosseini SA, Soltani F, Cheraghian B, Namjoonia M. The effects of Taurine supplementation on inflammatory markers and clinical outcomes in patients with traumatic brain injury: a double-blind randomized controlled trial. Nutr J 2021; 20(1): 53.
[http://dx.doi.org/10.1186/s12937-021-00712-6] [PMID: 34103066]

[93] Gu Y, Zhao Y, Qian K, Sun M. Taurine attenuates hippocampal and corpus callosum damage, and enhances neurological recovery after closed head injury in rats. Neuroscience 2015; 291: 331-40.
[http://dx.doi.org/10.1016/j.neuroscience.2014.09.073] [PMID: 25290011]

[94] Heidari R. Brain mitochondria as potential therapeutic targets for managing hepatic encephalopathy.

Life Sci 2019; 218: 65-80.
[http://dx.doi.org/10.1016/j.lfs.2018.12.030] [PMID: 30578865]

[95]   Roşca AE, Badiu C, Uscătescu V, *et al.* Influence of chronic administration of anabolic androgenic steroids and taurine on haemostasis profile in rats. Blood Coagul Fibrinolysis 2013; 24(3): 256-60.
[http://dx.doi.org/10.1097/MBC.0b013e32835b7611] [PMID: 23160242]

[96]   Miglis M, Wilder D, Reid T, Bakaltcheva I. Effect of taurine on platelets and the plasma coagulation system. Platelets 2002; 13(1): 5-10.
[http://dx.doi.org/10.1080/09537100120112558] [PMID: 11918831]

[97]   Lamade AM, Kenny EM, Anthonymuthu TS, *et al.* Aiming for the target: Mitochondrial drug delivery in traumatic brain injury. Neuropharmacology 2019; 145(Pt B): 209-19.
[http://dx.doi.org/10.1016/j.neuropharm.2018.07.014] [PMID: 30009835]

[98]   Blei AT, Córdoba J. Hepatic encephalopathy. Am J Gastroenterol 2001; 96(7): 1968-76.
[http://dx.doi.org/10.1111/j.1572-0241.2001.03964.x] [PMID: 11467622]

[99]   Felipo V. Hepatic encephalopathy: effects of liver failure on brain function. Nat Rev Neurosci 2013; 14(12): 851-8.
[http://dx.doi.org/10.1038/nrn3587] [PMID: 24149188]

[100] Cordoba J. Hepatic encephalopathy: From the pathogenesis to the new treatments. ISRN Hepatol 2014; 2014: 1-16.
[http://dx.doi.org/10.1155/2014/236268] [PMID: 27335836]

[101] Felipo V, Hermenegildo C, Montoliu C, Llansola M, Miñana MD. Neurotoxicity of ammonia and glutamate: molecular mechanisms and prevention. Neurotoxicology 1998; 19(4-5): 675-81.
[PMID: 9745928]

[102] Jamshidzadeh A, Heidari R, Abasvali M, *et al.* Taurine treatment preserves brain and liver mitochondrial function in a rat model of fulminant hepatic failure and hyperammonemia. Biomed Pharmacother 2017; 86: 514-20.
[http://dx.doi.org/10.1016/j.biopha.2016.11.095] [PMID: 28024286]

[103] Heidari R, Jamshidzadeh A, Ommati MM, *et al.* Ammonia-induced mitochondrial impairment is intensified by manganese co-exposure: relevance to the management of subclinical hepatic encephalopathy and cirrhosis-associated brain injury. Clin Exp Hepatol 2019; 5(2): 109-17.
[http://dx.doi.org/10.5114/ceh.2019.85071] [PMID: 31501786]

[104] Jamshidzadeh A, Niknahad H, Heidari R, Zarei M, Ommati MM, Khodaei F. Carnosine protects brain mitochondria under hyperammonemic conditions: Relevance to hepatic encephalopathy treatment. PharmaNutrition 2017; 5(2): 58-63.
[http://dx.doi.org/10.1016/j.phanu.2017.02.004]

[105] Weiss N, Barbier Saint Hilaire P, Colsch B, *et al.* Cerebrospinal fluid metabolomics highlights dysregulation of energy metabolism in overt hepatic encephalopathy. J Hepatol 2016; 65(6): 1120-30.
[http://dx.doi.org/10.1016/j.jhep.2016.07.046] [PMID: 27520878]

[106] Rao KVR, Norenberg MD. Cerebral energy metabolism in hepatic encephalopathy and hyperammonemia. Metab Brain Dis 2001; 16(1/2): 67-78.
[http://dx.doi.org/10.1023/A:1011666612822] [PMID: 11726090]

[107] Hertz L, Kala G. Energy metabolism in brain cells: effects of elevated ammonia concentrations. Metab Brain Dis 2007; 22(3-4): 199-218.
[http://dx.doi.org/10.1007/s11011-007-9068-z] [PMID: 17882538]

[108] Rama Rao KV, Norenberg MD. Brain energy metabolism and mitochondrial dysfunction in acute and chronic hepatic encephalopathy. Neurochem Int 2012; 60(7): 697-706.
[http://dx.doi.org/10.1016/j.neuint.2011.09.007] [PMID: 21989389]

[109] Dhanda S, Sunkaria A, Halder A, Sandhir R. Mitochondrial dysfunctions contribute to energy deficits in rodent model of hepatic encephalopathy. Metab Brain Dis 2018; 33(1): 209-23.

[http://dx.doi.org/10.1007/s11011-017-0136-8] [PMID: 29138968]

[110] Ramarao K, Jayakumar A, Norenberg M. Role of oxidative stress in the ammonia-induced mitochondrial permeability transition in cultured astrocytes. Neurochem Int 2005; 47(1-2): 31-8.
[http://dx.doi.org/10.1016/j.neuint.2005.04.004] [PMID: 15908047]

[111] Chepkova AN, Sergeeva OA, Haas HL. Taurine rescues hippocampal long-term potentiation from ammonia-induced impairment. Neurobiol Dis 2006; 23(3): 512-21.
[http://dx.doi.org/10.1016/j.nbd.2006.04.006] [PMID: 16766203]

[112] Boer LA, Panatto JP, Fagundes DA, *et al.* Inhibition of mitochondrial respiratory chain in the brain of rats after hepatic failure induced by carbon tetrachloride is reversed by antioxidants. Brain Res Bull 2009; 80(1-2): 75-8.
[http://dx.doi.org/10.1016/j.brainresbull.2009.04.009] [PMID: 19406217]

[113] Bobermin LD, Wartchow KM, Flores MP, Leite MC, Quincozes-Santos A, Gonçalves CA. Ammonia-induced oxidative damage in neurons is prevented by resveratrol and lipoic acid with participation of heme oxygenase 1. Neurotoxicology 2015; 49: 28-35.
[http://dx.doi.org/10.1016/j.neuro.2015.05.005] [PMID: 26003724]

[114] Butterworth RF. Taurine in hepatic encephalopathy. In: Huxtable RJ, Azuma J, Kuriyama K, Nakagawa M, Baba A, editors. Taurine 2. Advances in Experimental Medicine and Biology: Springer US; 1996. p. 601-6.
[http://dx.doi.org/10.1007/978-1-4899-0182-8_66]

[115] Jover R, Rodrigo R, Felipo V, *et al.* Brain edema and inflammatory activation in bile duct ligated rats with diet-induced hyperammonemia: A model of hepatic encephalopathy in cirrhosis. Hepatology 2006; 43(6): 1257-66.
[http://dx.doi.org/10.1002/hep.21180] [PMID: 16729306]

[116] Cudalbu C, Taylor-Robinson SD. Brain edema in chronic hepatic encephalopathy. J Clin Exp Hepatol 2019; 9(3): 362-82.
[http://dx.doi.org/10.1016/j.jceh.2019.02.003] [PMID: 31360029]

[117] Norenberg MD, Rao KVR, Jayakumar AR. Mechanisms of ammonia-induced astrocyte swelling. Metab Brain Dis 2005; 20(4): 303-18.
[http://dx.doi.org/10.1007/s11011-005-7911-7] [PMID: 16382341]

[118] Albrecht J, Norenberg MD. Glutamine: A Trojan horse in ammonia neurotoxicity. Hepatology 2006; 44(4): 788-94.
[http://dx.doi.org/10.1002/hep.21357] [PMID: 17006913]

[119] Jayakumar AR, Rao KVR, Murthy CRK, Norenberg MD. Glutamine in the mechanism of ammonia-induced astrocyte swelling. Neurochem Int 2006; 48(6-7): 623-8.
[http://dx.doi.org/10.1016/j.neuint.2005.11.017] [PMID: 16517020]

[120] Norenberg MD, Jayakumar AR, Rama Rao KV, Panickar KS. New concepts in the mechanism of ammonia-induced astrocyte swelling. Metab Brain Dis 2007; 22(3-4): 219-34.
[http://dx.doi.org/10.1007/s11011-007-9062-5] [PMID: 17823859]

[121] Rama Rao KV, Reddy PVB, Tong X, Norenberg MD. Brain edema in acute liver failure: inhibition by L-histidine. Am J Pathol 2010; 176(3): 1400-8.
[http://dx.doi.org/10.2353/ajpath.2010.090756] [PMID: 20075201]

[122] Butterworth RF. Pathogenesis of hepatic encephalopathy and brain edema in acute liver failure. J Clin Exp Hepatol 2015; 5 (Suppl. 1): S96-S103.
[http://dx.doi.org/10.1016/j.jceh.2014.02.004] [PMID: 26041966]

[123] Siracusa R, Fusco R, Cuzzocrea S. Astrocytes: Role and functions in brain pathologies. Front Pharmacol 2019; 10: 1114.
[http://dx.doi.org/10.3389/fphar.2019.01114] [PMID: 31611796]

[124] Rama Rao KV, Chen M, Simard JM, Norenberg MD. Suppression of ammonia-induced astrocyte

swelling by cyclosporin A. J Neurosci Res 2003; 74(6): 891-7.
[http://dx.doi.org/10.1002/jnr.10755] [PMID: 14648594]

[125] Reddy PVB, Rama Rao KV, Norenberg MD. Inhibitors of the mitochondrial permeability transition reduce ammonia-induced cell swelling in cultured astrocytes. J Neurosci Res 2009; 87(12): 2677-85.
[http://dx.doi.org/10.1002/jnr.22097] [PMID: 19382208]

[126] Jamshidzadeh A, Heidari R, Latifpour Z, *et al.* Carnosine ameliorates liver fibrosis and hyperammonemia in cirrhotic rats. Clin Res Hepatol Gastroenterol 2017; 41(4): 424-34.
[http://dx.doi.org/10.1016/j.clinre.2016.12.010] [PMID: 28283328]

[127] Heidari R, Jamshidzadeh A, Ghanbarinejad V, Ommati MM, Niknahad H. Taurine supplementation abates cirrhosis-associated locomotor dysfunction. Clin Exp Hepatol 2018; 4(2): 72-82.
[http://dx.doi.org/10.5114/ceh.2018.75956] [PMID: 29904723]

[128] Albrecht J, Zielińska M. The role of inhibitory amino acidergic neurotransmission in hepatic encephalopathy: a critical overview. Metab Brain Dis 2002; 17(4): 283-94.
[http://dx.doi.org/10.1023/A:1021901700493] [PMID: 12602505]

[129] Heidari R, Jamshidzadeh A, Niknahad H, *et al.* Effect of taurine on chronic and acute liver injury: Focus on blood and brain ammonia. Toxicol Rep 2016; 3: 870-9.
[http://dx.doi.org/10.1016/j.toxrep.2016.04.002] [PMID: 28959615]

[130] Niknahad H, Jamshidzadeh A, Heidari R, Zarei M, Ommati MM. Ammonia-induced mitochondrial dysfunction and energy metabolism disturbances in isolated brain and liver mitochondria, and the effect of taurine administration: relevance to hepatic encephalopathy treatment. Clin Exp Hepatol 2017; 3(3): 141-51.
[http://dx.doi.org/10.5114/ceh.2017.68833] [PMID: 29062904]

[131] Albrecht J, Wegrzynowicz M. Endogenous neuro-protectants in ammonia toxicity in the central nervous system: facts and hypotheses. Metab Brain Dis 2005; 20(4): 253-63.
[http://dx.doi.org/10.1007/s11011-005-7904-6] [PMID: 16382336]

[132] Schousboe A, Pasantes-Morales H. Role of taurine in neural cell volume regulation. Can J Physiol Pharmacol 1992; 70(S1) (Suppl.): S356-61.
[http://dx.doi.org/10.1139/y92-283] [PMID: 1295685]

[133] Pasantes Morales H, Schousboe A. Volume regulation in astrocytes: a role for taurine as an osmoeffector. J Neurosci Res 1988; 20(4): 503-9.
[PMID: 3184212]

[134] Vidot H, Cvejic E, Carey S, *et al.* Randomised clinical trial: oral taurine supplementation versus placebo reduces muscle cramps in patients with chronic liver disease. Aliment Pharmacol Ther 2018; 48(7): 704-12.
[http://dx.doi.org/10.1111/apt.14950] [PMID: 30136291]

[135] Singh A, Trevick S. The epidemiology of global epilepsy. Neurol Clin 2016; 34(4): 837-47.
[http://dx.doi.org/10.1016/j.ncl.2016.06.015] [PMID: 27719996]

[136] Kovac S, Dinkova Kostova A, Herrmann A, Melzer N, Meuth S, Gorji A. Metabolic and homeostatic changes in seizures and acquired epilepsy—mitochondria, calcium dynamics and reactive oxygen species. Int J Mol Sci 2017; 18(9): 1935.
[http://dx.doi.org/10.3390/ijms18091935] [PMID: 28885567]

[137] Bindoff LA, Engelsen BA. Mitochondrial diseases and epilepsy. Epilepsia 2012; 53 (Suppl. 4): 92-7.
[http://dx.doi.org/10.1111/j.1528-1167.2012.03618.x] [PMID: 22946726]

[138] Folbergrová J, Kunz WS. Mitochondrial dysfunction in epilepsy. Mitochondrion 2012; 12(1): 35-40.
[http://dx.doi.org/10.1016/j.mito.2011.04.004] [PMID: 21530687]

[139] Zsurka G, Kunz WS. Mitochondrial dysfunction and seizures: the neuronal energy crisis. Lancet Neurol 2015; 14(9): 956-66.
[http://dx.doi.org/10.1016/S1474-4422(15)00148-9] [PMID: 26293567]

[140] Mastrangelo M. Epilepsy in inherited neurotransmitter disorders: Spotlights on pathophysiology and clinical management. Metab Brain Dis 2021; 36(1): 29-43.
[http://dx.doi.org/10.1007/s11011-020-00635-x] [PMID: 33095372]

[141] Lee S, Na JH, Lee YM. Epilepsy in Leigh Syndrome with mitochondrial DNA mutations. Front Neurol 2019; 10: 496.
[http://dx.doi.org/10.3389/fneur.2019.00496] [PMID: 31139141]

[142] Wallace DC, Lott MT, Shoffner JM, Ballinger S. Mitochondrial DNA mutations in epilepsy and neurological disease. Epilepsia 1994; 35(s1) (Suppl. 1): S43-50.
[http://dx.doi.org/10.1111/j.1528-1157.1994.tb05928.x] [PMID: 8293723]

[143] Shen C, Xian W, Zhou H, Li X, Liang X, Chen L. Overlapping Leigh syndrome/myoclonic epilepsy eith ragged red fibres in an adolescent patient with a mitochondrial DNA A8344G mutation. Front Neurol 2018; 9: 724.
[http://dx.doi.org/10.3389/fneur.2018.00724] [PMID: 30271374]

[144] Shoffner JM, Lott MT, Lezza AMS, Seibel P, Ballinger SW, Wallace DC. Myoclonic epilepsy and ragged-red fiber disease (MERRF) is associated with a mitochondrial DNA tRNALys mutation. Cell 1990; 61(6): 931-7.
[http://dx.doi.org/10.1016/0092-8674(90)90059-N] [PMID: 2112427]

[145] Canafoglia L, Franceschetti S, Antozzi C, et al. Epileptic phenotypes associated with mitochondrial disorders. Neurology 2001; 56(10): 1340-6.
[http://dx.doi.org/10.1212/WNL.56.10.1340] [PMID: 11376185]

[146] Rahman S. Pathophysiology of mitochondrial disease causing epilepsy and status epilepticus. Epilepsy Behav 2015; 49: 71-5.
[http://dx.doi.org/10.1016/j.yebeh.2015.05.003] [PMID: 26162691]

[147] Pauletti A, Terrone G, Shekh-Ahmad T, Salamone A, Ravizza T, Rizzi M, et al. Targeting oxidative stress improves disease outcomes in a rat model of acquired epilepsy: Oxford University Press; 2019.

[148] Folbergrová J, Ješina P, Drahota Z, et al. Mitochondrial complex I inhibition in cerebral cortex of immature rats following homocysteic acid-induced seizures. Exp Neurol 2007; 204(2): 597-609.
[http://dx.doi.org/10.1016/j.expneurol.2006.12.010] [PMID: 17270175]

[149] Folbergrová J, Ješina P, Haugvicová R, Lisý V, Houštěk J. Sustained deficiency of mitochondrial complex I activity during long periods of survival after seizures induced in immature rats by homocysteic acid. Neurochem Int 2010; 56(3): 394-403.
[http://dx.doi.org/10.1016/j.neuint.2009.11.011] [PMID: 19931336]

[150] Sharma L, Lu J, Bai Y. Mitochondrial respiratory complex I: structure, function and implication in human diseases. Curr Med Chem 2009; 16(10): 1266-77.
[http://dx.doi.org/10.2174/092986709787846578] [PMID: 19355884]

[151] Jong C, Ito T, Prentice H, Wu JY, Schaffer S. Role of mtochondria and endoplasmic reticulum in taurine-deficiency-mediated apoptosis. Nutrients 2017; 9(8): 795.
[http://dx.doi.org/10.3390/nu9080795] [PMID: 28757580]

[152] Yamamoto A, Murphy N, Schindler CK, et al. Endoplasmic reticulum stress and apoptosis signaling in human temporal lobe epilepsy. J Neuropathol Exp Neurol 2006; 65(3): 217-25.
[http://dx.doi.org/10.1097/01.jnen.0000202886.22082.2a] [PMID: 16651883]

[153] Ochoa-de la Paz L, Zenteno E, Gulias-Cañizo R, Quiroz-Mercado H. Taurine and GABA neurotransmitter receptors, a relationship with therapeutic potential? Expert Rev Neurother 2019; 19(4): 289-91.
[http://dx.doi.org/10.1080/14737175.2019.1593827] [PMID: 30892104]

[154] Oja SS, Saransaari P. Taurine and epilepsy. Epilepsy Res 2013; 104(3): 187-94.
[http://dx.doi.org/10.1016/j.eplepsyres.2013.01.010] [PMID: 23410665]

[155] Bureau MH, Olsen RW. Taurine acts on a subclass of GABAa receptors in mammalian brain *in vitro*. Eur J Pharmacol (Mol Pharmacol Sect) 1991; 207(1): 9-16.
[http://dx.doi.org/10.1016/S0922-4106(05)80031-8] [PMID: 1655497]

[156] Oja SS, Saransaari P., Editors. Pharmacology of taurine 2007: [Western Pharmacology Society]; 1998.

[157] Song N, Shi H, Li C, Yin S. Interaction between taurine and GABAA/glycine receptors in neurons of the rat anteroventral cochlear nucleus. Brain Res 2012; 1472: 1-10.
[http://dx.doi.org/10.1016/j.brainres.2012.07.001] [PMID: 22796293]

[158] Ye GI, Tse ACO, Yung W. Taurine inhibits rat substantia nigra pars reticulata neurons by activation of GABA- and glycine-linked chloride conductance. Brain Res 1997; 749(1): 175-9.
[http://dx.doi.org/10.1016/S0006-8993(96)01427-8] [PMID: 9070647]

[159] Oja SS, Korpi ER, Saransaari P. Modification of chloride flux across brain membranes by inhibitory amino acids in developing and adult mice. Neurochem Res 1990; 15(8): 797-804.
[http://dx.doi.org/10.1007/BF00968557] [PMID: 2120601]

[160] Jia F, Yue M, Chandra D, *et al.* Taurine is a potent activator of extrasynaptic GABA(A) receptors in the thalamus. J Neurosci 2008; 28(1): 106-15.
[http://dx.doi.org/10.1523/JNEUROSCI.3996-07.2008] [PMID: 18171928]

[161] Nguyen TTH, Bhattarai JP, Park SJ, Han SK. Activation of glycine and extrasynaptic GABA(A) receptors by taurine on the substantia gelatinosa neurons of the trigeminal subnucleus caudalis. Neural Plast 2013; 2013: 1-12.
[http://dx.doi.org/10.1155/2013/740581] [PMID: 24379976]

[162] Singh S, Singh TG, Rehni AK, Sharma V, Singh M, Kaur R. Reviving mitochondrial bioenergetics: A relevant approach in epilepsy. Mitochondrion 2021; 58: 213-26.
[http://dx.doi.org/10.1016/j.mito.2021.03.009] [PMID: 33775871]

[163] Wesół-Kucharska D, Rokicki D, Jezela-Stanek A. Epilepsy in mitochondrial diseases-current state of knowledge on aetiology and treatment. Children (Basel) 2021; 8(7): 532.
[http://dx.doi.org/10.3390/children8070532] [PMID: 34206602]

[164] Suzuki T, Suzuki T, Wada T, Saigo K, Watanabe K. Taurine as a constituent of mitochondrial tRNAs: new insights into the functions of taurine and human mitochondrial diseases. EMBO J 2002; 21(23): 6581-9.
[http://dx.doi.org/10.1093/emboj/cdf656] [PMID: 12456664]

[165] Lin MT, Beal MF. Mitochondrial dysfunction and oxidative stress in neurodegenerative diseases. Nature 2006; 443(7113): 787-95.
[http://dx.doi.org/10.1038/nature05292] [PMID: 17051205]

[166] Golpich M, Amini E, Mohamed Z, Azman Ali R, Mohamed Ibrahim N, Ahmadiani A. Mitochondrial dysfunction and biogenesis in neurodegenerative diseases: pathogenesis and treatment. CNS Neurosci Ther 2017; 23(1): 5-22.
[http://dx.doi.org/10.1111/cns.12655] [PMID: 27873462]

[167] Gao J, Wang L, Liu J, Xie F, Su B, Wang X. Abnormalities of mitochondrial dynamics in neurodegenerative diseases. Antioxidants 2017; 6(2): 25.
[http://dx.doi.org/10.3390/antiox6020025] [PMID: 28379197]

[168] Francis PT. The interplay of neurotransmitters in Alzheimer's disease. CNS Spectr 2005; 10(S18): 6-9.
[http://dx.doi.org/10.1017/S1092852900014164] [PMID: 16273023]

[169] Ferreira-Vieira TH, Guimaraes IM, Silva FR, Ribeiro FM. Alzheimer's disease: Targeting the cholinergic system. Curr Neuropharmacol 2016; 14(1): 101-15.
[http://dx.doi.org/10.2174/1570159X13666150716165726] [PMID: 26813123]

[170] Kumar A, Singh A, Ekavali . A review on Alzheimer's disease pathophysiology and its management: an update. Pharmacol Rep 2015; 67(2): 195-203.

[http://dx.doi.org/10.1016/j.pharep.2014.09.004] [PMID: 25712639]

[171] Hardingham GE, Bading H. Synaptic versus extrasynaptic NMDA receptor signalling: implications for neurodegenerative disorders. Nat Rev Neurosci 2010; 11(10): 682-96.
[http://dx.doi.org/10.1038/nrn2911] [PMID: 20842175]

[172] Kamat PK, Kalani A, Rai S, *et al.* Mechanism of oxidative stress and synapse dysfunction in the pathogenesis of Alzheimer's disease: Understanding the therapeutics strategies. Mol Neurobiol 2016; 53(1): 648-61.
[http://dx.doi.org/10.1007/s12035-014-9053-6] [PMID: 25511446]

[173] Chen K, Zhang Q, Wang J, *et al.* Taurine protects transformed rat retinal ganglion cells from hypoxia-induced apoptosis by preventing mitochondrial dysfunction. Brain Res 2009; 1279: 131-8.
[http://dx.doi.org/10.1016/j.brainres.2009.04.054] [PMID: 19427840]

[174] Kim HY, Kim HV, Yoon JH, *et al.* Taurine in drinking water recovers learning and memory in the adult APP/PS1 mouse model of Alzheimer's disease. Sci Rep 2014; 4(1): 7467.
[http://dx.doi.org/10.1038/srep07467] [PMID: 25502280]

[175] Jang H, Lee S, Choi SL, Kim HY, Baek S, Kim Y. Taurine directly binds to oligomeric amyloid-β and recovers cognitive deficits in Alzheimer model mice. Adv Exp Med Biol 2017; 975(Pt 1): 233-41.
[http://dx.doi.org/10.1007/978-94-024-1079-2_21] [PMID: 28849459]

[176] Chen C, Xia S, He J, Lu G, Xie Z, Han H. Roles of taurine in cognitive function of physiology, pathologies and toxication. Life Sci 2019; 231: 116584.
[http://dx.doi.org/10.1016/j.lfs.2019.116584] [PMID: 31220527]

[177] van de Haar HJ, Burgmans S, Jansen JFA, *et al.* Blood-brain barrier leakage in patients with early Alzheimer disease. Radiology 2016; 281(2): 527-35.
[http://dx.doi.org/10.1148/radiol.2016152244] [PMID: 27243267]

[178] Gorgani S, Jahanshahi M, Elyasi L. Taurine prevents passive avoidance memory impairment, accumulation of amyloid-β plaques, and neuronal loss in the hippocampus of scopolamine-treated rats. Neurophysiology 2019; 51(3): 171-9.
[http://dx.doi.org/10.1007/s11062-019-09810-y]

[179] Ito T, Miyazaki N, Schaffer S, Azuma J. Potential anti-aging role of taurine via proper protein folding: a study from taurine transporter knockout mouse Taurine 9. Springer 2015; pp. 481-7.

[180] Chaturvedi SK, Alam P, Khan JM, *et al.* Biophysical insight into the anti-amyloidogenic behavior of taurine. Int J Biol Macromol 2015; 80: 375-84.
[http://dx.doi.org/10.1016/j.ijbiomac.2015.06.035] [PMID: 26111912]

[181] Schapira AHV, Tolosa E. Molecular and clinical prodrome of Parkinson disease: implications for treatment. Nat Rev Neurol 2010; 6(6): 309-17.
[http://dx.doi.org/10.1038/nrneurol.2010.52] [PMID: 20479780]

[182] Chaudhuri KR, Schapira AHV. Non-motor symptoms of Parkinson's disease: dopaminergic pathophysiology and treatment. Lancet Neurol 2009; 8(5): 464-74.
[http://dx.doi.org/10.1016/S1474-4422(09)70068-7] [PMID: 19375664]

[183] Perier C, Bové J, Vila M. Mitochondria and programmed cell death in Parkinson's disease: apoptosis and beyond. Antioxid Redox Signal 2012; 16(9): 883-95.
[http://dx.doi.org/10.1089/ars.2011.4074] [PMID: 21619488]

[184] Schapira AHV. Mitochondrial dysfunction in Parkinson's disease: Nature Publishing Group; 2007.

[185] Park JS, Davis RL, Sue CM. Mitochondrial dysfunction in Parkinson's disease: new mechanistic insights and therapeutic perspectives. Curr Neurol Neurosci Rep 2018; 18(5): 21.
[http://dx.doi.org/10.1007/s11910-018-0829-3] [PMID: 29616350]

[186] Porras G, Li Q, Bezard E. Modeling Parkinson's disease in primates: The MPTP model. Cold Spring Harb Perspect Med 2012; 2(3): a009308.

[http://dx.doi.org/10.1101/cshperspect.a009308] [PMID: 22393538]

[187] Blesa J, Phani S, Jackson-Lewis V, Przedborski S. Classic and new animal models of Parkinson's disease. BioMed Research International 2012.
[http://dx.doi.org/10.1155/2012/845618]

[188] Exner N, Lutz AK, Haass C, Winklhofer KF. Mitochondrial dysfunction in Parkinson's disease: molecular mechanisms and pathophysiological consequences. EMBO J 2012; 31(14): 3038-62.
[http://dx.doi.org/10.1038/emboj.2012.170] [PMID: 22735187]

[189] Camilleri A, Vassallo N. The centrality of mitochondria in the pathogenesis and treatment of Parkinson's disease. CNS Neurosci Ther 2014; 20(7): 591-602.
[http://dx.doi.org/10.1111/cns.12264] [PMID: 24703487]

[190] Stefanis L. α-Synuclein in Parkinson's disease. Cold Spring Harb Perspect Med 2012; 2(2): a009399.
[http://dx.doi.org/10.1101/cshperspect.a009399] [PMID: 22355802]

[191] Hsu LJ, Sagara Y, Arroyo A, *et al.* alpha-synuclein promotes mitochondrial deficit and oxidative stress. Am J Pathol 2000; 157(2): 401-10.
[http://dx.doi.org/10.1016/S0002-9440(10)64553-1] [PMID: 10934145]

[192] Smith WW, Jiang H, Pei Z, *et al.* Endoplasmic reticulum stress and mitochondrial cell death pathways mediate A53T mutant alpha-synuclein-induced toxicity. Hum Mol Genet 2005; 14(24): 3801-11.
[http://dx.doi.org/10.1093/hmg/ddi396] [PMID: 16239241]

[193] Calì T, Ottolini D, Brini M. Mitochondria, calcium, and endoplasmic reticulum stress in Parkinson's disease. Biofactors 2011; 37(3): 228-40.
[http://dx.doi.org/10.1002/biof.159] [PMID: 21674642]

[194] Subramaniam SR, Chesselet MF. Mitochondrial dysfunction and oxidative stress in Parkinson's disease. Prog Neurobiol 2013; 106-107: 17-32.
[http://dx.doi.org/10.1016/j.pneurobio.2013.04.004] [PMID: 23643800]

[195] Jin H, Kanthasamy A, Ghosh A, Anantharam V, Kalyanaraman B, Kanthasamy AG. Mitochondria-targeted antioxidants for treatment of Parkinson's disease: Preclinical and clinical outcomes. Biochim Biophys Acta Mol Basis Dis 2014; 1842(8): 1282-94.
[http://dx.doi.org/10.1016/j.bbadis.2013.09.007] [PMID: 24060637]

[196] Thomas B, Beal MF. Mitochondrial therapies for Parkinson's disease. Mov Disord 2010; 25(S1): S155-60.
[http://dx.doi.org/10.1002/mds.22781] [PMID: 20187246]

[197] Grünewald A, Kumar KR, Sue CM. New insights into the complex role of mitochondria in Parkinson's disease. Prog Neurobiol 2019; 177: 73-93.
[http://dx.doi.org/10.1016/j.pneurobio.2018.09.003] [PMID: 30219247]

[198] Prasuhn J, Davis RL, Kumar KR. Targeting mitochondrial impairment in Parkinson's Disease: Challenges and opportunities. Front Cell Dev Biol 2021; 8: 615461.
[http://dx.doi.org/10.3389/fcell.2020.615461] [PMID: 33469539]

[199] Morales I, Dopico JG, Sabate M, Gonzalez-Hernandez T, Rodriguez M. Substantia nigra osmoregulation: taurine and ATP involvement. Am J Physiol Cell Physiol 2007; 292(5): C1934-41.
[http://dx.doi.org/10.1152/ajpcell.00593.2006] [PMID: 17215320]

[200] Dawson R Jr, Pelleymounter MA, Cullen MJ, Gollub M. An age-related decline in striatal taurine is correlated with a loss of dopaminergic markers. 1999;48(3):319-24.

[201] Che Y, Hou L, Sun F, *et al.* Taurine protects dopaminergic neurons in a mouse Parkinson's disease model through inhibition of microglial M1 polarization. Cell Death Dis 2018; 9(4): 435.
[http://dx.doi.org/10.1038/s41419-018-0468-2] [PMID: 29568078]

[202] Castro-Caldas M, Carvalho AN, Rodrigues E, *et al.* Tauroursodeoxycholic acid prevents MPTP-induced dopaminergic cell death in a mouse model of Parkinson's disease. Mol Neurobiol 2012; 46(2):

475-86.
[http://dx.doi.org/10.1007/s12035-012-8295-4] [PMID: 22773138]

[203]   Pan C, Gupta A, Prentice H, Wu JY. Protection of taurine and granulocyte colony-stimulating factor against excitotoxicity induced by glutamate in primary cortical neurons. J Biomed Sci 2010; 17(Suppl 1): S18.
[http://dx.doi.org/10.1186/1423-0127-17-S1-S18] [PMID: 20804592]

[204]   Mizuno Y, Ohta S, Tanaka M, *et al.* Deficiencies in Complex I subunits of the respiratory chain in Parkinson's disease. Biochem Biophys Res Commun 1989; 163(3): 1450-5.
[http://dx.doi.org/10.1016/0006-291X(89)91141-8] [PMID: 2551290]

[205]   McColgan P, Tabrizi SJ. Huntington's disease: a clinical review. Eur J Neurol 2018; 25(1): 24-34.
[http://dx.doi.org/10.1111/ene.13413] [PMID: 28817209]

[206]   Damiano M, Galvan L, Déglon N, Brouillet E. Mitochondria in Huntington's disease. Biochim Biophys Acta Mol Basis Dis 2010; 1802(1): 52-61.
[http://dx.doi.org/10.1016/j.bbadis.2009.07.012] [PMID: 19682570]

[207]   Jodeiri Farshbaf M, Ghaedi K. Huntington's disease and mitochondria. Neurotox Res 2017; 32(3): 518-29.
[http://dx.doi.org/10.1007/s12640-017-9766-1] [PMID: 28639241]

[208]   Carmo C, Naia L, Lopes C, Rego AC. Mitochondrial dysfunction in Huntington's disease. Adv Exp Med Biol 2018; 1049: 59-83.
[http://dx.doi.org/10.1007/978-3-319-71779-1_3] [PMID: 29427098]

[209]   Kremer H, Roos R, Dingjan G, Marani E. Bots GTAJJon, neurology e. Atrophy of the hypothalamic lateral tuberal nucleus in Huntington's disease. 1990; 49(4): 371-82.

[210]   Stricker-Shaver J, Novati A, Yu-Taeger L, Nguyen HP. Genetic rodent models of Huntington disease. Adv Exp Med Biol 2018; 1049: 29-57.
[http://dx.doi.org/10.1007/978-3-319-71779-1_2] [PMID: 29427097]

[211]   Li XJ, Li S. Large animal models of Huntington's disease. Curr Top Behav Neurosci 2013; 22: 149-60.
[http://dx.doi.org/10.1007/7854_2013_246] [PMID: 24048953]

[212]   Askeland G, Rodinova M, Štufková H, *et al.* A transgenic minipig model of Huntington's disease shows early signs of behavioral and molecular pathologies. Dis Model Mech 2018; 11(10): dmm035949.
[http://dx.doi.org/10.1242/dmm.035949] [PMID: 30254085]

[213]   Chaturvedi RK, Flint Beal M. Mitochondrial diseases of the brain. Free Radic Biol Med 2013; 63: 1-29.
[http://dx.doi.org/10.1016/j.freeradbiomed.2013.03.018] [PMID: 23567191]

[214]   I Duarte A, Cristina Rego A. Mitochondrial-associated metabolic changes and neurodegeneration in Huntington's disease-from clinical features to the bench. Curr Drug Targets 2010; 11(10): 1218-36.
[http://dx.doi.org/10.2174/138945011007011218] [PMID: 20840066]

[215]   Brustovetsky N, LaFrance R, Purl KJ, *et al.* Age-dependent changes in the calcium sensitivity of striatal mitochondria in mouse models of Huntington's Disease. J Neurochem 2005; 93(6): 1361-70.
[http://dx.doi.org/10.1111/j.1471-4159.2005.03036.x] [PMID: 15935052]

[216]   Veldman MB. Yang XWJCoin. Molecular insights into cortico-striatal miscommunications in Huntington's disease. 2018;48:79-89.

[217]   Tabrizi SJ, Cleeter MWJ, Xuereb J, Taanman JW, Cooper JM, Schapira AHV. Biochemical abnormalities and excitotoxicity in Huntington's disease brain. Ann Neurol 1999; 45(1): 25-32.
[http://dx.doi.org/10.1002/1531-8249(199901)45:1<25::AID-ART6>3.0.CO;2-E] [PMID: 9894873]

[218]   Fan M, Raymond L. N-Methyl-d-aspartate (NMDA) receptor function and excitotoxicity in

Huntington's disease. Prog Neurobiol 2007; 81(5-6): 272-93.
[http://dx.doi.org/10.1016/j.pneurobio.2006.11.003] [PMID: 17188796]

[219] Portera-Cailliau C, Hedreen JC, Price DL, Koliatsos VE. Evidence for apoptotic cell death in Huntington disease and excitotoxic animal models. J Neurosci 1995; 15(5): 3775-87.
[http://dx.doi.org/10.1523/JNEUROSCI.15-05-03775.1995] [PMID: 7751945]

[220] Tadros MG, Khalifa AE, Abdel-Naim AB, Arafa HMM. Neuroprotective effect of taurine in 3-nitropropionic acid-induced experimental animal model of Huntington's disease phenotype. Pharmacol Biochem Behav 2005; 82(3): 574-82.
[http://dx.doi.org/10.1016/j.pbb.2005.10.018] [PMID: 16337998]

[221] Rivas-arancibia S, Rodríguez AI, Zigova T, *et al.* Taurine increases rat survival and reduces striatal damage caused by 3-nitropropionic acid. Int J Neurosci 2001; 108(1-2): 55-67.
[http://dx.doi.org/10.3109/00207450108986505] [PMID: 11328702]

[222] El Idrissi A, Trenkner E. Taurine as a modulator of excitatory and inhibitory neurotransmission. Neurochem Res 2004; 29(1): 189-97.
[http://dx.doi.org/10.1023/B:NERE.0000010448.17740.6e] [PMID: 14992278]

[223] Morris G, Berk M. The many roads to mitochondrial dysfunction in neuroimmune and neuropsychiatric disorders. BMC Med 2015; 13(1): 68.
[http://dx.doi.org/10.1186/s12916-015-0310-y] [PMID: 25889215]

[224] Angebault C, Charif M, Guegen N, *et al.* Mutation in NDUFA13/GRIM19 leads to early onset hypotonia, dyskinesia and sensorial deficiencies, and mitochondrial complex I instability. Hum Mol Genet 2015; 24(14): 3948-55.
[http://dx.doi.org/10.1093/hmg/ddv133] [PMID: 25901006]

CHAPTER 4

Taurine and the Cardiovascular System: Focus on Mitochondrial-related Pathologies

Abstract: It is well-known that taurine (TAU) concentration in the excitable tissues, such as the myocardium is exceptionally high (up to 30 mM). TAU accumulation in the cardiomyocytes is a transporter-mediated process. Therefore, this amino acid should play a critical role in cardiac tissue. Several studies revealed that a decrease in cardiac TAU could lead to atrophic cardiomyopathy and impaired cardiac function. At subcellular levels, the effects of TAU on mitochondria and energy metabolism are an essential part of its function in the heart. Besides, it has been found that exogenous TAU supplementation significantly enhanced cardiac mitochondrial function and ATP levels. In the current chapter, the effects of TAU on cardiovascular diseases linked with mitochondrial impairment are highlighted, and the role of TAU as a cardioprotective agent is discussed. The data collected here could provide clues in managing a wide range of cardiovascular complications connected with the energy crisis and mitochondrial dysfunction.

Keywords: Arrhythmia, Cardiovascular diseases, Cardiomyopathy, Energy Crisis, Heart disease, Mitochondrial impairment.

INTRODUCTION

Cardiovascular diseases (CVDs) refer to a wide range of complications that could severely affect patients' quality of life [1, 2]. More importantly, CVDs are among the leading cause of mortality worldwide [3]. Several pathological conditions, including disturbed plasma lipids, formation of atherosclerotic plaques, hypertension, and congenital heart tissue defects, could contribute to CVDs [4, 5]. On the other hand, heart tissue demands an immense energy value daily to properly pump enough blood through the body [6 - 8]. Actually, heart tissue contains numerous mitochondria that make this process possible [6 - 8].

It is well-established that cardiac tissue has a very high level of taurine (TAU) [9 - 12]. It seems that TAU plays a pivotal role in regulating cardiac tissues mitochondrial function and energy metabolism since TAU depleted models revealed deleterious cardiac defects, which finally lead to animals' death [13 - 15]. TAU depletion could also cause various disorders in other organs [16]. Most

Reza Heidari and M. Mehdi Ommati

of the cardiac TAU content is localized in the cellular mitochondria. It is well-known that TAU regulates mitochondrial respiratory chain activity, decreases mitochondria-mediated reactive oxygen species formation, blunts mitochondria-mediated cell death, and enhances mitochondrial energy metabolism in the heart [17 - 23]. These features make TAU an ideal cardioprotective for a wide range of CVDs.

Interestingly, many clinical studies revealed the positive effects of TAU in CVDs. It seems that cardiomyocytes' mitochondria are the primary place for the cardioprotective mechanisms of action of TAU. The current chapter describes the effects of TAU on mitochondrial function as a plausible mechanism of its action. Then, the application of this amino acid in a variety of CVDs is highlighted. The data collected in this chapter could develop safe and clinically applicable therapeutic options in CVDs.

TAURINE AND THE CARDIOVASCULAR SYSTEM

The effects of TAU on the cardiovascular system are one of the most investigated biological properties of this amino acid [9, 11, 24 - 28]. Several studies mentioned the positive effects of TAU in the cardiovascular system [9]. Antihypertensive, anti-atherosclerotic plaque formation and anti-hyperlipidemia properties of TAU are repeatedly reported in experimental models and clinical trials [9, 29 - 33]. The effects of TAU on cardiac complications such as arrhythmia, myocardial infarction, and heart failure have also been widely investigated [34 - 37].

A high level of taurine (TAU) is found in cardiomyocytes (up to 30 mM). TAU uptake by cardiomyocytes is a transporter-mediated process [38, 39]. Several physiological roles have been proposed for TAU in the heart tissue [9, 27, 32, 40 - 43]. It has been mentioned that TAU could act as a vital osmoregulator in the heart [9, 27, 32, 40 - 43]. Moreover, TAU regulates the proteins phosphorylation process and cytoplasmic calcium (Ca^{2+}) levels in cardiomyocytes [44]. The increase in Ca^{2+}-ATPase activity plays a pivotal role in the effects of TAU on cardiomyocytes' Ca^{2+} levels [21, 45] (Fig. **1**). It is well-known that Ca^{2+} signaling plays a fundamental action in the excitation-contraction coupling of the cardiac muscle. Therefore, enough TAU concentration guarantees proper cardiac contraction and preserves cardiac output. Based on these data, TAU could regulate various basic parameters in the cardiovascular system (Fig. **1**). Therefore, it is important to investigate the molecular mechanisms of TAU action in cardiovascular diseases.

Previous studies have repeatedly mentioned the effects of TAU deficiency on cardiac function [9, 35, 46, 47]. It is well-known that TAU deprivation severely impaired cardiac function in some species, such as foxes, cats, and dogs [14, 48,

49]. Cardiomyopathy is a common pathological change associated with TAU deficiency [50 - 53]. Investigations in different experimental models also revealed that the inhibition of TAU transport to cardiomyocytes significantly influenced myocardial energy metabolism and led to impaired cardiac function [53]. Therefore, the regulation of ATP metabolism is one of the basic functions of TAU in the cardiac tissue [22, 54] (Fig. **1**). All these data indicate an essential role for TAU in normal cardiac function and highlight the importance of this amino acid in mitochondrial function as a primary mechanism for its cardioprotective properties (Fig. **1**).

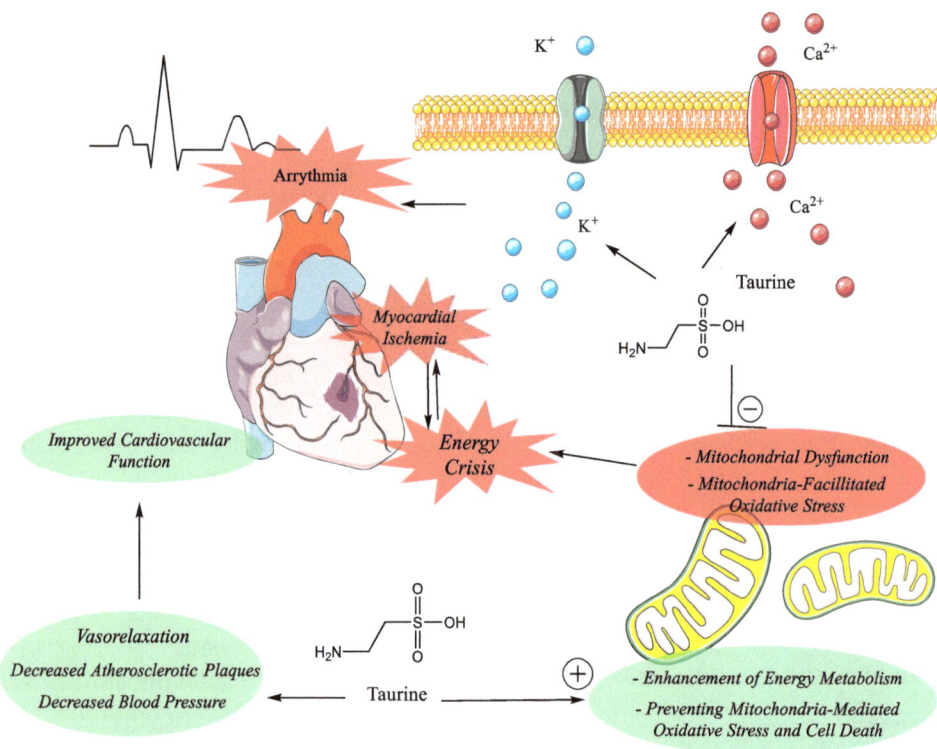

Fig. (1). Taurine regulates different parameters in the cardiovascular system. The effects of TAU on mitochondrial function and cardiomyocytes' energy status play a pivotal role in the effects of this amino acid in the cardiovascular system. TAU also regulates the level of crucial ions such as Ca^{2+} in cardiomyocytes. Ca^{2+} dyshomeostasis is associated with complications such as arrhythmia. The effects of TAU on parameters such as the formation of atherosclerotic plaques or decreasing blood pressure could also eventually decrease the risk of cardiovascular disease.

Cardiovascular diseases (CVDs) are the leading cause of morbidity and mortality worldwide [55]. Arrhythmia, myocardial infarction, high blood pressure, atherosclerosis, and cerebrovascular disorders are examples of CVDs. Although several pharmacological and surgical innovations have been developed against CVDs, there are challenges for using these approaches so far. Therefore, finding safe and clinically applicable agents with low adverse effects is favorable.

A plethora of investigations has been carried out to identify mechanisms of heart and vessels damage induced by CVDs. In this context, oxidative stress and its linked complications are well-investigated mechanisms involved in the pathogenesis of CVDs [56 - 59]. As functional units of the heart tissue, cardiomyocytes possess a strong enzymatic and non-enzymatic defense system [56 - 59]. However, it has been found that cardiomyocytes' antioxidant systems are interrupted in many CVDs [56 - 59]. This notion provides the idea of developing antioxidant molecules as protective agents against CVDs [60, 61]. The current chapter discusses the effects of TAU on oxidative stress biomarkers in CVDs.

Mitochondrial impairment is another critical mechanism involved in the pathogenesis of CVDs [3, 6, 62, 63] (Fig. **1**). Several heart diseases or xenobiotics-induced heart injuries are associated with mitochondrial impairment [64 - 66]. The mitochondrial injury could entail cardiomyocytes injury and various types of heart disease. Besides, the heart is a high-energy demand organ. Thus, any significant changes in mitochondrial function and energy metabolism could lead to severe cardiac events [3, 6, 62, 63]. On the other hand, mitochondria are the major sites of intracellular ROS formation [67]. It is well-known that mitochondrial dysfunction could facilitate mitochondria-mediated ROS generation [67] (Fig. **1**). Oxidative stress could also deteriorate mitochondrial injury [67], thus, targeting cardiomyocytes mitochondria could serve as a potential point of intervention against CVDs. The role of mitochondrial impairment in the pathogenesis of CVDs will be discussed in this chapter.

In the forthcoming sections, the molecular mechanisms of the effects of TAU in cardiomyocytes are highlighted. Then, the application of TAU in CVDs focusing on the effects of this amino acid on mitochondrial function is reviewed.

MOLECULAR MECHANISMS OF TAURINE ACTION IN CARDIOMYOCYTES

As mentioned, TAU concentration in the cardiac tissue is very high [52]. Therefore, TAU might play a crucial physiological role in the heart. In this context, several studies have been conducted to evaluate the pathological consequences of TAU depletion in the cardiac tissue [23, 38, 42, 47, 68 - 70]. Severe cardiomyopathy that finally entails animal death occurred in most TAU deprivation experimental models [38, 69, 70].

Several mechanisms have been identified for TAU deficiency-associated cardiac injury. In investigations that evaluated the effects of endoplasmic reticulum (ER) damage and disturbed cytoplasmic Ca^{2+} homeostasis, severe oxidative stress, mitochondrial impairment, energy crisis, and the activation of mitochondria-mediated cell death pathways have been reported of TAU deficiency in cardiomyocytes [20 - 23]. Besides, several investigations mentioned that TAU supplementation could alleviate cardiomyocytes injury in experimental models of heart damage by blunting oxidative stress, preventing mitochondrial impairment, and decreasing cell death [71 - 73]. Based on these data, several major mechanisms could be delineated for the positive effects of TAU in cardiac tissue. These mechanisms are highlighted in the following sections.

Many investigations indicated the pivotal role of TAU in the mitochondrial protein synthesis process [17 - 19]. This function of TAU could be critical in the heart as cardiac tissue continuously requires a high amount of ATP. As mentioned in previous chapters, TAU incorporates the mitochondrial tRNA structure and plays a significant role in synthesizing mitochondrial respiratory chain components [17 - 19]. Interestingly, it has been found that TAU could significantly alleviate cardiac dysfunction in diseases such as MELAS, which is associated with an impaired TAU-modified tRNA in the mitochondria [52, 74, 75]. On the other hand, it has been found that impaired tRNA function induced by TAU deficiency or genetic diseases could significantly enhance mitochondria-facilitated ROS formation and oxidative stress [52]. Therefore, a crucial mechanism for the protective role of TAU in heart tissue is its effects on mitochondrial protein synthesis, energy turnover, and alleviation of oxidative stress and its associated complications [52, 74, 75] (Fig. **2**). However, as mentioned in various chapters of this book, TAU is a weak radical scavenger and practically did not react with many ROS forms [76, 77], but it has been repeatedly reported that TAU could significantly enhance the expression of many enzymatic antioxidant defense systems in the heart tissue [47, 78 - 80]. Hence, a part of the antioxidative properties of TAU could be mediated through its effects on cellular antioxidant defense mechanisms (Fig. **2**). The effects of TAU and its derivatives on cellular antioxidant defense capacity could also be mediated through other mechanisms. For instance, some studies have found the effects of TAU and its derivatives on nuclear factor-E2-related factor-2 (Nrf2) signaling [81, 82] (Fig. **2**). Nrf2 activation and the translocation of this protein to the nucleus could induce the transcription of various genes involved in the expression of antioxidant enzymes [83, 84]. The effect of TAU on the Nrf2 pathway could lead to an increased level of cellular enzymatic antioxidant defense [81, 82] (Fig. **2**). Moreover, as previously mentioned, mitochondria-mediated ROS formation also plays a pivotal role in the pathogenesis of heart injury with different etiologies [6, 85]. It has been revealed that TAU could ameliorate mitochondria-originated ROS and prevent oxidative stress [86 - 88]. Thus, the mitigation of mitochondria-mediated ROS formation could also play a critical role in the antioxidative properties of TAU in cardiac tissue (Fig. **2**).

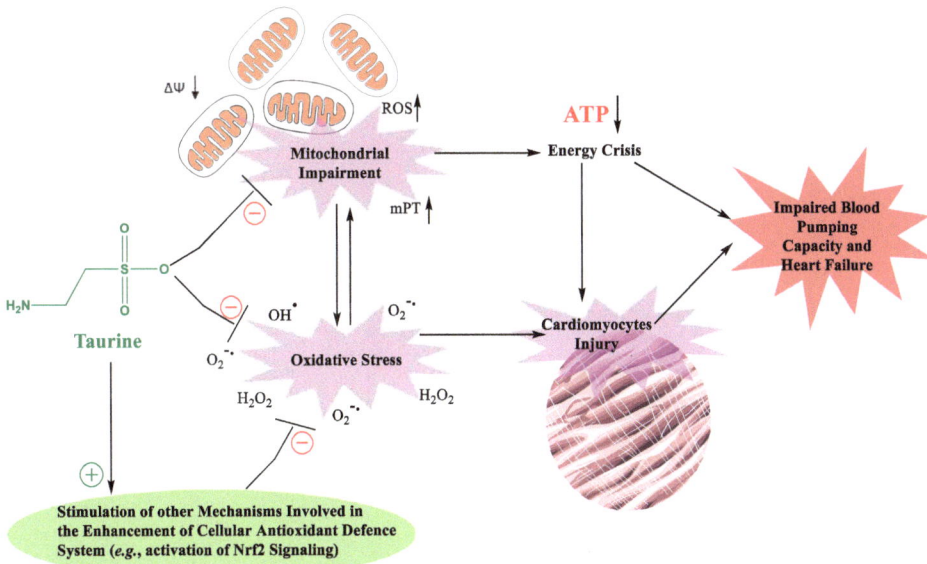

Fig. (2). Mitochondrial impairment and oxidative stress play a crucial role in the pathogenesis of heart failure and impaired blood pumping by this organ. Several investigations mentioned that taurine could alleviate heart failure with different etiologies. The effects of taurine on oxidative stress markers, mitochondrial function, and energy metabolism seem to play a pivotal role in its cardioprotective properties. $\Delta\Psi$: mitochondrial membrane potential; mPT: mitochondrial permeability transition; ATP: adenosine triphosphate; ROS: Reactive oxygen Species; OH$^\cdot$: Hydroxyl radical; O$_2^{\cdot-}$: Superoxide anion; H$_2$O$_2$: Hydrogen peroxide; Nrf2: erythroid 2–related nuclear factor 2.

Cytoplasmic calcium (Ca^{2+}) homeostasis is another critical parameter tightly connected with oxidative stress, mitochondrial impairment, and cell death [67]. The smooth endoplasmic reticulum (ER or the sarcoplasmic reticulum; SR; in the cardiac tissue) is the primary site of Ca^{2+} storage. Several investigations revealed that ER stress and Ca^{2+} dyshomeostasis could occur in the association of cardiac diseases or xenobiotics-induced heart injury [89 - 93] (Fig. **3**). ER stress and cytoplasmic Ca^{2+} overload could activate cell death signaling [67, 89, 90]. It has been revealed that TAU could play a crucial role in cytoplasmic Ca^{2+} homeostasis and its compartmentalization [94, 95]. It should be mentioned that mitochondria act as "safety valves" when cytoplasmic Ca^{2+} is mildly increased [96]. However, when cytoplasmic Ca^{2+} overload is severe, this mechanism does not work properly. A crucial mechanism for the cytoplasmic Ca^{2+} regulating properties of

TAU is mediated through the effects of this amino acid on mitochondria [97, 98]. Some studies revealed that TAU could significantly enhance the Ca^{2+} sequestering capability of mitochondria [97, 98] (Fig. **3**). Therefore, Ca^{2+}-induced activation of cell death signaling is blunted. Previous studies have also mentioned the effects of TAU on cardiomyocytes Ca^{2+} dys-homeostasis and its related cell death [21, 99, 100]. Based on these data, the effects of TAU on cellular Ca^{2+} could play a critical role in its cardioprotective properties (Fig. **3**).

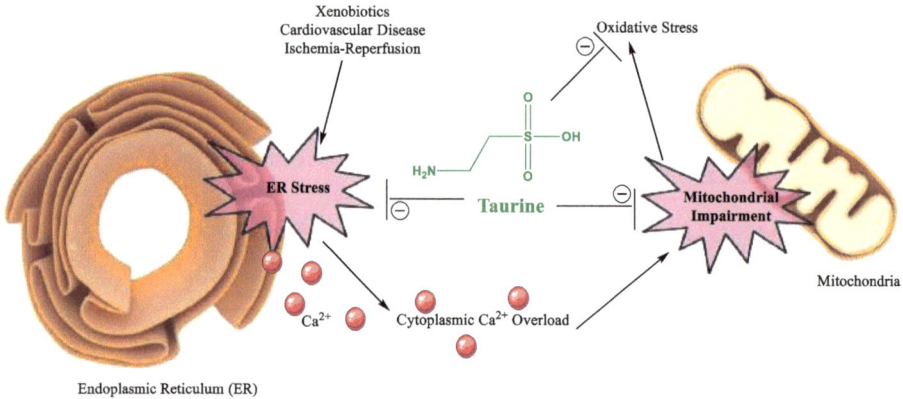

Fig. (3). Schematic representation of endoplasmic reticulum (ER) stress and cytoplasmic Ca^{2+} overload and its connection to mitochondrial impairment and energy crisis. The effects of TAU on Ca^{2+} homeostasis seem to play a critical role in its cardioprotective properties.

The effects of TAU on mitochondrial permeability and the release of cell death mediators is another important mechanism for the cardioprotective properties of this compound [20, 101] (Fig. **4**). The induction of mitochondrial permeability is a common mechanism of cytotoxicity induced by xenobiotics or diseases [102, 103]. Mitochondrial transition permeability (mPT) and mitochondria-mediated cell death have also been repeatedly mentioned in the pathogenesis of CVDs [102, 104 - 107]. The induction of mPT is recognized as a critical mechanism involved in different modes of cell death (necrosis, apoptosis, and autophagy) [108] (Fig. **3**). The mode of cell death induced by mPT induction depends on several parameters, including ATP availability [108]. In cases such as cardiac ischemia (MI), heart failure, or ischemia/reperfusion-induced heart injury, severe mPT induction, mitochondrial swelling, and finally, necrotic mode of cell death could occur [109 - 111] (Fig. **4**). Interestingly, several studies revealed that TAU could ameliorate cardiomyocyte death mainly by inhibiting mPT and preventing different types of cell death [10, 20, 72, 112] (Fig. **4**). All the data represented in this section indicate that the role of TAU in sealing mPT and preventing mitochondria-mediated cell death could play a vital role in its cardioprotective mechanisms (Fig. **4**).

Fig. (4). Induction of mitochondrial permeability (mPT) and the release of cell death mediators from this organelle has been repeatedly mentioned in various cardiovascular diseases and xenobiotics-induced cardiomyocytes injury. In this context, several studies revealed that taurine could act as an mPT sealing agent and significantly blunt mitochondria-mediated cell death.

In the forthcoming parts, the effects of TAU on some common CVDs are described. It highlights the mitochondria-mediated mechanisms associated with TAU effects in these complications. These data could provide clues on developing new therapeutic strategies in CVDs.

MYOCARDIAL INFARCTION AND ISCHEMIA-REPERFUSION INJURY

Myocardial infarction (MI) is the foremost cause of mortality among CVDs [113]. MI is connected to coronary heart disease that could occur in the association of a wide range of etiologies, including atherosclerosis [114]. Ischemia-reperfusion injury is also a major complication, especially in cases such as organ transplantation. The effects of TAU on MI and ischemia-reperfusion injury are represented in the forthcoming sections, focusing on the effects of this amino acid on cardiomyocytes' mitochondrial function.

Cellular hypoxia is an important factor that could induce mitochondrial depolarization and the induction of mitochondrial permeability and swelling [115]. These events have been repeatedly mentioned in experimental models of cardiomyocytes ischemia and are implicated in cell death and organ injury [115]. Therefore, the effects of TAU on mitochondrial permeabilization and depolarization could play a pivotal role in its protective properties against heart injury in complications such as MI. The effects of TAU on mitochondrial permeabilization and depolarization have been repeatedly mentioned in experimental models of isolated cardiomyocytes and/or *in vivo* heart injury [10, 20, 72, 112].

Several other molecular mechanisms have also been identified that could be involved in the response of heart tissue to ischemia and the mechanisms of cytoprotection provided by TAU [112]. For instance, an important pathway involved in cytoprotection during heart tissue ischemia-reperfusion is mediated through the activation of Akt [112]. Akt is a kinase enzyme involved in the phosphorylation of many proteins [116, 117]. In the heart ischemia-induced injury models, it has been found that Akt phosphorylates glycogen synthase kinase-3β (GSK-3β) [112, 118 - 120]. GSK-3β is inactivated in its phosphorylated form. Hence, Akt signaling inactivates GSK-3β. It is well-established that GSK-3β could impair mitochondrial function by inducing mPT and cell death [121 - 124]. Many cytoprotective agents have been identified that mediate their positive effects by activating Akt and phosphorylation of GSK-3β [125 - 129]. The effects of TAU on Akt signaling are also the subject of many studies [130 - 136]. TAU also enhances the phosphorylation of GSK-3β and decreases its activity [131]. In an interesting paper by Schaffer *et al.*, the authors described that the effects of TAU on Akt signaling could effectively prevent mitochondria injury, oxidative stress, and cellular energy crisis in ischemia-reperfusion conditions [112]. Based on these data, the activation of Akt signaling could serve as an important pathway for TAU to induce its protective properties in CVDs such as ischemia-reperfusion and MI.

Interestingly, TAU has been successfully tested in experimental animals and human cases of MI [36, 37]. It has been revealed that TAU significantly improved patients' survival and ameliorated post-MI complications [36, 37]. Thus, TAU could consider as a clinically applicable therapeutic option in MI. The effects of this amino acid on mitochondrial function, energy metabolism, and oxidative stress biomarkers seem to play a fundamental role in its protective effects in cardiac ischemia [21, 79, 135, 137]. Indeed, further mechanistic and epidemiologic studies along with the development of efficient drug delivery systems could enhance the therapeutic efficacy of TAU in complications such as MI. On the other hand, there is a plethora of evidence indicating the pathogenic role of oxidative stress in MI [138 - 140]. MI-linked severe oxidative stress could lead to cardiomyocytes injury, cardiac remodeling, and heart failure [138]. As mentioned, it has been found that TAU could blunt oxidative stress in cardiomyocytes ischemia models [21, 79, 137]. Hence, the effects of TAU on oxidative stress could prevent further complications such as cardiac remodeling and heart failure.

Based on the data provided in this section, TAU could be a promising therapeutic agent in MI and ischemia-reperfusion injury since it could significantly mitigate oxidative stress, prevent cardiac remodeling and anatomical changes, enhance cardiac tissue ATP levels and finally improve its contractile function and the ability for pumping enough blood. The effects of TAU on cardiomyocytes' mitochondria seem to play a pivotal role in its protective mechanisms in ischemia-reperfusion injury and MI.

HEART FAILURE

Heart failure (HF) is a chronic and degenerative condition that impairs the heart's capacity to pump an appropriate blood volume [141]. HF develops in the association of a wide range of pathologies [141]. Several pharmacological interventions have been developed (*e.g.*, digoxin) for managing HF [142]. However, the development of safe agents with lower adverse effects is always favorable. Interestingly, the positive effects of TAU on HF have been mentioned in both experimental and clinical studies [22, 143 - 146]. Therefore, the role of TAU in the management of HF and its potential mechanisms of action are discussed in the current section.

Several investigations mentioned the pivotal role of mitochondrial impairment in the pathogenesis of heart failure [7, 147 - 149]. An impaired mitochondrial function could induce heart failure through the induction of energy crisis and myocardium contractile failure [7, 147 - 149]. Moreover, mitochondria-mediated ROS formation and oxidative stress are also involved in HF's pathophysiology [7]. The role of oxidative stress in HF has repeatedly been mentioned in experimental and clinical studies [150 - 152]. Oxidative stress could be a fundamental factor for cardiac remodeling in HF [153 - 156]. Other mitochondria-related complications, including the dysregulation of mitochondrial biogenesis, the enhanced release of cell death mediators from cardiomyocytes mitochondria, and changes in mitochondrial structure and number, are all involved in the mechanisms of mitochondrial impairment-induced cardiac injury during HF [7]. Therefore, targeting mitochondria is a reasonable choice for ameliorating HF-associated complications [7].

Interestingly, the positive effects of TAU on myocardial mitochondria have been revealed in several investigations [21, 86, 101, 157]. These studies mentioned that TAU could enhance mitochondrial membrane potential, increase ATP production, and blunt mitochondria-mediated cell death in the myocardium [86, 101]. Moreover, TAU could significantly abrogate mitochondria-mediated ROS formation and oxidative stress in the heart [86]. The positive effects of TAU on mitochondria could provide enough ATP levels needed for efficient cardiac contraction. These data suggest the effects of TAU on cardiomyocytes' mitochondria as a potential mechanism for its positive effects in HF.

An interesting point indicating the effectiveness of TAU in HF is the approval of this compound for the treatment of HF in some countries such as Japan [34, 35]. This mentions the clinical value of TAU in managing CVDs such as HF. More epidemiological studies and finding the optimum dose of TAU in the management of HF could lead to the clinical use of this amino acid. Conclusively, it seems that TAU could be used as a safe and effective therapeutic agent in HF. Clearly, more studies, especially clinical trials, are needed to establish the effectiveness of TAU against HF and, finally, its application against this disease worldwide.

ROLE OF TAURINE IN THE MANAGEMENT OF ARRHYTHMIA

The arrhythmia occurs when there is a lack of coordination between the electrical signals that regulate the heartbeat. Although many forms of arrhythmia are harmless, some severe forms could lead to serious complications such as heart failure and death. Some forms of arrhythmia that need therapeutic interventions are bradycardia, tachycardia, fibrillation (atrial or ventricular), flutter, QT prolongation syndrome, and premature cardiac contraction. Arrhythmia could evolve in the association of a wide range of etiologies. Generally, any interruption in the heart's electrical impulse could result in arrhythmia. Xenobiotics (*e.g.,* alcohol, caffeine, several drugs), diseases (*e.g.,* diabetes, high blood pressure, hyperthyroidism), or environmental factors (*e.g.,* stress, smoking) could cause arrhythmia. Despite the etiology of arrhythmia, medical intervention is needed in conditions with an increased risk of more severe complications. Surgical intervention, electric shock, or a wide range of drugs could be used against various forms of arrhythmia.

In the current section, we will focus on oxidative stress and mitochondrial dysfunction in the pathogenesis of arrhythmia. Afterward, the role of TAU in the management of arrhythmia is discussed, focusing on the effects of this amino acid on mitochondrial function and oxidative stress biomarkers. These data could lead to the development of safe therapeutic strategies against different forms of arrhythmia.

The role of mitochondria in the pathogenesis of various forms of arrhythmia is the subject of many investigations [158 - 163]. The connection between mitochondrial impairment and deterioration of arrhythmia seems to be mediated through several mechanisms, including the role of mitochondria in the regulation of intracellular ion homeostasis, ATP metabolism, and oxidative stress [159]. These mechanisms are discussed below, and their relevance to the antiarrhythmic properties of TAU is highlighted.

The interconnection between mitochondrial function and sarcoplasmic reticulum (SR) is one of the most investigated subjects which correlates mitochondrial impairment with various types of arrhythmia [164]. It is estimated that a large amount of ATP produced by cardiomyocytes' mitochondria is consumed to regulate SR ion channels which play a crucial role in the electrical activity of these cells [159, 165]. Therefore, proper mitochondrial function and ATP metabolism guarantee appropriate cardiac function. The Ca^{2+} ion concentration in cardiomyocytes plays a crucial role in cardiac excitability [164, 166]. On the other hand, Ca^{2+} is vital for proper cardiac contraction, and any disturbances in its homeostasis could lead to arrhythmia [164]. Cardiomyocytes SR is in close proximity to mitochondria, and several proteins and transporters have been identified that connect these two organelles [164]. It has been found that mitochondrial impairment could lead to disruption of cardiac rhythm through the depletion of ATP supply for ion channels in cardiomyocytes [159, 167]. These data mention the crucial role of mitochondrial function in the pathogenesis of cardiac arrhythmias [164]. Thus, mitochondrial impairment could lead to impaired cardiac excitability and arrhythmia [158, 164, 166].

As repeatedly mentioned in this chapter, an exciting and crucial function of TAU that has been mentioned in various experimental models is its effect on cytoplasmic Ca^{2+} homeostasis and mitochondrial sequestration of Ca^{2+} [168]. TAU increases the Ca^{2+} buffering capability of mitochondria [168, 169]. This interesting feature of TAU prevents the activation of cell death pathways induced by cytoplasmic Ca^{2+} overload [86, 168 - 181]. Moreover, this feature of TAU could prevent electrophysiological disturbances induced by Ca^{2+} overload and consequently prevent ATP crisis and cardiac rhythm abnormalities.

Oxidative stress is a joint event linked with the pathogenesis of heart injury in various types of arrhythmia [182, 183]. Although the exact mechanisms leading to severe oxidative stress remain to be more investigated, it is well known that a big part of ROS and the occurrence of oxidative stress in arrhythmia is associated with cardiomyocytes mitochondria [182] (Fig. **2**). Arrhythmia-linked oxidative stress could affect various intracellular targets, including DNA, proteins, lipids, and the mitochondria itself [184]. Moreover, emerging evidence indicates that mitochondria-mediated ROS formation and oxidative stress play an essential role in the function of cardiac transporters and ion channels [159]. Therefore, oxidative stress could be involved in the dyshomeostasis of important ions such as Ca^{2+} in cardiomyocytes. Several studies mentioned the importance of mitochondria-targeted agents (*e.g.*, antioxidants) as therapeutic strategies in arrhythmia [183, 185]. In this context, several powerful antioxidants such as coenzyme Q and 4-Hydroxy-2,2,6,6-tetramethylpiperidine-1-oxy (TEMPO) have been targeted to cardiac mitochondria for alleviating signs and symptoms of various types of arrhythmia [183, 185]. These studies mention mitochondria-targeted antioxidant therapies as "innovative concepts "for managing arrhythmia and its complications [183, 185]. Liu *et al.* suggested that antioxidants not only abrogate the severity of different types of arrhythmia but also their regular consumption might be effective for disease prevention [183, 185]. Sovari *et al.* also mentioned that mitochondria-targeted antioxidants could increase connexin43 (Cx43) [183]. It is well-established that Cx43 is the major ventricular gap junctions protein, and any factor that suppresses Cx43 could induce sudden arrhythmic death [183]. It has been found that a part of oxidative stress-induced arrhythmia could also be mediated through the suppression of Cx43 [183]. All these data mention the importance of oxidative stress in the pathogenesis of cardiac arrhythmias. As repeatedly mentioned in the current book, a big part of the antioxidant properties of TAU is mediated through the effects of this amino acid on oxidative stress biomarkers and mitochondria-facilitated ROS formation [86, 172 - 174, 176, 178, 181, 186 - 192]. Thus, the effect of TAU on oxidative stress biomarkers could play a tremendous role in its antiarhythmogenic properties (Fig. **1**). Interestingly, cardiac electrophysiological abnormalities have been reported in TAU deficiency [46]. These data could mention the importance of this amino acid in preventing different types of arrhythmia. On the other hand, designing a cardiac targeted formulation of TAU and enhancing its effects on cardiomyocytes' mitochondria may also enhance its anti-arrhythmogenic properties.

Another important factor identified in the mechanism of arrhythmia is its connection to mitochondrial permeability [193, 194]. As repeatedly mentioned in the current chapter, mitochondria play a significant role in the cellular Ca^{2+} homeostasis in cardiomyocytes. Cytoplasmic Ca^{2+} influx to the mitochondrial matrix is mediated through the mitochondrial Ca^{2+} uniporter (mCU) [193, 195]. On the other hand, some mechanisms have been identified for mitochondrial efflux of Ca^{2+} [193]. The Na^+/Ca^{2+} exchanger (mitochondrial NCX) are also involved in mitochondrial Ca^{2+} efflux [193]. Interestingly, it is well-established that the perseverance of mitochondrial membrane potential ($\Delta\Psi_m$) plays a vital role in the mitochondrial Ca^{2+} transports and channels [196]. It has been found that mitochondrial depolarization leads to the significant release of Ca^{2+}via mPT pore [196]. Subsequently, the release of Ca^{2+} could promote the release of more Ca^{2+} from cardiomyocytes SR [196]. Significant anti-arrhythmogenic effects have been demonstrated in cyclophilin D, an mPT component, knockout models [193]. These data confirm the importance of mPT in cellular Ca^{2+} signaling and its relevance to cardiac arrhythmia [193].

The effect of TAU on mPT and the prevention of mitochondria permeability induced by various etiologies is the subject of many investigations [170, 172, 197,

198]. Therefore, a significant part of the anti-arrhythmogenic properties of TAU could be mediated through the effects of this amino acid on mitochondrial permeabilization in cardiomyocytes (Fig. **4**). Interestingly, it has been revealed that a modest increase in mitochondrial Ca^{2+} uptake could enhance the capability of this organelle for ATP synthesis [199 - 201]. It has been shown that several enzymes such as Krebs cycle dehydrogenases are in a more active state by increasing mitochondrial Ca^{2+} levels [199 - 201]. Therefore, more substrates (NADH and FADH2) are produced and utilized by the electron transport chain for ATP production. A part of the produced ATP is used for Ca^{2+} uptake pumps, transporting this ion from the cytosol to the SR [199 - 201]. This is just an example of mitochondrial and SR interconnection in the heart and its relevance to various forms of arrhythmia. As mentioned, TAU is able to change the mitochondria sequestrating capability of Ca^{2+}. Hence, this amino acid could affect arrhythmia through this mechanism too. Clearly, further investigations are needed to connect the mPT inhibitory properties of TAU to its antiarhythmogenic properties.

All data provided in this section offer targeting cardiomyocytes mitochondria as an opportunity to develop new therapeutic options aimed at managing different types of cardiac arrhythmias. As TAU is safe and clinically applicable and its antiarrhythmic effects have been tested [202 - 208], this amino acid could be a potential anti-arrhythmogenic agent for more investigations in clinical trials.

TAURINE AND OTHER CARDIOVASCULAR DISORDERS

Although it may not be directly related to mitochondria-regulating properties of TAU, the effects of this amino acid on the vascular system, lipid profile, and blood pressure is another widely investigated field [27, 209 - 212]. Several mechanisms have been proposed for the positive effects of TAU on vascular disorders. The effects of TAU on lipid profile, the anti-inflammatory properties of this amino acid, the antihypertensive effects of TAU, and the action of TAU as an antioxidant are proposed to be involved in its effects on cardiovascular disorders (*e.g.*, coronary heart disease) [9].

The effects of TAU on lipid profile is an essential feature of this amino acid which could be related to its protective effects in CVDs [27]. It is well-known that TAU could enhance cholesterol solubility and excretion [27]. The effects of TAU on cholesterol metabolism are mediated through the enzyme 7-α-hydroxylase (CYP7A1) [213 - 215]. CYP7A1 is a rate-limiting enzyme that produces bile acids [213 - 215]. Many investigations indicate that TAU could significantly decrease cholesterol levels in experimental models and clinical studies [212, 216 - 220]. As high cholesterol level is a significant risk factor for CVDs, the cholesterol-lowering property of TAU could play a pivotal role in its protective effects.

The effects of TAU in decreasing blood pressure (BP) are another interesting feature of this compound [210, 211] (Fig. **1**). An important mechanism for the antihypertensive properties of TAU is mediated through its effects on the renin-angiotensin system [221]. It has been found that TAU could significantly attenuate the vaso-constrictive properties of angiotensin II [221] (Fig. **1**). The effect of TAU on the renal system of kinin-kallikrein could also play a role in its antihypertensive properties [222, 223]. Moreover, some studies indicate that the decrease in norepinephrine and epinephrine levels by TAU could also be involved in its antihypertensive effects [224, 225]. In addition to experimental data, several clinical studies revealed the role of TAU in regulating BP [24, 209, 210, 226 - 229]. TAU has been administered at high doses (*e.g.*, 6g/day) without significant adverse effects in patients with CVDs [226]. These data suggest TAU as a safe and effective agent to attenuate high BP and associated cardiovascular complications.

Atherosclerosis is another complication involved in the pathogenesis of many CVDs, including coronary heart disease, MI, and high blood pressure [230, 231]. It has been well-known that oxidative stress plays a crucial role in the pathophysiology of damage induced by atherosclerotic plaques [232, 233]. On the other hand, several studies mentioned the anti-atherosclerotic properties of TAU [11, 37, 234]. It has been found that the antioxidant properties of TAU could play a fundamental role in its anti-atherogenic properties [234, 235]. Several experimental data indicate a significant decrease in the plasma biomarkers of oxidative stress upon TAU supplementation [9, 236, 237].

The role of inflammatory cells in the pathogenesis of sclerotic lesions has been well-investigated [238, 239]. The adhesion of inflammatory cells to the endothelium and their trans-endothelial migration is critical in atherosclerosis [238, 239]. Several mediators, including cytokines, are involved in the inflammatory response-induced deterioration of atherosclerosis [238 - 240]. Interestingly, it has been found that TAU could significantly decrease the activation of inflammatory cells and the release of inflammatory cytokines [11, 240]. TAU is reacted with hypochlorous acid (HClO), produced by inflammatory cells, to form taurochloramine (TauCl) [241]. TauCl is well-known for its anti-inflammatory properties [241, 242]. These data indicate that the anti-inflammatory effect of TAU could play a crucial role in decreasing atherosclerosis lesions formation and its associated cardiovascular complications.

CONCLUSION

As CVDs are the leading cause of mortality and morbidity worldwide, finding safe and clinically applicable therapeutic options against these disorders is always plausible. In this regard, it should be mentioned that many interesting clinical studies indicate the beneficial role of TAU in CVDs. Many studies revealed the beneficial effects of this amino acid in CVDs. TAU is generally well-tolerated with minimal and/or no adverse effects. However, it seems that very high doses of this amino acid (*e.g.*, 5 g before artery bypass surgery or 3-6 g/day for its antihypertensive effects) [226, 243] are needed for its positive effects in CVDs. This point could mention the importance of further studies for identifying the exact targets of TAU responsible for the cardiovascular effects of this amino acid. Moreover, preparing appropriate formulations of TAU could increase its effectiveness in cardiovascular complications. Further intervention and epidemiologic studies could provide a better insight into the effectiveness of TAU in CVDs.

REFERENCES

[1]   Komalasari R, Nurjanah N, Yoche MM. Nurjanah, Yoche MM. Quality of life of people with cardiovascular disease: A descriptive study. Asian Pac Isl Nurs J 2019; 4(2): 92-6.
        [http://dx.doi.org/10.31372/20190402.1045]

[2]   Mayou R, Bryant B. Quality of life in cardiovascular disease. Heart 1993; 69(5): 460-6.
        [http://dx.doi.org/10.1136/hrt.69.5.460]

[3]   Chistiakov DA, Shkurat TP, Melnichenko AA, Grechko AV, Orekhov AN. The role of mitochondrial dysfunction in cardiovascular disease: a brief review. Ann Med 2018; 50(2): 121-7.
        [http://dx.doi.org/10.1080/07853890.2017.1417631]

[4]   Sayols-Baixeras S, Lluís-Ganella C, Lucas G, Elosua R. Pathogenesis of coronary artery disease: focus on genetic risk factors and identification of genetic variants. Appl Clin Genet 2014; 7: 15-32.

[5]   Amin MN, Siddiqui SA, Ibrahim M, *et al.* Inflammatory cytokines in the pathogenesis of cardiovascular disease and cancer. SAGE Open Med 2020; 8
        [http://dx.doi.org/10.1177/2050312120965752]

[6]   Peoples JN, Saraf A, Ghazal N, Pham TT, Kwong JQ. Mitochondrial dysfunction and oxidative stress in heart disease. Exp Mol Med 2019; 51(12): 1-13.
        [http://dx.doi.org/10.1038/s12276-019-0355-7]

[7]   Zhou B, Tian R. Mitochondrial dysfunction in pathophysiology of heart failure. J Clin Invest 2018; 128(9): 3716-26.
        [http://dx.doi.org/10.1172/JCI120849]

[8]   Huss JM, Kelly DP. Mitochondrial energy metabolism in heart failure: a question of balance. J Clin Invest 2005; 115(3): 547-55.
        [http://dx.doi.org/10.1172/JCI24405]

[9]   Xu Y-J, Arneja AS, Tappia PS, Dhalla NS. The potential health benefits of taurine in cardiovascular disease. Exp Clin Cardiol 2008; 13(2): 57-65.

[10]   Roysommuti S, Wyss Jm. Taurine exposure affects cardiac function and disease Handbook of nutrition in heart health Human Health Handbooks 14. Wageningen Academic Publishers 2017; pp. 231-47.

[11] Qaradakhi T, Gadanec LK, McSweeney KR, Abraham JR, Apostolopoulos V, Zulli A. The anti-inflammatory effect of taurine on cardiovascular disease. Nutrients 2020; 12(9): 2847.
[http://dx.doi.org/10.3390/nu12092847]

[12] Militante J, Lombardini JB, Schaffer SW. The role of taurine in the pathogenesis of the cardiomyopathy of insulin-dependent diabetes mellitus. Cardiovasc Res 2000; 46(3): 393-402.
[http://dx.doi.org/10.1016/S0008-6363(00)00025-0]

[13] Dow SW, Fettman MJ, Smith KR, Ching SV, Hamar DW, Rogers QR. Taurine depletion and cardiovascular disease in adult cats fed a potassium-depleted acidified diet. Am J Vet Res 1992; 53(3): 402-5.

[14] Moise NS, Pacioretty LM, Kallfelz FA, Stipanuk MH, King JM, Gilmour RF Jr. Dietary taurine deficiency and dilated cardiomyopathy in the fox. Am Heart J 1991; 121(2): 541-7.
[http://dx.doi.org/10.1016/0002-8703(91)90724-V]

[15] Ito T, Yoshikawa N, Inui T, Miyazaki N, Schaffer SW, Azuma J. Tissue depletion of taurine accelerates skeletal muscle senescence and leads to early death in mice. PLoS One 2014; 9(9): e107409.
[http://dx.doi.org/10.1371/journal.pone.0107409]

[16] Najibi A, Rezaei H, Kumar Manthari R, *et al.* Cellular and mitochondrial taurine depletion in bile duct ligated rats: a justification for taurine supplementation in cholestasis/cirrhosis. Clin Exp Hepatol 2022; 8(3): 195-210.
[http://dx.doi.org/10.5114/ceh.2022.119216]

[17] Fakruddin M, Wei FY, Suzuki T, *et al.* Defective mitochondrial tRNA taurine modification activates global proteostress and leads to mitochondrial disease. Cell Rep 2018; 22(2): 482-96.
[http://dx.doi.org/10.1016/j.celrep.2017.12.051]

[18] Tsutomu S, Asuteka N, Takeo S. Human mitochondrial diseases caused by lack of taurine modification in mitochondrial tRNAs. Wiley Interdiscip Rev RNA 2011; 2(3): 376-86.
[http://dx.doi.org/10.1002/wrna.65]

[19] Suzuki T, Suzuki T, Wada T, Saigo K, Watanabe K. Taurine as a constituent of mitochondrial tRNAs: new insights into the functions of taurine and human mitochondrial diseases. EMBO J 2002; 21(23): 6581-9.
[http://dx.doi.org/10.1093/emboj/cdf656]

[20] Jong CJ, Azuma J, Schaffer SW. Role of mitochondrial permeability transition in taurine deficiency-induced apoptosis. Exp Clin Cardiol 2011; 16(4): 125-8.

[21] Yang Y, Zhang Y, Liu X, *et al.* Exogenous taurine attenuates mitochondrial oxidative stress and endoplasmic reticulum stress in rat cardiomyocytes. Acta Biochim Biophys Sin (Shanghai) 2013; 45(5): 359-67.
[http://dx.doi.org/10.1093/abbs/gmt034]

[22] Schaffer S, Kim HW. Effects and mechanisms of taurine as a therapeutic agent. Biomol Ther (Seoul) 2018; 26(3): 225-41.
[http://dx.doi.org/10.4062/biomolther.2017.251]

[23] Jong C, Ito T, Prentice H, Wu JY, Schaffer S. Role of mitochondria and endoplasmic reticulum in taurine-deficiency-mediated apoptosis. Nutrients 2017; 9(8): 795.
[http://dx.doi.org/10.3390/nu9080795]

[24] Zulli A. Taurine in cardiovascular disease. Curr Opin Clin Nutr Metab Care 2011; 14(1): 57-60.
[http://dx.doi.org/10.1097/MCO.0b013e328340d863]

[25] Niittynen L, Nurminen ML, Korpela R, Vapaatalo H. Role of arginine, taurine 4 and homocysteine in cardiovascular diseases. Ann Med 1999; 31(5): 318-26.
[http://dx.doi.org/10.3109/07853899908995898]

[26]   Oudit GY, Trivieri MG, Khaper N, *et al.* Taurine supplementation reduces oxidative stress and improves cardiovascular function in an iron-overload murine model. Circulation 2004; 109(15): 1877-85.
[http://dx.doi.org/10.1161/01.CIR.0000124229.40424.80]

[27]   Wójcik OP, Koenig KL, Zeleniuch-Jacquotte A, Costa M, Chen Y. The potential protective effects of taurine on coronary heart disease. Atherosclerosis 2010; 208(1): 19-25.
[http://dx.doi.org/10.1016/j.atherosclerosis.2009.06.002]

[28]   Sahin MA, Yucel O, Guler A, *et al.* Is there any cardioprotective role of Taurine during cold ischemic period following global myocardial ischemia? J Cardiothorac Surg 2011; 6(1): 31.
[http://dx.doi.org/10.1186/1749-8090-6-31]

[29]   Kim KS, You JS, Kim JY, Chang KJ, Yoo MC, Song R, Eds. Taurine ameliorates hypercholesterolemia but not obesity in rats fed a lard-based, high-fat diet2015. Springer International Publishing 2015.

[30]   Hagar HH, El Etter E, Arafa M. Taurine attenuates hypertension and renal dysfunction induced by cyclosporine A in rats. Clin Exp Pharmacol Physiol 2006; 33(3): 189-96.
[http://dx.doi.org/10.1111/j.1440-1681.2006.04345.x]

[31]   Hu J, Xu X, Yang J, Wu G, Sun C, Lv Q. Antihypertensive effect of taurine in rat. Adv Exp Med Biol 2009; 643: 75-84.
[http://dx.doi.org/10.1007/978-0-387-75681-3_8]

[32]   Yamori Y, Taguchi T, Hamada A, Kunimasa K, Mori H, Mori M. Taurine in health and diseases: consistent evidence from experimental and epidemiological studies. J Biomed Sci 2010; 17(1) (Suppl. 1): S6.
[http://dx.doi.org/10.1186/1423-0127-17-S1-S6]

[33]   Matsui S, Maruyama C, Arai H, Hashimoto S, Asakusa T, Yoshida H, *et al.* Effects of taurine intake on serum lipids in young women. Functional Foods in Health and Disease. 2015;5(5):155-64-64.
[http://dx.doi.org/10.31989/ffhd.v5i5.180]

[34]   Azuma J, Sawamura A, Awata N, *et al.* Therapeutic effect of taurine in congestive heart failure: A double-blind crossover trial. Clin Cardiol 1985; 8(5): 276-82.
[http://dx.doi.org/10.1002/clc.4960080507]

[35]   Azuma J, Sawamura A, Awata N. Usefulness of taurine in chronic congestive heart failure and its prospective application: Current Therapy of intractable heart failure. Jpn Circ J 1992; 56(1): 95-9.
[http://dx.doi.org/10.1253/jcj.56.95]

[36]   Ardisson LP, Rafacho BPM, Santos PP, *et al.* Taurine attenuates cardiac remodeling after myocardial infarction. Int J Cardiol 2013; 168(5): 4925-6.
[http://dx.doi.org/10.1016/j.ijcard.2013.07.091]

[37]   Ahmadian M, Roshan VD, Aslani E, Stannard SR. Taurine supplementation has anti-atherogenic and anti-inflammatory effects before and after incremental exercise in heart failure. Ther Adv Cardiovasc Dis 2017; 11(7): 185-94.
[http://dx.doi.org/10.1177/1753944717711138]

[38]   Ito T, Oishi S, Takai M, *et al.* Cardiac and skeletal muscle abnormality in taurine transporter-knockout mice. J Biomed Sci 2010; 17 (Suppl. 1): S20.
[http://dx.doi.org/10.1186/1423-0127-17-S1-S20]

[39]   Baliou S, Kyriakopoulos A, Goulielmaki M, Panayiotidis M, Spandidos D, Zoumpourlis V. Significance of taurine transporter (TauT) in homeostasis and its layers of regulation (Review). Mol Med Rep 2020; 22(3): 2163-73.
[http://dx.doi.org/10.3892/mmr.2020.11321]

[40]   Pasantes-Morales H, Quesada O, Morán J. Taurine: An osmolyte in mammalian tissues.Taurine 3: Cellular and Regulatory Mechanisms Advances in Experimental Medicine and Biology. Boston, MA:

Springer US 1998; pp. 209-17.
[http://dx.doi.org/10.1007/978-1-4899-0117-0_27]

[41] Schuller-Levis GB, Park E. Taurine: new implications for an old amino acid. FEMS Microbiol Lett 2003; 226(2): 195-202.
[http://dx.doi.org/10.1016/S0378-1097(03)00611-6]

[42] Ito T, Kimura Y, Uozumi Y, *et al.* Taurine depletion caused by knocking out the taurine transporter gene leads to cardiomyopathy with cardiac atrophy. J Mol Cell Cardiol 2008; 44(5): 927-37.
[http://dx.doi.org/10.1016/j.yjmcc.2008.03.001]

[43] Li Y, Arnold J, Pampillo M, Babwah A, Peng T. Taurine prevents cardiomyocyte death by inhibiting NADPH oxidase-mediated calpain activation. Free Radic Biol Med 2009; 46(1): 51-61.
[http://dx.doi.org/10.1016/j.freeradbiomed.2008.09.025]

[44] Bkaily G, Jazzar A, Normand A, Simon Y, Al-Khoury J, Jacques D. Taurine and cardiac disease: state of the art and perspectives. Can J Physiol Pharmacol 2019.

[45] Chang L, Xu J, Yu F, Zhao J, Tang X, Tang C. Taurine protected myocardial mitochondria injury induced by hyperhomocysteinemia in rats. Amino Acids 2004; 27(1): 37-48.
[http://dx.doi.org/10.1007/s00726-004-0096-2]

[46] Lake N. Effects of taurine deficiency on arrhythmogenesis and excitation-contraction coupling in cardiac tissue.Taurine: Nutritional Value and Mechanisms of Action Advances in Experimental Medicine and Biology. Boston, MA: Springer US 1992; pp. 173-9.
[http://dx.doi.org/10.1007/978-1-4615-3436-5_19]

[47] Pansani MC, Azevedo PS, Rafacho BPM, *et al.* Atrophic cardiac remodeling induced by taurine deficiency in Wistar rats. PLoS One 2012; 7(7): e41439.
[http://dx.doi.org/10.1371/journal.pone.0041439]

[48] Larsen JA, Fascetti AJ. The role of taurine in cardiac health in dogs and cats. Advances in Small Animal Care 2020; 1: 227-38.
[http://dx.doi.org/10.1016/j.yasa.2020.07.015]

[49] Morris JG, Rogers QR, Pacioretty LM. Taurine: an essential nutrient for cats. J Small Anim Pract 1990; 31(10): 502-9.
[http://dx.doi.org/10.1111/j.1748-5827.1990.tb00672.x]

[50] Kaplan JL, Stern JA, Fascetti AJ, *et al.* Taurine deficiency and dilated cardiomyopathy in golden retrievers fed commercial diets. PLoS One 2018; 13(12): e0209112.
[http://dx.doi.org/10.1371/journal.pone.0209112]

[51] Schaffer S, Solodushko V, Azuma J. Taurine-deficient cardiomyopathy: Role of phospholipids, calcium and osmotic stress.Taurine 4: Taurine and Excitable Tissues Advances in Experimental Medicine and Biology. Boston, MA: Springer US 2002; pp. 57-69.
[http://dx.doi.org/10.1007/0-306-46838-7_6]

[52] Schaffer S, Ito T, Azuma J, Jong C, Kramer J. Mechanisms underlying development of taurine-deficient cardiomyopathy. Hearts 2020; 1(2): 86-98.
[http://dx.doi.org/10.3390/hearts1020010]

[53] Jong CJ, Ito T, Schaffer SW. The ubiquitin–proteasome system and autophagy are defective in the taurine-deficient heart. Amino Acids 2015; 47(12): 2609-22.
[http://dx.doi.org/10.1007/s00726-015-2053-7]

[54] Yang YJ, Han YY, Chen K, Zhang Y, Liu X, Li S, *et al.* TonEBP modulates the protective effect of taurine in ischemia-induced cytotoxicity in cardiomyocytes. Cell Death Dis. 2015;6(12):e2025-e.
[http://dx.doi.org/10.1038/cddis.2015.372]

[55] Mc Namara K, Alzubaidi H, Jackson JK. Cardiovascular disease as a leading cause of death: how are pharmacists getting involved? Integr Pharm Res Pract 2019; 8: 1-11.
[http://dx.doi.org/10.2147/IPRP.S133088]

[56]   Senoner T, Dichtl W. Oxidative stress in cardiovascular diseases: Still a therapeutic target? Nutrients 2019; 11(9): 2090.
        [http://dx.doi.org/10.3390/nu11092090]

[57]   Rodrigo R, González J, Paoletto F. The role of oxidative stress in the pathophysiology of hypertension. Hypertens Res 2011; 34(4): 431-40.
        [http://dx.doi.org/10.1038/hr.2010.264]

[58]   Münzel T, Camici GG, Maack C, Bonetti NR, Fuster V, Kovacic JC. Impact of oxidative stress on the heart and vasculature: Part 2 of a 3-Part Series. J Am Coll Cardiol 2017; 70(2): 212-29.
        [http://dx.doi.org/10.1016/j.jacc.2017.05.035]

[59]   Dubois-Deruy E, Peugnet V, Turkieh A, Pinet F. Oxidative stress in cardiovascular diseases. Antioxidants 2020; 9(9): 864.
        [http://dx.doi.org/10.3390/antiox9090864]

[60]   Jain A, Mehra N, Swarnakar N. Role of antioxidants for the treatment of cardiovascular diseases: Challenges and opportunities. Curr Pharm Des 2015; 21(30): 4441-55.
        [http://dx.doi.org/10.2174/1381612821666150803151758]

[61]   Mangge H, Becker K, Fuchs D, Gostner JM. Antioxidants, inflammation and cardiovascular disease. World J Cardiol 2014; 6(6): 462-77.
        [http://dx.doi.org/10.4330/wjc.v6.i6.462]

[62]   Zhunina OA, Yabbarov NG, Grechko AV, *et al.* The role of mitochondrial dysfunction in vascular disease, tumorigenesis, and diabetes. Front Mol Biosci 2021; 8: 671908.
        [http://dx.doi.org/10.3389/fmolb.2021.671908]

[63]   Poznyak AV, Ivanova EA, Sobenin IA, Yet SF, Orekhov AN. The role of mitochondria in cardiovascular diseases. Biology (Basel) 2020; 9(6): 137.
        [http://dx.doi.org/10.3390/biology9060137]

[64]   Rosca MG, Hoppel CL. Mitochondrial dysfunction in heart failure. Heart Fail Rev 2013; 18(5): 607-22.
        [http://dx.doi.org/10.1007/s10741-012-9340-0]

[65]   Varga ZV, Ferdinandy P, Liaudet L, Pacher P. Drug-induced mitochondrial dysfunction and cardiotoxicity. Am J Physiol Heart Circ Physiol 2015; 309(9): H1453-67.
        [http://dx.doi.org/10.1152/ajpheart.00554.2015]

[66]   Kiyuna LA, Albuquerque RP, Chen C-H, Mochly-Rosen D, Ferreira JCB. Targeting mitochondrial dysfunction and oxidative stress in heart failure: Challenges and opportunities. Free Radic Biol Med 2018; 129: 155-68.
        [http://dx.doi.org/10.1016/j.freeradbiomed.2018.09.019]

[67]   Brookes PS, Yoon Y, Robotham JL, Anders MW, Sheu SS. Calcium, ATP, and ROS: a mitochondrial love-hate triangle. Am J Physiol Cell Physiol 2004; 287(4): C817-33.
        [http://dx.doi.org/10.1152/ajpcell.00139.2004]

[68]   Harada H, Cusack BJ, Olson RD, *et al.* Taurine deficiency and doxorubicin: interaction with the cardiac sarcolemmal calcium pump. Biochem Pharmacol 1990; 39(4): 745-51.
        [http://dx.doi.org/10.1016/0006-2952(90)90154-D]

[69]   Pion PD, Kittleson MD, Thomas WP, Skiles ML, Rogers QR. Clinical findings in cats with dilated cardiomyopathy and relationship of findings to taurine deficiency. J Am Vet Med Assoc 1992; 201(2): 267-74.

[70]   Schaffer SW, Shimada-Takaura K, Jong CJ, Ito T, Takahashi K. Impaired energy metabolism of the taurine-deficient heart. Amino Acids 2016; 48(2): 549-58.
        [http://dx.doi.org/10.1007/s00726-015-2110-2]

[71]   Ghosh J, Das J, Manna P, Sil PC. Taurine prevents arsenic-induced cardiac oxidative stress and

apoptotic damage: Role of NF-κB, p38 and JNK MAPK pathway. Toxicol Appl Pharmacol 2009; 240(1): 73-87.
[http://dx.doi.org/10.1016/j.taap.2009.07.008]

[72]   Das J, Ghosh J, Manna P, Sil PC. Taurine suppresses doxorubicin-triggered oxidative stress and cardiac apoptosis in rat via up-regulation of PI3-K/Akt and inhibition of p53, p38-JNK. Biochem Pharmacol 2011; 81(7): 891-909.
[http://dx.doi.org/10.1016/j.bcp.2011.01.008]

[73]   Das J, Ghosh S, Sil PC. Taurine and cardiac oxidative stress in diabetes. Diabetes. 2nd ed. Academic Press 2020; pp. 361-72.
[http://dx.doi.org/10.1016/B978-0-12-815776-3.00037-1]

[74]   Meseguer S, Martínez-Zamora A, García-Arumí E, Andreu AL, Armengod ME. The ROS-sensitive microRNA-9/9* controls the expression of mitochondrial tRNA-modifying enzymes and is involved in the molecular mechanism of MELAS syndrome. Hum Mol Genet 2015; 24(1): 167-84.
[http://dx.doi.org/10.1093/hmg/ddu427]

[75]   Schaffer SW, Jong CJ, Ito T, Azuma J. Role of taurine in the pathologies of MELAS and MERRF. Amino Acids 2014; 46(1): 47-56.
[http://dx.doi.org/10.1007/s00726-012-1414-8]

[76]   Mehta TR, Dawson R Jr. Taurine is a weak scavenger of peroxynitrite and does not attenuate sodium nitroprusside toxicity to cells in culture. Amino Acids 2001; 20(4): 419-33.
[http://dx.doi.org/10.1007/s007260170038]

[77]   Jong CJ, Schaffer S. Mechanism underlying the antioxidant activity of taurine. The FASEB Journal. 2013;27(S1):1086.1-.1.
[http://dx.doi.org/10.1096/fasebj.27.1_supplement.1086.1]

[78]   Parildar H, Dogru-Abbasoglu S, Mehmetçik G, Özdemirler G, Koçak-Toker N, Uysal M. Lipid peroxidation potential and antioxidants in the heart tissue of beta-alanine- or taurine-treated old rats. J Nutr Sci Vitaminol (Tokyo) 2008; 54(1): 61-5.
[http://dx.doi.org/10.3177/jnsv.54.61]

[79]   Shiny KS, Kumar SHS, Farvin KHS, Anandan R, Devadasan K. Protective effect of taurine on myocardial antioxidant status in isoprenaline-induced myocardial infarction in rats. J Pharm Pharmacol 2010; 57(10): 1313-7.
[http://dx.doi.org/10.1211/jpp.57.10.0010]

[80]   Sochor J, Nejdl L, Ruttkay-Nedecky B, *et al.* Investigating the influence of taurine on thiol antioxidant status in Wistar rats with a multi-analytical approach. J Appl Biomed 2014; 12(2): 97-110.
[http://dx.doi.org/10.1016/j.jab.2013.01.002]

[81]   Sun Jang J, Piao S, Cha YN, Kim C. Taurine chloramine activates Nrf2, increases HO-1 expression and protects cells from death caused by hydrogen peroxide. J Clin Biochem Nutr 2009; 45(1): 37-43.
[http://dx.doi.org/10.3164/jcbn.08-262]

[82]   Agca CA, Tuzcu M, Hayirli A, Sahin K. Taurine ameliorates neuropathy *via* regulating NF-κB and Nrf2/HO-1 signaling cascades in diabetic rats. Food Chem Toxicol 2014; 71: 116-21.
[http://dx.doi.org/10.1016/j.fct.2014.05.023]

[83]   Nguyen T, Nioi P, Pickett CB. The Nrf2-antioxidant response element signaling pathway and Its activation by oxidative stress. J Biol Chem 2009; 284(20): 13291-5.
[http://dx.doi.org/10.1074/jbc.R900010200]

[84]   Mousavi K, Niknahad H, Li H, *et al.* The activation of nuclear factor-E2-related factor 2 (Nrf2)/heme oxygenase-1 (HO-1) signaling blunts cholestasis-induced liver and kidney injury. Toxicol Res (Camb) 2021; 10(4): 911-27.
[http://dx.doi.org/10.1093/toxres/tfab073]

[85]   Tsutsui H, Kinugawa S, Matsushima S. Mitochondrial oxidative stress and dysfunction in myocardial

remodelling. Cardiovasc Res 2008; 81(3): 449-56.
[http://dx.doi.org/10.1093/cvr/cvn280]

[86]   Mousavi K, Niknahad H, Ghalamfarsa A, *et al.* Taurine mitigates cirrhosis-associated heart injury through mitochondrial-dependent and antioxidative mechanisms. Clin Exp Hepatol 2020; 6(3): 207-19.
[http://dx.doi.org/10.5114/ceh.2020.99513]

[87]   Schaffer SW, Ju Jong C, Kc R, Azuma J. Physiological roles of taurine in heart and muscle. J Biomed Sci 2010; 17(1) (Suppl. 1): S2.
[http://dx.doi.org/10.1186/1423-0127-17-S1-S2]

[88]   Shimada K, Jong CJ, Takahashi K, Schaffer SW. Role of ROS production and turnover in the antioxidant activity of taurine Taurine 9. Springer 2015; pp. 581-96.
[http://dx.doi.org/10.1007/978-3-319-15126-7_47]

[89]   Ruan Y, Zeng J, Jin Q, *et al.* Endoplasmic reticulum stress serves an important role in cardiac ischemia/reperfusion injury (Review). Exp Ther Med 2020; 20(6): 1.
[http://dx.doi.org/10.3892/etm.2020.9398]

[90]   Zhang C, Syed TW, Liu R, Yu J. Role of endoplasmic reticulum stress, autophagy, and inflammation in cardiovascular disease. Front Cardiovasc Med 2017; 4: 29.
[http://dx.doi.org/10.3389/fcvm.2017.00029]

[91]   Hong J, Kim K, Kim JH, Park Y. The role of endoplasmic reticulum stress in cardiovascular disease and exercise. Int J Vasc Med 2017; 2017: 1-9.
[http://dx.doi.org/10.1155/2017/2049217]

[92]   Minamino T, Kitakaze M. ER stress in cardiovascular disease. J Mol Cell Cardiol 2010; 48(6): 1105-10.
[http://dx.doi.org/10.1016/j.yjmcc.2009.10.026]

[93]   Ren J, Bi Y, Sowers JR, Hetz C, Zhang Y. Endoplasmic reticulum stress and unfolded protein response in cardiovascular diseases. Nat Rev Cardiol 2021; 18(7): 499-521.
[http://dx.doi.org/10.1038/s41569-021-00511-w]

[94]   Chen WQ, Jin H, Nguyen M, *et al.* Role of taurine in regulation of intracellular calcium level and neuroprotective function in cultured neurons. J Neurosci Res 2001; 66(4): 612-9.
[http://dx.doi.org/10.1002/jnr.10027]

[95]   Menzie J, Prentice H, Wu JY. Neuroprotective mechanisms of taurine against ischemic stroke. Brain Sci 2013; 3(4): 877-907.
[http://dx.doi.org/10.3390/brainsci3020877]

[96]   Giorgi C, Marchi S, Pinton P. The machineries, regulation and cellular functions of mitochondrial calcium. Nat Rev Mol Cell Biol 2018; 19(11): 713-30.
[http://dx.doi.org/10.1038/s41580-018-0052-8]

[97]   El Idrissi A, Trenkner E. Taurine regulates mitochondrial calcium homeostasis. Adv Exp Med Biol 2003; 526: 527-36.
[http://dx.doi.org/10.1007/978-1-4615-0077-3_63]

[98]   El Idrissi A. Taurine increases mitochondrial buffering of calcium: role in neuroprotection. Amino Acids 2008; 34(2): 321-8.
[http://dx.doi.org/10.1007/s00726-006-0396-9]

[99]   Chowdhury S, Sinha K, Banerjee S, Sil PC. Taurine protects cisplatin induced cardiotoxicity by modulating inflammatory and endoplasmic reticulum stress responses. Biofactors 2016; 42(6): 647-64.
[http://dx.doi.org/10.1002/biof.1301]

[100]   Nonaka H, Tsujino T, Watari Y, Emoto N, Yokoyama M. Taurine prevents the decrease in expression and secretion of extracellular superoxide dismutase induced by homocysteine. Circulation 2001; 104(10): 1165-70.

[http://dx.doi.org/10.1161/hc3601.093976]

[101] Takatani T, Takahashi K, Uozumi Y, *et al.* Taurine inhibits apoptosis by preventing formation of the Apaf-1/caspase-9 apoptosome. Am J Physiol Cell Physiol 2004; 287(4): C949-53.
        [http://dx.doi.org/10.1152/ajpcell.00042.2004]

[102] Javadov S, Karmazyn M. Mitochondrial permeability transition pore opening as an endpoint to initiate cell death and as a putative target for cardioprotection. Cell Physiol Biochem 2007; 20(1-4): 1-22.
        [http://dx.doi.org/10.1159/000103747]

[103] Tsujimoto Y, Shimizu S. Role of the mitochondrial membrane permeability transition in cell death. Apoptosis. An International Journal on Programmed Cell Death 2007; 12(5): 835-40.

[104] Pritzwald-Stegmann P, Hoyer A, Kempfert J, Dhein S, Mohr FW. Cardioprotective effects of low-dose cyclosporin A added to histidine-tryptophan-ketoglutarate cardioplegia solution prior to total myocardial ischemia: An *in vitro* rabbit heart study. Pharmacology 2011; 88(3-4): 167-73.
        [http://dx.doi.org/10.1159/000330099]

[105] Javadov S, Hunter JC, Barreto-Torres G, Parodi-Rullan R. Targeting the mitochondrial permeability transition: Cardiac ischemia-reperfusion versus carcinogenesis. Cell Physiol Biochem 2011; 27(3-4): 179-90.
        [http://dx.doi.org/10.1159/000327943]

[106] Javadov S, Karmazyn M, Escobales N. Mitochondrial permeability transition pore opening as a promising therapeutic target in cardiac diseases. J Pharmacol Exp Ther 2009; 330(3): 670-8.
        [http://dx.doi.org/10.1124/jpet.109.153213]

[107] Halestrap AP, Pasdois P. The role of the mitochondrial permeability transition pore in heart disease. Biochim Biophys Acta Bioenerg 2009; 1787(11): 1402-15.
        [http://dx.doi.org/10.1016/j.bbabio.2008.12.017]

[108] Lemasters JJ, Nieminen AL, Qian T, *et al.* The mitochondrial permeability transition in cell death: a common mechanism in necrosis, apoptosis and autophagy. Biochim Biophys Acta Bioenerg 1998; 1366(1-2): 177-96.
        [http://dx.doi.org/10.1016/S0005-2728(98)00112-1]

[109] Webster KA. Mitochondrial membrane permeabilization and cell death during myocardial infarction: roles of calcium and reactive oxygen species. Future Cardiol 2012; 8(6): 863-84.
        [http://dx.doi.org/10.2217/fca.12.58]

[110] Honda HM, Ping P. Mitochondrial permeability transition in cardiac cell injury and death. Cardiovasc Drugs Ther 2006; 20(6): 425-32.
        [http://dx.doi.org/10.1007/s10557-006-0642-0]

[111] Zhu H, Sun A. Programmed necrosis in heart disease: Molecular mechanisms and clinical implications. J Mol Cell Cardiol 2018; 116: 125-34.
        [http://dx.doi.org/10.1016/j.yjmcc.2018.01.018]

[112] Schaffer SW, Jong CJ, Ito T, Azuma J. Effect of taurine on ischemia–reperfusion injury. Amino Acids 2014; 46(1): 21-30.
        [http://dx.doi.org/10.1007/s00726-012-1378-8]

[113] Roger VL. Epidemiology of myocardial infarction. Med Clin North Am 2007; 91(4): 537-52.
        [http://dx.doi.org/10.1016/j.mcna.2007.03.007]

[114] White AD, Folsom AR, Chambless LE, *et al.* Community surveillance of coronary heart disease in the Atherosclerosis Risk in Communities (ARIC) Study: Methods and initial two years' experience. J Clin Epidemiol 1996; 49(2): 223-33.
        [http://dx.doi.org/10.1016/0895-4356(95)00041-0]

[115] Kim JS, He L, Lemasters JJ. Mitochondrial permeability transition: a common pathway to necrosis and apoptosis. Biochem Biophys Res Commun 2003; 304(3): 463-70.
        [http://dx.doi.org/10.1016/S0006-291X(03)00618-1]

[116] Zhao Y, Hu X, Liu Y, *et al.* ROS signaling under metabolic stress: cross-talk between AMPK and AKT pathway. Mol Cancer 2017; 16(1): 79.
[http://dx.doi.org/10.1186/s12943-017-0648-1]

[117] Koundouros N, Poulogiannis G. Phosphoinositide 3-kinase/Akt signaling and redox metabolism in cancer. Front Oncol 2018; 8: 160.
[http://dx.doi.org/10.3389/fonc.2018.00160]

[118] Bharti S, Golechha M, Kumari S, Siddiqui KM, Arya DS. Akt/GSK-3β/eNOS phosphorylation arbitrates safranal-induced myocardial protection against ischemia–reperfusion injury in rats. Eur J Nutr 2012; 51(6): 719-27.
[http://dx.doi.org/10.1007/s00394-011-0251-y]

[119] Zhai P, Sciarretta S, Galeotti J, Volpe M, Sadoshima J. Differential roles of GSK-3β during myocardial ischemia and ischemia/reperfusion. Circ Res 2011; 109(5): 502-11.
[http://dx.doi.org/10.1161/CIRCRESAHA.111.249532]

[120] Wang Y, Ge C, Chen J, Tang K, Liu J. GSK-3β inhibition confers cardioprotection associated with the restoration of mitochondrial function and suppression of endoplasmic reticulum stress in sevoflurane preconditioned rats following ischemia/reperfusion injury. Perfusion 2018; 33(8): 679-86.
[http://dx.doi.org/10.1177/0267659118787143]

[121] Juhaszova M, Zorov DB, Kim SH, *et al.* Glycogen synthase kinase-3β mediates convergence of protection signaling to inhibit the mitochondrial permeability transition pore. J Clin Invest 2004; 113(11): 1535-49.
[http://dx.doi.org/10.1172/JCI19906]

[122] Yang K, Chen Z, Gao J, *et al.* The key roles of GSK-3β in regulating mitochondrial activity. Cell Physiol Biochem 2017; 44(4): 1445-59.
[http://dx.doi.org/10.1159/000485580]

[123] Tanno M, Kuno A, Ishikawa S, *et al.* Translocation of glycogen synthase kinase-3β (GSK-3β), a trigger of permeability transition, is kinase activity-dependent and mediated by interaction with voltage-dependent anion channel 2 (VDAC2). J Biol Chem 2014; 289(42): 29285-96.
[http://dx.doi.org/10.1074/jbc.M114.563924]

[124] Petit-Paitel A, Brau F, Cazareth J, Chabry J. Involvment of cytosolic and mitochondrial GSK-3β in mitochondrial dysfunction and neuronal cell death of MPTP/MPP+-treated neurons. PLoS One 2009; 4(5): e5491.
[http://dx.doi.org/10.1371/journal.pone.0005491]

[125] Wang D, Zhang X, Li D, *et al.* Kaempferide protects against myocardial ischemia/reperfusion injury through activation of the PI3K/Akt/GSK-3β pathway. Mediators Inflamm 2017; 2017: 1-11.
[http://dx.doi.org/10.1155/2017/5278218]

[126] Duan J, Guan Y, Mu F, *et al.* Protective effect of butin against ischemia/reperfusion-induced myocardial injury in diabetic mice: involvement of the AMPK/GSK-3β/Nrf2 signaling pathway. Sci Rep 2017; 7(1): 41491.
[http://dx.doi.org/10.1038/srep41491]

[127] Ucar BI, Ucar G, Saha S, Buttari B, Profumo E, Saso L. Pharmacological protection against ischemia-reperfusion injury by regulating the Nrf2-Keap1-ARE signaling pathway. Antioxidants 2021; 10(6): 823.
[http://dx.doi.org/10.3390/antiox10060823]

[128] Yang Q, Huang DD, Li DG, *et al.* Tetramethylpyrazine exerts a protective effect against injury from acute myocardial ischemia by regulating the PI3K/Akt/GSK-3β signaling pathway. Cell Mol Biol Lett 2019; 24(1): 17.
[http://dx.doi.org/10.1186/s11658-019-0141-5]

[129] Chen ZQ, Zhou Y, Chen F, *et al.* Breviscapine pretreatment inhibits myocardial inflammation and

apoptosis in rats after coronary microembolization by activating the PI3K/Akt/GSK-3β signaling pathway. Drug Des Devel Ther 2021; 15: 843-55.
[http://dx.doi.org/10.2147/DDDT.S293382]

[130] Baek YY, Cho DH, Choe J, *et al.* Extracellular taurine induces angiogenesis by activating ERK-, Akt-, and FAK-dependent signal pathways. Eur J Pharmacol 2012; 674(2-3): 188-99.
[http://dx.doi.org/10.1016/j.ejphar.2011.11.022]

[131] Sun G, Qu S, Wang S, Shao Y, Sun J. Taurine attenuates acrylamide-induced axonal and myelinated damage through the Akt/GSK3β-dependent pathway. Int J Immunopathol Pharmacol 2018; 32: 2058738418805322.

[132] Chen B, Abaydula Y, Li D, Tan H, Ma X. Taurine ameliorates oxidative stress by regulating PI3K/Akt/GLUT4 pathway in HepG2 cells and diabetic rats. J Funct Foods 2021; 85: 104629.
[http://dx.doi.org/10.1016/j.jff.2021.104629]

[133] Sun Y, Dai S, Tao J, *et al.* Taurine suppresses ROS-dependent autophagy via activating Akt/mTOR signaling pathway in calcium oxalate crystals-induced renal tubular epithelial cell injury. Aging (Albany NY) 2020; 12(17): 17353-66.
[http://dx.doi.org/10.18632/aging.103730]

[134] Barbiera A, Sorrentino S, Lepore E, *et al.* Taurine attenuates catabolic processes related to the onset of sarcopenia. Int J Mol Sci 2020; 21(22): 8865.
[http://dx.doi.org/10.3390/ijms21228865]

[135] Takatani T, Takahashi K, Uozumi Y, *et al.* Taurine prevents the ischemia-induced apoptosis in cultured neonatal rat cardiomyocytes through Akt/caspase-9 pathway. Biochem Biophys Res Commun 2004; 316(2): 484-9.
[http://dx.doi.org/10.1016/j.bbrc.2004.02.066]

[136] Jia N, Sun Q, Su Q, Dang S, Chen G. Taurine promotes cognitive function in prenatally stressed juvenile rats via activating the Akt-CREB-PGC1α pathway. Redox Biol 2016; 10: 179-90.
[http://dx.doi.org/10.1016/j.redox.2016.10.004]

[137] Oriyanhan W, Yamazaki K, Miwa S, Takaba K, Ikeda T, Komeda M. Taurine prevents myocardial ischemia/reperfusion-induced oxidative stress and apoptosis in prolonged hypothermic rat heart preservation. Heart Vessels 2005; 20(6): 278-85.
[http://dx.doi.org/10.1007/s00380-005-0841-9]

[138] Kurian GA, Rajagopal R, Vedantham S, Rajesh M. The role of oxidative stress in myocardial ischemia and reperfusion injury and remodeling: Revisited. Oxid Med Cell Longev 2016; 2016: 1-14.
[http://dx.doi.org/10.1155/2016/1656450]

[139] Tomandlova M, Parenica J, Lokaj P, *et al.* Prognostic value of oxidative stress in patients with acute myocardial infarction complicated by cardiogenic shock: A prospective cohort study. Free Radic Biol Med 2021; 174: 66-72.
[http://dx.doi.org/10.1016/j.freeradbiomed.2021.07.040]

[140] Neri M, Fineschi V, Paolo M, *et al.* Cardiac oxidative stress and inflammatory cytokines response after myocardial infarction. Curr Vasc Pharmacol 2015; 13(1): 26-36.
[http://dx.doi.org/10.2174/15701611113119990003]

[141] Groenewegen A, Rutten FH, Mosterd A, Hoes AW. Epidemiology of heart failure. Eur J Heart Fail 2020; 22(8): 1342-56.
[http://dx.doi.org/10.1002/ejhf.1858]

[142] Konstantinou DM, Karvounis H, Giannakoulas G. Digoxin in heart failure with a reduced ejection fraction: A risk factor or a risk marker? Cardiology 2016; 134(3): 311-9.
[http://dx.doi.org/10.1159/000444078]

[143] Ito T, Schaffer S, Azuma J. The effect of taurine on chronic heart failure: actions of taurine against catecholamine and angiotensin II. Amino Acids 2014; 46(1): 111-9.

[http://dx.doi.org/10.1007/s00726-013-1507-z]

[144]   Takihara K, Azuma J, Awata N, *et al.* Beneficial effect of taurine in rabbits with chronic congestive heart failure. Am Heart J 1986; 112(6): 1278-84.
[http://dx.doi.org/10.1016/0002-8703(86)90360-1]

[145]   Huxtable R, Bressler R. Elevation of taurine in human congestive heart failure. Life Sci 1974; 14(7): 1353-9.
[http://dx.doi.org/10.1016/0024-3205(74)90444-5]

[146]   Liu J, Ai Y, Niu X, *et al.* Taurine protects against cardiac dysfunction induced by pressure overload through SIRT1–p53 activation. Chem Biol Interact 2020; 317: 108972.
[http://dx.doi.org/10.1016/j.cbi.2020.108972]

[147]   Sabbah HN. Targeting the mitochondria in heart failure: A translational perspective. JACC Basic Transl Sci 2020; 5(1): 88-106.
[http://dx.doi.org/10.1016/j.jacbts.2019.07.009]

[148]   Marin-Garcia J, Goldenthal MJ, Moe GW. Mitochondrial pathology in cardiac failure. Cardiovasc Res 2001; 49(1): 17-26.
[http://dx.doi.org/10.1016/S0008-6363(00)00241-8]

[149]   Bisaccia G, Ricci F, Gallina S, Di Baldassarre A, Ghinassi B. Mitochondrial dysfunction and heart disease: Critical appraisal of an overlooked association. Int J Mol Sci 2021; 22(2): 614.
[http://dx.doi.org/10.3390/ijms22020614]

[150]   Ide T, Tsutsui H, Kinugawa S, *et al.* Direct evidence for increased hydroxyl radicals originating from superoxide in the failing myocardium. Circ Res 2000; 86(2): 152-7.
[http://dx.doi.org/10.1161/01.RES.86.2.152]

[151]   Belch JJ, Bridges AB, Scott N, Chopra M. Oxygen free radicals and congestive heart failure. Heart 1991; 65(5): 245-8.
[http://dx.doi.org/10.1136/hrt.65.5.245]

[152]   Tsutsui H, Kinugawa S, Matsushima S. Oxidative stress and mitochondrial DNA damage in heart failure. Circulation Journal: Official Journal of the Japanese Circulation Society. 2008;72 Suppl A:A31-7.
[http://dx.doi.org/10.1253/circj.CJ-08-0014]

[153]   Huo S, Shi W, Ma H, Yan D, Luo P, Guo J, *et al.* Alleviation of inflammation and oxidative stress in pressure overload-induced cardiac remodeling and heart failure *via* IL-6/STAT3 inhibition by raloxifene. Oxid Med Cell Longev 2021; 2021: 6699054.

[154]   Rababa'h AM, Guillory AN, Mustafa R, Hijjawi T. Oxidative stress and cardiac remodeling: An updated edge. Curr Cardiol Rev 2018; 14(1): 53-9.
[http://dx.doi.org/10.2174/1573403X14666180111145207]

[155]   Takano H, Hasegawa H, Nagai T, Komuro I. Implication of cardiac remodeling in heart failure: Mechanisms and therapeutic strategies. Intern Med 2003; 42(6): 465-9.
[http://dx.doi.org/10.2169/internalmedicine.42.465]

[156]   Tsutsui H, Kinugawa S, Matsushima S. Oxidative stress and heart failure. Am J Physiol Heart Circ Physiol 2011; 301(6): H2181-90.
[http://dx.doi.org/10.1152/ajpheart.00554.2011]

[157]   Lv Q, Yang J, Wang Y, Liu M, Feng Y, Wu G, Eds. Taurine prevented hypoxia induced chicken cardiomyocyte apoptosis through the inhibition of mitochondrial pathway activated by calpain-12019. Singapore: Springer 2019.

[158]   van Opbergen CJM, den Braven L, Delmar M, van Veen TAB. Mitochondrial dysfunction as substrate for arrhythmogenic cardiomyopathy: A search for new disease mechanisms. Front Physiol 2019; 10: 1496.
[http://dx.doi.org/10.3389/fphys.2019.01496]

[159] Yang KC, Bonini MG, Dudley SC Jr. Mitochondria and arrhythmias. Free Radic Biol Med 2014; 71: 351-61.
[http://dx.doi.org/10.1016/j.freeradbiomed.2014.03.033]

[160] Pool L, Wijdeveld LFJM, de Groot NMS, Brundel BJJM. The role of mitochondrial dysfunction in atrial fibrillation: Translation to druggable target and biomarker discovery. Int J Mol Sci 2021; 22(16): 8463.
[http://dx.doi.org/10.3390/ijms22168463]

[161] Brown DA, O'Rourke B. Cardiac mitochondria and arrhythmias. Cardiovasc Res 2010; 88(2): 241-9.
[http://dx.doi.org/10.1093/cvr/cvq231]

[162] Liu C, Bai J, Dan Q, *et al.* Mitochondrial dysfunction contributes to aging-related atrial fibrillation. Oxid Med Cell Longev 2021; 2021: 1-13.
[http://dx.doi.org/10.1155/2021/5530293]

[163] Joseph LC, Reyes MV, Homan EA, *et al.* The mitochondrial calcium uniporter promotes arrhythmias caused by high-fat diet. Sci Rep 2021; 11(1): 17808.
[http://dx.doi.org/10.1038/s41598-021-97449-3]

[164] Salazar-Ramírez F, Ramos-Mondragón R, García-Rivas G. Mitochondrial and sarcoplasmic reticulum interconnection in cardiac arrhythmia. Front Cell Dev Biol 2021; 8: 623381.
[http://dx.doi.org/10.3389/fcell.2020.623381]

[165] Schramm M, Klieber HG, Daut J. The energy expenditure of actomyosin-ATPase, Ca(2+)-ATPase and Na+,K(+)-ATPase in guinea-pig cardiac ventricular muscle. The Journal of physiology. 1994;481 (Pt 3)(Pt 3):647-62.

[166] Gambardella J, Sorriento D, Ciccarelli M, *et al.* Functional role of mitochondria in arrhythmogenesis. Adv Exp Med Biol 2017; 982: 191-202.
[http://dx.doi.org/10.1007/978-3-319-55330-6_10]

[167] Overend CL, Eisner DA, O'Neill SC. Altered cardiac sarcoplasmic reticulum function of intact myocytes of rat ventricle during metabolic inhibition. Circ Res 2001; 88(2): 181-7.
[http://dx.doi.org/10.1161/01.RES.88.2.181]

[168] Palmi M, Youmbi GT, Fusi F, *et al.* Potentiation of mitochondrial Ca^{2+} sequestration by taurine. Biochem Pharmacol 1999; 58(7): 1123-31.
[http://dx.doi.org/10.1016/S0006-2952(99)00183-5]

[169] Palmi M, Youmbi GT, Sgaragli G, Meini A, Benocci A, Fusi F, *et al.* The mitochondrial permeability transition and taurine.Taurine 4: Taurine and Excitable Tissues Advances in Experimental Medicine and Biology. Boston, MA: Springer US 2002; pp. 87-96.
[http://dx.doi.org/10.1007/0-306-46838-7_8]

[170] Heidari R, Babaei H, Eghbal MA. Ameliorative effects of taurine against methimazole-induced cytotoxicity in isolated rat hepatocytes. Sci Pharm 2012; 80(4): 987-99.
[http://dx.doi.org/10.3797/scipharm.1205-16]

[171] Heidari R, Babaei H, Eghbal MA. Cytoprotective effects of taurine against toxicity induced by isoniazid and hydrazine in isolated rat hepatocytes. Arh Hig Rada Toksikol 2013; 64(2): 201-10.
[http://dx.doi.org/10.2478/10004-1254-64-2013-2297]

[172] Heidari R, Babaei H, Eghbal MA. Amodiaquine-induced toxicity in isolated rat hepatocytes and the cytoprotective effects of taurine and/or N-acetyl cysteine. Res Pharm Sci 2014; 9(2): 97-105.

[173] Jamshidzadeh A, Heidari R, Abasvali M, *et al.* Taurine treatment preserves brain and liver mitochondrial function in a rat model of fulminant hepatic failure and hyperammonemia. Biomed Pharmacother 2017; 86: 514-20.
[http://dx.doi.org/10.1016/j.biopha.2016.11.095]

[174] Niknahad H, Jamshidzadeh A, Heidari R, Zarei M, Ommati MM. Ammonia-induced mitochondrial

dysfunction and energy metabolism disturbances in isolated brain and liver mitochondria, and the effect of taurine administration: relevance to hepatic encephalopathy treatment. Clin Exp Hepatol 2017; 3(3): 141-51.
[http://dx.doi.org/10.5114/ceh.2017.68833]

[175]   Ahmadi N, Ghanbarinejad V, Ommati MM, Jamshidzadeh A, Heidari R. Taurine prevents mitochondrial membrane permeabilization and swelling upon interaction with manganese: Implication in the treatment of cirrhosis-associated central nervous system complications. J Biochem Mol Toxicol 2018; 32(11): e22216.
[http://dx.doi.org/10.1002/jbt.22216]

[176]   Heidari R, Abdoli N, Ommati MM, Jamshidzadeh A, Niknahad H. Mitochondrial impairment induced by chenodeoxycholic acid: The protective effect of taurine and carnosine supplementation. Trends in Pharmaceutical Sciences. 2018;4(2).

[177]   Heidari R, Ghanbarinejad V, Ommati MM, Jamshidzadeh A, Niknahad H. Mitochondria protecting amino acids: Application against a wide range of mitochondria-linked complications. PharmaNutrition 2018; 6(4): 180-90.
[http://dx.doi.org/10.1016/j.phanu.2018.09.001]

[178]   Heidari R, Behnamrad S, Khodami Z, Ommati MM, Azarpira N, Vazin A. The nephroprotective properties of taurine in colistin-treated mice is mediated through the regulation of mitochondrial function and mitigation of oxidative stress. Biomed Pharmacother 2019; 109: 103-11.
[http://dx.doi.org/10.1016/j.biopha.2018.10.093]

[179]   Mohammadi H, Ommati MM, Farshad O, Jamshidzadeh A, Nikbakht MR, Niknahad H, *et al.* Taurine and isolated mitochondria: A concentration-response study. Trends Pharmacol Sci 2019; 5(4): 197-206.

[180]   Ommati MM, Farshad O, Jamshidzadeh A, Heidari R. Taurine enhances skeletal muscle mitochondrial function in a rat model of resistance training. PharmaNutrition 2019; 9: 100161.
[http://dx.doi.org/10.1016/j.phanu.2019.100161]

[181]   Ommati MM, Heidari R, Ghanbarinejad V, Abdoli N, Niknahad H. Taurine Treatment Provides Neuroprotection in a Mouse Model of Manganism. Biol Trace Elem Res 2019; 190(2): 384-95.
[http://dx.doi.org/10.1007/s12011-018-1552-2]

[182]   Xie W, Santulli G, Reiken SR, *et al.* Mitochondrial oxidative stress promotes atrial fibrillation. Sci Rep 2015; 5(1): 11427.
[http://dx.doi.org/10.1038/srep11427]

[183]   Sovari AA, Rutledge CA, Jeong EM, *et al.* Mitochondria oxidative stress, connexin43 remodeling, and sudden arrhythmic death. Circ Arrhythm Electrophysiol 2013; 6(3): 623-31.
[http://dx.doi.org/10.1161/CIRCEP.112.976787]

[184]   Sovari AA. Cellular and molecular mechanisms of arrhythmia by oxidative stress. Cardiol Res Pract 2016; 2016: 1-7.
[http://dx.doi.org/10.1155/2016/9656078]

[185]   Liu C, Ma N, Guo Z, *et al.* Relevance of mitochondrial oxidative stress to arrhythmias: Innovative concepts to target treatments. Pharmacol Res 2022; 175: 106027.
[http://dx.doi.org/10.1016/j.phrs.2021.106027]

[186]   Heidari R, Jamshidzadeh A, Ghanbarinejad V, Ommati MM, Niknahad H. Taurine supplementation abates cirrhosis-associated locomotor dysfunction. Clin Exp Hepatol 2018; 4(2): 72-82.
[http://dx.doi.org/10.5114/ceh.2018.75956]

[187]   Jamshidzadeh A, Abdoli N, Niknahad H, Azarpira N, Mardani E, Mousavi S, *et al.* Taurine alleviates brain tissue markers of oxidative stress in a rat model of hepatic encephalopathy. Trends Pharmacol Sci 2017; 3(3): 181-92.

[188]   Heidari R, Jamshidzadeh A, Niknahad H, Safari F, Azizi H, Abdoli N, *et al.* The hepatoprotection

provided by taurine and glycine against antineoplastic drugs induced liver injury in an ex vivo model of normothermic recirculating isolated perfused rat liver. Trends Pharmacol Sci 2016; 2(1): 59-76.

[189] Heidari R, Jamshidzadeh A, Niknahad H, *et al.* Effect of taurine on chronic and acute liver injury: Focus on blood and brain ammonia. Toxicol Rep 2016; 3: 870-9.
[http://dx.doi.org/10.1016/j.toxrep.2016.04.002]

[190] Heidari R, Rasti M, Shirazi Yeganeh B, Niknahad H, Saeedi A, Najibi A. Sulfasalazine-induced renal and hepatic injury in rats and the protective role of taurine. Bioimpacts 2016; 6(1): 3-8.
[http://dx.doi.org/10.15171/bi.2016.01]

[191] Heidari R, Sadeghi N, Azarpira N, Niknahad H. Sulfasalazine-induced hepatic injury in an ex vivo model of isolated perfused rat liver and the protective role of taurine. Pharm Sci 2015; 21(4): 211-9.
[http://dx.doi.org/10.15171/PS.2015.39]

[192] Karamikhah R, Jamshidzadeh A, Azarpira N, Saeidi A, Heidari R. Propylthiouracil-induced liver injury in mice and the protective role of taurine. Pharm Sci 2015; 21(2): 94-101.
[http://dx.doi.org/10.15171/PS.2015.23]

[193] Gordan R, Fefelova N, Gwathmey JK, Xie LH. Involvement of mitochondrial permeability transition pore (mPTP) in cardiac arrhythmias: Evidence from cyclophilin D knockout mice. Cell Calcium 2016; 60(6): 363-72.
[http://dx.doi.org/10.1016/j.ceca.2016.09.001]

[194] Weiss JN, Korge P, Honda HM, Ping P. Role of the mitochondrial permeability transition in myocardial disease. Circ Res 2003; 93(4): 292-301.
[http://dx.doi.org/10.1161/01.RES.0000087542.26971.D4]

[195] Baughman JM, Perocchi F, Girgis HS, *et al.* Integrative genomics identifies MCU as an essential component of the mitochondrial calcium uniporter. Nature 2011; 476(7360): 341-5.
[http://dx.doi.org/10.1038/nature10234]

[196] Griffiths EJ. Mitochondrial calcium transport in the heart: Physiological and pathological roles. J Mol Cell Cardiol 2009; 46(6): 789-803.
[http://dx.doi.org/10.1016/j.yjmcc.2009.03.001]

[197] Heidari R, Jamshidzadeh A, Keshavarz N, Azarpira N. Mitigation of methimazole-induced hepatic injury by taurine in mice. Sci Pharm 2015; 83(1): 143-58.
[http://dx.doi.org/10.3797/scipharm.1408-04]

[198] Abdoli N, Sadeghian I, Azarpira N, Ommati MM, Heidari R. Taurine mitigates bile duct obstruction-associated cholemic nephropathy: effect on oxidative stress and mitochondrial parameters. Clin Exp Hepatol 2021; 7(1): 30-40.
[http://dx.doi.org/10.5114/ceh.2021.104675]

[199] Fernández-Sada E, Silva-Platas C, Villegas CA, *et al.* Cardiac responses to β-adrenoceptor stimulation is partly dependent on mitochondrial calcium uniporter activity. Br J Pharmacol 2014; 171(18): 4207-21.
[http://dx.doi.org/10.1111/bph.12684]

[200] Kwong JQ, Lu X, Correll RN, *et al.* The mitochondrial calcium uniporter selectively matches metabolic output to acute contractile stress in the heart. Cell Rep 2015; 12(1): 15-22.
[http://dx.doi.org/10.1016/j.celrep.2015.06.002]

[201] Kwong JQ. The mitochondrial calcium uniporter in the heart: energetics and beyond. J Physiol 2017; 595(12): 3743-51.
[http://dx.doi.org/10.1113/JP273059]

[202] Chahine R, Feng J. Protective effects of taurine against reperfusion-induced arrhythmias in isolated ischemic rat heart. Arzneimittelforschung 1998; 48(4): 360-4.

[203] Eby G, Halcomb WW. Elimination of cardiac arrhythmias using oral taurine with l-arginine with case histories: Hypothesis for nitric oxide stabilization of the sinus node. Med Hypotheses 2006; 67(5):

1200-4.
[http://dx.doi.org/10.1016/j.mehy.2006.04.055]

[204] Hernández J, Artillo S, Serrano MI, Serrano JS. Further evidence of the antiarrhythmic efficacy of taurine in the rat heart. Res Commun Chem Pathol Pharmacol 1984; 43(2): 343-6.

[205] Takahashi K, Azuma J, Awata N, *et al.* Protective effect of taurine on the irregular beating pattern of cultured myocardial cells induced by high and low extracellular calcium ion. J Mol Cell Cardiol 1988; 20(5): 397-403.
[http://dx.doi.org/10.1016/S0022-2828(88)80131-7]

[206] An M, Sun K, Li Y, *et al.* Therapeutic effects of a taurine-magnesium coordination compound on experimental models of type 2 short QT syndrome. Acta Pharmacol Sin 2018; 39(3): 382-92.
[http://dx.doi.org/10.1038/aps.2017.86]

[207] Lee CC, Chen WT, Chen S, Lee TM. Taurine alleviates sympathetic innervation by inhibiting NLRP3 inflammasome in postinfarcted rats. J Cardiovasc Pharmacol 2021; 77(6): 745-55.
[http://dx.doi.org/10.1097/FJC.0000000000001005]

[208] Zhao L, Yang XX, Yin YQ, Wu H, Kang Y, Lou JS. Acute and chronic effects of taurine magnesium coordination compound on cardiac sodium channel Nav1.5. Mol Med Rep 2017; 16(4): 4259-64.
[http://dx.doi.org/10.3892/mmr.2017.7117]

[209] Idrissi AE, Okeke E, Yan X, Sidime F, Neuwirth LS. Taurine regulation of blood pressure and vasoactivity. Adv Exp Med Biol 2013; 775: 407-25.
[http://dx.doi.org/10.1007/978-1-4614-6130-2_31]

[210] Sun Q, Wang B, Li Y, *et al.* Taurine supplementation lowers blood pressure and improves vascular function in prehypertension: Randomized, double-blind, placebo-controlled study. Hypertension 2016; 67(3): 541-9.
[http://dx.doi.org/10.1161/HYPERTENSIONAHA.115.06624]

[211] Waldron M, Patterson SD, Tallent J, Jeffries O. The effects of oral taurine on resting blood pressure in humans: A meta-analysis. Curr Hypertens Rep 2018; 20(9): 81.
[http://dx.doi.org/10.1007/s11906-018-0881-z]

[212] Yokogoshi H, Mochizuki H, Nanami K, Hida Y, Miyachi F, Oda H. Dietary taurine enhances cholesterol degradation and reduces serum and liver cholesterol concentrations in rats fed a high-cholesterol diet. J Nutr 1999; 129(9): 1706-13.
[http://dx.doi.org/10.1093/jn/129.9.1705]

[213] Lam NV, Chen W, Suruga K, Nishimura N, Goda T, Yokogoshi H. Enhancing effect of taurine on CYP7A1 mRNA expression in Hep G2 cells. Amino Acids 2006; 30(1): 43-8.
[http://dx.doi.org/10.1007/s00726-005-0244-3]

[214] Chen W, Guo JX, Chang P. The effect of taurine on cholesterol metabolism. Mol Nutr Food Res 2012; 56(5): 681-90.
[http://dx.doi.org/10.1002/mnfr.201100799]

[215] Nishimura N, Umeda C, Oda H, Yokogoshi H. The effect of taurine on the cholesterol metabolism in rats fed diets supplemented with cholestyramine or high amounts of bile acid. J Nutr Sci Vitaminol (Tokyo) 2003; 49(1): 21-6.
[http://dx.doi.org/10.3177/jnsv.49.21]

[216] Guo J, Gao Y, Cao X, Zhang J, Chen W. Cholesterol-lowing effect of taurine in HepG2 cell. Lipids Health Dis 2017; 16(1): 56.
[http://dx.doi.org/10.1186/s12944-017-0444-3]

[217] Murakami S, Kondo Y, Toda Y, *et al.* Effect of taurine on cholesterol metabolism in hamsters: Up-regulation of low density lipoprotein (LDL) receptor by taurine. Life Sci 2002; 70(20): 2355-66.
[http://dx.doi.org/10.1016/S0024-3205(02)01507-2]

[218] Chen W, Matuda K, Nishimura N, Yokogoshi H. The effect of taurine on cholesterol degradation in

mice fed a high-cholesterol diet. Life Sci 2004; 74(15): 1889-98.
[http://dx.doi.org/10.1016/j.lfs.2003.08.041]

[219] Zhang M, Bi LF, Fang JH, *et al.* Beneficial effects of taurine on serum lipids in overweight or obese non-diabetic subjects. Amino Acids 2004; 26(3): 267-71.
[http://dx.doi.org/10.1007/s00726-003-0059-z]

[220] Maleki V, Alizadeh M, Esmaeili F, Mahdavi R. The effects of taurine supplementation on glycemic control and serum lipid profile in patients with type 2 diabetes: a randomized, double-blind, placebo-controlled trial. Amino Acids 2020; 52(6-7): 905-14.
[http://dx.doi.org/10.1007/s00726-020-02859-8]

[221] Schaffer SW, Lombardini JB, Azuma J. Interaction between the actions of taurine and angiotensin II. Amino Acids 2000; 18(4): 305-18.
[http://dx.doi.org/10.1007/PL00010320]

[222] Nandhini ATA, Thirunavukkarasu V, Anuradha CV. Potential role of kinins in the effects of taurine in high-fructose-fed rats. Can J Physiol Pharmacol 2004; 82(1): 1-8.
[http://dx.doi.org/10.1139/y03-118]

[223] Ideishi M, Miura S, Sakai T, Sasaguri M, Misumi Y, Arakawa K. Taurine amplifies renal kallikrein and prevents salt-induced hypertension in Dahl rats. J Hypertens 1994; 12(6): 653-62.
[http://dx.doi.org/10.1097/00004872-199406000-00005]

[224] Li N, Sawamura M, Nara Y, Ikeda K, Yamori Y. Direct inhibitory effects of taurine on norepinephrine-induced contraction in mesenteric artery of stroke-prone spontaneously hypertensive rats.Taurine 2: Basic and Clinical Aspects Advances in Experimental Medicine and Biology. Boston, MA: Springer US 1996; pp. 257-62.
[http://dx.doi.org/10.1007/978-1-4899-0182-8_27]

[225] Fujita T, Ando K, Noda H, Ito Y, Sato Y. Effects of increased adrenomedullary activity and taurine in young patients with borderline hypertension. Circulation 1987; 75(3): 525-32.
[http://dx.doi.org/10.1161/01.CIR.75.3.525]

[226] Militante JD, Lombardini JB. Treatment of hypertension with oral taurine: experimental and clinical studies. Amino Acids 2002; 23(4): 381-93.
[http://dx.doi.org/10.1007/s00726-002-0212-0]

[227] Scabora JE. Impact of taurine supplementation on blood pressure in gestational protein-restricted offspring: Effect on the medial solitary tract nucleus cell numbers, angiotensin receptors, and renal sodium handling. J Renin Angiotensin Aldosterone Syst 2013.

[228] Schwarzer R, Kivaranovic D, Mandorfer M, *et al.* Randomised clinical study: the effects of oral taurine 6g/day vs placebo on portal hypertension. Aliment Pharmacol Ther 2018; 47(1): 86-94.
[http://dx.doi.org/10.1111/apt.14377]

[229] Guan L, Miao P. The effects of taurine supplementation on obesity, blood pressure and lipid profile: A meta-analysis of randomized controlled trials. Eur J Pharmacol 2020; 885: 173533.
[http://dx.doi.org/10.1016/j.ejphar.2020.173533]

[230] Singh RB, Mengi SA, Xu Y-J, Arneja AS, Dhalla NS. Pathogenesis of atherosclerosis: A multifactorial process. Exp Clin Cardiol 2002; 7(1): 40-53.

[231] Bergheanu SC, Bodde MC, Jukema JW. Pathophysiology and treatment of atherosclerosis. Neth Heart J 2017; 25(4): 231-42.
[http://dx.doi.org/10.1007/s12471-017-0959-2]

[232] Fatkhullina AR, Peshkova IO, Koltsova EK. The role of cytokines in the development of atherosclerosis. Biochemistry 2016; 81(11): 1358-70.

[233] Tousoulis D, Oikonomou E, Economou EK, Crea F, Kaski JC. Inflammatory cytokines in atherosclerosis: current therapeutic approaches. Eur Heart J 2016; 37(22): 1723-32.
[http://dx.doi.org/10.1093/eurheartj/ehv759]

[234] Petty MA, Kintz J, DiFrancesco GF. The effects of taurine on atherosclerosis development in cholesterol-fed rabbits. Eur J Pharmacol 1990; 180(1): 119-27.
[http://dx.doi.org/10.1016/0014-2999(90)90599-2]

[235] Zulli A, Lau E, Wijaya BPP, *et al.* High dietary taurine reduces apoptosis and atherosclerosis in the left main coronary artery. Hypertension 2009; 53(6): 1017-22.
[http://dx.doi.org/10.1161/HYPERTENSIONAHA.109.129924]

[236] Sethupathy S, Elanchezhiyan C, Vasudevan K, Rajagopal G. Antiatherogenic effect of taurine in high fat diet fed rats. Indian J Exp Biol 2002; 40(10): 1169-72.

[237] Kondo Y, Toda Y, Kitajima H, *et al.* Taurine inhibits development of atherosclerotic lesions in apolipoprotein E-deficient mice. Clin Exp Pharmacol Physiol 2001; 28(10): 809-15.
[http://dx.doi.org/10.1046/j.1440-1681.2001.03527.x]

[238] Conti P, Shaik-Dasthagirisaeb Y. Atherosclerosis: a chronic inflammatory disease mediated by mast cells. Cent Eur J Immunol 2015; 3(3): 380-6.
[http://dx.doi.org/10.5114/ceji.2015.54603]

[239] Raggi P, Genest J, Giles JT, *et al.* Role of inflammation in the pathogenesis of atherosclerosis and therapeutic interventions. Atherosclerosis 2018; 276: 98-108.
[http://dx.doi.org/10.1016/j.atherosclerosis.2018.07.014]

[240] Murakami S. Taurine and atherosclerosis. Amino Acids 2014; 46(1): 73-80.
[http://dx.doi.org/10.1007/s00726-012-1432-6]

[241] Kontny E, Maśliński W, Marcinkiewicz J. Anti-inflammatory activities of taurine chloramine.Taurine 5: Beginning the 21st Century. Advances in Experimental Medicine and Biology.. Boston, MA: Springer US 2003; pp. 329-40.
[http://dx.doi.org/10.1007/978-1-4615-0077-3_41]

[242] Dall'igna DM, Luz JMD, Vuolo F, Michels M, Dal-Pizzol F. Taurine Chloramine decreases cell viability and cytokine production in blood and spleen lymphocytes from septic rats. An Acad Bras Cienc. 2020; 92.
[http://dx.doi.org/10.1590/0001-3765202020191311]

[243] Milei J, Ferreira R, Llesuy S, Forcada P, Covarrubias J, Boveris A. Reduction of reperfusion injury with preoperative rapid intravenous infusion of taurine during myocardial revascularization. Am Heart J 1992; 123(2): 339-45.
[http://dx.doi.org/10.1016/0002-8703(92)90644-B]

CHAPTER 5

Taurine and the Liver: A Focus on Mitochondria-related Liver Disease

Abstract: Although the liver is the leading site for taurine (TAU) synthesis, the level of this amino acid in hepatic tissue is relatively low. It is well-known that TAU is efficiently redistributed from hepatocytes to the circulation. However, the human body's capacity for TAU synthesis is negligible, and we receive a very high percentage of our body TAU from exogenous sources. Plasma TAU is taken up by several tissues, such as the skeletal muscle and the heart. The roles of TAU in liver function are the subject of many investigations. It has been found that TAU could have beneficial effects against xenobiotics-induced liver injury, alcoholism-associated hepatic damage, non-alcoholic fatty liver disease (NAFLD), non-alcoholic steatohepatitis (NASH), or even viral hepatitis infections. The inhibition of cytochrome P450, alleviation of oxidative stress, inhibition of inflammatory reactions, and the mitigation of tissue fibrosis are fundamental mechanisms proposed for the hepatoprotective properties of TAU. On the other hand, many studies indicate that hepatocytes' mitochondria are essential targets for the cytoprotective properties of TAU. The current chapter reviews the beneficial role of TAU on the most common liver disorders, focusing on the effects of this amino acid on mitochondrial function and energy metabolism.

Keywords: Hepatoprotection, Hepatotoxicity, Liver disease, Liver injury, Mitochondria, Oxidative stress.

INTRODUCTION

Although the liver is the main organ responsible for taurine (TAU) biosynthesis, the hepatic concentration of this amino acid is relatively low [1]. On the other hand, the TAU synthesis capacity of hepatic tissue is extremely variable between species [2, 3]. Some species such as foxes and felines are entirely dependent on the dietary sources of TAU [2, 3]. On the other hand, TAU is readily from the amino acids cysteine and methionine in the liver of dogs and rats [4 - 6]. The capability of a human liver for TAU synthesis is scarce and we receive almost all body TAU from dietary sources [7 - 10].

It has been found that TAU could play several pivotal roles in the liver. Many investigations revealed that TAU could effectively act as an antidote and protect

Reza Heidari and M. Mehdi Ommati

the liver against xenobiotics such as drugs, alcohol, or a wide range of other toxicants [11 - 16]. Nowadays, it is well-known that TAU is a robust inhibitor of the enzyme CYP2E1 [11, 17 - 20]. CYP2E1 is an important liver enzyme responsible for the bioactivation of many hepatotoxicants such as ethanol, carbon tetrachloride, and thioacetamide [11, 17 - 20]. Therefore, the inhibitory effects of TAU on CYP2E1 play a fundamental role in its hepatoprotective properties. Moreover, it has been found that TAU activates basic metabolic pathways, for example, long-chain fatty acids metabolism, in the liver [21 - 23]. Hence, this amino acid could act as a good candidate for liver diseases such as fatty liver.

More interestingly, TAU revealed potent antifibrotic properties in the liver and many other organs [14, 24 - 35]. Several hepatic disorders have been identified which could entail liver fibrosis and organ failure [32, 33]. Actually, hepatic fibrosis is the leading cause of liver transplantation worldwide [36, 37]. Hence, finding chemicals that could blunt or even prevent this process has a huge clinical value. It has been found that TAU possesses antifibrotic properties by inhibiting stellate cell activation, decreasing the release of pro-inflammatory mediators, and blunting oxidative stress and its associated complications [14, 24 - 35].

The effect of TAU on hepatocytes mitochondria is one of the most interesting features of this amino acid. Several experimental models revealed that TAU could significantly enhance mitochondrial membrane potential ($\Delta\Psi_m$), decrease mitochondrial release of cell death mediators, blunt mitochondria-mediated ROS formation and oxidative stress, and finally enhance the ATP level [38 - 55].

In the current chapter, the effects of TAU on several fundamental mechanisms involved in the pathogenesis of hepatic disorders are discussed. In this context, the antifibrotic properties of TAU (*e.g.*, in diseases such as alcoholism) are widely described. Moreover, the therapeutic potential of TAU on other common liver disorders such as non-alcoholic fatty liver disease (NAFLD) and non-alcoholic steatohepatitis (NASH) are discussed. Finally, the potential application of TAU against xenobiotics-induced liver injury is highlighted. In all these parts, the connection between the effects of TAU on mitochondrial indices and its relevance to these pathologies is considered.

TAURINE AND THE LIVER

The liver is the main organ responsible for TAU synthesis [6, 20, 41, 56]. However, the liver capacity for TAU synthesis is considerably variable between species [2, 3]. TAU is readily synthesized from the amino acid cysteine in the liver of dogs, rats, and Guinea pigs [57, 58]. However, some species, such as foxes and felines, are entirely dependent on the dietary sources of TAU [2, 3, 59 -

61]. The TAU synthesizing capability of the human liver is also negligible, and we receive a high percentage of our body TAU from exogenous sources [7 - 10, 20, 62 - 65]. As mentioned in chapter 1, TAU is abundantly found in foods such as meat (*e.g.*, turkey meat) and seafood (*e.g.*, oyster and muscles) [7, 8, 10, 65].

Hepatocytes contain lower TAU concentrations in comparison with other tissues such as skeletal muscle, cardiomyocytes, and the brain [6, 20, 41, 56]. As mentioned, endogenous TAU synthesis of the human liver is low, and a considerable portion of body TAU is provided through dietary sources [6, 20, 41, 56]. However, a lower concentration of TAU in hepatocytes could also be connected to the transport systems responsible for distributing this compound from hepatocytes and its uptake from the bloodstream [6, 20, 41, 56]. It is well-known that TAU transporters (TauT) expression is highly variable between different tissues [4, 21, 66, 67]. When TAU reaches the bloodstream, its uptake by tissues with more TauT is fast and high. Skeletal muscles and cardiomyocytes express a very high level of TauT [21, 58, 67, 68]. Hepatocytes have a lower level of transporters for TAU uptake. Hence, the level of this amino acid could be lower due to this issue, especially in species dependent on its exogenous sources.

TAU plays several essential physiological roles in the liver [20, 69 - 72]. TAU could also play a role in detoxifying xenobiotics from the liver and protecting hepatic tissue against their harmful effects, such as oxidative stress [71]. Bile acid conjugation is one of the most established physiologic roles of TAU in the liver [20, 73]. TAU-conjugated bile acids are secreted to the intestine, where they could be excreted through the feces or degraded by gut bacteria. The osmoregulatory properties of TAU in hepatocytes, its role in regulating cytoplasmic Ca^{2+} homeostasis, and the effects of TAU on mitochondrial function and energy metabolism are also important roles attributed to this amino acid in hepatocytes [20, 69 - 72]. In the current chapter, the role of TAU in common liver disease, as well as xenobiotics-induced hepatotoxicity, is discussed, focusing on the effects of this amino acid on mitochondrial function and its linked events. The data collected here could help the development of therapeutic strategies against liver disease as one of the most common causes of morbidity and mortality worldwide.

TAURINE AND LIVER FIBROSIS

Tissue fibrosis is a complicated process that could occur in response to a wide range of stimuli [74]. Several liver diseases have been identified in this context, which could entail liver fibrosis, dysfunction, and finally, hepatic failure [75 - 79]. Alcoholism, infectious liver disease, metabolism disorders, and a wide range of xenobiotics could induce liver fibrosis [80, 81]. There is no pharmacological intervention for reversing the function of the fibrotic area in the liver to date.

However, several strategies have been developed to prevent or blunt hepatic fibrosis [82 - 86].

Many factors have been identified to be involved in the mechanism of tissue fibrosis [87, 88]. Oxidative stress is a primary event involved in the mechanism of liver fibrosis [88, 89]. However, there is no clear idea of the source of ROS in fibrotic liver disease. ROS could derive from stellate cells, infiltrated neutrophils, Kupffer cells, or mitochondria [87, 90 - 92] (Fig. **1**). Therefore, many investigations focused on the role of antioxidants in the alleviation of liver fibrosis in different experimental models or clinical trials [93 - 106]. As repeatedly mentioned in various chapters of this book, TAU could significantly blunt oxidative stress and its linked complications in different experimental models [48, 51, 53, 107 - 113]. It is also well-known that a big part of the antioxidant properties of TAU is mediated through the effects of this amino acid on mitochondria [48, 51, 53, 107 - 113].

Several studies mentioned the antifibrotic properties of TAU not only in the liver but also in other tissues such as the lung and kidneys [32, 33, 114 - 117]. These investigations mentioned that the effects of TAU on oxidative stress and its associated events are critical for its antifibrotic properties [32, 33]. As previously mentioned, TAU is a weak radical scavenger [118], and the antioxidant properties of this amino acid are mainly mediated through regulating mitochondria-facilitated ROS formation [118]. Therefore, the antioxidative and antifibrotic effects of TAU might be mediated through a mitochondria-dependent pathway.

It has been well-documented that oxidative stress is tightly connected to the tissue fibrosis process in various experimental moles of liver disease [119 - 121]. Interestingly some studies mentioned the connection between mitochondrial impairment and liver fibrosis [122, 123]. Mitchell *et al.* reported that protecting hepatocytes mitochondria significantly decreased biomarkers of liver fibrosis [123]. Based on such studies, we might be able to emphasize that mitochondria-facilitated ROS formation could play a role in the liver fibrosis process [123]. However, Mitchell *et al.* mentioned that mitochondria-derived ROS might only play a partial role in the pathogenesis of liver fibrosis since mitochondrial protection did not prevent tissue fibrosis at later stages of their cirrhosis model [123]. Hence, the role of other factors involved in liver fibrosis (*e.g.,* inflammatory factors) could not be ignored (Fig. **1**). Pérez *et al.* also reported that protecting cellular mitochondria could play a significant role in preventing liver injury and fibrosis in an experimental model of cirrhosis [122]. In a study by Pérez *et al.*, administration of insulin-like growth factor provided significant mitochondrial protection by inhibiting mitochondrial membrane dissipation, increasing ATP production, preventing mitochondrial permeabilization, and inhibiting cell death mediators released from this organelle [122]. They concluded that mitochondria-mediated cell death could play a crucial role in liver injury and fibrosis [122]. These investigations highlight the importance of mitochondrial impairment in liver disease, which could lead to fibrotic lesions (Fig. **1**).

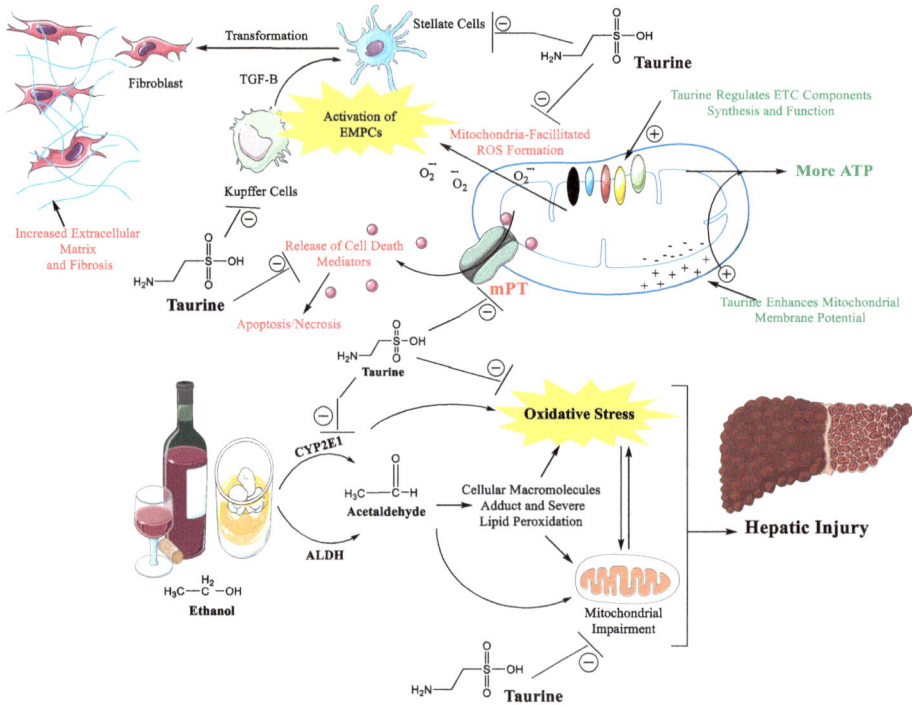

Fig. (1). Inhibition of CYP2E1 plays a pivotal role in the hepatoprotective effects of taurine (TAU) against different xenobiotics metabolized by this enzyme (*e.g.,* ethanol). On the other hand, the effect of taurine on mitochondrial impairment, mitochondria-facilitated oxidative stress, mitochondria-mediated cell death, and energy metabolism play a fundamental role in the hepatoprotective effects of this amino acid. Besides, it has been found that TAU plays a crucial role in Kupffer cell activation and their transformation to fibroblasts. Fibroblasts play a significant role in tissue fibrosis. ALDH: Aldehyde dehydrogenase; EMPCs: Extracellular matrix producing cells; TGF-β: Transforming growth factor-β; mPT: Mitochondrial permeability transition.

The positive effects of TAU on the hepatocyte's mitochondria have been repeatedly investigated [48, 54, 124 - 127]. Previous investigations indicated that liver mitochondrial function was severely impaired in an experimental model of liver fibrosis [103, 128 - 130]. An important notion about the role of mitochondrial impairment in different models of liver fibrosis is this point that mitochondrial impairment could be induced by different hepatotoxins used as the experimental models or endogenous cytotoxic compounds (*e.g.,* bilirubin and hydrophobic bile acids) accumulated in the liver (*e.g.*, in bile duct ligated rat model of cholestasis) as well as many other organs [53, 92, 96 - 98, 102, 103, 131 - 137]. On the other hand, it has been found that TAU could significantly enhance mitochondrial function and prevent mitochondria-facilitated ROS formation and oxidative stress in the liver [53] (Fig. **1**). Therefore, we could hypothesize that a part of the antifibrotic effects of TAU might be mediated through a mitochondria-dependent mechanism (Fig. **1**).

Some investigations mentioned the effects of TAU on cells involved in the progression of tissue fibrosis [32, 33, 138]. Hepatic Stellate (Ito) cells and Kupffer cells are key players in extracellular matrix production and fibrosis in the liver [138, 139] (Fig. **1**). It has also been found that TAU can suppress stellate cells' proliferation and activity and promote their apoptosis [140]. Besides, it has been revealed that TAU significantly blunted Kupffer cells' activity and cytokine production in different experimental models [138, 141] (Fig. **1**). Transforming growth factor-β (TGF-β) is an important cytokine secreted from Kupffer cells. It is well-known that TGF-β is responsible for transforming stellate cells into myofibroblasts [142] (Fig. **1**). Some studies reported that TAU suppresses TGF-β levels in different experimental models of liver fibrosis [143]. It has also been found that TAU can suppress stellate cells' proliferation and activity and promote their apoptosis [29, 140, 144]. All these data indicate that TAU could act as an excellent anti-fibrotic agent. Therefore, TAU could be reliably used in liver disease associated with tissue fibrosis (Fig. **1**). However, the effects of TAU on cellular mitochondria and its relevance to the tissue fibrosis process warranted further studies to be precisely cleared.

Several lines of evidence mentioned the positive effects of TAU on anti-apoptotic genes such as Bcl-2 in various experimental models [57, 145, 146]. Interestingly, it has been found that proteins like Bcl-2 could act as an antioxidant molecule at the mitochondrial level [123, 147, 148]. Bcl-2 protein is a well-known regulator of cell death that its major target is cellular mitochondria [149]. TAU also prevents the increase in pro-apoptotic proteins such as Bax [57]. Proteins such as Bax could severely facilitate the release of cell death mediators from mitochondria [57] (Fig. **1**). Interestingly, some studies mentioned the effects of TAU on the downregulation of the Bcl-2 gene [150]. The controversies in the effects of TAU on the apoptosis process and its related genes could be associated with the concentration of this amino acid used in each investigation, as well as the differences between the applied experimental models (*in vitro* or *in vivo*). For example, studies that reported the downregulation of Bcl-2 protein in an *in vitro* model of cancer cell line culture applied high and supraphysiological concentrations of TAU (*e.g.*, 160 mM) in their experiments [150, 151]. Recently, our research team also found that a high concentration of TAU could deteriorate mitochondrial function [55]. On the other hand, most *in vivo* models revealed the antiapoptotic effect and upregulation of Bcl-2 after TAU treatment [145]. Hence, the effect of TAU on mitochondrial function and mitochondria-mediated apoptosis could be concentration and model-dependent.

Previous sections discussed the effects of TAU on liver fibrosis as a primary mechanism involved in the pathogenesis of a wide range of liver diseases. In the following parts of this chapter, the effects of TAU on several liver diseases, which also could lead to tissue fibrosis and hepatic failure, are discussed, focusing on the role of TAU on mitochondrial function and its relevance to the pathogenesis of these disorders.

TAURINE AND ALCOHOL-INDUCED LIVER INJURY

Alcoholism plays a major role in hepatic injury and failure worldwide [152]. Alcohol (Ethanol)-induced liver injury involves several pathological changes including fatty liver, high serum markers of liver injury (*e.g.*, bilirubin and ALT), progressive inflammatory response in the liver, and finally tissue fibrosis and hepatic failure [152 - 154]. Alcoholism and its linked adverse effects impose a tremendous economic burden on the health care system. Therefore, finding therapeutic agents against alcohol-associated liver diseases could have significant clinical, economic, and even social value.

It has been found that TAU could significantly alleviate ethanol-induced fatty liver and steatohepatitis in different experimental models [155, 156]. Interestingly, in clinical settings, it has also been found that TAU significantly improved liver function in alcoholic patients [157]. Several mechanisms have been proposed for the positive effects of TAU against alcohol-induced liver injury. These mechanisms include the inhibition of hepatic enzymes (*e.g.*, CYP2E1), prevention of oxidative stress, alleviation of the inflammatory response, and prevention of mitochondrial impairment and its associated events [15, 54, 156, 158 - 163] (Fig. **1**).

The effects of TAU on CYP2E1 is a fundamental mechanism involved in its hepatoprotective properties [11, 17 - 20] (Fig. **1**). This enzyme is involved in the metabolism and bio-activation of several hepatotoxic agents. It has been revealed that TAU could effectively inhibit CYP2E1 [11, 17 - 20]. Therefore, the hepatotoxicity induced by xenobiotics that are metabolized by CYP2E1 (*e.g.*, ethanol and acetaminophen) is significantly suppressed by TAU treatment [11, 17 - 20]. Ethanol is converted into potentially cytotoxic agents such as acetaldehyde in the liver (Fig. **1**). These mediators are able to target cellular macromolecules (*e.g.*, lipids, DNA, and proteins), impair mitochondrial function, and induce oxidative stress (Fig. **1**). Hence, a major part of the hepatoprotective effects of

TAU in alcohol-induced liver injury is mediated through the inhibitory effect of this amino acid on the CYP2E1 enzyme (Fig. **1**).

Alcohol-induced oxidative stress is a well-known phenomenon in the liver tissue [164 - 168]. Severe ROS formation, lipid peroxidation, depletion of cellular antioxidant capacity, and proteins adducts have been detected in the liver in various experimental models as well as in human studies [164 - 170]. Ethanol-induced oxidative stress in the liver could be mediated through several mechanisms. Foremost, ethanol metabolites such as acetaldehyde could directly affect proteins, including antioxidant enzymes [165]. Moreover, acetaldehyde could induce significant lipid peroxidation in the liver [165]. Alcohol metabolism could also enhance mitochondria-facilitated ROS formation by providing excessive reducing equivalents (NADH) for the mitochondrial electron chain activity [165]. As mentioned, TAU could significantly inhibit ethanol metabolism and its conversion to reactive metabolites (Fig. **1**). TAU is also able to efficiently subside mitochondria-mediated ROS formation [7, 41, 65, 109, 171 - 175]. Thus, alcohol-induced oxidative stress could be significantly abrogated by TAU (Fig. **1**).

Inflammatory cells are also potential sources of ROS formation in alcohol-induced liver injury [166, 176, 177]. Infiltrated inflammatory cells such as neutrophils or Kupffer cells, as resident macrophages in the liver, could produce a high amount of ROS through the activity of enzymes such as NADPH oxidase [176, 177]. On the other hand, TAU is well-known for its anti-inflammatory properties in experimental models of alcohol-induced liver injury [156, 178]. Inhibition of the production of inflammatory cytokines is a well-investigated mechanism for the anti-inflammatory effects of TAU in alcohol-induced liver injury [33, 156, 178]. However, TAU can also inhibit NADPH oxidase and myeloperoxidase enzymes' activity and ROS formation [161, 179]. Based on these data, a part of the antioxidant properties of TAU in the alcohol-exposed liver could be mediated through its inhibitory effects on the inflammatory response.

Hepatocytes mitochondria are also well-investigated as sources of ROS in alcohol-induced liver injury [180 - 182]. In both experimental models and human cases, significant changes in mitochondrial morphology and function have been repeatedly mentioned in the liver during alcohol exposure [183]. Significant increases in mitochondrial DNA damage, enhancement of mitochondria-facilitated ROS formation, impaired mitochondrial biogenesis, induction of mitochondrial permeability, and elevation in mitochondria-mediated cell death have been reported in alcohol-induced liver injury [180 - 183]. These investigations suggest hepatocytes mitochondria as novel therapeutic targets for preventing alcohol-induced liver injury. In this context, the effects of TAU on mitochondrial indices have been investigated in alcohol-induced liver injury [54, 124]. It is reported that TAU could significantly alleviate mitochondria-mediated ROS formation, oxidative stress, and cell death in the liver [54]. Moreover, Lakshmi Devi *et al.* found a significant decrease in mitochondrial respiratory chain activity, along with decreased mitochondrial antioxidant capacity and mitochondrial swelling in an animal model of alcoholic liver fibrosis [124]. They found that TAU could significantly restore mitochondrial function and diminish oxidative stress biomarkers in the liver [124]. In another study by Shim *et al.*, the authors revealed a significant decrease in hepatocytes' mitochondrial respiratory chain activity in ethanol-exposed rats [184]. It was found that TAU could significantly abrogate ethanol-induced suppression of mitochondrial respiratory chain activity and energy metabolism [184]. All these data provide clues about the significant hepatoprotective properties of TAU against alcohol-induced liver injury. Interestingly, it has also been found that TAU protects the liver tissue and could significantly protect other organs such as the brain against the adverse effects of ethanol [185, 186].

The data provided in this section mention TUA as a viable hepatoprotective agent against alcohol-induced liver injury. As TAU is a safe and clinically applicable agent, this amino acid could readily find application against alcoholism in clinical settings.

TAURINE AND NON-ALCOHOLIC FATTY LIVER

Fatty liver is a complication that affects a large population's health status worldwide [187 - 189]. Changes in dietary habits and high fat and calorie diet intake lead to a higher rate of fatty liver [190]. Non-alcoholic fatty liver disease (NAFLD) and non-alcoholic steatohepatitis (NASH) are two forms of fatty liver that could lead to hepatic fibrosis and liver failure [191]. NASH is associated with a significant inflammatory response, where NAFLD is linked to fatty acids accumulation without inflammation [191]. It is well-known that NAFLD might progress to NASH [191]. Fatty acids changes in the liver, inflammatory response, severe oxidative stress, and hepatocytes necrosis/apoptosis occur in various stages of the fatty liver [191 - 194].

Several mechanisms have been proposed to be involved in the pathogenesis of fatty liver disease [191, 192, 195]. The "two-hit" theory is the most accepted mechanism for fatty liver-induced liver injury [196]. This mechanism mentions that the accumulation of fatty acids in the liver is the first step. Then the occurrence of oxidative stress, which could lead to severe lipid peroxidation (Lipotoxixicty) in the hepatic tissue, is the next step [196]. Inflammatory cells infiltrated into the hepatic tissue of NASH patients could play a pivotal role in ROS formation and oxidative stress [197, 198]. The enzyme nicotinamide adenine dinucleotide phosphate (NADPH) oxidase in inflammatory cells such as neutrophils could produce high ROS [199, 200]. Inflammation-linked ROS formation and oxidative stress could affect several targets such as the lipid membrane bilayer, mitochondria, proteins, DNA, and many other targets [201].

Strong evidence indicates that NAFLD and NASH are mitochondria-related disorders [202 - 205]. Different mechanisms could be involved in the pathogenesis of NAFLD/NASH-linked mitochondrial impairment [206]. It is well-established that NAFLD/NASH could induce impaired mitochondrial biogenesis and deteriorate mitochondrial respiratory chain complexes function and energy metabolism [206]. Mitochondria could also act as a major source of ROS in NFLD/NASH [195, 196, 207]. Other mechanisms such as ER stress and disturbances of cytoplasmic Ca^{2+} homeostasis are also involved in the mechanism of hepatocytes injury in NAFLD/NASH [190]. All the mentioned parameters (Oxidative stress, mitochondrial impairment, and ER stress; Fig. **1**) could be restrained by TAU. Hence, this amino acid might play a role in ameliorating NAFLD/NASH. Several experimental models mentioned the beneficial effects of TAU in NAFLD and NASH [208 - 210]. TAU has been supposed to provide hepatoprotection in NASH and NAFLD by regulating oxidative stress and its consequences [208 - 210]. The effect of TAU on the inflammatory response in the liver of NASH cases is also an interesting mechanism for hepatoprotective properties of this amino acid [208, 209]. It has also been reported that CYP2E1 activity is increased in experimental models or patients with NASH [211, 212]. Hence, CYP2E1 overactivity could play a pathogenic role in fatty liver disease [211, 212]. As mentioned, TAU is a CYP2E1 inhibitor (Fig. **1**). Hence, a part of hepatoprotective effects of TAU in fatty liver disease could be mediated through the effects of this amino acid on CYP2E1 activity.

Fatty acids metabolism has occurred in hepatocytes' mitochondria through the β-oxidation process. Interestingly, a recent study by Bonfleur *et al.* revealed that TAU administration significantly enhanced the expression of genes involved in the metabolism of fatty acids in the liver tissue (*e.g.*, carnitine palmitoyl transferase) [23]. Therefore, improvement in the mitochondrial β-oxidation of fatty acids could play a significant role in the positive effects of TAU in NAFL and NASH (Fig. **2**). Unfortunately, there is a lack of clinical studies on the effects of TAU in patients with fatty liver. Meanwhile, Obinata *et al.* found that TAU administration could significantly decrease fatty liver in children with simple obesity [22]. Obviously, more studies are needed to conclude the efficacy of TAU against different forms of fatty liver in clinical settings.

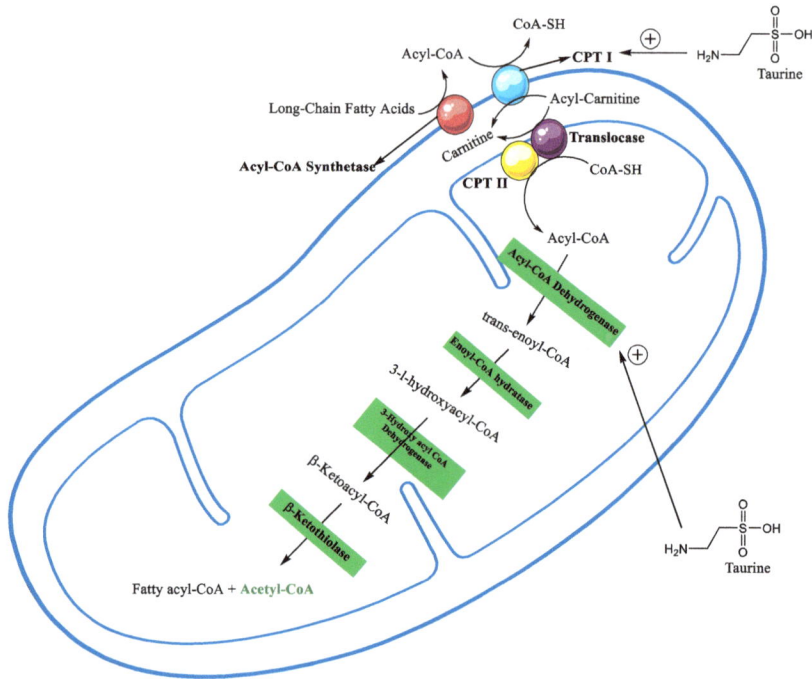

Fig. (2). The effects of taurine on the β-oxidation process in cellular mitochondria could play a fundamental role in the hepatoprotective properties of this amino acid (*e.g.*, in the fatty liver). CPT: Carnitine palmitoyltransferase.

As previously mentioned, a mildly alkaline pH is an essential factor for the activity of enzymes such as acyl-CoA dehydrogenase [21]. Acyl-CoA dehydrogenase is responsible for fatty acids β-oxidation (Fig. **2**). It has been found that the TAU buffering capacity of the mitochondrial matrix could enhance acyl-CoA dehydrogenase activity and probably fatty acids metabolism [21] (Fig. **2**). These data indicate the importance of TAU in fatty acid metabolism and preventing these compounds' accumulation in tissues such as the liver.

Although the hepatoprotective properties of TAU have been investigated in several forms of fatty liver diseases (*e.g.*, NASH), there is a lack of evidence on the role of this amino acid in hepatocytes' mitochondrial function. Therefore, further investigations are warranted to reveal the effects of TAU on mitochondrial function and its relevance to the pathophysiology of hepatic diseases.

TAURINE PREVENTS XENOBIOTICS-INDUCED LIVER INJURY: A FOCUS ON MITOCHONDRIAL-DEPENDENT MECHANISMS

A wide range of xenobiotics, including several drugs, could induce liver injury. Actually, drug-induced liver injury is the major cause of drug withdrawal from the market and a big challenge in developing new drug candidates [213 - 220]. Hepatocytes mitochondria are crucial targets affected by xenobiotics [213 - 222]. Xenobiotics affect mitochondrial function through various mechanisms [221, 222]. The inhibition of electron transport chain, the dissipation of mitochondrial membrane potential, the opening of mitochondrial permeability pore, induction of mitochondrial membranes disintegrity and disruption, and the inhibition of enzymes involved in the mitochondrial function have been studied as mechanisms of xenobiotics-induced mitochondrial impairment in the liver [48, 221 - 225] (Fig. 3).

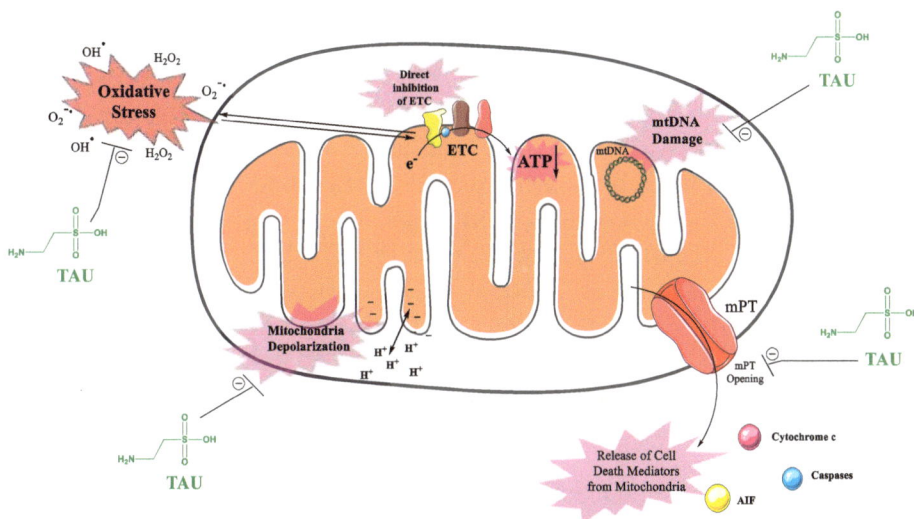

Fig. (3). Many xenobiotics, including drugs, could affect several points in hepatocytes' mitochondria and deteriorate the functionality of this organelle. Xenobiotics-induced mitochondrial dysfunction could lead to cell death and liver injury. Taurine (TAU) could interfere with several points in mitochondrial function and alleviate xenobiotics-induced mitochondrial injury in the liver.

The effects of TAU on mitochondria-mediated cell death and its relevance to xenobiotics-induced liver injury have been revealed in several studies [11, 41, 143]. Many other investigations mentioned the ameliorative effects of TAU on oxidative stress biomarkers in xenobiotics-induced liver injury [32, 51, 110, 113, 226 - 228]. As mentioned, the effect of TAU on mitochondria-facilitated ROS formation is a crucial mechanism for this compound's antioxidative stress properties [51, 118] (Fig. **3**). Hence, a big part of the antioxidant properties of TAU in the liver could be mediated through modulating mitochondrial function in hepatocytes (Fig. **3**). It has also been found that TAU significantly suppressed the release of cell death mediators from mitochondria and decreased the expression of apoptosis-related factors in the liver [4] (Fig. **3**).

Based on the data provided in this section, TAU could be readily used as a hepatoprotective agent against xenobiotics-induced liver injury. The positive effects of TAU on mitochondrial indices seem to play a significant role in its hepatoprotective properties.

CONCLUSION

The hepatoprotective properties of TUA are the subject of a plethora of investigations. It has been found that TAU can protect the liver from many toxic insults as well as diseases. On the other hand, TAU is a safe compound even at very high doses (*e.g.*, 3-4 g/day). Therefore, several brands of TAU-containing hepatoprotective supplementary agents have been developed. However, the amount of TAU in these products seems to be negligible (*e.g.*, 200 mg TAU/tab in the LiverCare®-Health Aid® company, as a TAU-containing product available in the market) when compared with the experimental models that investigated the hepatoprotective properties of this amino acid (*e.g.*, 1 g/day). This issue might mention the importance of revisiting the effects of TAU doses on liver function in controlled trials. On the other hand, it could also mention the significance of effective formulation and drug delivery techniques to enhance the concentration of TUA in hepatocytes. It could be concluded that the effects of TAU on mitochondrial function could be significantly involved in the hepatoprotective properties of this amino acid.

All data provided in the current chapter could indicate TAU as a promising pharmacological intervention against liver disease. Indeed, more clinical trials could help the administration of this amino acid in clinical settings as a hepatoprotective agent.

REFERENCES

[1]   Bouckenooghe T, Remacle C, Reusens B. Is taurine a functional nutrient? Curr Opin Clin Nutr Metab Care 2006; 9(6): 728-33.
[http://dx.doi.org/10.1097/01.mco.0000247469.26414.55] [PMID: 17053427]

[2]   Moise NS, Pacioretty LM, Kallfelz FA, Stipanuk MH, King JM, Gilmour RF Jr. Dietary taurine deficiency and dilated cardiomyopathy in the fox. Am Heart J 1991; 121(2): 541-7.
[http://dx.doi.org/10.1016/0002-8703(91)90724-V] [PMID: 1990761]

[3]   Pion PD, Kittleson MD, Skiles ML, Rogers QR, Morris JG. Dilated cardiomyopathy associated with taurine deficiency in the domestic cat: relationship to diet and myocardial taurine content Taurine. Springer 1992; pp. 63-73.

[4]   Lambert IH, Kristensen DM, Holm JB, Mortensen OH. Physiological role of taurine - from organism to organelle. Acta Physiol (Oxf) 2015; 213(1): 191-212.
[http://dx.doi.org/10.1111/apha.12365] [PMID: 25142161]

[5]   Bella DL, Hirschberger LL, Kwon YH, Stipanuk MH. Cysteine metabolism in periportal and perivenous hepatocytes: perivenous cells have greater capacity for glutathione production and taurine synthesis but not for cysteine catabolism. Amino Acids 2002; 23(4): 453-8.
[http://dx.doi.org/10.1007/s00726-002-0213-z] [PMID: 12436215]

[6]   Stipanuk MH. Role of the liver in regulation of body cysteine and taurine levels: a brief review. Neurochem Res 2004; 29(1): 105-10.
[http://dx.doi.org/10.1023/B:NERE.0000010438.40376.c9] [PMID: 14992268]

[7]   Hansen SH, Grunnet N. Taurine, glutathione and bioenergetics.Taurine 8 Advances in Experimental Medicine and Biology: Springer New York. 2013; pp. 3-12.

[8]   Huxtable RJ. Taurine in nutrition and neurology: Springer Science & Business Media; 2013.

[9]   Laidlaw SA, Grosvenor M, Kopple JD. The taurine content of common foodstuffs. JPEN J Parenter Enteral Nutr 1990; 14(2): 183-8.
[http://dx.doi.org/10.1177/0148607190014002183] [PMID: 2352336]

[10]   Xu Y-J, Arneja AS, Tappia PS, Dhalla NS. The potential health benefits of taurine in cardiovascular disease. Exp Clin Cardiol 2008; 13(2): 57-65.
[PMID: 19343117]

[11]   Heidari R, Jamshidzadeh A, Niknahad H, *et al*. Effect of taurine on chronic and acute liver injury: Focus on blood and brain ammonia. Toxicol Rep 2016; 3: 870-9.
[http://dx.doi.org/10.1016/j.toxrep.2016.04.002] [PMID: 28959615]

[12]   Jagadeesan G, Sankarsami Pillai S. Hepatoprotective effects of taurine against mercury induced toxicity in rats. J Environ Biol 2007; 28(4): 753-6.
[PMID: 18405108]

[13]   Fang YJ, Chiu CH, Chang YY, *et al*. Taurine ameliorates alcoholic steatohepatitis via enhancing self-antioxidant capacity and alcohol metabolism. Food Res Int 2011; 44(9): 3105-10.
[http://dx.doi.org/10.1016/j.foodres.2011.08.004]

[14]   Abdel-Moneim AM, Al-Kahtani MA, El-Kersh MA, Al-Omair MA. Free radical-scavenging, anti-inflammatory/anti-fibrotic and hepatoprotective actions of taurine and silymarin against CCl4 induced rat liver damage. PLoS One 2015; 10(12): e0144509.
[http://dx.doi.org/10.1371/journal.pone.0144509] [PMID: 26659465]

[15]   Lee SY, Ko KS. Effects of S-adenosylmethionine and its combinations with taurine and/or betaine on glutathione homeostasis in ethanol-induced acute hepatotoxicity. J Cancer Prev 2016; 21(3): 164-72.
[http://dx.doi.org/10.15430/JCP.2016.21.3.164] [PMID: 27722142]

[16]   Heidari R, Ommati MM, Alahyari S, Azarpira N, Niknahad H. Amino acid-containing Krebs-Henseleit buffer protects rat liver in a long-term organ perfusion model. Ulum-i Daruyi 2018; 24(3): 168-79.
[http://dx.doi.org/10.15171/PS.2018.25]

[17]   Yao HT, Lin P, Chang YW, *et al*. Effect of taurine supplementation on cytochrome P450 2E1 and oxidative stress in the liver and kidneys of rats with streptozotocin-induced diabetes. Food Chem Toxicol 2009; 47(7): 1703-9.
[http://dx.doi.org/10.1016/j.fct.2009.04.030] [PMID: 19406192]

[18]   Das J, Ghosh J, Manna P, Sil PC. Taurine protects acetaminophen-induced oxidative damage in mice kidney through APAP urinary excretion and CYP2E1 inactivation. Toxicology 2010; 269(1): 24-34.
[http://dx.doi.org/10.1016/j.tox.2010.01.003] [PMID: 20067817]

[19]   Das J, Ghosh J, Manna P, Sil PC. Acetaminophen induced acute liver failure via oxidative stress and

JNK activation: Protective role of taurine by the suppression of cytochrome P450 2E1. Free Radic Res 2010; 44(3): 340-55.
[http://dx.doi.org/10.3109/10715760903513017] [PMID: 20166895]

[20]   Miyazaki T, Matsuzaki Y. Taurine and liver diseases: a focus on the heterogeneous protective properties of taurine. Amino Acids 2014; 46(1): 101-10.
[http://dx.doi.org/10.1007/s00726-012-1381-0] [PMID: 22918604]

[21]   Hansen SH, Andersen ML, Birkedal H, Cornett C, Wibrand F. The important role of taurine in oxidative metabolism. Adv Exp Med Biol 2006; 583: 129-35.
[http://dx.doi.org/10.1007/978-0-387-33504-9_13] [PMID: 17153596]

[22]   Obinata K, Maruyama T, Hayashi M, Watanabe T, Nittono H. Effect of taurine on the fatty liver of children with simple obesity. Adv Exp Med Biol 1996; 403: 607-13.
[http://dx.doi.org/10.1007/978-1-4899-0182-8_67] [PMID: 8915401]

[23]   Bonfleur ML, Borck PC, Ribeiro RA, *et al.* Improvement in the expression of hepatic genes involved in fatty acid metabolism in obese rats supplemented with taurine. Life Sci 2015; 135: 15-21.
[http://dx.doi.org/10.1016/j.lfs.2015.05.019] [PMID: 26092479]

[24]   Mas MR, Isik AT, Yamanel L, *et al.* Antioxidant treatment with taurine ameliorates chronic pancreatitis in an experimental rat model. Pancreas 2006; 33(1): 77-81.
[http://dx.doi.org/10.1097/01.mpa.0000222316.74607.07] [PMID: 16804416]

[25]   Ohta H, Azuma J, Onishi S, Awata N, Takihara K, Kishimoto S. Protective effect of taurine against isoprenaline-induced myocardial damage. Basic Res Cardiol 1986; 81(5): 473-81.
[http://dx.doi.org/10.1007/BF01907753] [PMID: 3800845]

[26]   Gurujeyalakshmi G, Hollinger MA, Giri SN. Regulation of transforming growth factor-β1 mRNA expression by taurine and niacin in the bleomycin hamster model of lung fibrosis. Am J Respir Cell Mol Biol 1998; 18(3): 334-42.
[http://dx.doi.org/10.1165/ajrcmb.18.3.2867] [PMID: 9490651]

[27]   Schuller-Levis GB, Gordon RE, Wang C, Park E. Taurine reduces lung inflammation and fibrosis caused by bleomycin.Taurine 5: Beginning the 21st Century. Advances in Experimental Medicine and Biology.. Boston, MA: Springer US 2003; pp. 395-402.
[http://dx.doi.org/10.1007/978-1-4615-0077-3_48]

[28]   Schuller-Levis GB, Gordon RE, Wang C, Park E. Taurine reduces lung inflammation and fibrosis caused by bleomycin. Adv Exp Med Biol 2003; 526: 395-402.
[http://dx.doi.org/10.1007/978-1-4615-0077-3_48] [PMID: 12908624]

[29]   Kato J, Ido A, Hasuike S, *et al.* Transforming growth factor-?-induced stimulation of formation of collagen fiber network and anti-fibrotic effect of taurine in an *in vitro* model of hepatic fibrosis. Hepatol Res 2004; 30(1): 34-41.
[http://dx.doi.org/10.1016/j.hepres.2004.04.006] [PMID: 15341772]

[30]   Oudit GY, Trivieri MG, Khaper N, *et al.* Taurine supplementation reduces oxidative stress and improves cardiovascular function in an iron-overload murine model. Circulation 2004; 109(15): 1877-85.
[http://dx.doi.org/10.1161/01.CIR.0000124229.40424.80] [PMID: 15037530]

[31]   Refik Mas M, Comert B, Oncu K, *et al.* The effect of taurine treatment on oxidative stress in experimental liver fibrosis. Hepatol Res 2004; 28(4): 207-15.
[http://dx.doi.org/10.1016/j.hepres.2003.11.012] [PMID: 15040961]

[32]   Miyazaki T, Karube M, Matsuzaki Y, *et al.* Taurine inhibits oxidative damage and prevents fibrosis in carbon tetrachloride-induced hepatic fibrosis. J Hepatol 2005; 43(1): 117-25.
[http://dx.doi.org/10.1016/j.jhep.2005.01.033] [PMID: 15893842]

[33]   Devi SL, Viswanathan P, Anuradha CV. Regression of liver fibrosis by taurine in rats fed alcohol: Effects on collagen accumulation, selected cytokines and stellate cell activation. Eur J Pharmacol

2010; 647(1-3): 161-70.
[http://dx.doi.org/10.1016/j.ejphar.2010.08.011] [PMID: 20813107]

[34] Yang L, Tang J, Chen H, *et al.* Taurine reduced epidural fibrosis in rat models after laminectomy *via* downregulating EGR1. Cell Physiol Biochem 2016; 38(6): 2261-71.
[http://dx.doi.org/10.1159/000445581] [PMID: 27188306]

[35] Liu J, Ai Y, Niu X, *et al.* Taurine protects against cardiac dysfunction induced by pressure overload through SIRT1–p53 activation. Chem Biol Interact 2020; 317108972
[http://dx.doi.org/10.1016/j.cbi.2020.108972] [PMID: 32017914]

[36] Tabatabai L, Lewis W, Gordon F, Jenkins R, Khettry U. Fibrosis/cirrhosis after orthotopic liver transplantation*1. Hum Pathol 1999; 30(1): 39-47.
[http://dx.doi.org/10.1016/S0046-8177(99)90298-8] [PMID: 9923925]

[37] Berumen J, Baglieri J, Kisseleva T, Mekeel K. Liver fibrosis: Pathophysiology and clinical implications. WIREs Mech Dis 2021; 13(1): e1499.
[http://dx.doi.org/10.1002/wsbm.1499] [PMID: 32713091]

[38] You JS, Chang KJ. Taurine protects the liver against lipid peroxidation and membrane disintegration during rat hepatocarcinogenesis. Adv Exp Med Biol 1998; 442: 105-12.
[http://dx.doi.org/10.1007/978-1-4899-0117-0_14] [PMID: 9635021]

[39] Palmi M, Youmbi GT, Fusi F, *et al.* Potentiation of mitochondrial Ca^{2+} sequestration by taurine. Biochem Pharmacol 1999; 58(7): 1123-31.
[http://dx.doi.org/10.1016/S0006-2952(99)00183-5] [PMID: 10484070]

[40] Palmi M, Youmbi GT, Sgaragli G, Meini A, Benocci A, Fusi F, *et al.* The mitochondrial permeability transition and taurine.Taurine 4: Taurine and Excitable Tissues Advances in Experimental Medicine and Biology. Boston, MA: Springer US 2002; pp. 87-96.
[http://dx.doi.org/10.1007/0-306-46838-7_8]

[41] Schuller-Levis GB, Park E. Taurine: new implications for an old amino acid. FEMS Microbiol Lett 2003; 226(2): 195-202.
[http://dx.doi.org/10.1016/S0378-1097(03)00611-6] [PMID: 14553911]

[42] Park S-H, Lee H, Park KK, Kim HW, Lee DH, Park T, Eds. Taurine-induced changes in transcription profiling of metabolism-related genes in human hepatoma cells HepG22006. Springer US 2006.

[43] Warskulat U, Borsch E, Reinehr R, *et al.* Chronic liver disease is triggered by taurine transporter knockout in the mouse. FASEB J 2006; 20(3): 574-6.
[http://dx.doi.org/10.1096/fj.05-5016fje] [PMID: 16421246]

[44] Parvez S, Tabassum H, Banerjee BD, Raisuddin S. Taurine prevents tamoxifen-induced mitochondrial oxidative damage in mice. Basic Clin Pharmacol Toxicol 2008; 102(4): 382-7.
[http://dx.doi.org/10.1111/j.1742-7843.2008.00208.x] [PMID: 18312495]

[45] Ubuka T, Okada A, Nakamura H. Production of hypotaurine from l-cysteinesulfinate by rat liver mitochondria. Amino Acids 2008; 35(1): 53-8.
[http://dx.doi.org/10.1007/s00726-007-0633-x] [PMID: 18219548]

[46] Mortensen O, Olsen H, Frandsen L, *et al.* A maternal low protein diet has pronounced effects on mitochondrial gene expression in offspring liver and skeletal muscle; protective effect of taurine. J Biomed Sci 2010; 17(Suppl 1): S38.
[http://dx.doi.org/10.1186/1423-0127-17-S1-S38] [PMID: 20804614]

[47] El-Sayed WM, Al-Kahtani MA, Abdel-Moneim AM. Prophylactic and therapeutic effects of taurine against aluminum-induced acute hepatotoxicity in mice. J Hazard Mater 2011; 192(2): 880-6.
[http://dx.doi.org/10.1016/j.jhazmat.2011.05.100] [PMID: 21703760]

[48] Heidari R, Babaei H, Eghbal MA. Amodiaquine-induced toxicity in isolated rat hepatocytes and the cytoprotective effects of taurine and/or N-acetyl cysteine. Res Pharm Sci 2014; 9(2): 97-105.
[PMID: 25657778]

[49] Zhang Z, Liu D, Yi B, *et al.* Taurine supplementation reduces oxidative stress and protects the liver in an iron-overload murine model. Mol Med Rep 2014; 10(5): 2255-62.
[http://dx.doi.org/10.3892/mmr.2014.2544] [PMID: 25201602]

[50] Ahmadian E, Babaei H, Mohajjel Nayebi A, Eftekhari A, Eghbal MA. Venlafaxine-induced cytotoxicity towards isolated rat hepatocytes involves oxidative stress and mitochondrial/lysosomal dysfunction. Adv Pharm Bull 2016; 6(4): 521-30.
[http://dx.doi.org/10.15171/apb.2016.066] [PMID: 28101459]

[51] Jamshidzadeh A, Heidari R, Abasvali M, *et al.* Taurine treatment preserves brain and liver mitochondrial function in a rat model of fulminant hepatic failure and hyperammonemia. Biomed Pharmacother 2017; 86: 514-20.
[http://dx.doi.org/10.1016/j.biopha.2016.11.095] [PMID: 28024286]

[52] Eftekhari A, Ahmadian E, Azarmi Y, Parvizpur A, Fard JK, Eghbal MA. The effects of cimetidine, N-acetylcysteine, and taurine on thioridazine metabolic activation and induction of oxidative stress in isolated rat hepatocytes. Pharm Chem J 2018; 51(11): 965-9.
[http://dx.doi.org/10.1007/s11094-018-1724-6]

[53] Heidari R, Abdoli N, Ommati MM, Jamshidzadeh A, Niknahad H. Mitochondrial impairment induced by chenodeoxycholic acid: The protective effect of taurine and carnosine supplementation. Trends in Pharmaceutical Sciences. 2018;4(2).

[54] Wu G, Yang J, Lv H, *et al.* Taurine prevents ethanol-induced apoptosis mediated by mitochondrial or death receptor pathways in liver cells. Amino Acids 2018; 50(7): 863-75.
[http://dx.doi.org/10.1007/s00726-018-2561-3] [PMID: 29626300]

[55] Mohammadi H, Ommati MM, Farshad O, Jamshidzadeh A, Nikbakht MR, Niknahad H, *et al.* Taurine and isolated mitochondria: A concentration-response study. Trends Pharmacol Sci 2019; 5(4): 197-206.

[56] Butterworth RF. Taurine in Hepatic Encephalopathy. In: Huxtable RJ, Azuma J, Kuriyama K, Nakagawa M, Baba A, editors. Taurine 2. Advances in Experimental Medicine and Biology: Springer US; 1996. p. 601-6.
[http://dx.doi.org/10.1007/978-1-4899-0182-8_66]

[57] Ripps H, Shen W. Review: taurine: a "very essential" amino acid. Mol Vis 2012; 18: 2673-86.
[PMID: 23170060]

[58] Jacobsen JG, Smith LH. Biochemistry and physiology of taurine and taurine derivatives. Physiol Rev 1968; 48(2): 424-511.
[http://dx.doi.org/10.1152/physrev.1968.48.2.424] [PMID: 4297098]

[59] Hayes KC, Trautwein EA. Taurine deficiency syndrome in cats. Vet Clin North Am Small Anim Pract 1989; 19(3): 403-13.
[http://dx.doi.org/10.1016/S0195-5616(89)50052-4] [PMID: 2658282]

[60] Pion PD, Kittleson MD, Thomas WP, Skiles ML, Rogers QR. Clinical findings in cats with dilated cardiomyopathy and relationship of findings to taurine deficiency. J Am Vet Med Assoc 1992; 201(2): 267-74.
[PMID: 1500323]

[61] Dow SW, Fettman MJ, Smith KR, Ching SV, Hamar DW, Rogers QR. Taurine depletion and cardiovascular disease in adult cats fed a potassium-depleted acidified diet. Am J Vet Res 1992; 53(3): 402-5.
[PMID: 1534475]

[62] Lourenço R, Camilo ME. Taurine: a conditionally essential amino acid in humans? An overview in health and disease. Nutr Hosp 2002; 17(6): 262-70.
[PMID: 12514918]

[63] Stapleton PP, Charles RP, Redmond HP, Bouchier-Hayes DJ. Taurine and human nutrition. Clin Nutr

1997; 16(3): 103-8.
[http://dx.doi.org/10.1016/S0261-5614(97)80234-8] [PMID: 16844580]

[64] Yamori Y, Taguchi T, Hamada A, Kunimasa K, Mori H, Mori M. Taurine in health and diseases: consistent evidence from experimental and epidemiological studies. J Biomed Sci 2010; 17(Suppl 1): S6.
[http://dx.doi.org/10.1186/1423-0127-17-S1-S6] [PMID: 20804626]

[65] Seidel U, Huebbe P, Rimbach G. Taurine: A regulator of cellular redox homeostasis and skeletal muscle function. Mol Nutr Food Res 2019; 63(16): 1800569.
[http://dx.doi.org/10.1002/mnfr.201800569] [PMID: 30211983]

[66] De Luca A, Pierno S, Camerino DC. Taurine: the appeal of a safe amino acid for skeletal muscle disorders. J Transl Med 2015; 13(1): 243.
[http://dx.doi.org/10.1186/s12967-015-0610-1] [PMID: 26208967]

[67] Ito T, Oishi S, Takai M, *et al.* Cardiac and skeletal muscle abnormality in taurine transporter-knockout mice. J Biomed Sci 2010; 17(Suppl 1): S20.
[http://dx.doi.org/10.1186/1423-0127-17-S1-S20] [PMID: 20804595]

[68] Baliou S, Kyriakopoulos A, Goulielmaki M, Panayiotidis M, Spandidos D, Zoumpourlis V. Significance of taurine transporter (TauT) in homeostasis and its layers of regulation (Review). Mol Med Rep 2020; 22(3): 2163-73.
[http://dx.doi.org/10.3892/mmr.2020.11321] [PMID: 32705197]

[69] Pasantes-Morales H, Wright CE, Gaull GE. Taurine protection of lymphoblastoid cells from iron-ascorbate induced damage. Biochem Pharmacol 1985; 34(12): 2205-7.
[http://dx.doi.org/10.1016/0006-2952(85)90419-8] [PMID: 4004939]

[70] Nieminen ML, Tuomisto L, Solatunturi E, Eriksson L, Paasonen MK. Taurine in the osmoregulation of the Brattleboro rat. Life Sci 1988; 42(21): 2137-43.
[http://dx.doi.org/10.1016/0024-3205(88)90128-2] [PMID: 3386398]

[71] Nakamura T, Ogasawara M, Koyama I, Nemoto M, Yoshida T. The protective effect of taurine on the biomembrane against damage produced by oxygen radicals. Biol Pharm Bull 1993; 16(10): 970-2.
[http://dx.doi.org/10.1248/bpb.16.970] [PMID: 8287047]

[72] Huxtable RJ. Physiological actions of taurine. Physiol Rev 1992; 72(1): 101-63.
[http://dx.doi.org/10.1152/physrev.1992.72.1.101] [PMID: 1731369]

[73] Schaffer S, Azuma J, Takahashi K, Mozaffari M. Why is taurine cytoprotective? Taurine 5. Springer 2003; pp. 307-12.

[74] Wynn TA. Cellular and molecular mechanisms of fibrosis. J Pathol 2008; 214(2): 199-210.
[http://dx.doi.org/10.1002/path.2277] [PMID: 18161745]

[75] Lim YS, Kim WR. The global impact of hepatic fibrosis and end-stage liver disease. Clin Liver Dis 2008; 12(4): 733-46.
[http://dx.doi.org/10.1016/j.cld.2008.07.007] [PMID: 18984463]

[76] Angulo P, Kleiner DE, Dam-Larsen S, *et al.* Liver Fibrosis, but no other histologic features, is associated with long-term outcomes of patients with nonalcoholic fatty liver disease. Gastroenterology 2015; 149(2): 389-397.e10.
[http://dx.doi.org/10.1053/j.gastro.2015.04.043] [PMID: 25935633]

[77] Albanis E, Friedman SL. Hepatic fibrosis. Pathogenesis and principles of therapy. Clin Liver Dis 2001; 5(2): 315-34.
[http://dx.doi.org/10.1016/S1089-3261(05)70168-9] [PMID: 11385966]

[78] Benyon RC, Arthur MJP. Mechanisms of hepatic fibrosis. J Pediatr Gastroenterol Nutr 1998; 27(1): 75-85.
[http://dx.doi.org/10.1097/00005176-199807000-00013] [PMID: 9669730]

[79]   Trautwein C, Friedman SL, Schuppan D, Pinzani M. Hepatic fibrosis: Concept to treatment. J Hepatol 2015; 62(1) (Suppl.): S15-24.
[http://dx.doi.org/10.1016/j.jhep.2015.02.039] [PMID: 25920084]

[80]   Zhang CY, Yuan WG, He P, Lei JH, Wang CX. Liver fibrosis and hepatic stellate cells: Etiology, pathological hallmarks and therapeutic targets. World J Gastroenterol 2016; 22(48): 10512-22.
[http://dx.doi.org/10.3748/wjg.v22.i48.10512] [PMID: 28082803]

[81]   Wiegand J, Berg T. The etiology, diagnosis and prevention of liver cirrhosis: part 1 of a series on liver cirrhosis. Dtsch Arztebl Int 2013; 110(6): 85-91.
[PMID: 23451000]

[82]   Koyama Y, Xu J, Liu X, Brenner DA. New developments on the treatment of liver fibrosis. Dig Dis 2016; 34(5): 589-96.
[http://dx.doi.org/10.1159/000445269] [PMID: 27332862]

[83]   Schon HT, Bartneck M, Borkham-Kamphorst E, *et al.* Pharmacological intervention in hepatic Stellate cell activation and hepatic fibrosis. Front Pharmacol 2016; 7: 33.
[http://dx.doi.org/10.3389/fphar.2016.00033] [PMID: 26941644]

[84]   Bansal R, Nagórniewicz B, Prakash J. Clinical advancements in the targeted therapies against liver fibrosis. Mediators Inflamm 2016; 2016: 1-16.
[http://dx.doi.org/10.1155/2016/7629724] [PMID: 27999454]

[85]   Fallowfield JA, Jimenez-Ramos M, Robertson A. Emerging synthetic drugs for the treatment of liver cirrhosis. Expert Opin Emerg Drugs 2021; 26(2): 149-63.
[http://dx.doi.org/10.1080/14728214.2021.1918099] [PMID: 33856246]

[86]   Ahmadian E, Pennefather PS, Eftekhari A, Heidari R, Eghbal MA. Role of renin-angiotensin system in liver diseases: an outline on the potential therapeutic points of intervention. Expert Rev Gastroenterol Hepatol 2016; 10(11): 1279-88.
[http://dx.doi.org/10.1080/17474124.2016.1207523] [PMID: 27352778]

[87]   Moreira RK. Hepatic stellate cells and liver fibrosis. Arch Pathol Lab Med 2007; 131(11): 1728-34.
[http://dx.doi.org/10.5858/2007-131-1728-HSCALF] [PMID: 17979495]

[88]   Parola M, Robino G. Oxidative stress-related molecules and liver fibrosis. J Hepatol 2001; 35(2): 297-306.
[http://dx.doi.org/10.1016/S0168-8278(01)00142-8] [PMID: 11580156]

[89]   Tsukada S, Parsons CJ, Rippe RA. Mechanisms of liver fibrosis. Clin Chim Acta 2006; 364(1-2): 33-60.
[http://dx.doi.org/10.1016/j.cca.2005.06.014] [PMID: 16139830]

[90]   Sánchez-Valle V, Chávez-Tapia NC, Uribe M, Méndez-Sánchez N. Role of oxidative stress and molecular changes in liver fibrosis: a review. Curr Med Chem 2012; 19(28): 4850-60.
[http://dx.doi.org/10.2174/092986712803341520] [PMID: 22709007]

[91]   Tsukamoto H, Rippe R, Niemelä O, Lin M. Roles of oxidative stress in activation of Kupffer and Ito cells in liver fibrogenesis. J Gastroenterol Hepatol 1995; 10(S1): S50-3.
[http://dx.doi.org/10.1111/j.1440-1746.1995.tb01798.x] [PMID: 8589343]

[92]   Ghanbarinejad V, Ommati MM, Jia Z, Farshad O, Jamshidzadeh A, Heidari R. Disturbed mitochondrial redox state and tissue energy charge in cholestasis. J Biochem Mol Toxicol 2021; 35(9): e22846.
[http://dx.doi.org/10.1002/jbt.22846] [PMID: 34250697]

[93]   Ramos-Tovar E, Muriel P. Molecular mechanisms that link oxidative stress, inflammation, and fibrosis in the liver. Antioxidants 2020; 9(12): 1279.
[http://dx.doi.org/10.3390/antiox9121279] [PMID: 33333846]

[94]   Mousavi K, Niknahad H, Li H, *et al.* The activation of nuclear factor-E2-related factor 2 (Nrf2)/heme

oxygenase-1 (HO-1) signaling blunts cholestasis-induced liver and kidney injury. Toxicol Res (Camb) 2021; 10(4): 911-27.
[http://dx.doi.org/10.1093/toxres/tfab073] [PMID: 34484683]

[95]   Ahmadi A, Niknahad H, Li H, *et al*. The inhibition of NFκB signaling and inflammatory response as a strategy for blunting bile acid-induced hepatic and renal toxicity. Toxicol Lett 2021; 349: 12-29.
[http://dx.doi.org/10.1016/j.toxlet.2021.05.012] [PMID: 34089816]

[96]   Siavashpour A, Khalvati B, Azarpira N, Mohammadi H, Niknahad H, Heidari R. Poly (ADP-Ribose) polymerase-1 (PARP-1) overactivity plays a pathogenic role in bile acids-induced nephrotoxicity in cholestatic rats. Toxicol Lett 2020; 330: 144-58.
[http://dx.doi.org/10.1016/j.toxlet.2020.05.012] [PMID: 32422328]

[97]   Ommati MM, Mohammadi H, Mousavi K, Azarpira N, Farshad O, Dehghani R, *et al*. Metformin alleviates cholestasis-associated nephropathy through regulating oxidative stress and mitochondrial function. Liver Res 2020.

[98]   Ommati MM, Farshad O, Mousavi K, *et al*. Agmatine alleviates hepatic and renal injury in a rat model of obstructive jaundice. PharmaNutrition 2020; 13: 100212.
[http://dx.doi.org/10.1016/j.phanu.2020.100212]

[99]   Ommati MM, Attari H, Siavashpour A, Shafaghat M, Azarpira N, Ghaffari H, *et al*. Mitigation of cholestasis-associated hepatic and renal injury by edaravone treatment: Evaluation of its effects on oxidative stress and mitochondrial function. Liver Res 2020.

[100]   Farshad O, Ommati MM, Yüzügülen J, *et al*. Carnosine mitigates biomarkers of oxidative stress, improves mitochondrial function, and alleviates histopathological alterations in the renal tissue of cholestatic rats. Ulum-i Daruyi 2020; 27(1): 32-45.
[http://dx.doi.org/10.34172/PS.2020.60]

[101]   Heidari R, Mohammadi H, Ghanbarinejad V, *et al*. Proline supplementation mitigates the early stage of liver injury in bile duct ligated rats. J Basic Clin Physiol Pharmacol 2018; 30(1): 91-101.
[http://dx.doi.org/10.1515/jbcpp-2017-0221] [PMID: 30205645]

[102]   Heidari R, Mandegani L, Ghanbarinejad V, *et al*. Mitochondrial dysfunction as a mechanism involved in the pathogenesis of cirrhosis-associated cholemic nephropathy. Biomed Pharmacother 2019; 109: 271-80.
[http://dx.doi.org/10.1016/j.biopha.2018.10.104] [PMID: 30396085]

[103]   Heidari R, Ghanbarinejad V, Mohammadi H, *et al*. Mitochondria protection as a mechanism underlying the hepatoprotective effects of glycine in cholestatic mice. Biomed Pharmacother 2018; 97: 1086-95.
[http://dx.doi.org/10.1016/j.biopha.2017.10.166] [PMID: 29136945]

[104]   Heidari R, Ghanbarinejad V, Mohammadi H, *et al*. Dithiothreitol supplementation mitigates hepatic and renal injury in bile duct ligated mice: Potential application in the treatment of cholestasis-associated complications. Biomed Pharmacother 2018; 99: 1022-32.
[http://dx.doi.org/10.1016/j.biopha.2018.01.018] [PMID: 29307496]

[105]   Jamshidzadeh A, Heidari R, Latifpour Z, *et al*. Carnosine ameliorates liver fibrosis and hyperammonemia in cirrhotic rats. Clin Res Hepatol Gastroenterol 2017; 41(4): 424-34.
[http://dx.doi.org/10.1016/j.clinre.2016.12.010] [PMID: 28283328]

[106]   Heidari R, Moezi L, Asadi B, Ommati MM, Azarpira N. Hepatoprotective effect of boldine in a bile duct ligated rat model of cholestasis/cirrhosis. PharmaNutrition 2017; 5(3): 109-17.
[http://dx.doi.org/10.1016/j.phanu.2017.07.001]

[107]   Mousavi K, Niknahad H, Ghalamfarsa A, *et al*. Taurine mitigates cirrhosis-associated heart injury through mitochondrial-dependent and antioxidative mechanisms. Clin Exp Hepatol 2020; 6(3): 207-19.
[http://dx.doi.org/10.5114/ceh.2020.99513] [PMID: 33145427]

[108] Ommati MM, Heidari R, Ghanbarinejad V, Abdoli N, Niknahad H. Taurine treatment provides neuroprotection in a mouse model of manganism. Biol Trace Elem Res 2019; 190(2): 384-95.
[http://dx.doi.org/10.1007/s12011-018-1552-2] [PMID: 30357569]

[109] Heidari R, Behnamrad S, Khodami Z, Ommati MM, Azarpira N, Vazin A. The nephroprotective properties of taurine in colistin-treated mice is mediated through the regulation of mitochondrial function and mitigation of oxidative stress. Biomed Pharmacother 2019; 109: 103-11.
[http://dx.doi.org/10.1016/j.biopha.2018.10.093] [PMID: 30396066]

[110] Heidari R, Jamshidzadeh A, Ghanbarinejad V, Ommati MM, Niknahad H. Taurine supplementation abates cirrhosis-associated locomotor dysfunction. Clin Exp Hepatol 2018; 4(2): 72-82.
[http://dx.doi.org/10.5114/ceh.2018.75956] [PMID: 29904723]

[111] Niknahad H, Jamshidzadeh A, Heidari R, Zarei M, Ommati MM. Ammonia-induced mitochondrial dysfunction and energy metabolism disturbances in isolated brain and liver mitochondria, and the effect of taurine administration: relevance to hepatic encephalopathy treatment. Clin Exp Hepatol 2017; 3(3): 141-51.
[http://dx.doi.org/10.5114/ceh.2017.68833] [PMID: 29062904]

[112] Jamshidzadeh A, Abdoli N, Niknahad H, Azarpira N, Mardani E, Mousavi S, et al. Taurine alleviates brain tissue markers of oxidative stress in a rat model of hepatic encephalopathy. Trends Pharmacol Sci 2017; 3(3): 181-92.

[113] Heidari R, Jamshidzadeh A, Niknahad H, Safari F, Azizi H, Abdoli N, et al. The hepatoprotection provided by taurine and glycine against antineoplastic drugs induced liver injury in an ex vivo model of normothermic recirculating isolated perfused rat liver. Trends Pharmacol Sci 2016; 2(1): 59-76.

[114] Wang Q, Hollinger MA, Giri SN. Attenuation of amiodarone-induced lung fibrosis and phospholipidosis in hamsters by taurine and/or niacin treatment. J Pharmacol Exp Ther 1992; 262(1): 127-32.
[PMID: 1625191]

[115] Robb WB, Condron C, Moriarty M, Walsh TN, Bouchier-Hayes DJ. Taurine attenuates radiation-induced lung fibrosis in C57/Bl6 fibrosis prone mice. Ir J Med Sci 2010; 179(1): 99-105.
[http://dx.doi.org/10.1007/s11845-009-0389-2] [PMID: 19609640]

[116] Das J, Sil PC. Taurine ameliorates alloxan-induced diabetic renal injury, oxidative stress-related signaling pathways and apoptosis in rats. Amino Acids 2012; 43(4): 1509-23.
[http://dx.doi.org/10.1007/s00726-012-1225-y] [PMID: 22302365]

[117] Sato S, Yamate J, Saito T, Hosokawa T, Saito S, Kurasaki M. Protective effect of taurine against renal interstitial fibrosis of rats induced by cisplatin. Naunyn Schmiedebergs Arch Pharmacol 2002; 365(4): 277-83.
[http://dx.doi.org/10.1007/s00210-001-0524-8] [PMID: 11919651]

[118] Jong CJ, Azuma J, Schaffer S. Mechanism underlying the antioxidant activity of taurine: prevention of mitochondrial oxidant production. Amino Acids 2012; 42(6): 2223-32.
[http://dx.doi.org/10.1007/s00726-011-0962-7] [PMID: 21691752]

[119] Ljubuncic P, Tanne Z, Bomzon A. Evidence of a systemic phenomenon for oxidative stress in cholestatic liver disease. Gut 2000; 47(5): 710-6.
[http://dx.doi.org/10.1136/gut.47.5.710] [PMID: 11034590]

[120] Lizana P, Galdames M, Rodrigo R. Oxidative stress and endoplasmic reticulum stress as potential therapeutic targets in non-alcoholic fatty liver disease. Reactive Oxygen Species. 2017;4(10):266-7-74.
[http://dx.doi.org/10.20455/ros.2017.847]

[121] Camini FC, da Silva Caetano CC, Almeida LT, de Brito Magalhães CL. Implications of oxidative stress on viral pathogenesis. Arch Virol 2017; 162(4): 907-17.
[http://dx.doi.org/10.1007/s00705-016-3187-y] [PMID: 28039563]

[122] Pérez R, García-Fernández M, Díaz-Sánchez M, *et al.* Mitochondrial protection by low doses of insulin-like growth factor-Iin experimental cirrhosis. World J Gastroenterol 2008; 14(17): 2731-9.
[http://dx.doi.org/10.3748/wjg.14.2731] [PMID: 18461658]

[123] Mitchell C, Robin MA, Mayeuf A, *et al.* Protection against hepatocyte mitochondrial dysfunction delays fibrosis progression in mice. Am J Pathol 2009; 175(5): 1929-37.
[http://dx.doi.org/10.2353/ajpath.2009.090332] [PMID: 19808650]

[124] Lakshmi Devi S, Anuradha CV. Mitochondrial damage, cytotoxicity and apoptosis in iron-potentiated alcoholic liver fibrosis: amelioration by taurine. Amino Acids 2010; 38(3): 869-79.
[http://dx.doi.org/10.1007/s00726-009-0293-0] [PMID: 19381777]

[125] Feng X, Hu W, Hong Y, Ruan L, Hu Y, Liu D. Taurine ameliorates iron overload-induced hepatocyte injury via the Bcl-2/VDAC1-mediated mitochondrial apoptosis pathway. Oxid Med Cell Longev 2022; 2022: 1-14.
[http://dx.doi.org/10.1155/2022/4135752] [PMID: 35879990]

[126] Wu G, San J, Pang H, *et al.* Taurine attenuates AFB1-induced liver injury by alleviating oxidative stress and regulating mitochondria-mediated apoptosis. Toxicon 2022; 215: 17-27.
[http://dx.doi.org/10.1016/j.toxicon.2022.06.003] [PMID: 35688267]

[127] Zheng J, Qiu G, Zhou Y, Ma K, Cui S. Hepatoprotective effects of taurine against cadmium-induced liver injury in female mice. Biol Trace Elem Res 2022.
[PMID: 35581430]

[128] Heidari R, Niknahad H, Sadeghi A, *et al.* Betaine treatment protects liver through regulating mitochondrial function and counteracting oxidative stress in acute and chronic animal models of hepatic injury. Biomed Pharmacother 2018; 103: 75-86.
[http://dx.doi.org/10.1016/j.biopha.2018.04.010] [PMID: 29635131]

[129] Krähenbühl S, Talos C, Lauterburg BH, Reichen J. Reduced antioxidative capacity in liver mitochondria from bile duct ligated rats*1. Hepatology 1995; 22(2): 607-12.
[http://dx.doi.org/10.1016/0270-9139(95)90586-3] [PMID: 7635430]

[130] Sastre J, Serviddio G, Tormos AM, Monsalve M, Sastre J. Mitochondrial dysfunction in cholestatic liver diseases. Front Biosci (Elite Ed) 2012; E4(6): 2233-52.
[http://dx.doi.org/10.2741/e539] [PMID: 22202034]

[131] Heidari R, Niknahad H. The role and study of mitochondrial impairment and oxidative stress in cholestasis.Experimental Cholestasis Research Methods in Molecular Biology. New York, NY: Springer 2019; pp. 117-32.
[http://dx.doi.org/10.1007/978-1-4939-9420-5_8]

[132] Ommati MM, Farshad O, Niknahad H, *et al.* Cholestasis-associated reproductive toxicity in male and female rats: The fundamental role of mitochondrial impairment and oxidative stress. Toxicol Lett 2019; 316: 60-72.
[http://dx.doi.org/10.1016/j.toxlet.2019.09.009] [PMID: 31520699]

[133] Abdoli N, Sadeghian I, Mousavi K, Azarpira N, Ommati MM, Heidari R. Suppression of cirrhosis-related renal injury by N-acetyl cysteine. Current Research in Pharmacology and Drug Discovery 2020; 1: 30-8.
[http://dx.doi.org/10.1016/j.crphar.2020.100006] [PMID: 34909640]

[134] Heidari R, Ahmadi A, Ommati MM, Niknahad H. Methylene blue improves mitochondrial function in the liver of cholestatic rats. Trends Pharmacol Sci 2020; 6(2): 73-86.

[135] Ommati MM, Farshad O, Mousavi K, *et al.* Betaine supplementation mitigates intestinal damage and decreases serum bacterial endotoxin in cirrhotic rats. PharmaNutrition 2020; 12: 100179.
[http://dx.doi.org/10.1016/j.phanu.2020.100179]

[136] Ghanbarinejad V, Jamshidzadeh A, Khalvati B, *et al.* Apoptosis-inducing factor plays a role in the pathogenesis of hepatic and renal injury during cholestasis. Naunyn Schmiedebergs Arch Pharmacol

2021; 394(6): 1191-203.
[http://dx.doi.org/10.1007/s00210-020-02041-7] [PMID: 33527194]

[137]   Ommati MM, Farshad O, Azarpira N, Ghazanfari E, Niknahad H, Heidari R. Silymarin mitigates bile duct obstruction-induced cholemic nephropathy. Naunyn Schmiedebergs Arch Pharmacol 2021; 394(6): 1301-14.
[http://dx.doi.org/10.1007/s00210-020-02040-8] [PMID: 33538845]

[138]   Seabra V, Stachlewitz RF, Thurman RG. Taurine blunts LPS-induced increases in intracellular calcium and TNF-α production by Kupffer cells. J Leukoc Biol 1998; 64(5): 615-21.
[http://dx.doi.org/10.1002/jlb.64.5.615] [PMID: 9823766]

[139]   Kisseleva T, Brenner DA. Role of hepatic stellate cells in fibrogenesis and the reversal of fibrosis. J Gastroenterol Hepatol 2007; 22(s1): S73-8.
[http://dx.doi.org/10.1111/j.1440-1746.2006.04658.x] [PMID: 17567473]

[140]   Deng X, Liang J, Lin Z-X, Wu F-S, Zhang Y-P, Zhang Z-W. Natural taurine promotes apoptosis of human hepatic stellate cells in proteomics analysis. World J Gastroenterol 2010; 16(15): 1916-23.
[http://dx.doi.org/10.3748/wjg.v16.i15.1916] [PMID: 20397272]

[141]   Wei S, Huang Q, Li J, *et al.* Taurine attenuates liver injury by downregulating phosphorylated p38 MAPK of Kupffer cells in rats with severe acute pancreatitis. Inflammation 2012; 35(2): 690-701.
[http://dx.doi.org/10.1007/s10753-011-9362-0] [PMID: 21833764]

[142]   Kolios G, Valatas V, Kouroumalis E. Role of Kupffer cells in the pathogenesis of liver disease. World J Gastroenterol 2006; 12(46): 7413-20.
[http://dx.doi.org/10.3748/wjg.v12.i46.7413] [PMID: 17167827]

[143]   Miyazaki T, Bouscarel B, Ikegami T, Honda A, Matsuzaki Y. The protective effect of taurine against hepatic damage in a model of liver disease and hepatic stellate cells Taurine 7. Springer 2009; pp. 293-303.
[http://dx.doi.org/10.1007/978-0-387-75681-3_30]

[144]   Chen YX, Zhang XR, Xie WF, Li S. Effects of taurine on proliferation and apoptosis of hepatic stellate cells in vitro. Hepatobiliary Pancreat Dis Int 2004; 3(1): 106-9.
[PMID: 14969850]

[145]   Niu X, Zheng S, Liu H, Li S. Protective effects of taurine against inflammation, apoptosis, and oxidative stress in brain injury. Mol Med Rep 2018; 18(5): 4516-22.
[http://dx.doi.org/10.3892/mmr.2018.9465] [PMID: 30221665]

[146]   Giriş M, Depboylu B, Doğru-Abbasoğlu S, *et al.* Effect of taurine on oxidative stress and apoptosis-related protein expression in trinitrobenzene sulphonic acid-induced colitis. Clin Exp Immunol 2008; 152(1): 102-10.
[http://dx.doi.org/10.1111/j.1365-2249.2008.03599.x] [PMID: 18241224]

[147]   Hockenbery DM, Oltvai ZN, Yin XM, Milliman CL, Korsmeyer SJ. Bcl-2 functions in an antioxidant pathway to prevent apoptosis. Cell 1993; 75(2): 241-51.
[http://dx.doi.org/10.1016/0092-8674(93)80066-N] [PMID: 7503812]

[148]   Kane D, Sarafian T, Anton R, *et al.* Bcl-2 inhibition of neural death: decreased generation of reactive oxygen species. Science 1993; 262(5137): 1274-7.
[http://dx.doi.org/10.1126/science.8235659] [PMID: 8235659]

[149]   Gross A. BCL-2 family proteins as regulators of mitochondria metabolism. Biochim Biophys Acta Bioenerg 2016; 1857(8): 1243-6.
[http://dx.doi.org/10.1016/j.bbabio.2016.01.017] [PMID: 26827940]

[150]   Tu S, Zhang XL, Wan HF, *et al.* Effect of taurine on cell proliferation and apoptosis human lung cancer A549 cells. Oncol Lett 2018; 15(4): 5473-80.
[http://dx.doi.org/10.3892/ol.2018.8036] [PMID: 29552188]

[151]   Zhang X, Tu S, Wang Y, Xu B, Wan F. Mechanism of taurine-induced apoptosis in human colon

cancer cells. Acta Biochim Biophys Sin (Shanghai) 2014; 46(4): 261-72.
[http://dx.doi.org/10.1093/abbs/gmu004] [PMID: 24610575]

[152]   Szabo G, Kamath PS, Shah VH, Thursz M, Mathurin P, Meeting E-AJ, *et al.* Alcohol-related liver disease: areas of consensus, unmet needs and opportunities for further study. Hepatology 2019; 69(5): 2271-83.
[http://dx.doi.org/10.1002/hep.30369] [PMID: 30645002]

[153]   Arab JP, Roblero JP, Altamirano J, *et al.* Alcohol-related liver disease: Clinical practice guidelines by the Latin American Association for the Study of the Liver (ALEH). Ann Hepatol 2019; 18(3): 518-35.
[http://dx.doi.org/10.1016/j.aohep.2019.04.005] [PMID: 31053546]

[154]   Gustot T, Jalan R. Acute-on-chronic liver failure in patients with alcohol-related liver disease. J Hepatol 2019; 70(2): 319-27.
[http://dx.doi.org/10.1016/j.jhep.2018.12.008] [PMID: 30658733]

[155]   Kerai MDJ, Waterfield CJ, Kenyon SH, Asker DS, Timbrell JA. Reversal of ethanol-induced hepatic steatosis and lipid peroxidation by taurine: a study in rats. Alcohol Alcohol 1999; 34(4): 529-41.
[http://dx.doi.org/10.1093/alcalc/34.4.529] [PMID: 10456581]

[156]   Lin CJ, Chiu CC, Chen YC, Chen ML, Hsu TC, Tzang BS. Taurine attenuates hepatic inflammation in chronic alcohol-fed rats through inhibition of TLR4/MyD88 signaling. J Med Food 2015; 18(12): 1291-8.
[http://dx.doi.org/10.1089/jmf.2014.3408] [PMID: 26090712]

[157]   Hsieh YL, Yeh YH, Lee YT, Huang CY. Effect of taurine in chronic alcoholic patients. Food Funct 2014; 5(7): 1529-35.
[http://dx.doi.org/10.1039/C3FO60597C] [PMID: 24841875]

[158]   Chen X, Sebastian BM, Tang H, *et al.* Taurine supplementation prevents ethanol-induced decrease in serum adiponectin and reduces hepatic steatosis in rats. Hepatology 2009; 49(5): 1554-62.
[http://dx.doi.org/10.1002/hep.22811] [PMID: 19296466]

[159]   Kerai MDJ, Waterfield CJ, Kenyon SH, Asker DS, Timbrell JA. Taurine: Protective properties against ethanol-induced hepatic steatosis and lipid peroxidation during chronic ethanol consumption in rats. Amino Acids 1998; 15(1-2): 53-76.
[http://dx.doi.org/10.1007/BF01345280] [PMID: 9871487]

[160]   Pushpakiran G, Mahalakshmi K, Anuradha CV. Taurine restores ethanol-induced depletion of antioxidants and attenuates oxidative stress in rat tissues. Amino Acids 2004; 27(1): 91-6.
[http://dx.doi.org/10.1007/s00726-004-0066-8] [PMID: 15309576]

[161]   Goc Z, Kapusta E, Formicki G, Martiniaková M, Omelka R. Effect of taurine on ethanol-induced oxidative stress in mouse liver and kidney. Chin J Physiol 2019; 62(4): 148-56.
[http://dx.doi.org/10.4103/CJP.CJP_28_19] [PMID: 31535630]

[162]   Balkan J, Kanbağli Ö, Aykaç-Toker G, Uysal M. Taurine treatment reduces hepatic lipids and oxidative stress in chronically ethanol-treated rats. Biol Pharm Bull 2002; 25(9): 1231-3.
[http://dx.doi.org/10.1248/bpb.25.1231] [PMID: 12230126]

[163]   Kerai MDJ, Waterfield CJ, Kenyon SH, Asker DS, Timbrell JA. The effect of taurine depletion by β-alanine treatment on the susceptibility to ethanol-induced hepatic dysfunction in rats. Alcohol Alcohol 2001; 36(1): 29-38.
[http://dx.doi.org/10.1093/alcalc/36.1.29] [PMID: 11139413]

[164]   Wu D, Cederbaum A. Oxidative stress and alcoholic liver disease. Semin Liver Dis 2009; 29(2): 141-54.
[http://dx.doi.org/10.1055/s-0029-1214370] [PMID: 19387914]

[165]   Tan HK, Yates E, Lilly K, Dhanda AD. Oxidative stress in alcohol-related liver disease. World J Hepatol 2020; 12(7): 332-49.
[http://dx.doi.org/10.4254/wjh.v12.i7.332] [PMID: 32821333]

[166] Ambade A, Mandrekar P. Oxidative stress and inflammation: essential partners in alcoholic liver disease. Int J Hepatol 2012; 2012: 1-9.
       [http://dx.doi.org/10.1155/2012/853175] [PMID: 22500241]

[167] Albano E. Alcohol, oxidative stress and free radical damage. Proc Nutr Soc 2006; 65(3): 278-90.
       [http://dx.doi.org/10.1079/PNS2006496] [PMID: 16923312]

[168] Tsedensodnom O, Vacaru AM, Howarth DL, Yin C, Sadler KC. Ethanol metabolism and oxidative stress are required for unfolded protein response activation and steatosis in zebrafish with alcoholic liver disease. Dis Model Mech 2013; 6(5): 1213-26.
       [PMID: 23798569]

[169] Han KH, Hashimoto N, Fukushima M. Relationships among alcoholic liver disease, antioxidants, and antioxidant enzymes. World J Gastroenterol 2016; 22(1): 37-49.
       [http://dx.doi.org/10.3748/wjg.v22.i1.37] [PMID: 26755859]

[170] Galicia-Moreno M, Rosique-Oramas D, Medina-Avila Z, *et al.* Behavior of oxidative stress markers in alcoholic liver cirrhosis patients. Oxid Med Cell Longev 2016; 2016: 1-10.
       [http://dx.doi.org/10.1155/2016/9370565] [PMID: 28074118]

[171] Palmi M, Youmbi GT, Sgaragli G, Meini A, Benocci A, Fusi F, *et al.* The mitochondrial permeability transition and taurine Taurine 4. Springer 2002; pp. 87-96.

[172] Schaffer S, Azuma J, Takahashi K, Mozaffari M. Why Is Taurine Cytoprotective?Taurine 5: Beginning the 21st Century. Advances in Experimental Medicine and Biology.. Boston, MA: Springer US 2003; pp. 307-21.
       [http://dx.doi.org/10.1007/978-1-4615-0077-3_39]

[173] Hansen S, Andersen M, Cornett C, Gradinaru R, Grunnet N. A role for taurine in mitochondrial function. J Biomed Sci 2010; 17(Suppl 1): S23.
       [http://dx.doi.org/10.1186/1423-0127-17-S1-S23] [PMID: 20804598]

[174] Shimada K, Jong CJ, Takahashi K, Schaffer SW, Eds. Role of ROS production and turnover in the antioxidant activity of taurine2015. Cham: Springer International Publishing 2015.

[175] Jong C, Ito T, Prentice H, Wu JY, Schaffer S. Role of mitochondria and endoplasmic reticulum in taurine-deficiency-mediated apoptosis. Nutrients 2017; 9(8): 795.
       [http://dx.doi.org/10.3390/nu9080795] [PMID: 28757580]

[176] Kono H, Rusyn I, Yin M, *et al.* NADPH oxidase–derived free radicals are key oxidants in alcohol-induced liver disease. J Clin Invest 2000; 106(7): 867-72.
       [http://dx.doi.org/10.1172/JCI9020] [PMID: 11018074]

[177] De Minicis S, Brenner DA. Oxidative stress in alcoholic liver disease: Role of NADPH oxidase complex. J Gastroenterol Hepatol 2008; 23(s1): S98-S103.
       [http://dx.doi.org/10.1111/j.1440-1746.2007.05277.x] [PMID: 18336675]

[178] Wu G, Yang J, Sun C, Luan X, Shi J, Hu J. Effect of taurine on alcoholic liver disease in rats. Amino Acids 2009; 36(3): 457-64.
       [http://dx.doi.org/10.1007/s00726-008-0101-2] [PMID: 18509591]

[179] Latchoumycandane C, Nagy LE, McIntyre TM. Chronic ethanol ingestion induces oxidative kidney injury through taurine-inhibitable inflammation. Free Radic Biol Med 2014; 69: 403-16.
       [http://dx.doi.org/10.1016/j.freeradbiomed.2014.01.001] [PMID: 24412858]

[180] Bailey SM, Cunningham CC. Contribution of mitochondria to oxidative stress associated with alcoholic liver disease1 1This article is part of a series of reviews on "Alcohol, Oxidative Stress and Cell Injury". The full list of papers may be found on the homepage of the journal. Free Radic Biol Med 2002; 32(1): 11-6.
       [http://dx.doi.org/10.1016/S0891-5849(01)00769-9] [PMID: 11755312]

[181] Adachi M, Ishii H. Role of mitochondria in alcoholic liver injury. Free Radic Biol Med 2002; 32(6):

487-91.
[http://dx.doi.org/10.1016/S0891-5849(02)00740-2] [PMID: 11958949]

[182]   Hoek JB, Cahill A, Pastorino JG. Alcohol and mitochondria: A dysfunctional relationship. Gastroenterology 2002; 122(7): 2049-63.
[http://dx.doi.org/10.1053/gast.2002.33613] [PMID: 12055609]

[183]   Abdallah MA, Singal AK. Mitochondrial dysfunction and alcohol-associated liver disease: a novel pathway and therapeutic target. Signal Transduct Target Ther 2020; 5(1): 26.
[http://dx.doi.org/10.1038/s41392-020-0128-8] [PMID: 32296016]

[184]   Shim K, Park G, Kim S-B. Effects of taurine supplementation on mitochondrial function in chronic ethanol administered rats. J Community Nutr 2005; 7(3): 163-8.

[185]   Olive MF. Interactions between taurine and ethanol in the central nervous system. Amino Acids 2002; 23(4): 345-57.
[http://dx.doi.org/10.1007/s00726-002-0203-1] [PMID: 12436202]

[186]   Hansen AW, Almeida FB, Bandiera S, *et al.* Taurine restores the exploratory behavior following alcohol withdrawal and decreases BDNF mRNA expression in the frontal cortex of chronic alcohol-treated rats. Pharmacol Biochem Behav 2017; 161: 6-12.
[http://dx.doi.org/10.1016/j.pbb.2017.09.001] [PMID: 28882570]

[187]   Bhala N, Angulo P, van der Poorten D, *et al.* The natural history of nonalcoholic fatty liver disease with advanced fibrosis or cirrhosis: An international collaborative study. Hepatology 2011; 54(4): 1208-16.
[http://dx.doi.org/10.1002/hep.24491] [PMID: 21688282]

[188]   Angulo P. Nonalcoholic fatty liver disease and liver transplantation. Liver Transpl 2006; 12(4): 523-34.
[http://dx.doi.org/10.1002/lt.20738] [PMID: 16555318]

[189]   Huang TD, Behary J, Zekry A. Non-alcoholic fatty liver disease: a review of epidemiology, risk factors, diagnosis and management. Intern Med J 2020; 50(9): 1038-47.
[http://dx.doi.org/10.1111/imj.14709] [PMID: 31760676]

[190]   Kutlu O, Kaleli HN, Ozer E. Molecular pathogenesis of nonalcoholic steatohepatitis- (NASH-) related hepatocellular carcinoma. Can J Gastroenterol Hepatol. 2018.

[191]   Bugianesi E, Marzocchi R, Villanova N, Marchesini G. Non-alcoholic fatty liver disease/non-alcoholic steatohepatitis (NAFLD/NASH): treatment. Best Pract Res Clin Gastroenterol 2004; 18(6): 1105-16.
[http://dx.doi.org/10.1016/S1521-6918(04)00086-1] [PMID: 15561641]

[192]   Videla LA, Rodrigo R, Araya J, Poniachik J. Insulin resistance and oxidative stress interdependency in non-alcoholic fatty liver disease. Trends Mol Med 2006; 12(12): 555-8.
[http://dx.doi.org/10.1016/j.molmed.2006.10.001] [PMID: 17049925]

[193]   Azarang A, Farshad O, Ommati MM, *et al.* Protective role of probiotic supplements in hepatic steatosis: A rat model study. BioMed Res Int 2020; 2020: 1-15.
[http://dx.doi.org/10.1155/2020/5487659] [PMID: 33299871]

[194]   Ommati MM, Li H, Jamshidzadeh A, Khoshghadam F, Retana-Márquez S, Lu Y, *et al.* The crucial role of oxidative stress in non-alcoholic fatty liver disease-induced male reproductive toxicity: the ameliorative effects of Iranian indigenous probiotics. Naunyn Schmiedebergs Arch Pharmacol 2022; 395(2): 247-65.
[http://dx.doi.org/10.1007/s00210-021-02177-0]

[195]   Satapati S, Kucejova B, Duarte JAG, *et al.* Mitochondrial metabolism mediates oxidative stress and inflammation in fatty liver. J Clin Invest 2015; 125(12): 4447-62.
[http://dx.doi.org/10.1172/JCI82204] [PMID: 26571396]

[196]   Mantena SK, King AL, Andringa KK, Eccleston HB, Bailey SM. Mitochondrial dysfunction and oxidative stress in the pathogenesis of alcohol- and obesity-induced fatty liver diseases. Free Radic

Biol Med 2008; 44(7): 1259-72.
[http://dx.doi.org/10.1016/j.freeradbiomed.2007.12.029] [PMID: 18242193]

[197] Sumida Y, Niki E, Naito Y, Yoshikawa T. Involvement of free radicals and oxidative stress in NAFLD/NASH. Free Radic Res 2013; 47(11): 869-80.
[http://dx.doi.org/10.3109/10715762.2013.837577] [PMID: 24004441]

[198] Farrell GC, Rooyen D, Gan L, Chitturi S. NASH is an inflammatory disorder: pathogenic, prognostic and therapeutic implications. Gut Liver 2012; 6(2): 149-71.
[http://dx.doi.org/10.5009/gnl.2012.6.2.149] [PMID: 22570745]

[199] Gujral JS, Hinson JA, Farhood A, Jaeschke H. NADPH oxidase-derived oxidant stress is critical for neutrophil cytotoxicity during endotoxemia. Am J Physiol Gastrointest Liver Physiol 2004; 287(1): G243-52.
[http://dx.doi.org/10.1152/ajpgi.00287.2003] [PMID: 15044177]

[200] Liang S, Kisseleva T, Brenner DA. The role of NADPH oxidases (NOXs) in liver fibrosis and the activation of myofibroblasts. Front Physiol 2016; 7: 17.
[http://dx.doi.org/10.3389/fphys.2016.00017] [PMID: 26869935]

[201] Mittal M, Siddiqui MR, Tran K, Reddy SP, Malik AB. Reactive oxygen species in inflammation and tissue injury. Antioxid Redox Signal 2014; 20(7): 1126-67.
[http://dx.doi.org/10.1089/ars.2012.5149] [PMID: 23991888]

[202] Fromenty B, Robin MA, Igoudjil A, Mansouri A, Pessayre D. The ins and outs of mitochondrial dysfunction in NASH. Diabetes Metab 2004; 30(2): 121-38.
[http://dx.doi.org/10.1016/S1262-3636(07)70098-8] [PMID: 15223984]

[203] Begriche K, Igoudjil A, Pessayre D, Fromenty B. Mitochondrial dysfunction in NASH: Causes, consequences and possible means to prevent it. Mitochondrion 2006; 6(1): 1-28.
[http://dx.doi.org/10.1016/j.mito.2005.10.004] [PMID: 16406828]

[204] Pessayre D, Fromenty B. NASH: a mitochondrial disease. J Hepatol 2005; 42(6): 928-40.
[http://dx.doi.org/10.1016/j.jhep.2005.03.004] [PMID: 15885365]

[205] Nassir F, Ibdah J. Role of mitochondria in nonalcoholic fatty liver disease. Int J Mol Sci 2014; 15(5): 8713-42.
[http://dx.doi.org/10.3390/ijms15058713] [PMID: 24837835]

[206] Dornas W, Schuppan D. Mitochondrial oxidative injury: a key player in nonalcoholic fatty liver disease. Am J Physiol Gastrointest Liver Physiol 2020; 319(3): G400-11.
[http://dx.doi.org/10.1152/ajpgi.00121.2020] [PMID: 32597705]

[207] García-Ruiz C, Fernández-Checa JC. Mitochondrial oxidative stress and antioxidants balance in fatty liver disease. Hepatol Commun 2018; 2(12): 1425-39.
[http://dx.doi.org/10.1002/hep4.1271] [PMID: 30556032]

[208] Chen SW, Chen YX, Shi J, Lin Y, Xie WF. The restorative effect of taurine on experimental nonalcoholic steatohepatitis. Dig Dis Sci 2006; 51(12): 2225-34.
[http://dx.doi.org/10.1007/s10620-006-9359-y] [PMID: 17080243]

[209] Gentile CL, Nivala AM, Gonzales JC, *et al.* Experimental evidence for therapeutic potential of taurine in the treatment of nonalcoholic fatty liver disease. Am J Physiol Regul Integr Comp Physiol 2011; 301(6): R1710-22.
[http://dx.doi.org/10.1152/ajpregu.00677.2010] [PMID: 21957160]

[210] Murakami S, Ono A, Kawasaki A, Takenaga T, Ito T. Taurine attenuates the development of hepatic steatosis through the inhibition of oxidative stress in a model of nonalcoholic fatty liver disease *in vivo* and *in vitro*. Amino Acids 2018; 50(9): 1279-88.
[http://dx.doi.org/10.1007/s00726-018-2605-8] [PMID: 29946793]

[211] Weltman MD, Farrell GC, Hall P, Ingelman-Sundberg M, Liddle C. Hepatic cytochrome P450 2E1 is increased in patients with nonalcoholic steatohepatitis. Hepatology 1998; 27(1): 128-33.

[http://dx.doi.org/10.1002/hep.510270121] [PMID: 9425928]

[212] Weltman MD, Farrell GC, Liddle C. Increased hepatocyte CYP2E1 expression in a rat nutritional model of hepatic steatosis with inflammation. Gastroenterology 1996; 111(6): 1645-53.
[http://dx.doi.org/10.1016/S0016-5085(96)70028-8] [PMID: 8942745]

[213] Heidari R, Niknahad H, Jamshidzadeh A, Abdoli N. Factors affecting drug-induced liver injury: antithyroid drugs as instances. Clin Mol Hepatol 2014; 20(3): 237-48.
[http://dx.doi.org/10.3350/cmh.2014.20.3.237] [PMID: 25320726]

[214] Heidari R, Niknahad H, Jamshidzadeh A, Eghbal MA, Abdoli N. An overview on the proposed mechanisms of antithyroid drugs-induced liver injury. Adv Pharm Bull 2015; 5(1): 1-11.
[PMID: 25789213]

[215] Wang Q, Huang A, Wang JB, Zou Z. Chronic drug-induced liver injury: Updates and future challenges. Front Pharmacol 2021; 12: 627133.
[http://dx.doi.org/10.3389/fphar.2021.627133] [PMID: 33762948]

[216] Gerbes AL. Drug-induced liver injury (DILI): A major challenge. Drug Res. 2021;71(S 1):S7-S.

[217] Heidari R, Babaei H, Eghbal MA. Ameliorative effects of taurine against methimazole-induced cytotoxicity in isolated rat hepatocytes. Sci Pharm 2012; 80(4): 987-99.
[http://dx.doi.org/10.3797/scipharm.1205-16] [PMID: 23264945]

[218] Heidari R, Babaei H, Eghbal M. Mechanisms of methimazole cytotoxicity in isolated rat hepatocytes. Drug Chem Toxicol 2013; 36(4): 403-11.
[http://dx.doi.org/10.3109/01480545.2012.749272] [PMID: 23256569]

[219] Heidari R, Babaei H, Eghbal MA. Cytoprotective effects of organosulfur compounds against methimazole induced toxicity in isolated rat hepatocytes. Adv Pharm Bull 2013; 3(1): 135-42.
[PMID: 24312826]

[220] Abdoli N, Heidari R, Azarmi Y, Eghbal MA. Mechanisms of the statins cytotoxicity in freshly isolated rat hepatocytes. J Biochem Mol Toxicol 2013; 27(6): 287-94.
[http://dx.doi.org/10.1002/jbt.21485] [PMID: 23761184]

[221] Ramachandran A, Visschers RGJ, Duan L, Akakpo JY, Jaeschke H. Mitochondrial dysfunction as a mechanism of drug-induced hepatotoxicity: current understanding and future perspectives. J Clin Transl Res 2018; 4(1): 75-100.
[PMID: 30873497]

[222] Labbe G, Pessayre D, Fromenty B. Drug-induced liver injury through mitochondrial dysfunction: mechanisms and detection during preclinical safety studies. Fundam Clin Pharmacol 2008; 22(4): 335-53.
[http://dx.doi.org/10.1111/j.1472-8206.2008.00608.x] [PMID: 18705745]

[223] Jamshidzadeh A, Niknahad H, Heidari R, *et al.* Propylthiouracil-induced mitochondrial dysfunction in liver and its relevance to drug-induced hepatotoxicity. Ulum-i Daruyi 2017; 23(2): 95-102.
[http://dx.doi.org/10.15171/PS.2017.15]

[224] Niknahad H, Heidari R, Alzuhairi AM, Najibi A. Mitochondrial dysfunction as a mechanism for pioglitazone-induced injury toward HepG2 cell line. Pharm Sci 2015; 20(4): 169-74.

[225] Niknahad H, Jamshidzadeh A, Heidari R, *et al.* Paradoxical effect of methimazole on liver mitochondria: *In vitro* and *in vivo*. Toxicol Lett 2016; 259: 108-15.
[http://dx.doi.org/10.1016/j.toxlet.2016.08.003] [PMID: 27506418]

[226] Balkan J, Doğğru-Abbasoğlul S, Kanbaglil , Çevikbas U, Aykaç-Toker G, Uysal M. Taurine has a protective effect against thioacetamide-induced liver cirrhosis by decreasing oxidative stress. Hum Exp Toxicol 2001; 20(5): 251-4.
[http://dx.doi.org/10.1191/096032701678227758] [PMID: 11476157]

[227] Erman F, Balkan J, Çevikbaş U, Koçak-Toker N, Uysal M. Betaine or taurine administration prevents

fibrosis and lipid peroxidation induced by rat liver by ethanol plus carbon tetrachloride intoxication. Amino Acids 2004; 27(2): 199-205.
[http://dx.doi.org/10.1007/s00726-004-0105-5] [PMID: 15338317]

[228] Boşgelmez İİ, Söylemezoğlu T, Güvendik G. The protective and antidotal effects of taurine on hexavalent chromium-induced oxidative stress in mice liver tissue. Biol Trace Elem Res 2008; 125(1): 46-58.
[http://dx.doi.org/10.1007/s12011-008-8154-3] [PMID: 18528645]

CHAPTER 6

Taurine as an Anti-aging Compound: Focus on Mitochondria-related Mechanisms

Abstract: It has been well-established that mitochondria play a crucial role in aging. Thus, targeting mitochondria is a leading approach for anti-aging pharmacological interventions. On the other hand, the anti-aging effect of taurine (TAU) is an exciting feature of this amino acid. Effects of TAU on mitochondria-facilitated oxidative stress as well as mitochondria-mediated cell death, seem to play a pivotal role in its antiaging properties. The current chapter will discuss a good body of investigations that have converged at a consensus regarding mitochondria (dynamics and functionality) and oxidative stress as essential mechanisms involved in the aging process. In each part, the potential antiaging properties of TAU and its mechanisms of action are also highlighted. Finally, in the last section of this chapter, we described the possible role of recently-discovered signaling pathways (*i.e.*, aryl hydrocarbon receptors; AhR) on mitochondria and their relevance to senescence.

Keywords: Cell death, Endoplasmic reticulum stress, Oxidative stress, Reproduction, Senescence.

INTRODUCTION

There are many definitions of aging in various organs. As a general definition, aging could be interpreted as "a multifaceted event described by a typical time-dependent decline in physiological performances of creatures (human, animals, plants), interconnected with a rising risk of illness and death rate which eventually corresponded in the lifespan of organisms, and in which multi-factorial elements of genetic/hereditary and environmental components play a crucial moderating role in this phenomenon".

However, as mentioned, aging in various organs has a specific description. For instance, brain aging is described by several neurochemical alterations, comprising variations in the levels of structural proteins, neurotransmitters, and neuropeptides (*i.e.*, decrement in glutamate decarboxylase and somatostatinergic subpopulations of GABAergic neurons), as well as associated receptors (decrements in ionotropic GABA receptors). Changes in neurochemical parameters of the synaptic function associated with aging-related central

Reza Heidari and M. Mehdi Ommati

function impairments (*i.e.*, memory and sensory performances and locomotion). Hence, Idrissi *et al.* have highlighted the crucial role of GABA inhibitory neurotransmission in the age-related decline in cognitive functions [1]. In the same vein, it has been shown that ionotropic GABA receptors, glutamate decarboxylase (GAD), and somatostatinergic subpopulations of GABAergic neurons considerably declined in the aged animal's brain. Several studies demonstrate that ionotropic GABA receptors, glutamate decarboxylase (GAD), and somatostatinergic subpopulations of GABAergic neurons are markedly decreased in experimental animal brains during aging. Hence, a decrement in cognition functionality in aging animals might be caused (at least in part) due to decreases in GABA inhibitory neurotransmission.

On the other hand, there are specific definitions for reproductive aging of both genders. A considerable reduction could occur in reproductive indices in a species- and sex-dependent manner. For instance, the reproductive functionality of females halts with the beginning of the menopause (menstrual cycle pauses in women reaching about 45 to 60 years old). In males, it is also defined as any decrement in androgen formation, sperm production, and sexual desire or function being the major phenotypes or reasons of aging that might be ascribed to impairments of male gonad. Hence, in men, this phenomenon initiates with a decline in male gonad activity and subsequently neuroendocrine alterations impacting on some indices of physiology and psychology, a natural manner well-known as andropause[1]. Hence, aging in the male reproduction system initiates with a combination of morphological and endocrinological alterations. However, reproductive aging happens gradually in men, and they also do not undergo a whole termination of reproductive ability. Hence, males could maintain their reproductive capacity through proper spermatogenesis and steroidogenesis until the approximate end of life [2 - 7].

Nevertheless, it has been well reported that the alterations in the reproductive capacity of aged men are individually erratic and depend on the daily life patterns and other xenobiotics, such as environmental elements [2, 6 - 8]. Meanwhile, it is getting progressively clear that one of the well-known indices for reproductive aging in men is the continuing decrement in biosynthesis and secretion of testosterone that initiates around 30- years old and gradually continues time-dependently [4, 5, 9 - 11]. Because of this alteration in steroidogenesis performance, hormone replacement therapy in aged men (testosterone therapy) and women (estrogen replacement therapy) is recommended. It has been a valuable target for in-depth studies in the last decades. Nevertheless, their risks and benefits remain enigmatic to this day. As mentioned, there are various definitions for aging in different endogenous systems. Approximately, all these investigations agreed on a general theory that aging occurs based on the two crucial hypotheses. The first assumes that the lifespan is regulated by the expression of some specific genes *via* controlling of neuroendocrine system (hormone secretion) and consequent signaling routes. The second postulates a close relation between oxidative stress induction in various organs with enhancing age [12 - 15]. Meanwhile, these two routes are possibly more associated and will be discussed in detail in the following sections.

Cells aging occurs with apparent symptoms. For instance, it has been shown that aged cells are often larger as compared with the fresh and young cells; it could be interpreted that aged cells have more waste materials as a result of progressive degeneration of various organelles (*e.g.*, formation of large-double membrane vacuoles containing damaged mitochondrial during autophagy process, called autophagosomes). Meanwhile, the nuclei of aged cells could be detected easily due to the high levels of heterochromatin, damaged DNA, and nuclear proteins. These alterations are not distinguishable in nuclear levels; because both proteins and lipids within the cytoplasm and cellular plasma membrane could be damaged, which could eventually lead to substantial alterations in membrane permeability and fluidity, subsequent molecular transport, and cellular signaling. Intracellular accumulation of these unwanted proteins and lipids in aged cells could increase the generation of reactive oxygen species (ROS) and consequently increase the risk of oxidative stress induction (as mentioned above; for details, see sections 2 to 4). Mitochondrial impairment is one of the hallmarks of aging. In this view, many in-depth investigations highlighted that the most noticeable feature in these aging cells and the aging process is recorded alterations in the structure and functionality of mitochondria (and their association with stem cell fate, innate immune system, inflammation, metabolic status, age-dependent pathology, and nuclear signaling) [2, 13, 16 - 22]. By aging the cells, mitochondria will also be senescent, which has characteristics such as structural damages (ranging from swelling and loss of cristae to the destruction of the matrix and membrane structure), which eventually lead to the generation of intracellular amorphous elements. These senescent mitochondria are generally known as giant mitochondria because they are larger than younger ones.

Meanwhile, it has been well reported that mitochondrial genome mutation and mitochondrial proteins alteration progressively increase in the aging process [23]. In the next section, we will discuss the relation between oxidative stress and aging-induced mitochondrial injury, as well as the ameliorative role of taurine (TAU) on these processes. For instance, it has been shown that because of the specific features of TAU (such as antioxidant properties), it has a crucial role on reproductive indices (as a testosterone stimulating factor, a sperm membrane stabilizer and motility factor, an anti-apoptotic and anti-autophagic agent) and anti-aging through mitochondrial-dependent and -independent signal pathways.

THE RELEVANCE OF MITOCHONDRIA-ORIGINATED OXIDATIVE STRESS AND AGING

For many years, mitochondria have been thought to be the center of intracellular events during the aging process; however, some investigations have challenged this hypothesis [24 - 27]. It was not until the mid-1990s that Harman proposed that ROS produced during the normal process of cell metabolism could cause cumulative oxidative stress, which eventually led to physiological anomalies. This diminishing process of physiological responses can finally lead to aging and death; a process is called the free radical theory of aging [28] (Fig. **1**). After a while, Harman highlighted an essential issue: mitochondria are the leading producers of ROS (through the accumulation of aging-related mutations in mitochondrial DNA; mtDNA) and the main target of oxidative stress. This physiological status represents a defective cell cycle in which injured mitochondria produced a high amount of ROS, leading to the progressive, cumulative effect of cell damage, which peaks in the aging process and is called the mitochondrial theory of aging [29] (Fig. **1** and **2-A**). Following this hypothesis, several studies were conducted to complete it, which eventually addressed the role of all forms of ROS in this phenomenon. This polished hypothesis is now known as oxidative stress theory in aging [27] (Fig. **1, 2-A**, and **3**). Aging-related mtDNA mutations could cause increased ROS formation and consequently enhanced levels of oxidative stress in mitochondria [30] (Fig. **3**). In the last century, comprehensive studies on the crucial role of oxidative stress in longevity, aging, and death have been published, which led to this theory being recognized as one of the main hypotheses of aging [27, 31 - 33]. In recent years, the mitochondrial-lysosomal axis theory (*i.e.*, mitophagy: autophagy of mitochondria; Fig. **2-B**) has again put mitochondria at the forefront of the aging process [34].

Nevertheless, although the correlation between oxidative stress and aging has been well established, contradictory observations have also been reported. Several alternative hypotheses have questioned the validity of the theory of "oxidative stress/damage accumulation" with aging; and or have claimed that this cumulative effect of oxidative stress-induced injuries is closely associated with the occurrence of degenerative disorders, such as neurodegenerative diseases and cancer, which in turn reduce life expectancy and the quality of life. These alternative theories ultimately claimed that the oxidative damage accumulation was not necessarily and directly related to the aging process itself [24 - 27]. Meanwhile, it should also be noted that discrepancies in published observations extracted from these alternative theories could be due to the existence of various co-factors, including different considered experimental methods (*i.e.*, mitochondrial isolation methods, *in-vitro*) or various cell types used [36]. In comparison, it is also important to note that oxidative stress theory does not ignore that other key factors could play a crucial role in the aging process. Hence, a good body of literature is continuously published in favor of this theory of oxidative stress in aging [37, 38]. Recently, several new intracellular players are regularly being proposed, as are the fingerprints of autophagic related routes (*i.e.*, AMPK/mTOR/ULK1 pathway) [39, 40] and apoptosis (*i.e.*, activated by cytochrome *c*) [41, 42] in the aging as a physiological event. Therefore, it is evident that a multi-factorial approach should be accepted in future researches. Based on the above literature, it will be improbable that a single-factorial approach could provide reliable results in aging research. Then in the following sentences, we have tried to point out and discuss some of the well-known and proven approaches involved in the triple-axis of oxidative stress-mitochondrion-aging.

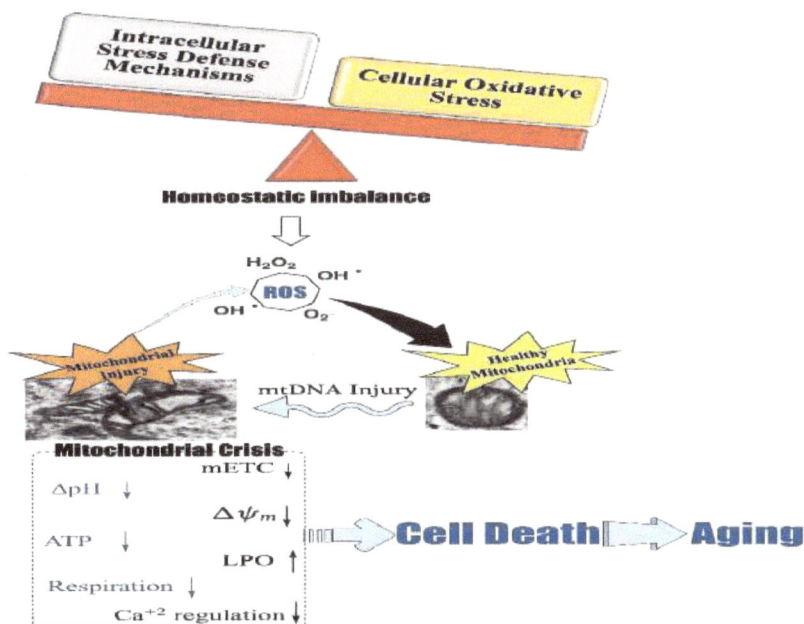

Fig. (1). A schematic model for the free radical theory and the mitochondrial theory of aging. Oxidative stress-induced ROS over-formation impairs cellular homeostatic pathways and consequently mitochondria function. Oxidative stress induces mitochondria impairments by influencing the organelle's life-sustaining functions, including alterations in the bioenergetics pathway, biogenesis of metabolites, Ca^{2+} homeostasis, and regulation of redox biology. These alterations finally result in cell death and aging. The above schematic illustration of the mitochondrial theory of aging is inspired by an in-depth investigation in this field (DOI: 10.1242/jcs.070490). Meanwhile, the TEM- recorded mitochondria are inserted from our recent publication (Fig. 1; DOI: 10.1016/j.ecoenv.2020.110973) [35].

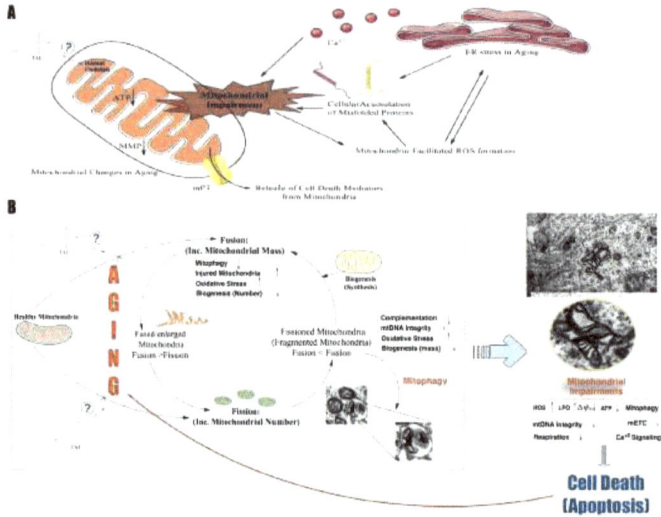

Fig. (2). Taurine might provide anti-aging effects through a mitochondria-dependent mechanism. It has been well-documented that mitochondrial functionality alterations play a critical role in aging. Mitochondrial changes in aging include enhanced mitochondria-facilitated ROS formation, decreased mitochondrial ATP, and induction of mPT (**A**). Another critical process involved in aging is ER stress. ER stress could further deteriorate mitochondrial impairment. Disturbances in mitochondrial fusion and fission (**B**) also play a crucial role in aging. The above TEM- mitophagy images are extracted from a recent study of authors (DOI: 10.1016/j.ecoenv.2020.110973) [35].

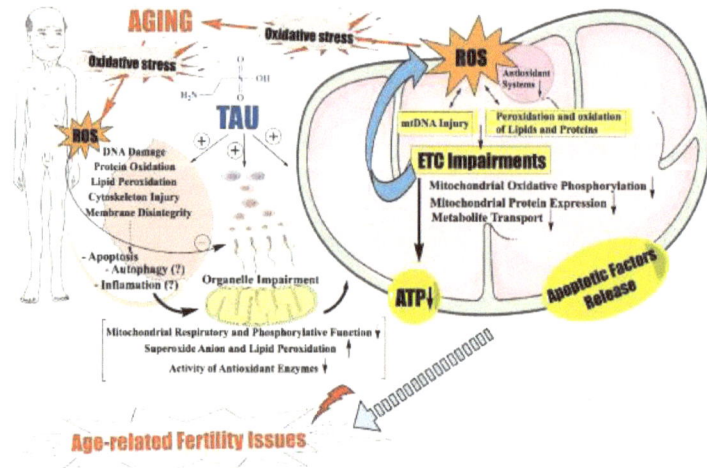

Fig. (3). Ameliorative effects of taurine (TAU) against aging-induced mitochondrial impairment in male gonads. Electron transport chain (ETC) defects-induced ROS overproduction could induce injuries in mtDNA and subsequently to a general mitochondrial dysfunction, ultimately leading to more oxidative stress. Mitochondrial injuries and oxidative stress responses are two important and well-known events in age-associated reproductive impairments, primarily due to the consequential energy crisis. UCP2- mediated proton leak increment might be considered a well adaptive strategy against ROS formation (Refer to test; adopted from Amaral *et al.*, 2013). Hence, it could be assumed that mitochondria are a critical link between aging and age-related decline in reproduction functionality (For more information, see chapter 10).

It has been well established that age-related mitochondria-facilitated ROS formation could be a significant source of oxidative lesions. However, we should not overlook that other cellular enzyme systems can produce ROS. The common belief is that ROS could be produced as by-products in complexes I and III of the mitochondrial electron transfer chain (mETC) [43]. On the other hand, Ago and colleagues (2010) showed that ROS are also generated in the heart by cardiac mitochondrial NADPH oxidases (such as NADPH oxidase-4l; NOX4) in an age-dependent manner [44]. Moreover, it has also been claimed that neutrophils are critical resources for ROS generation (through the NADPH oxidase activity) [45]. As a breach of an old-fashioned Iranian proverb, "A knife does not cut its own handle"; therefore, as the well-known major fact of the intracellular ROS supplier, mitochondria are not immune to the imminent attack by their ROS (Fig. **3**).

Under normal intracellular circumstances, ROS are trapped and inactivated by multiple antioxidant systems (*i.e.*, enzymatic and non-enzymatic) (Fig. **3**). However, it has been well established that several factors, including aging, could adversely affect these cellular balancing systems. To this end, in recent years, the role of natural antioxidants in the aging process has been the topic of much discussion in many scientific circles. Also, it has been the subject of extensive research, including research on knockout and transgenic laboratory rodents and aging-models animals exposed to natural antioxidants. Nonetheless, there are many contradictory observations in the literature, with either positive and negative statements or no association with lifespan and aging [24, 26, 27, 46, 47] questioning the oxidative stress theory in the aging process. For this reason, the identification of compounds with high antioxidative potency as antiaging options continues and could raise awareness of this hot topic of the day.

Over the years, the authors of this book have focused on the antioxidant role of various compounds (*e.g.*, silymarin, carnosine, histidine, betaine, boldine, glycine, proline, chlorogenic acid, N-acetyl cysteine, cimetidine, sulfasalazine, methylene blue, metformin, edaravone, glycyrrhizic acid, vitamins, hormones, probiotic supplements, herbal extracts, natural products and compounds, and TAU) in different experimental models of oxidative stress in various organs (*i.e.*, reproductive related organs, liver, kidney, brain, intestine, and isolated cells) [48 - 93]. Among these antioxidant compounds, TAU, as the most abundant amino acid with high physiological and pharmacological roles in the human body, has attracted the attention of many researchers due to its unique properties and beneficial functions. Hence, in several studies, we have also highlighted the antioxidative and mitochondrial protective roles of TAU in various tissues [54, 62, 71 - 75, 94 - 99]. Based on our observations, it could be assumed that a big part of the cytoprotective properties of TAU is mediated through targeting cellular mitochondria and oxidative stress in various complications. As mentioned, aging is one of the most prominent mitochondria-linked events [16]. Several chemicals have been tested to blunt or reverse the cellular aging process [100, 101]. Targeting cellular mitochondria and oxidative stress is the leading approach for anti-aging pharmacological interventions [13, 17, 31, 43, 100, 101]. Interestingly, it has been found that the consumption of TAU-rich diets is directly related to a broader life span [102, 103]. Hence, the antioxidative and mitochondria protecting effects of TAU can be considered as a fundamental role in moderating the aging process.

AGE-ASSOCIATED OXIDATIVE STRESS TO MITOCHONDRIAL STRUCTURE AND FUNCTION

Whether mutations in mtDNA play a vital role in the aging process is still a matter of debate. However, there is no doubt that a considerable decrease in the functionality of mitochondria occurs with aging. Meanwhile, the proper functioning of mitochondria to improve longevity and mitigate age-associated anomalies could not be negated.

There is a positive correlation between aging and the level of oxidative stress-induced protein carbonylation, lipid peroxidation, and ROS biosynthesis in mitochondria [104, 105]. To fulfill the above scenario, because of the high polyunsaturated fatty acid (PUFA) levels in the mitochondria membrane, mitochondrial membrane lipids (main cardiolipin in the inner layer of mitochondrial membrane) are predominantly under the risk of irreversible damages induced by oxidative stress in an age-dependent manner. Cardiolipin is a unique mitochondrial inner membrane-localized phospholipid containing three glycerol backbones, four acyl chains, and a polar head group catching protons for the action of oxidative phosphorylation [106]. The primary role of cardiolipin is preserving the integrity of the mitochondrial membrane's structure [107, 108], along with maintaining the proper function of proteins and enzyme complexes participating in oxidative phosphorylation [109 - 111]. Then, this unique phospholipid specifically cooperates with the proteins of the ETC. On the other hand, the high-values existent of cardiolipin in PUFA (*i.e.*, linoleic acid) and its proximal location to the ROS biosynthesis sites in the mitochondrial ETC make it the primary target for ROS action.

A review of the published literature showed the crucial role of cardiolipin in the functionality of the mitochondrial membrane. Thus, it could be assumed that this lipid is vital for mitochondrial bioenergetics. Multiple *in-vitro* studies have revealed that cardiolipin oxidation causes mitochondrial dysfunction (Fig. **2-A**). Accumulating evidence indicates a time-dependent decrement for cardiolipin in various tissues [2, 112]. Hence, it should not come as a wonder that aging-induced oxidative stress is interconnected with a substantial decrement of phospholipids and proteins content and functionality of the inner membrane by increasing the sensitivity of this membrane to oxidative stress [2, 112]. On the other hand, as mentioned in the previous section, we have frequently shown the protective role of TAU in mitochondrial functionality against oxidative stress-induced adverse effects. To the best of our knowledge, there have been no studies to date dedicated to the influence of TAU on this unique phospholipid (Fig. **2-A**).

Except for cardiolipin, multiple lines of research have revealed that other mitochondrial components, such as ATP synthase, the adenine nucleotide transporter, and the matrix enzyme aconitase, could be considerably affected by oxidative stress [113 - 115]. It has also been shown that the entry and exit of metabolites to or from mitochondria could also be adversely affected by aging [116]. The xenobiotics-induced oxidative stress through ROS could considerably induce the oxidation of mitochondrial mtDNA and proteins, as well as peroxidation of PUFA in mitochondria, which ultimately causes abnormalities in the morphological indices and functionality of the mitochondria. Due to the proximity of the mitochondrial genome (mtDNA) to ETC (the place of ROS biogenesis), it could be an easy target for ROS-associated injury [117 - 120]. mtDNA damage could induce more ROS formation through impaired synthesis of ETC components (Fig. **2-A** and **3**).

Substantial evidence exists that any anomaly in aging-associated mtDNA accumulation possibly decreases or inhibits the protein's renewal of mitochondria [31, 34]. mtDNA damage and mutations could occur at any cell and/or mitochondrial division stage. These anomalies can lead to an overall decrease in the respiratory capacity, disruption of ATP biosynthesis, and ultimately increased levels of ROS, all of which could lead to a considerable increment of mtDNA mutation and subsequent oxidative stress [120, 121] (Fig. **2-B**). However, Xu *et al.* (2015) have shown that TAU pretreatment could efficiently maintain the functionality of mitochondria in nickel-treated nerve cells through increment of the mtDNA [122]. A similar observation was found by Chou and colleagues (2015), who reported that arsenite-triggered oxidative stress, mitochondrial impairments, and degradation of mtDNA were significantly mitigated by co-treatment of TAU [123]. However, except for lipid peroxidation and the mitochondrial permeability transition, mtDNA damage could be considered one of the primary stimulators for apoptosis and autophagy induction, specifically mitophagy [124].

Moreover, oxidative stress-related mitochondrial impairments stimulated by aging are assumed to have a crucial impact on triggering the other essential intrinsic-related routes (such as apoptosis and autophagy) in the early hours of the onset of oxidative stress, which needs further research to complete our acknowledgment in this field. Because of the occurrence of oxidative stress in both events, aging, and apoptosis, they have many mutual countenances, including decreased mitochondrial membrane potential ($\Delta\Psi_m$), higher peroxidation of lipids (TBARS content and lipid peroxidation levels), and oxidation of proteins (protein carbonylation), more elevated and decreased levels of oxidized (GSSG) and reduced (GSH) forms of glutathione, respectively, and finally mtDNA oxidative damage [33, 120, 125]; where, all these injured or dysfunctional organelles, such as mitochondria (called mitophagy) will be eliminated by autophagy [35, 126 - 129]. There is a good body of literature proofing the association between all above-highlighted factors with mitochondrial respiratory dysfunctionality (*i.e.*, decrements in respiratory control, oxidative phosphorylation efficiency, the rates of resting (State 4) and ADP-stimulated (State 3) respiration, as well as the activities of respiratory enzyme complexes [43, 120]) in a time-dependent manner (aging). However, it should be noted that, like other scientific issues, there are some contradicting opinions and interpretations in the above factors and their relations with mitochondrial functionality and aging [24, 27] that leave the researches' windows open for further studies, so that we can reach to a final and precise decision.

The high level of DNA mutations, deficiency of protein functions, genomic instability, and impairments in metabolic and signaling related routes, could be induced through oxidative stress-triggered ROS formation, have been reported in various organs or cells challenging with different pathological conditions, including aging, neurodegenerative disorders, and cancer [13]. Based on the above literature, it could be concluded that mitochondrial impairments and oxidative damage unavoidably happen in the aging process and could induce age-related neurodegenerative disorders and might be a risk factor for carcinogenesis. In this view, it has been well shown that TAU may have a high potential of pharmacological aspects to mitigate the side effects of xenobiotics targeting the mitochondria in various tissues [54, 62, 73, 94 - 99, 122, 130] and aging [131, 132]. Meanwhile, Aydin *et al.* (2016) have reported that TAU significantly attenuated the occurrence of oxidative stress, apoptosis, and histopathological alterations in the brain of the rats challenged with D-galactose (a valid animal model for brain aging and anti-aging studies). Yildirim *et al.* (2007) have shown that TAU has a crucial role in aging through decreasing the free radical levels and increasing the antioxidant capacity [133].

Apart from the mentioned factors above, fortunately, progress in the field has revealed that there is a close relation between aging and some intrinsic elements, such as decrements in the LON protease expression (an essential gene involved in the biogenesis of mitochondria) and genes involved in fatty acids, cholesterol synthesis, protein turnover, the subunits of ATP synthesize, and NADP transhydrogenase [31, 32, 120]. Ultimately, all these altered indices can lead to a considerable decline in ATP formation. Lee and colleagues (2001) have shown that the observed decline in ATP biosynthesis because of an aging-dependent mitochondrial impairment could ultimately cause an intracellular energy crisis impacting numerous energy-dependent cellular routes [15]. In this regard, we have recently reported that exogenous TAU (5 and 10 mM) attenuated xenobiotic-caused mitochondrial dysfunction by mitigating energy metabolism disturbances [74].

THE ROLE OF UNCOUPLING PROTEINS AND ROS FORMATION IN AGING: NON-INVESTIGATED ROLE OF TAURINE

The previous section shows the adverse effects of oxidative stress in aging through mitochondrial-related pathways. This section will highlight the crucial roles of mitochondrial uncoupling proteins on ROS formation and its consequent adverse effects; ROS- stimulated damages have been highlighted as one of the principal routes involved in aging. Another influential intracellular factor affecting ROS synthesis is the proton motive force launch throughout the inner membrane of mitochondria. It has been well shown that uncoupling proteins (UCPs) could trigger a mid-uncoupling inducing a proton motive force decrement resulting in a decrement of mitochondrial ROS generation and subsequently protecting the organelles- or cells- associated damages against ROS [134, 135]. Recently, the innovation of specific proteins in the inner membrane of mitochondria, responsible for increasing the uncoupling of proton flux, called UCPs, from the ATP synthase, shed light on possible mechanisms involved in the ROS buffering, and subsequently in the senescence process. Hence, these UCPs have a crucial role in physiological uncoupling leading to a reduction in ROS formation inside the mitochondria.

In this regard, in-depth investigations have monitored the deletion and over-expression of UCPs on lifespan and aging. For instance, Fridell *et al.* have reported that life expectancy could be increased by 10-30% through increasing the expression of human-UCP2 (hUCP2) in the nervous system of fruit flies, which resulted in a considerable reduction in the ROS formation in these hUCP2 expressing flies [136]. They also pointed out that Knockout flies for the UCP5 gene had a longer lifespan when fed with a low-calorie diet. However, the same flies' survival was remarkably reduced during starvation [137]. In the same vein, a considerable increment of ATP level in the UCP4-like protein knockout *C. elegans* nematodes is reported. However, there was no significant difference in life expectancy compared with the control group [138].

Moreover, there is a good body of evidence in mammals (such as rodents) proving the potential role of UCPs in longevity and aging. For example, a substantial increment of proton leak rate in the inner membrane along with a decrement of ATP turnover reactions in the hepatic cells of mice was observed in a time-dependent manner [139]. In addition, it is shown that skeletal muscle respiratory uncoupling due to the UCP1 gene expression appears to reduce age-related maladies in laboratory animal models [140]; meanwhile, excessive UCP3 expression in rats has also been shown to reduce the formation of age-related ROS significantly [141]. Another study revealed that decreased UCP1 gene expression could reduce mitochondrial superoxide generation in brown adipose tissue; this reduction might have been due to the suppression of cold-induced substrate oxidation; though these researchers have not reported the effect of this expression reduction on longevity [142]. In an interesting study, researchers examined the effects of different diets on the life expectancy of two different mouse types (wild type and transgenic type for high levels of skeletal muscle UCP1); they showed that mitochondrial uncoupling significantly reduced the destructive effects of high-fat diets, causing to expand the longevity of transgenic mice [143].

As a general result of this section, it could be assumed that any alteration in the expression of these UCPs, for induction of uncoupling, could reduce cellular damage during the aging process, which is caused by the excessive formation of ROS. On the other hand, just as we know, it seems that no comprehensive research has been reported on the possible role of TAU on the functionality of these UCPs and remains enigmatic to this day. Therefore, investigating the role of TAU on mitochondrial UCPs may open new doors in senescence-related researches.

IMPAIRED EXTRA-MITOCHONDRIAL BIOMOLECULES TURN-OVER AND AGING

The destructive effects of oxidative stress affect mitochondria and other cellular biomolecules, such as proteins, lipids, and DNA [144 - 148]. As noted earlier, the aging process is characterized by intracellular changes, such as the accumulation of damaged proteins, lipids, and impaired mitochondria in the post-meiotic cells, reflecting age-associated alterations through degradation-related pathways [23, 34]. It has been well shown that the aging-associated increased content of mtDNA could cause modifications in cell-signaling related routes triggering cell dysfunction and initiating some important intracellular routes, including autophagy and apoptosis, regardless of increased ROS formation and oxidative stress in mitochondria [149].

There are several vital intracellular mechanisms to digest the injured intracellular components, some of which are activated due to xenobiotics-induced oxidative stress [35, 126 - 129]. One of the critical degradation intracellular routes is autophagy, which has been discussed in detail in previous sections (see sections 1 and 3 of this chapter), as well as highlighted in the chapter "Reproduction and Taurine," where we tried to discuss this crucial route and the vitally related genes and proteins comprehensively. Briefly, it should be highlighted that autophagy will present different responses under different physiological conditions (depending on the intensity of oxidative stress). Regarding aging, it has been shown that downregulation of autophagy could increase the half-lives of long-lived proteins, lipids, and intracellular organelles, leading to conditions in which cells are forced to perform their characteristic functions under sub-optimal circumstances [23, 34].

Except for mitophagy (removal of dysfunctional mitochondria through autophagy), another pathway is also involved in removing the injured mitochondria, such as the mitochondrial proteolytic machinery, consisting of the ATP-dependent matrix proteases (such as LON, Clp-like, and AAA proteases). Meanwhile, it is reported that the activity of these enzymes was decreased in the aged rodents [34]. Therefore, it could be imagined that the decrease in autophagy capacity in aged cells, along with alterations in the mitochondrial proteolytic machinery activity, could lead to the decrement in mitochondrial turnover and consequently accumulation of damaged organelles during the aging process. Regarding the relation between aging and cell death, it could be conveyed (as mentioned) that senescent mitochondria produce almost less ATP and generate more ROS, which could increase oxidative stress, impeding mitochondrial turnover. Eventually, it may lead to apoptotic cell death [23, 34], which could be considered testimony of aging.

On the other hand, it is well shown that the over-expression of autophagy is closely related to the induction of apoptotic or necrotic cell death, speciously *via* regulators of Bcl-2 family members. Oxidative and nitrosative stresses, endoplasmic reticulum (ER) stress, excitotoxicity-induced cellular injury progresses, ionic imbalance, and subsequent mitochondrial disturbances, eventually could induce programmed cell death and necrosis [150] (Fig. **2-A**).

However, the role of cell death in aging needs further discussions and studies. Moreover, due to the elimination of dysfunctional or damaged mitochondria by autophagy, mitochondrial biogenesis is a crucial intracellular process essential for maintaining energy production and cellular homeostasis. However, it has been well demonstrated that this crucial intracellular process loses its effectiveness with the aging process by reducing the functionality of many intracellular factors involved in this process [34]. One of the critical elements in various significant pathologies and or anomalies related to aging is mitochondrial morphology's functional and structural changes through the balance between mitochondrial fusion and fission [149].

It is getting progressively clear that these intracellular organelles are substantially mobile and functionally plastic organelles that incessantly experience fusion and fission events; hence, they dynamically could change their morphology depending on the cellular circumstances. These days, a hot topic is the existence of an equilibrium between mitochondrial fusion and fission in this process (Fig. **2-B**). This balance is vital for maintaining mitochondria dynamics (such as morphology, distribution, function, and inheritance). However, accumulating evidence revealed the pleiotropic role of fusion and fission in various cellular routes (*i.e.*, cellular redox status, metabolism of mitochondria, the maintenance of mtDNA integrity, organelle function, and cellular death signaling) [151]. Hence, the action of mitochondria and subsequent cells functions will be seriously compromised upon alterations of this balance. Moreover, a recent wave of evidence has revealed that vital cellular-related routes, including mitochondrial fusion and fission, as well as autophagy, could be considered as a quality-maintenance mechanism accelerating the elimination of injured mitochondria from the cells affected by numerous types of stress (*i.e.*, various xenobiotics and/or aging process), a multiple intracellular processes that are predominantly crucial to hinder aging.

Additionally, it has been reported that the vital components of the fusion/fission system (*i.e.*, OPA1 or Drp1) are prone to significant changes with the aging process [2]. Changes in the fission machinery could have adverse effects; because it has been shown that although alterations in the fusion machinery didn't cause mitochondrial damage between senescent mitochondria and normal ones; however, dysfunction of the fission machinery could cause abnormalities in the destruction of damaged mitochondria (For more information see reference [34]). To read more about the recent studies that have converged at a consensus regarding the involvement of mitochondrial dynamics in vital cellular routes (*i.e.*, mitochondrial biogenesis, mtDNA homeostasis, autophagy, and cell death), and announce a potential link between atypical mitochondrial dynamics and aging, as well as mechanisms underlying mitochondrial dynamics, refer to the commentary conducted by Seo and colleagues (2010); who claimed the consequences of mitochondrial fusion and fission on aging-associated intracellular mechanisms had not been completely understood, maybe partially due to the aging-related molecular events that have not yet been fully revealed. The conspicuous signs of mitochondrial dynamics in the aging process are tried to illustrate in Fig. (**2B**).

As a result of this section, it could be stated that the functionality of mitochondria could be considerably affected by aging; as it has been shown that during the aging process, a significant decrease in mitochondrial bioenergetics indices, mitochondrial protein synthesis, and expression of mitochondrial turnover- related genes, along with an increment in peroxide formation and mitochondrial size, as well as considerable changes in mtDNA, were recorded [15, 17]. However, more researches are needed to clarify the ameliorative role of TAU, more than just an antioxidant, on aging through the mentioned parameters.

PARTICIPATION OF MITOCHONDRIA IN AGE-RELATED SUB-/IN-FERTILITY?

The role of TAU on reproductive parameters through alterations of mitochondrial functionality is discussed in chapter 10. This section will look at the role of the aging process on mitochondrial-related indices in the reproductive system. In the next step, we will discuss the ameliorative role of TAU against aging-induced reproductive impairments.

The need for energy in the male and female reproductive systems is different. It has been shown that the male gonads (testis; plural form: testes) need more energy than the female ones in the early stages of development. The number of active mitochondria varies depending on the development stage of the spermatogonia stem cells. On the other hand, the high number of efficient mitochondria in sperm (spermatozoa (singular form: spermatozoon), male germ cells, or gametes; both singular and plural forms: sperm) highlights the importance of this organelle in the metabolism of the testis [2]. It has been well established that although spermatogonia, mature sperm, and Sertoli cells are highly dependent on glycolytic activity; nevertheless, spermatocytes, spermatids, and hyperactive sperm in the female reproductive tract, are highly reliant on the mitochondrial oxidative phosphorylation to produce ATP [152 - 154]. In addition, several studies have pointed out mitochondria's unique features in testis compared to other organs, as these testicular organelles seem to generate the maximum electric potential compared to mitochondria of other tissues by consuming the least amount of oxygen [155, 156].

A significant point in the role and function of mitochondria in various reproductive-related cells might be due to the mitochondrial diversity in these cells. For instance, it has been well-established that three different types of mitochondria (orthodox-type, intermediate, and condensed form) are involved in the process of spermatogenesis. The orthodox-type in spermatogonia, preleptotene, and leptotene spermatocytes, Sertoli cells; the intermediate mitochondria in zygotene spermatocytes; and the condensed form of mitochondria are presented in the pachytene and secondary spermatocytes, as well as in early spermatids (for review see [157, 158]). Thus, it is not far-fetched to understand that the alterations in metabolic dynamics during spermatogenesis, other than Sertoli cells secretions [159], might be due to these mitochondrial structural changes.

We have frequently presented the relation between mitochondrial functionality and oxidative stress. Oxidative stress is one of the well-known reasons (about 50%) of men's sub-/in-fertility cases. There are two crucial sources of ROS in semen, which include leukocytes and sperm. It should be considered that ROS plays as a double-edged sword. This means that the low concentrations are helpful in the reproductive process, fertilization (specifically in the capacitation process). In contrast, high concentrations have destructive effects on sperm parameters and functionality through affecting both sperm membranes and DNA [160, 161], as follow:

- By the first mechanism (membrane integrity), ROS can reduce the motility of male gametes and their abilities to fuse with female gametes, ovum (egg or oocyte).
- Through sperm DNA alterations: ROS cooperates paternal genomic contribution to the next generation.

Mitochondrial respiratory dysfunction in spermatogenic cells could occur with a high accumulation of pathogenic mutant mtDNA in the male gonad, resulting in a considerable decrement of energy formation in these germ cells that finally causes meiotic arrest to increase the percentage of sperm abnormality. These alterations emphasized the importance of mitochondrial respiratory function in the spermatogenesis of mammals.

Meanwhile, we have frequently reported that various xenobiotics, including environmental pollutants, chemicals and drugs, pathologies of the reproductive system, and chronic diseases, could be the primary sources of sperm oxidative damage [35, 48, 53, 76, 128, 129, 146, 148, 162]. Similar to what happened in the inner membrane of mitochondria, sperm are also prone to oxidative stress-induced severe damages due to the high percentage of PUFA and their weak antioxidant system. These factors have been reported in defective sperm function of most infertile patients (for review, see [160]). On the other hand, many factors, such as environmental toxicants, reproductive related anomalies (*i.e.*, varicocele, orchitis, cryptorchidism), and aging, have been reported as inducers of testicular oxidative stress through triggering of apoptosis in germ cells, hypo-spermatogenesis, and primary hypogonadism (reviewed in [2, 163]). Meanwhile, multiple lines of research have revealed that in germ cells, apoptosis can be triggered through

ROS-caused DNA injuries, which could consequently cause a considerable decrement in sperm concentration resulting in a decline in semen quality. Both defects are correlated with sub-/in-fertility in males [160] (Fig. **3**).

As mentioned above, there are a considerable number of factors affecting fertility. One of the well-known factors is aging. The aging-induced reproductive failure happens in a species and sex-specific manner. Although the reproductive activity of females/women ends with the arrival of menopause, in males/men, this process of infertility is gradual and prolonged so that they do not experience a complete cessation of fertility during their lifetime. Therefore, they could maintain the process of spermatogenesis for the rest of their lives [3 - 7]. However, this gradual decrement in male fertility involves a combination of alterations in the morphological features of reproductive-related organs and neuroendocrine-related routes. It has been shown that these alterations are incredibly unpredictable from person to person and seem to be affected by standards of living and environmental elements [6 - 8]. Furthermore, an interruption in communication between nurse cells (Sertoli cells) and germ cells was also reported [164], resulting in an impairment of spermatogenesis in the aged testis [7, 8, 165].

Another notable feature of reproductive aging is a gradual and continuing decrease in steroidogenesis, especially testosterone levels and dehydroepiandrosterone (DHEA; an adrenal precursor of estrogenic steroids). This decrement could be instigated around 30 years old in humans and continued in an age-dependent manner through compromised cholesterol transport and Leydig cell mitochondrial steroidogenesis [9 - 11]. Moreover, this decrement in steroidogenesis might be clarified by alterations in the hypothalamus-pituitar- -gonadal axis (HPG) functionality [35, 128, 129]. Concurrent with their decrements, many other biological elements, such as tumor necrosis factor, cytokines, transforming growth factor-b1, interleukins, and ROS, affect steroidogenesis by increasing in aged subjects [11]. In the same vein, comprehensive research has been conducted on replacement therapies for testosterone and other crucial reproductive hormones in elderly guys [4 - 6, 166 - 168]. However, investigating the interaction of different hormones and their risk/benefit assessments is still a controversial issue that needs further investigation in both sexes. The age-related decline in spermatogenesis may be explained by any interruption in communication between nurse- and germ cells. On the other hand, an in-depth investigation highlighted the role of mitochondrial dysfunction in the aging epididymis. Hence, the question arises: "are mitochondria reliable connections between aging and sub-/in- fertility?".

Indeed, a recent wave of studies has revealed the role of mitochondria in aging and age-related men's fertility loss. In the same vein, assessing the aged male gonad's mitochondria has revealed a considerable decline in their functionality. For instance, it has been shown that fatty acid composition was tangibly changed in an age-dependent manner, ultimately affecting mitochondrial complex activity and fluidity [169]. In aged mitochondria, a high production rate of superoxide anion and lipid peroxidation, along with the reduced activity of antioxidant enzymes, has been shown [170, 171] (Fig. **3**). However, it has been demonstrated that in aging male gonad's mitochondria, the equilibrium between pro- and antioxidative elements notably changed, especially with a shift in the glutathione redox state towards the pro-oxidizing condition [172].

Amaral *et al.* (2008) reported mitochondrial functionality (*i.e.*, bioenergetics characteristics) of different aged rats, who reported the correlation between rats' reproductive cycle with mitochondrial respiratory and oxidative phosphorylation function. They showed these indices were significantly increased and decreased in mature and older animals, respectively [155]. Although reduced mitochondrial activity has been well demonstrated in older animals, it should be noted that there are always protective mechanisms in these cases. For instance, the role of mitochondrial UCP2, which has been shown to increase significantly with age, in content and function. This event could promote proton leakage and ultimately attenuate ROS production by reducing mitochondrial membrane potential.

Based on the evidence available at present, it could be concluded that any alteration in reproductive function induced by aging might be caused due to abnormalities in the function of testicular mitochondria, which in turn reduces ATP formation and subsequent energy crisis to maintain testicular homeostasis [155] (Fig. **3**). The role of TAU in improving sub/in-fertility is tried to describe comprehensively in chapter 10. Meanwhile, it has been reported that TAU could considerably improve testicular injury induced by senescent through recovering antioxidant systems [131, 173], triggering the luteinizing hormone and testosterone secretion, increasing the testicular marker enzymes levels and testicular antioxidation (increased levels of superoxide dismutase (SOD), acid phosphatase (ACP), lactate dehydrogenase [174], sorbitol dehydrogenase (SDH), nitric oxide synthase (NOS), nitric oxide (NO), and reduced glutathione hormone (GSH), concomitant with a decrement in aspartate aminotransferase (AST) and alanine aminotransferase (ALT) levels), and improving sperm quality (*i.e.*, sperm concentration, motility, and the viability) [173], mitigating the apoptotic [131]. Meanwhile, Yang *et al.* (2013) have reported that TAU considerably improved the sexual response and mating ability in aged rodents *via* increasing the testosterone and NO level [175]. Hence, TAU plays a crucial role in male reproduction, particularly in aging animals or humans. However, it sounds that further studies are needed to support the ameliorative role of TAU against aging-induced reproductive toxicity through autophagic and inflammatory-related routes.

AHR- ASSOCIATED AGING: AHR-MITOCHONDRIA CROSSTALK

As mentioned in previous sections, almost all aging-triggering factors could induce adverse effects through the functionality of mitochondria. Hence, mitochondria are claimed to play a central role in the senescence and aging process; where, their dysfunctionality is well-known as one of the aging hallmarks. Despite several lines of converging evidence and scientific arguments linking oxidative stress-induced senescence through mitochondrial impairments and subsequent cellular events (such as apoptosis, autophagy, and inflammation), there is a new-growing body of literature on the role of an evolutionarily conserved over 600-million-year-old transcription factor, Aryl hydrocarbon Receptor (AhR), on aging that could be considered as "Another Puzzling Role for This Highly Conserved Transcription Factor," as Brinkmann *et al.* (2020) claimed.

Fascinatingly, various kinds of xenobiotics, including environmental toxicants and nutritional elements, affect the aging process and mitochondrial functionality through the activity of AhR (*via* direct or indirect related routes). Hence, recent years have witnessed the growing body of evidence of this versatile transcription factor through mitochondrial related routes on the senescence in laboratory animals [176 - 178] and humans [179].

There are few studies about the role of AhR on human-related *in-vivo* and *in-vitro* subjects. Most of these investigations were aimed to assess the specific AhR modulators on senescence and/or aging-associated indices. For instance, Qiao and colleagues (2017) have shown that airborne polycyclic aromatic hydrocarbons-activated AhR caused cellular aging in human skin cells through up-regulation of important aging-related genes [180]. They have also demonstrated that this up-regulation was interestingly restrained upon exposure of an AhR antagonist [180]. In human retinal pigment epithelial cells, it has also shown that AhR activity was considerably declined with age [181]. Meanwhile, these authors have also reported that the protein levels of AhR were tangibly decreased on old donors-extracted cells than young donors- cells. Finally, they confirmed their observation by a laboratory animal model, where they proved a considerable mitigated AhR activity in the age-related macular degeneration-like pathology [181].

The role of AhR in other aging-related tissue pathologies are also considered; for instance, a study from 2016 claimed that AhR expression level could be regarded as a precise indicator for vessel functionality in humans due to the recorded high correlation between AhR expression and cardiovascular aging (Eckers *et al.*, 2016). In fact, pulse wave velocity, as a well-known marker for vascular aging, is intensified in an age-dependent manner and is highly associated with the expression of AhR. Hence, it could be assumed that up-regulation of AhR seems to be correlated with aging in humans. In the same vein, Huang and colleagues (2015) have found a positive correlation between AhR mRNA levels and the incidence of coronary arterial disease in Chinese patients [182]. Hence, they proposed this versatile transcription factor, AhR, as a diagnostic biomarker for coronary arterial disease [182].

Altogether, there is a lack of investigation on the role of AhR in various tissues or organs of humans or laboratory animals aging, demonstrating a multifaceted role of the AhR in this phenomenon. However, Brinkmann *et al.* (2020) have established that aging-related AhR activity is possibly tissue or environmental dependent (Table 1). Hence, multiple lines of research in various tissues, organs, and or in the whole organism are needed to uncover the pathophysiological role of AhR in aging.

Table 1. Age-associated AhR alterations in various species and tissues.

Species	Foundations	AhR Activity	DOI
Human	In the cardiovascular system: A Positive relation between AhR and coronary arterial disease	Stimulates aging	10.1038/srep08022
Human and Mice	In the cardiovascular system: A positive relation between AhR and vessel stiffness/aging	Stimulates aging	10.1038/srep19618
Human and Mice	In Muscular system: Positive correlation between AhR and macular degeneration.	Prevents aging	10.1073/pnas.1307574110
Mice AhR $^{\Delta 3/\Delta 3}$	Hepatic fibrosis; Cardiac hypertrophy, kyphosis	Prevents aging	10.1096/fj.201901333R
Mice B6.129 AhR $^{\Delta 1/\Delta 1F}$	Bladder cancer in aged animals; degeneration of seminal vesicles	Prevents aging	10.1159/000117714; 10.1073/pnas.1120581109
Mice B6.129 AhR $^{\Delta 2/\Delta 2}$	No significant difference in survival rate than wild type mice till 15 months of age	No aging phenotype	10.1089/scd.2013.0346
Mice B6.129 AhR $^{\Delta G/\Delta 1G}$	Skin lesions; cardiac hypertrophy; hepatocellular tumours; Pyloric hyperplasia; macular degeneration	Prevents aging	10.1126/science.7732381; 10.1177/030098589703400609

Species	Foundations	AhR Activity	DOI
C. elegansAhR1(ju145) and & AhR-1(ia03)	Improved lifespan, heat stress resistance and Pharyngeal pumping, and movement	Stimulates aging	10.1038/srep19618; 10.1371/journal.pgen.1004673; 10.1073/pnas.1706464114
Stimulates aging through decrement in AhR expression. Prevents aging through increment in AhR expression.			

The current chapter repeatedly highlights the critical role of mitochondria, as a central hub in nutrient metabolism, in the aging process. Meanwhile, it is also mentioned that these vital organelles could be targeted by various kinds of xenobiotics, including environmental toxicants, dietary factors (*e.g.*, polyphenols), and endogenous parameters. On the other hand, it has been well shown that these xenobiotics could also affect the AhR transcriptional activity. For this reason, more scholarly reports have envisioned possible crosstalk between this internal organelle and AhR [183].

Between 1913 and the first days of 2022, more than 230,000 studies focused on mitochondria (pubmed.ncbi.nlm.nih.gov). There is a good body of literature among these studies assessing the impact of various AhR modulators on mitochondria; meanwhile, in the meantime, only less than 100 studies have directly linked mitochondria with AhR. Except for the general influence of natural polyphenols on mitochondria, such as their impacts on mitochondrial biogenesis, mitochondrial membrane potential, and mitochondrial electron transport chain activity [184], these dietary factors are considered a well-known ROS scavenger and thereby impact on mitochondria. On the other hand, it showed that this ROS scavenging role could be crucial for the influence of these dietary factors on the activity of AhR. Smirnova and colleagues (2016) have reported that ROS could activate AhR *via* the conversion of tryptophan to 6-formylindolo [3,2b] carbazole (FICZ) [185]. Hence, it could be concluded that these features of polyphenols (ROS-scavenging properties) could considerably mitigate this activation (AhR activation) and thus connect AhR with mitochondria.

There are also scholarly reports on the possible crosstalk between AhR and mitochondria associated with the aging process through SIRT1 activation. Given the pivotal role of SIRT1 in senescence, an exciting route of the independent action of polyphenols on mitochondria to inhibit ROS formation is to trigger mitochondrial biogenesis through SIRT1. On the other hand, several polyphenols have been reported to trigger SIRT1 [186]. Altogether, considering the influence of polyphenols on mitochondria [184], the interaction between AhR and SIRT1 [187 - 189], and activation of AhR by ROS [185], it could be assumed that there is a possible crosstalk between AhR, SIRT1, and mitochondria of relevance for the senescence.

Senft and co-workers were the first researchers who claimed the possible link between mitochondria and AhR in 2002 [190]. Their report focused on the role of AhR signaling and showed a considerable increment of hepatic mitochondrial ROS level in the wild-type mice exposed to dioxin, but not in AhR-/- mice whose basal mitochondrial ROS levels were lower (Senft *et al.*, 2002). Their observations proposed the possible role of AhR on mitochondria, not only in the presence of ligands but also under normal conditions. In this regard, Fisher *et al.* (2005) have reported a decrement in male gametes mitochondrial membrane potential of mice exposed to dioxin in an AhR dependent manner [176]. Based on the above literature, it could be suggested that AhR facilitates mitochondrial impairment in response to dioxin. On the other hand, Das and co-investigators (2017) have reported that the elimination of injured mitochondria by mitophagy (the autophagy of mitochondria) was significantly reduced in AhR and CYP1B1 (an AhR target gene) knockdown HaCaT cells; however, a direct link between AhR and mitophagy has not yet been established. Similarly, Carreira and colleagues have shown that any interruption in AhR signaling (the harmful effect of AhR function loss) can cause an embryonic cardiac mitochondrial dysfunction in mice [191].

Except for the influence of AhR on mitochondrial functionality, it has also been shown in two in-depth studies that AhR is localized into the mitochondria inside the intermembrane space [192, 193]. In this regard, Tappenden and colleagues were the first researchers who claimed an interaction between this highly conserved transcription factor and the ATP5a1 subunit of the ATP synthase complex in various cell lines. In these studies, authors showed that upon exposure to dioxin, localization of AhR in mitochondria and its interaction with ATP5a1 were lost [192, 193]. Based on their observations, it could be assumed that in the absence of ligands, AhR only localized into the mitochondria and bound with AhR-interacting protein [AIP (also XAP2)] [194], suggesting that AIP might be considered as the crucial mediator of AhR localization inside the mitochondria. In this way, it is shown that using siRNA against TOMM20, a mitochondrial import receptor subunit could significantly decrease mitochondrial AhR by 70%, but not cytoplasmic or nuclear AhR [193]. Similarly, they suggested that AIP and heat shock protein 90 (Hsp90) might be involved in the mitochondrial localization of AhR through TOMM20 interaction, which ultimately imports AhR into the intermembrane space of mitochondria. On the other hand, the increased levels of target genes of the AhR, including cyps, ugts, and gsts, in long-lived mitochondrial mutants in *C. elegans* have been shown [195 - 197].

To sum up, the mentioned literature comprehensively proposed that the influences of AhR on the functionality of mitochondria are probably sex-, age-, and tissue-dependent; therefore, there is a need to assess the possible crosstalk between AhR and mitochondria in appropriate *in-vivo* model systems which will certainly guarantee to uncover the potential role of this receptor in various pathophysiological situations, such as aging and related pathologies. However, because of the novelty of this route, there is a need to investigate the ameliorative role of TAU on mitochondrial functions involved in aging through this highly conserved transcription factor and/or other AhR-interacting elements.

CONCLUSION

Some well-known theories are involved in the aging process in the current chapter, including the free radical theory of aging, oxidative stress theory (oxidative stress/damage accumulation), the mitochondrial theory of aging, and the mitochondrial-lysosomal axis theory. Meanwhile, we have shown that mitochondria could be assumed as the primary target in this process. Aging-induced mitochondrial impairments (*i.e.*, enhanced mitochondria-facilitated ROS formation, decreased mitochondrial ATP, induction of mPT, and subsequently release of cell death mediators) could occur in reproductive and non-reproductive organs. Meanwhile, each section tries to highlight the ameliorative and protective role of TAU in mentioned involved pathways. The data gleaned hitherto show that TAU could reverse approximately all mentioned adverse effects collectively. However, there are still some gaps to support the crucial role of TAU against aging-induced organs toxicity through some intracellular pathways (including autophagic and inflammatory routes) and its effect on the content of lipids in the mitochondrial membrane (cardiolipin). In summary, additional studies are needed to understand better the TAU performance on other critical aspects of aging through different crucial unwell-known intracellular routes.

REFERENCES

[1] El Idrissi A, Shen CH, L'Amoreaux WJ. Neuroprotective role of taurine during aging. Amino Acids 2013; 45(4): 735-50.
[http://dx.doi.org/10.1007/s00726-013-1544-7] [PMID: 23963537]

[2] Amaral S, Amaral A, Ramalho-Santos J. Aging and male reproductive function A mitochondrial perspective. Front Biosci (Schol Ed) 2013; S5(1): 181-97.
[http://dx.doi.org/10.2741/S365] [PMID: 23277044]

[3] Sitzmann BD, Urbanski HF, Ottinger MA. Aging in male primates: reproductive decline, effects of calorie restriction and future research potential. Age (Omaha) 2008; 30(2-3): 157-68.
[http://dx.doi.org/10.1007/s11357-008-9065-0] [PMID: 19424865]

[4] Swerdloff RS, Wang C. Androgens and the ageing male. Best Pract Res Clin Endocrinol Metab 2004; 18(3): 349-62.
[http://dx.doi.org/10.1016/j.beem.2004.03.011] [PMID: 15261842]

[5]   Tenover JS. Declining testicular function in aging men. Int J Impot Res 2003; 15(S4) (Suppl. 4): S3-8.
        [http://dx.doi.org/10.1038/sj.ijir.3901029] [PMID: 12934044]

[6]   Matsumoto AM. Andropause: clinical implications of the decline in serum testosterone levels with
        aging in men. J Gerontol A Biol Sci Med Sci 2002; 57(2): M76-99.
        [http://dx.doi.org/10.1093/gerona/57.2.M76] [PMID: 11818427]

[7]   Hermann M, Untergasser G, Rumpold H, Berger P. Aging of the male reproductive system. Exp
        Gerontol 2000; 35(9-10): 1267-79.
        [http://dx.doi.org/10.1016/S0531-5565(00)00159-5] [PMID: 11113607]

[8]   Sampson N, Untergasser G, Plas E, Berger P. The ageing male reproductive tract. J Pathol 2007;
        211(2): 206-18.
        [http://dx.doi.org/10.1002/path.2077] [PMID: 17200938]

[9]   Morley JE, Kaiser FE, Perry HM III, *et al.* Longitudinal changes in testosterone, luteinizing hormone,
        and follicle-stimulating hormone in healthy older men. Metabolism 1997; 46(4): 410-3.
        [http://dx.doi.org/10.1016/S0026-0495(97)90057-3] [PMID: 9109845]

[10]   Harman SM, Metter EJ, Tobin JD, Pearson J, Blackman MR. Longitudinal effects of aging on serum
        total and free testosterone levels in healthy men. J Clin Endocrinol Metab 2001; 86(2): 724-31.
        [http://dx.doi.org/10.1210/jcem.86.2.7219] [PMID: 11158037]

[11]   Wang X, Stocco DM. The decline in testosterone biosynthesis during male aging: A consequence of
        multiple alterations. Mol Cell Endocrinol 2005; 238(1-2): 1-7.
        [http://dx.doi.org/10.1016/j.mce.2005.04.009] [PMID: 15939533]

[12]   Zhang H, Davies KJA, Forman HJ. Oxidative stress response and Nrf2 signaling in aging. Free Radic
        Biol Med. 2015;88(Pt B):314-36.
        [http://dx.doi.org/10.1016/j.freeradbiomed.2015.05.036]

[13]   Kudryavtseva AV, Krasnov GS, Dmitriev AA, *et al.* Mitochondrial dysfunction and oxidative stress in
        aging and cancer. Oncotarget 2016; 7(29): 44879-905.
        [http://dx.doi.org/10.18632/oncotarget.9821] [PMID: 27270647]

[14]   Cabello-Verrugio C, Simon F, Trollet C, Santibañez JF. Oxidative stress in disease and aging:
        Mechanisms and therapies. Oxid Med Cell Longev 2017; 2017: 1-2.
        [http://dx.doi.org/10.1155/2017/4310469] [PMID: 28246551]

[15]   Vatner SF, Zhang J, Oydanich M, Berkman T, Naftalovich R, Vatner DE. Healthful aging mediated by
        inhibition of oxidative stress. Ageing Res Rev 2020; 64: 101194.
        [http://dx.doi.org/10.1016/j.arr.2020.101194] [PMID: 33091597]

[16]   Chan DC. Mitochondria: dynamic organelles in disease, aging, and development. Cell 2006; 125(7):
        1241-52.
        [http://dx.doi.org/10.1016/j.cell.2006.06.010] [PMID: 16814712]

[17]   Jang JY, Blum A, Liu J, Finkel T. The role of mitochondria in aging. J Clin Invest 2018; 128(9):
        3662-70.
        [http://dx.doi.org/10.1172/JCI120842] [PMID: 30059016]

[18]   Zhang H, Menzies KJ, Auwerx J. The role of mitochondria in stem cell fate and aging. Development
        2018; 145(8): dev143420.
        [http://dx.doi.org/10.1242/dev.143420] [PMID: 29654217]

[19]   Janikiewicz J, Szymański J, Malinska D, *et al.* Mitochondria-associated membranes in aging and
        senescence: structure, function, and dynamics. Cell Death Dis 2018; 9(3): 332.
        [http://dx.doi.org/10.1038/s41419-017-0105-5] [PMID: 29491385]

[20]   Hood DA, Memme JM, Oliveira AN, Triolo M. Maintenance of skeletal muscle mitochondria in
        health, exercise, and aging. Annu Rev Physiol 2019; 81(1): 19-41.
        [http://dx.doi.org/10.1146/annurev-physiol-020518-114310] [PMID: 30216742]

[21]   Son JM, Lee C. Mitochondria: multifaceted regulators of aging. BMB Rep 2019; 52(1): 13-23.
         [http://dx.doi.org/10.5483/BMBRep.2019.52.1.300] [PMID: 30545443]

[22]   Chiang JL, Shukla P, Pagidas K, *et al.* Mitochondria in ovarian aging and reproductive longevity.
         Ageing Res Rev 2020; 63: 101168.
         [http://dx.doi.org/10.1016/j.arr.2020.101168] [PMID: 32896666]

[23]   Terman A, Gustafsson B, Brunk UT. Autophagy, organelles and ageing. J Pathol 2007; 211(2): 134-
         43.
         [http://dx.doi.org/10.1002/path.2094] [PMID: 17200947]

[24]   Buffenstein R, Edrey YH, Yang T, Mele J. The oxidative stress theory of aging: embattled or
         invincible? Insights from non-traditional model organisms. Age (Omaha) 2008; 30(2-3): 99-109.
         [http://dx.doi.org/10.1007/s11357-008-9058-z] [PMID: 19424860]

[25]   Van Remmen H, Jones DP. Current thoughts on the role of mitochondria and free radicals in the
         biology of aging. J Gerontol A Biol Sci Med Sci 2009; 64A(2): 171-4.
         [http://dx.doi.org/10.1093/gerona/gln058] [PMID: 19181714]

[26]   Alexeyev MF. Is there more to aging than mitochondrial DNA and reactive oxygen species? FEBS J
         2009; 276(20): 5768-87.
         [http://dx.doi.org/10.1111/j.1742-4658.2009.07269.x] [PMID: 19796285]

[27]   Salmon AB, Richardson A, Pérez VI. Update on the oxidative stress theory of aging: Does oxidative
         stress play a role in aging or healthy aging? Free Radic Biol Med 2010; 48(5): 642-55.
         [http://dx.doi.org/10.1016/j.freeradbiomed.2009.12.015] [PMID: 20036736]

[28]   Harman D. Aging: a theory based on free radical and radiation chemistry. J Gerontol 1956; 11(3):
         298-300.
         [http://dx.doi.org/10.1093/geronj/11.3.298] [PMID: 13332224]

[29]   Harman D. The biologic clock: the mitochondria? J Am Geriatr Soc 1972; 20(4): 145-7.
         [http://dx.doi.org/10.1111/j.1532-5415.1972.tb00787.x] [PMID: 5016631]

[30]   Sinha K, Das J, Pal PB, Sil PC. Oxidative stress: the mitochondria-dependent and mitochondria-
         independent pathways of apoptosis. Arch Toxicol 2013; 87(7): 1157-80.
         [http://dx.doi.org/10.1007/s00204-013-1034-4] [PMID: 23543009]

[31]   Lee HC, Wei YH. Mitochondrial alterations, cellular response to oxidative stress and defective
         degradation of proteins in aging. Biogerontology 2001; 2(4): 231-44.
         [http://dx.doi.org/10.1023/A:1013270512172] [PMID: 11868898]

[32]   Harper ME, Bevilacqua L, Hagopian K, Weindruch R, Ramsey JJ. Ageing, oxidative stress, and
         mitochondrial uncoupling. Acta Physiol Scand 2004; 182(4): 321-31.
         [http://dx.doi.org/10.1111/j.1365-201X.2004.01370.x] [PMID: 15569093]

[33]   Sastre J, Pallardó FV, Viña J. The role of mitochondrial oxidative stress in aging. Free Radic Biol Med
         2003; 35(1): 1-8.
         [http://dx.doi.org/10.1016/S0891-5849(03)00184-9] [PMID: 12826250]

[34]   Terman A, Kurz T, Navratil M, Arriaga EA, Brunk UT. Mitochondrial turnover and aging of long-
         lived postmitotic cells: the mitochondrial-lysosomal axis theory of aging. Antioxid Redox Signal
         2010; 12(4): 503-35.
         [http://dx.doi.org/10.1089/ars.2009.2598] [PMID: 19650712]

[35]   Ommati MM, Shi X, Li H, *et al.* The mechanisms of arsenic-induced ovotoxicity, ultrastructural
         alterations, and autophagic related paths: An enduring developmental study in folliculogenesis of
         mice. Ecotoxicol Environ Saf 2020; 204: 110973.
         [http://dx.doi.org/10.1016/j.ecoenv.2020.110973] [PMID: 32781346]

[36]   Ratajczak MZ, Shin DM, Ratajczak J, Kucia M, Bartke A. A novel insight into aging: are there
         pluripotent very small embryonic-like stem cells (VSELs) in adult tissues overtime depleted in an Igf-

1-dependent manner? Aging (Albany NY) 2010; 2(11): 875-83.
[http://dx.doi.org/10.18632/aging.100231] [PMID: 21084728]

[37]   Legan SK, Rebrin I, Mockett RJ, *et al.* Overexpression of glucose-6-phosphate dehydrogenase extends the life span of Drosophila melanogaster. J Biol Chem 2008; 283(47): 32492-9.
[http://dx.doi.org/10.1074/jbc.M805832200] [PMID: 18809674]

[38]   Sadoshima J. Sirt3 targets mPTP and prevents aging in the heart. Aging (Albany NY) 2011; 3(1): 12-3.
[http://dx.doi.org/10.18632/aging.100266] [PMID: 21248376]

[39]   Zheng J, Hu S, Wang J, *et al.* Icariin improves brain function decline in aging rats by enhancing neuronal autophagy through the AMPK/mTOR/ULK1 pathway. Pharm Biol 2021; 59(1): 181-9.
[http://dx.doi.org/10.1080/13880209.2021.1878238] [PMID: 33556283]

[40]   Aman Y, Schmauck-Medina T, Hansen M, *et al.* Autophagy in healthy aging and disease. Nature Aging 2021; 1(8): 634-50.
[http://dx.doi.org/10.1038/s43587-021-00098-4] [PMID: 34901876]

[41]   Yoo H, Kim HS. Cacao powder supplementation attenuates oxidative stress, cholinergic impairment, and apoptosis in d-galactose-induced aging rat brain. Sci Rep 2021; 11(1): 17914.
[http://dx.doi.org/10.1038/s41598-021-96800-y] [PMID: 34504131]

[42]   Chen F, Lei J, Wang G, Zhou B. The gut microbiota metabolite urolithin B improves cognitive deficits by inhibiting Cyt c-mediated apoptosis and promoting the survival of neurons through the PI3K pathway in aging mice. Front Pharmacol 2021; 12: 768097.
[http://dx.doi.org/10.3389/fphar.2021.768097]

[43]   Shigenaga MK, Hagen TM, Ames BN. Oxidative damage and mitochondrial decay in aging. Proc Natl Acad Sci USA 1994; 91(23): 10771-8.
[http://dx.doi.org/10.1073/pnas.91.23.10771] [PMID: 7971961]

[44]   Ago T, Matsushima S, Kuroda J, Zablocki D, Kitazono T, Sadoshima J. The NADPH oxidase Nox4 and aging in the heart. Aging (Albany NY) 2010; 2(12): 1012-6.
[http://dx.doi.org/10.18632/aging.100261] [PMID: 21212466]

[45]   Babior BM, Peters WA. The O_2-producing enzyme of human neutrophils. Further properties. J Biol Chem 1981; 256(5): 2321-3.
[http://dx.doi.org/10.1016/S0021-9258(19)69781-4] [PMID: 7462239]

[46]   Jang YC, Pérez VI, Song W, *et al.* Overexpression of Mn superoxide dismutase does not increase life span in mice. J Gerontol A Biol Sci Med Sci 2009; 64A(11): 1114-25.
[http://dx.doi.org/10.1093/gerona/glp100] [PMID: 19633237]

[47]   Dai DF, Santana LF, Vermulst M, *et al.* Overexpression of catalase targeted to mitochondria attenuates murine cardiac aging. Circulation 2009; 119(21): 2789-97.
[http://dx.doi.org/10.1161/CIRCULATIONAHA.108.822403] [PMID: 19451351]

[48]   Ommati MM, Heidari R. Amino acids ameliorate heavy metals-induced oxidative stress in male/female reproductive tissue.Toxicology. Academic Press 2021; pp. 371-86.
[http://dx.doi.org/10.1016/B978-0-12-819092-0.00037-6]

[49]   Ommati MM, Heidari R. Betaine, heavy metal protection, oxidative stress, and the liver.Toxicology. Academic Press 2021; pp. 387-95.
[http://dx.doi.org/10.1016/B978-0-12-819092-0.00038-8]

[50]   Ommati MM, Farshad O, Azarpira N, Ghazanfari E, Niknahad H, Heidari R. Silymarin mitigates bile duct obstruction-induced cholemic nephropathy. Naunyn Schmiedebergs Arch Pharmacol 2021; 394(6): 1301-14.
[http://dx.doi.org/10.1007/s00210-020-02040-8] [PMID: 33538845]

[51]   Ommati MM, Farshad O, Ghanbarinejad V, *et al.* The nephroprotective role of carnosine against ifosfamide-induced renal injury and electrolytes imbalance is mediated *via* the regulation of

mitochondrial function and alleviation of oxidative stress. Drug Res (Stuttg) 2020; 70(1): 49-56.
[http://dx.doi.org/10.1055/a-1017-5085] [PMID: 31671464]

[52] Ommati MM, Heidari R, Ghanbarinejad V, Aminian A, Abdoli N, Niknahad H. The neuroprotective
properties of carnosine in a mouse model of manganism is mediated *via* mitochondria regulating and
antioxidative mechanisms. Nutr Neurosci 2020; 23(9): 731-43.
[http://dx.doi.org/10.1080/1028415X.2018.1552399] [PMID: 30856059]

[53] Ommati MM, Jamshidzadeh A, Heidari R, *et al.* Carnosine and histidine supplementation blunt lead-
induced reproductive toxicity through antioxidative and mitochondria-dependent mechanisms. Biol
Trace Elem Res 2019; 187(1): 151-62.
[http://dx.doi.org/10.1007/s12011-018-1358-2] [PMID: 29767280]

[54] Heidari R, Abdoli N, Ommati MM, Jamshidzadeh A, Niknahad H. Mitochondrial impairment induced
by chenodeoxycholic acid: The protective effect of taurine and carnosine supplementation. Trends in
Pharmaceutical Sciences. 2018;4(2).

[55] Heidari R, Ghanbarinejad V, Ommati MM, Jamshidzadeh A, Niknahad H. Regulation of
mitochondrial function and energy metabolism: A primary mechanism of cytoprotection provided by
carnosine. Trends in Pharmaceutical Sciences. 2018;4(1).

[56] Jamshidzadeh A, Heidari R, Latifpour Z, *et al.* Carnosine ameliorates liver fibrosis and
hyperammonemia in cirrhotic rats. Clin Res Hepatol Gastroenterol 2017; 41(4): 424-34.
[http://dx.doi.org/10.1016/j.clinre.2016.12.010] [PMID: 28283328]

[57] Jamshidzadeh A, Niknahad H, Heidari R, Zarei M, Ommati MM, Khodaei F. Carnosine protects brain
mitochondria under hyperammonemic conditions: Relevance to hepatic encephalopathy treatment.
PharmaNutrition 2017; 5(2): 58-63.
[http://dx.doi.org/10.1016/j.phanu.2017.02.004]

[58] Jamshidzadeh A, Heidari R, Abazari F, *et al.* Antimalarial drugs-induced hepatic injury in rats and the
protective role of carnosine. Ulum-i Daruyi 2016; 22(3): 170-80.
[http://dx.doi.org/10.15171/PS.2016.27]

[59] Ommati MM, Farshad O, Azarpira N, Shafaghat M, Niknahad H, Heidari R. Betaine alleviates
cholestasis-associated renal injury by mitigating oxidative stress and enhancing mitochondrial
function. Biologia (Bratisl) 2021; 76(1): 351-65.
[http://dx.doi.org/10.2478/s11756-020-00576-x]

[60] Ommati MM, Farshad O, Mousavi K, *et al.* Betaine supplementation mitigates intestinal damage and
decreases serum bacterial endotoxin in cirrhotic rats. PharmaNutrition 2020; 12: 100179.
[http://dx.doi.org/10.1016/j.phanu.2020.100179]

[61] Heidari R, Niknahad H, Sadeghi A, *et al.* Betaine treatment protects liver through regulating
mitochondrial function and counteracting oxidative stress in acute and chronic animal models of
hepatic injury. Biomed Pharmacother 2018; 103: 75-86.
[http://dx.doi.org/10.1016/j.biopha.2018.04.010] [PMID: 29635131]

[62] Heidari R, Ghanbarinejad V, Ommati MM, Jamshidzadeh A, Niknahad H. Mitochondria protecting
amino acids: Application against a wide range of mitochondria-linked complications. PharmaNutrition
2018; 6(4): 180-90.
[http://dx.doi.org/10.1016/j.phanu.2018.09.001]

[63] Ommati MM, Farshad O, Mousavi K, Khalili M, Jamshidzadeh A, Heidari R. Chlorogenic acid
supplementation improves skeletal muscle mitochondrial function in a rat model of resistance training.
Biologia (Bratisl) 2020; 75(8): 1221-30.
[http://dx.doi.org/10.2478/s11756-020-00429-7]

[64] Ommati MM, Amjadinia A, Mousavi K, Azarpira N, Jamshidzadeh A, Heidari R. N-acetyl cysteine
treatment mitigates biomarkers of oxidative stress in different tissues of bile duct ligated rats. Stress
2021; 24(2): 213-28.
[http://dx.doi.org/10.1080/10253890.2020.1777970] [PMID: 32510264]

[65]   Abdoli N, Sadeghian I, Mousavi K, Azarpira N, Ommati MM, Heidari R. Suppression of cirrhosis-related renal injury by N-acetyl cysteine. Current Research in Pharmacology and Drug Discovery 2020; 1: 30-8.
[http://dx.doi.org/10.1016/j.crphar.2020.100006] [PMID: 34909640]

[66]   Farshad O, Heidari R, Zare F, *et al.* Effects of cimetidine and N-acetylcysteine on paraquat-induced acute lung injury in rats: a preliminary study. Toxicol Environ Chem 2018; 100(8-10): 785-93.
[http://dx.doi.org/10.1080/02772248.2019.1606225]

[67]   Ommati MM, Jamshidzadeh A, Niknahad H, *et al.* N-acetylcysteine treatment blunts liver failure-associated impairment of locomotor activity. PharmaNutrition 2017; 5(4): 141-7.
[http://dx.doi.org/10.1016/j.phanu.2017.10.003]

[68]   Ommati MM, Azarpira N, Khodaei F, Niknahad H, Gozashtegan V, Heidari R. Methylene blue treatment enhances mitochondrial function and locomotor activity in a C57BL/6 mouse model of multiple sclerosis. Trends Pharmacol Sci 2020; 6(1): 29-42.

[69]   Ommati MM, Mohammadi H, Mousavi K, Azarpira N, Farshad O, Dehghani R, *et al.* Metformin alleviates cholestasis-associated nephropathy through regulating oxidative stress and mitochondrial function. Liver Research 2021; 5(3): 171-180.

[70]   Ommati MM, Attari H, Siavashpour A, Shafaghat M, Azarpira N, Ghaffari H, *et al.* Mitigation of cholestasis-associated hepatic and renal injury by edaravone treatment: Evaluation of its effects on oxidative stress and mitochondrial function. Liver Research 2021; 5(3): 181-193.

[71]   Mohammadi H, Ommati MM, Farshad O, Jamshidzadeh A, Niknahad H, Heidari R. Taurine and isolated mitochondria: A concentration-response study. Trends Pharmacol Sci 2019; 5(4): 5-6.

[72]   Heidari R, Jamshidzadeh A, Ghanbarinejad V, Ommati MM, Niknahad H. Taurine supplementation abates cirrhosis-associated locomotor dysfunction. Clin Exp Hepatol 2018; 4(2): 72-82.
[http://dx.doi.org/10.5114/ceh.2018.75956] [PMID: 29904723]

[73]   Jamshidzadeh A, Heidari R, Abasvali M, *et al.* Taurine treatment preserves brain and liver mitochondrial function in a rat model of fulminant hepatic failure and hyperammonemia. Biomed Pharmacother 2017; 86: 514-20.
[http://dx.doi.org/10.1016/j.biopha.2016.11.095] [PMID: 28024286]

[74]   Niknahad H, Jamshidzadeh A, Heidari R, Zarei M, Ommati MM. Ammonia-induced mitochondrial dysfunction and energy metabolism disturbances in isolated brain and liver mitochondria, and the effect of taurine administration: relevance to hepatic encephalopathy treatment. Clin Exp Hepatol 2017; 3(3): 141-51.
[http://dx.doi.org/10.5114/ceh.2017.68833] [PMID: 29062904]

[75]   Heidari R, Jamshidzadeh A, Niknahad H, *et al.* Effect of taurine on chronic and acute liver injury: Focus on blood and brain ammonia. Toxicol Rep 2016; 3: 870-9.
[http://dx.doi.org/10.1016/j.toxrep.2016.04.002] [PMID: 28959615]

[76]   Ommati MM, Heidari R, Jamshidzadeh A, *et al.* Dual effects of sulfasalazine on rat sperm characteristics, spermatogenesis, and steroidogenesis in two experimental models. Toxicol Lett 2018; 284: 46-55.
[http://dx.doi.org/10.1016/j.toxlet.2017.11.034] [PMID: 29197623]

[77]   Yu Y, Han Y, Niu R, *et al.* Ameliorative effect of VE, IGF-I, and hCG on the fluoride-induced testosterone release suppression in mice Leydig cells. Biol Trace Elem Res 2018; 181(1): 95-103.
[http://dx.doi.org/10.1007/s12011-017-1023-1] [PMID: 28462439]

[78]   Niknahad H, Ommati MM, Sookhak N, Hajihashemi F, Azarpira N, Heidari R. Glycyrrhizic acid and the aqueous extract of Glycyrrhiza glabra attenuate hepatotoxicity in mice. Trends Pharmacol Sci 2021; 7(1): 59-72.

[79]   Azarang A, Farshad O, Ommati MM, *et al.* Protective role of probiotic supplements in hepatic steatosis: A rat model study. BioMed Res Int 2020; 2020: 1-15.

[http://dx.doi.org/10.1155/2020/5487659] [PMID: 33299871]

[80] Heidari R, Arabnezhad MR, Ommati MM, Azarpira N, Ghodsimanesh E, Niknahad H. Boldine supplementation regulates mitochondrial function and oxidative stress in a rat model of hepatotoxicity. Ulum-i Daruyi 2019; 25(1): 1-10.
[http://dx.doi.org/10.15171/PS.2019.1]

[81] Shafiekhani M, Ommati MM, Azarpira N, Heidari R, Salarian AA. Glycine supplementation mitigates lead-induced renal injury in mice. J Exp Pharmacol 2019; 11: 15-22.
[http://dx.doi.org/10.2147/JEP.S190846] [PMID: 30858736]

[82] Heidari R, Mohammadi H, Ghanbarinejad V, *et al.* Proline supplementation mitigates the early stage of liver injury in bile duct ligated rats. J Basic Clin Physiol Pharmacol 2018; 30(1): 91-101.
[http://dx.doi.org/10.1515/jbcpp-2017-0221] [PMID: 30205645]

[83] Ommati MM, Zamiri MJ, Akhlaghi A, *et al.* Seminal characteristics, sperm fatty acids, and blood biochemical attributes in breeder roosters orally administered with sage (Salvia officinalis) extract. Anim Prod Sci 2013; 53(6): 548-54.
[http://dx.doi.org/10.1071/AN12257]

[84] Saemi F, Zamiri MJ, Akhlaghi A, Niakousari M, Dadpasand M, Ommati MM. Dietary inclusion of dried tomato pomace improves the seminal characteristics in Iranian native roosters. Poult Sci 2012; 91(9): 2310-5.
[http://dx.doi.org/10.3382/ps.2012-02304] [PMID: 22912468]

[85] Jamshidzadeh A, Heidari R, Golzar T, Derakhshanfar A. Effect of Eisenia foetida extract against cisplatin-induced kidney injury in rats. J Diet Suppl 2016; 13(5): 551-9.
[http://dx.doi.org/10.3109/19390211.2015.1124163] [PMID: 26864051]

[86] Jamshidzadeh A, Dabagh F, Farshad O, Ommat MM, Mahdavinia A, Azarpira N, *et al.* Hepatoprotective properties of the glycolipoprotein extract from Eisenia foetida. Trends Pharmacol Sci 2018; 4(3): 149-60.

[87] Heidari R, Ghanbarinejad V, Mohammadi H, *et al.* Mitochondria protection as a mechanism underlying the hepatoprotective effects of glycine in cholestatic mice. Biomed Pharmacother 2018; 97: 1086-95.
[http://dx.doi.org/10.1016/j.biopha.2017.10.166] [PMID: 29136945]

[88] Heidari R, Moezi L, Asadi B, Ommati MM, Azarpira N. Hepatoprotective effect of boldine in a bile duct ligated rat model of cholestasis/cirrhosis. PharmaNutrition 2017; 5(3): 109-17.
[http://dx.doi.org/10.1016/j.phanu.2017.07.001]

[89] Jamshidzadeh A, Heidari R, Razmjou M, *et al.* An *in vivo* and *in vitro* investigation on hepatoprotective effects of Pimpinella anisum seed essential oil and extracts against carbon tetrachloride-induced toxicity. Iran J Basic Med Sci 2015; 18(2): 205-11.
[PMID: 25825639]

[90] Heidari R, Jamshidzadeh A, Niknahad H, Safari F, Azizi H, Abdoli N, *et al.* The hepatoprotection provided by taurine and glycine against antineoplastic drugs induced liver injury in an *ex vivo* model of normothermic recirculating isolated perfused rat liver. Trends Pharmacol Sci 2016; 2(1): 59-76.

[91] Niknahad H, Hosseini H, Gozashtegan F, Ebrahimi F, Azarpira N, Abdoli N, *et al.* The hepatoprotective role of thiol reductants against mitoxantrone-induced liver injury. Trends Pharmacol Sci 2017; 3(2): 113-22.
[PMID: 27855993]

[92] Mobasher MA, Jamshidzadeh A, Heidari R, Ghahiri G, Mobasher N. Hepatoprotective effects of Artemia salina L. extract against carbon tetrachloride-induced toxicity. Trends Pharmacol Sci 2016; 2(4): 259-64.

[93] Farshad O, Heidari R, Mohammadi H, Akbarizadeh AR, Zarshenas MM. Hepatoprotective effects of Avicennia Marina (Forssk.) Vierh. Trends Pharmacol Sci 2017; 3(4): 255-66.

[94]   Heidari R, Behnamrad S, Khodami Z, Ommati MM, Azarpira N, Vazin A. The nephroprotective properties of taurine in colistin-treated mice is mediated through the regulation of mitochondrial function and mitigation of oxidative stress. Biomed Pharmacother 2019; 109: 103-11.
        [http://dx.doi.org/10.1016/j.biopha.2018.10.093] [PMID: 30396066]

[95]   Abdoli N, Sadeghian I, Azarpira N, Ommati MM, Heidari R. Taurine mitigates bile duct obstruction-associated cholemic nephropathy: Effect on oxidative stress and mitochondrial parameters. Clin Exp Hepatol 2021; 7(1): 30–40.
        [PMID: 34027113]

[96]   Ommati MM, Farshad O, Jamshidzadeh A, Heidari R. Taurine enhances skeletal muscle mitochondrial function in a rat model of resistance training. PharmaNutrition 2019; 9: 100161.
        [http://dx.doi.org/10.1016/j.phanu.2019.100161]

[97]   Mousavi K, Niknahad H, Ghalamfarsa A, Mohammadi HR, Heidari R. Taurine mitigates cirrhosis-associated cardiac injury through mitochondrial-dependent and antioxidative mechanisms. Experimental and Clinical Hepatology. 2020;6(3).

[98]   Ommati MM, Heidari R, Ghanbarinejad V, Abdoli N, Niknahad H. Taurine treatment provides neuroprotection in a mouse model of manganism. Biol Trace Elem Res 2019; 190(2): 384-95.
        [http://dx.doi.org/10.1007/s12011-018-1552-2] [PMID: 30357569]

[99]   Ahmadi N, Ghanbarinejad V, Ommati MM, Jamshidzadeh A, Heidari R. Taurine prevents mitochondrial membrane permeabilization and swelling upon interaction with manganese: Implication in the treatment of cirrhosis-associated central nervous system complications. J Biochem Mol Toxicol 2018; 32(11): e22216.
        [http://dx.doi.org/10.1002/jbt.22216] [PMID: 30152904]

[100]   Oyewole AO, Birch-Machin MA. Mitochondria-targeted antioxidants. FASEB J 2015; 29(12): 4766-71.
        [http://dx.doi.org/10.1096/fj.15-275404] [PMID: 26253366]

[101]   Gruber J, Fong S, Chen CB, *et al.* Mitochondria-targeted antioxidants and metabolic modulators as pharmacological interventions to slow ageing. Biotechnol Adv 2013; 31(5): 563-92.
        [http://dx.doi.org/10.1016/j.biotechadv.2012.09.005] [PMID: 23022622]

[102]   Yamori Y, Liu L, Mori M, *et al.* Taurine as the nutritional factor for the longevity of the Japanese revealed by a world-wide epidemiological survey. Adv Exp Med Biol 2009; 643: 13-25.
        [http://dx.doi.org/10.1007/978-0-387-75681-3_2] [PMID: 19239132]

[103]   Yamori Y, Taguchi T, Hamada A, Kunimasa K, Mori H, Mori M. Taurine in health and diseases: consistent evidence from experimental and epidemiological studies. J Biomed Sci 2010; 17(Suppl 1): S6.
        [http://dx.doi.org/10.1186/1423-0127-17-S1-S6] [PMID: 20804626]

[104]   Sohal RS, Ku HH, Agarwal S, Forster MJ, Lal H. Oxidative damage, mitochondrial oxidant generation and antioxidant defenses during aging and in response to food restriction in the mouse. Mech Ageing Dev 1994; 74(1-2): 121-33.
        [http://dx.doi.org/10.1016/0047-6374(94)90104-X] [PMID: 7934203]

[105]   Agarwal S, Sohal RS. Differential oxidative damage to mitochondrial proteins during aging. Mech Ageing Dev 1995; 85(1): 55-63.
        [http://dx.doi.org/10.1016/0047-6374(95)01655-4] [PMID: 8789255]

[106]   Houtkooper RH, Vaz FM. Cardiolipin, the heart of mitochondrial metabolism. Cell Mol Life Sci 2008; 65(16): 2493-506.
        [http://dx.doi.org/10.1007/s00018-008-8030-5] [PMID: 18425414]

[107]   Vähäheikkilä M, Peltomaa T, Róg T, Vazdar M, Pöyry S, Vattulainen I. How cardiolipin peroxidation alters the properties of the inner mitochondrial membrane? Chem Phys Lipids 2018; 214: 15-23.
        [http://dx.doi.org/10.1016/j.chemphyslip.2018.04.005] [PMID: 29723518]

[108] Wong-ekkabut J, Xu Z, Triampo W, Tang IM, Peter Tieleman D, Monticelli L. Effect of lipid peroxidation on the properties of lipid bilayers: a molecular dynamics study. Biophys J 2007; 93(12): 4225-36.
[http://dx.doi.org/10.1529/biophysj.107.112565] [PMID: 17766354]

[109] Paradies G, Petrosillo G, Pistolese M, Di Venosa N, Federici A, Ruggiero FM. Decrease in mitochondrial complex I activity in ischemic/reperfused rat heart: involvement of reactive oxygen species and cardiolipin. Circ Res 2004; 94(1): 53-9.
[http://dx.doi.org/10.1161/01.RES.0000109416.56608.64] [PMID: 14656928]

[110] Mileykovskaya E, Dowhan W. Cardiolipin-dependent formation of mitochondrial respiratory supercomplexes. Chem Phys Lipids 2014; 179: 42-8.
[http://dx.doi.org/10.1016/j.chemphyslip.2013.10.012] [PMID: 24220496]

[111] Oemer G, Koch J, Wohlfarter Y, Alam MT, Lackner K, Sailer S, *et al.* Phospholipid acyl chain diversity controls the tissue-specific assembly of mitochondrial cardiolipins. Cell Rep. 2020;30(12):4281-91.
[http://dx.doi.org/10.1016/j.celrep.2020.02.115]

[112] Hoch FL. Cardiolipins and biomembrane function. Biochim Biophys Acta Rev Biomembr 1992; 1113(1): 71-133.
[http://dx.doi.org/10.1016/0304-4157(92)90035-9] [PMID: 1550861]

[113] Yan LJ, Sohal RS. Mitochondrial adenine nucleotide translocase is modified oxidatively during aging. Proc Natl Acad Sci USA 1998; 95(22): 12896-901.
[http://dx.doi.org/10.1073/pnas.95.22.12896] [PMID: 9789011]

[114] Lippe G, Comelli M, Mazzilis D, Sala FD, Mavelli I. The inactivation of mitochondrial F1 ATPase by H2O2 is mediated by iron ions not tightly bound in the protein. Biochem Biophys Res Commun 1991; 181(2): 764-70.
[http://dx.doi.org/10.1016/0006-291X(91)91256-C] [PMID: 1836727]

[115] Yan LJ, Levine RL, Sohal RS. Oxidative damage during aging targets mitochondrial aconitase. Proc Natl Acad Sci USA 1997; 94(21): 11168-72.
[http://dx.doi.org/10.1073/pnas.94.21.11168] [PMID: 9326580]

[116] Sastre J, Pallardó FV, Plá R, *et al.* Aging of the liver: Age-associated mitochondrial damage in intact hepatocytes. Hepatology 1996; 24(5): 1199-205.
[http://dx.doi.org/10.1002/hep.510240536] [PMID: 8903398]

[117] Yakes FM, Van Houten B. Mitochondrial DNA damage is more extensive and persists longer than nuclear DNA damage in human cells following oxidative stress. Proc Natl Acad Sci USA 1997; 94(2): 514-9.
[http://dx.doi.org/10.1073/pnas.94.2.514] [PMID: 9012815]

[118] Barja G, Herrero A. Oxidative damage to mitochondrial DNA is inversely related to maximum life span in the heart and brain of mammals. FASEB J 2000; 14(2): 312-8.
[http://dx.doi.org/10.1096/fasebj.14.2.312] [PMID: 10657987]

[119] Linford NJ, Schriner SE, Rabinovitch PS. Oxidative damage and aging: spotlight on mitochondria. Cancer Res 2006; 66(5): 2497-9.
[http://dx.doi.org/10.1158/0008-5472.CAN-05-3163] [PMID: 16510562]

[120] Remmen H, Richardson A. Oxidative damage to mitochondria and aging. Exp Gerontol 2001; 36(7): 957-68.
[http://dx.doi.org/10.1016/S0531-5565(01)00093-6] [PMID: 11404044]

[121] Kakkar P, Singh BK. Mitochondria: a hub of redox activities and cellular distress control. Mol Cell Biochem 2007; 305(1-2): 235-53.
[http://dx.doi.org/10.1007/s11010-007-9520-8] [PMID: 17562131]

[122] Xu S, He M, Zhong M, *et al.* The neuroprotective effects of taurine against nickel by reducing

oxidative stress and maintaining mitochondrial function in cortical neurons. Neurosci Lett 2015; 590: 52-7.
[http://dx.doi.org/10.1016/j.neulet.2015.01.065] [PMID: 25637701]

[123]   Chou CT, Lin HT, Hwang PA, Wang ST, Hsieh CH, Hwang DF. Taurine resumed neuronal differentiation in arsenite-treated N2a cells through reducing oxidative stress, endoplasmic reticulum stress, and mitochondrial dysfunction. Amino Acids 2015; 47(4): 735-44.
[http://dx.doi.org/10.1007/s00726-014-1901-1] [PMID: 25547999]

[124]   Dirks AJ, Hofer T, Marzetti E, Pahor M, Leeuwenburgh C. Mitochondrial DNA mutations, energy metabolism and apoptosis in aging muscle. Ageing Res Rev 2006; 5(2): 179-95.
[http://dx.doi.org/10.1016/j.arr.2006.03.002] [PMID: 16647308]

[125]   Pollack M, Leeuwenburgh C. Apoptosis and aging: role of the mitochondria. J Gerontol A Biol Sci Med Sci 2001; 56(11): B475-82.
[http://dx.doi.org/10.1093/gerona/56.11.B475] [PMID: 11682568]

[126]   Manthari RK, Tikka C, Ommati MM, et al. Arsenic-induced autophagy in the developing mouse cerebellum: Involvement of the blood-brain barrier's tight-junction proteins and the PI3K-Akt-mTOR signaling pathway. J Agric Food Chem 2018; 66(32): 8602-14.
[http://dx.doi.org/10.1021/acs.jafc.8b02654] [PMID: 30032600]

[127]   Manthari RK, Tikka C, Ommati MM, et al. Arsenic induces autophagy in developmental mouse cerebral cortex and hippocampus by inhibiting PI3K/Akt/mTOR signaling pathway: involvement of blood-brain barrier's tight junction proteins. Arch Toxicol 2018; 92(11): 3255-75.
[http://dx.doi.org/10.1007/s00204-018-2304-y] [PMID: 30225639]

[128]   Ommati MM, Heidari R, Manthari RK, et al. Paternal exposure to arsenic resulted in oxidative stress, autophagy, and mitochondrial impairments in the HPG axis of pubertal male offspring. Chemosphere 2019; 236: 124325.
[http://dx.doi.org/10.1016/j.chemosphere.2019.07.056] [PMID: 31326754]

[129]   Ommati MM, Manthari RK, Tikka C, et al. Arsenic-induced autophagic alterations and mitochondrial impairments in HPG-S axis of mature male mice offspring (F1-generation): A persistent toxicity study. Toxicol Lett 2020; 326: 83-98.
[http://dx.doi.org/10.1016/j.toxlet.2020.02.013] [PMID: 32112876]

[130]   Najibi A, Rezaei H, Kumar Manthari R, et al. Cellular and mitochondrial taurine depletion in bile duct ligated rats: a justification for taurine supplementation in cholestasis/cirrhosis. Clin Exp Hepatol 2022; 8(3): 195-210.
[http://dx.doi.org/10.5114/ceh.2022.119216] [PMID: 36685263]

[131]   Yang J, Zong X, Wu G, Lin S, Feng Y, Hu J. Taurine increases testicular function in aged rats by inhibiting oxidative stress and apoptosis. Amino Acids 2015; 47(8): 1549-58.
[http://dx.doi.org/10.1007/s00726-015-1995-0] [PMID: 25957528]

[132]   Aydın AF, Çoban J, Doğan-Ekici I, Betül-Kalaz E, Doğru-Abbasoğlu S, Uysal M. Carnosine and taurine treatments diminished brain oxidative stress and apoptosis in D-galactose aging model. Metab Brain Dis 2016; 31(2): 337-45.
[http://dx.doi.org/10.1007/s11011-015-9755-0] [PMID: 26518192]

[133]   Yildirim Z, Kiliç N, Ozer C, Babul A, Take G, Erdogan D. Effects of taurine in cellular responses to oxidative stress in young and middle-aged rat liver. Ann N Y Acad Sci 2007; 1100(1): 553-61.
[http://dx.doi.org/10.1196/annals.1395.061] [PMID: 17460221]

[134]   Klaus S, Ost M. Mitochondrial uncoupling and longevity - A role for mitokines? Exp Gerontol 2020; 130: 110796.
[http://dx.doi.org/10.1016/j.exger.2019.110796] [PMID: 31786315]

[135]   Mookerjee SA, Divakaruni AS, Jastroch M, Brand MD. Mitochondrial uncoupling and lifespan. Mech Ageing Dev 2010; 131(7-8): 463-72.
[http://dx.doi.org/10.1016/j.mad.2010.03.010] [PMID: 20363244]

[136] Fridell YWC, Sánchez-Blanco A, Silvia BA, Helfand SL. Targeted expression of the human uncoupling protein 2 (hUCP2) to adult neurons extends life span in the fly. Cell Metab 2005; 1(2): 145-52.
[http://dx.doi.org/10.1016/j.cmet.2005.01.005] [PMID: 16054055]

[137] Sánchez-Blanco A, Fridell YWC, Helfand SL. Involvement of Drosophila uncoupling protein 5 in metabolism and aging. Genetics 2006; 172(3): 1699-710.
[http://dx.doi.org/10.1534/genetics.105.053389] [PMID: 16387864]

[138] Iser WB, Kim D, Bachman E, Wolkow C. Examination of the requirement for ucp-4, a putative homolog of mammalian uncoupling proteins, for stress tolerance and longevity in C. elegans. Mech Ageing Dev 2005; 126(10): 1090-6.
[http://dx.doi.org/10.1016/j.mad.2005.04.002] [PMID: 15893362]

[139] Harper M-E, Monemdjou S, Ramsey JJ, Weindruch R. Age-related increase in mitochondrial proton leak and decrease in ATP turnover reactions in mouse hepatocytes. Am J Physiol 1998; 275(2): E197-206.
[PMID: 9688619]

[140] Gates AC, Bernal-Mizrachi C, Chinault SL, et al. Respiratory uncoupling in skeletal muscle delays death and diminishes age-related disease. Cell Metab 2007; 6(6): 497-505.
[http://dx.doi.org/10.1016/j.cmet.2007.10.010] [PMID: 18054318]

[141] Nabben M, Hoeks J, Briedé JJ, et al. The effect of UCP3 overexpression on mitochondrial ROS production in skeletal muscle of young versus aged mice. FEBS Lett 2008; 582(30): 4147-52.
[http://dx.doi.org/10.1016/j.febslet.2008.11.016] [PMID: 19041310]

[142] Oelkrug R, Kutschke M, Meyer CW, Heldmaier G, Jastroch M. Uncoupling protein 1 decreases superoxide production in brown adipose tissue mitochondria. J Biol Chem 2010; 285(29): 21961-8.
[http://dx.doi.org/10.1074/jbc.M110.122861] [PMID: 20466728]

[143] Keipert S, Voigt A, Klaus S. Dietary effects on body composition, glucose metabolism, and longevity are modulated by skeletal muscle mitochondrial uncoupling in mice. Aging Cell 2011; 10(1): 122-36.
[http://dx.doi.org/10.1111/j.1474-9726.2010.00648.x] [PMID: 21070590]

[144] Mousavi K, Manthari RK, Najibi A, Jia Z, Ommati MM, Heidari R. Mitochondrial dysfunction and oxidative stress are involved in the mechanism of tramadol-induced renal injury. Current Research in Pharmacology and Drug Discovery 2021; p. 100049.

[145] Ommati MM, Niknahad H, Farshad O, Azarpira N, Heidari R. In vitro and in vivo evidence on the role of mitochondrial impairment as a mechanism of lithium-induced nephrotoxicity. Biol Trace Elem Res 2021; 199(5): 1908-18.
[http://dx.doi.org/10.1007/s12011-020-02302-9] [PMID: 32712907]

[146] Ommati MM, Arabnezhad MR, Farshad O, et al. The role of mitochondrial impairment and oxidative stress in the pathogenesis of lithium-induced reproductive toxicity in male mice. Front Vet Sci 2021; 8(125): 603262.
[http://dx.doi.org/10.3389/fvets.2021.603262] [PMID: 33842567]

[147] Heidari R, Ommati MM, Niknahad H. Mitochondria as biosynthetic centers and targeted therapeutics Mitochondrial Metabolism. Elsevier 2021; pp. 19-47.

[148] Farshad O, Heidari R, Zamiri MJ, et al. Spermatotoxic effects of single-walled and multi-walled carbon nanotubes on male mice. Front Vet Sci 2020; 7(1007): 591558.
[http://dx.doi.org/10.3389/fvets.2020.591558] [PMID: 33392285]

[149] Seo AY, Joseph AM, Dutta D, Hwang JCY, Aris JP, Leeuwenburgh C. New insights into the role of mitochondria in aging: mitochondrial dynamics and more. J Cell Sci 2010; 123(15): 2533-42.
[http://dx.doi.org/10.1242/jcs.070490] [PMID: 20940129]

[150] Hossmann KA. Pathophysiology and therapy of experimental stroke. Cell Mol Neurobiol 2006; 26(7-8): 1055-81.

[http://dx.doi.org/10.1007/s10571-006-9008-1] [PMID: 16710759]

[151] Liesa M, Palacín M, Zorzano A. Mitochondrial dynamics in mammalian health and disease. Physiol Rev 2009; 89(3): 799-845.
[http://dx.doi.org/10.1152/physrev.00030.2008] [PMID: 19584314]

[152] Bajpai M, Gupta G, Setty BS. Changes in carbohydrate metabolism of testicular germ cells during meiosis in the rat. Eur J Endocrinol 1998; 138(3): 322-7.
[http://dx.doi.org/10.1530/eje.0.1380322] [PMID: 9539308]

[153] Boussouar F, Benahmed M. Lactate and energy metabolism in male germ cells. Trends Endocrinol Metab 2004; 15(7): 345-50.
[http://dx.doi.org/10.1016/j.tem.2004.07.003] [PMID: 15350607]

[154] Miki K, Qu W, Goulding EH, *et al.* Glyceraldehyde 3-phosphate dehydrogenase-S, a sperm-specific glycolytic enzyme, is required for sperm motility and male fertility. Proc Natl Acad Sci USA 2004; 101(47): 16501-6.
[http://dx.doi.org/10.1073/pnas.0407708101] [PMID: 15546993]

[155] Amaral S, Mota P, Rodrigues AS, Martins L, Oliveira PJ, Ramalho-Santos J. Testicular aging involves mitochondrial dysfunction as well as an increase in UCP2 levels and proton leak. FEBS Lett 2008; 582(30): 4191-6.
[http://dx.doi.org/10.1016/j.febslet.2008.11.020] [PMID: 19041646]

[156] Mota P, Amaral S, Martins L, de Lourdes Pereira M, Oliveira PJ, Ramalho-Santos J. Mitochondrial bioenergetics of testicular cells from the domestic cat (Felis catus)—A model for endangered species. Reprod Toxicol 2009; 27(2): 111-6.
[http://dx.doi.org/10.1016/j.reprotox.2009.01.008] [PMID: 19429391]

[157] Hess R. Spermatogenesis, overview.Encyclopedia of Reproduction: Academic Press, San Diego California pp. 1998.

[158] Holdcraft RW, Braun RE. Hormonal regulation of spermatogenesis. Int J Androl 2004; 27(6): 335-42.
[http://dx.doi.org/10.1111/j.1365-2605.2004.00502.x] [PMID: 15595952]

[159] Meinhardt A, McFarlane JR, Seitz J, de Kretser DM. Activin maintains the condensed type of mitochondria in germ cells. Mol Cell Endocrinol 2000; 168(1-2): 111-7.
[http://dx.doi.org/10.1016/S0303-7207(00)00308-7] [PMID: 11064157]

[160] Agarwal A, Saleh RA, Bedaiwy MA. Role of reactive oxygen species in the pathophysiology of human reproduction. Fertil Steril 2003; 79(4): 829-43.
[http://dx.doi.org/10.1016/S0015-0282(02)04948-8] [PMID: 12749418]

[161] Tremellen K. Oxidative stress and male infertility—a clinical perspective. Hum Reprod Update 2008; 14(3): 243-58.
[http://dx.doi.org/10.1093/humupd/dmn004] [PMID: 18281241]

[162] Ommati MM, Heidari R, Zamiri MJ, Shojaee S, Akhlaghi A, Sabouri S. Association of open field behavior with blood and semen characteristics in roosters: an alternative animal model. Rev Int Androl 2018; 16(2): 50-8.
[http://dx.doi.org/10.1016/j.androl.2017.02.002] [PMID: 30300125]

[163] Turner TT, Lysiak JJ. Oxidative stress: a common factor in testicular dysfunction. J Androl 2008; 29(5): 488-98.
[http://dx.doi.org/10.2164/jandrol.108.005132] [PMID: 18567643]

[164] Syed V, Hecht NB. Selective loss of Sertoli cell and germ cell function leads to a disruption in sertoli cell-germ cell communication during aging in the Brown Norway rat. Biol Reprod 2001; 64(1): 107-12.
[http://dx.doi.org/10.1095/biolreprod64.1.107] [PMID: 11133664]

[165] Levy S, Serre V, Hermo L, Robaire B. The effects of aging on the seminiferous epithelium and the blood-testis barrier of the Brown Norway rat. J Androl 1999; 20(3): 356-65.

[PMID: 10386815]

[166] Hijazi RA, Cunningham GR. Andropause: is androgen replacement therapy indicated for the aging male? Annu Rev Med 2005; 56(1): 117-37.
[http://dx.doi.org/10.1146/annurev.med.56.082103.104518] [PMID: 15660505]

[167] Hogervorst E, Williams J, Budge M, Riedel W, Jolles J. The nature of the effect of female gonadal hormone replacement therapy on cognitive function in post-menopausal women: a meta-analysis. Neuroscience 2000; 101(3): 485-512.
[http://dx.doi.org/10.1016/S0306-4522(00)00410-3] [PMID: 11113299]

[168] Markham JA, Pych JC, Juraska JM. Ovarian hormone replacement to aged ovariectomized female rats benefits acquisition of the morris water maze. Horm Behav 2002; 42(3): 284-93.
[http://dx.doi.org/10.1006/hbeh.2002.1819] [PMID: 12460588]

[169] Vázquez-Memije ME, Cárdenas-Méndez MJ, Tolosa A, Hafidi ME. Respiratory chain complexes and membrane fatty acids composition in rat testis mitochondria throughout development and ageing. Exp Gerontol 2005; 40(6): 482-90.
[http://dx.doi.org/10.1016/j.exger.2005.03.006] [PMID: 15972255]

[170] Vázquez-Memije ME, Capin R, Tolosa A, El-Hafidi M. Analysis of age-associated changes in mitochondrial free radical generation by rat testis. Mol Cell Biochem 2007; 307(1-2): 23-30.
[http://dx.doi.org/10.1007/s11010-007-9580-9] [PMID: 17805943]

[171] Sahoo D, Roy A, Chainy G. Rat testicular mitochondrial antioxidant defence system and its modulation by aging. Acta Biol Hung 2008; 59(4): 413-24.
[http://dx.doi.org/10.1556/ABiol.59.2008.4.3] [PMID: 19133498]

[172] Rebrin I, Kamzalov S, Sohal RS. Effects of age and caloric restriction on glutathione redox state in mice. Free Radic Biol Med 2003; 35(6): 626-35.
[http://dx.doi.org/10.1016/S0891-5849(03)00388-5] [PMID: 12957655]

[173] Yang J, Wu G, Feng Y, Lv Q, Lin S, Hu J. Effects of taurine on male reproduction in rats of different ages. J Biomed Sci 2010; 17(Suppl 1): S9.
[http://dx.doi.org/10.1186/1423-0127-17-S1-S9] [PMID: 20804629]

[174] Ahmad AA, Falla AM, Duffell E, *et al.* Estimating the scale of chronic hepatitis B virus infection among migrants in EU/EEA countries. BMC Infect Dis 2018; 18(1): 34.
[http://dx.doi.org/10.1186/s12879-017-2921-8] [PMID: 29325525]

[175] Yang J, Lin S, Feng Y, Wu G, Hu J, Eds. Taurine enhances the sexual response and mating ability in aged male rats. New York, NY: Springer New York 2013.
[http://dx.doi.org/10.1007/978-1-4614-6093-0_32]

[176] Fisher MT, Nagarkatti M, Nagarkatti PS. Aryl hydrocarbon receptor-dependent induction of loss of mitochondrial membrane potential in epididydimal spermatozoa by 2,3,7,8-tetrachlorodibenzo-p-dioxin (TCDD). Toxicol Lett 2005; 157(2): 99-107.
[http://dx.doi.org/10.1016/j.toxlet.2005.01.008] [PMID: 15836997]

[177] Wang Q, Kurita H, Carreira V, *et al.* Ah receptor activation by dioxin disrupts activin, BMP, and WNT signals during the early differentiation of mouse embryonic stem cells and inhibits cardiomyocyte functions. Toxicol Sci 2016; 149(2): 346-57.
[http://dx.doi.org/10.1093/toxsci/kfv246] [PMID: 26572662]

[178] Carreira VS, Fan Y, Kurita H, *et al.* Disruption of Ah receptor signaling during mouse development leads to abnormal cardiac structure and function in the adult. PLoS One 2015; 10(11): e0142440.
[http://dx.doi.org/10.1371/journal.pone.0142440] [PMID: 26555816]

[179] Das DN, Naik PP, Mukhopadhyay S, *et al.* Elimination of dysfunctional mitochondria through mitophagy suppresses benzo[a]pyrene-induced apoptosis. Free Radic Biol Med 2017; 112: 452-63.
[http://dx.doi.org/10.1016/j.freeradbiomed.2017.08.020] [PMID: 28843778]

[180] Qiao Y, Li Q, Du HY, Wang QW, Huang Y, Liu W. Airborne polycyclic aromatic hydrocarbons

trigger human skin cells aging through aryl hydrocarbon receptor. Biochem Biophys Res Commun 2017; 488(3): 445-52.
[http://dx.doi.org/10.1016/j.bbrc.2017.04.160] [PMID: 28526404]

[181] Hu P, Herrmann R, Bednar A, *et al.* Aryl hydrocarbon receptor deficiency causes dysregulated cellular matrix metabolism and age-related macular degeneration-like pathology. Proc Natl Acad Sci USA 2013; 110(43): E4069-78.
[http://dx.doi.org/10.1073/pnas.1307574110] [PMID: 24106308]

[182] Huang S, Shui X, He Y, *et al.* AhR expression and polymorphisms are associated with risk of coronary arterial disease in Chinese population. Sci Rep 2015; 5(1): 8022.
[http://dx.doi.org/10.1038/srep08022] [PMID: 25620626]

[183] Brinkmann V, Ale-Agha N, Haendeler J, Ventura N. The Aryl hydrocarbon receptor (AhR) in the aging process: Another puzzling role for this highly conserved transcription factor. Front Physiol 2020; 10: 1561.
[http://dx.doi.org/10.3389/fphys.2019.01561] [PMID: 32009975]

[184] Sandoval-Acuña C, Ferreira J, Speisky H. Polyphenols and mitochondria: An update on their increasingly emerging ROS-scavenging independent actions. Arch Biochem Biophys 2014; 559: 75-90.
[http://dx.doi.org/10.1016/j.abb.2014.05.017] [PMID: 24875147]

[185] Smirnova A, Wincent E, Vikström Bergander L, *et al.* Evidence for new light-independent pathways for generation of the endogenous aryl hydrocarbon receptor agonist FICZ. Chem Res Toxicol 2016; 29(1): 75-86.
[http://dx.doi.org/10.1021/acs.chemrestox.5b00416] [PMID: 26686552]

[186] Ajami M, Pazoki-Toroudi H, Amani H, *et al.* Therapeutic role of sirtuins in neurodegenerative disease and their modulation by polyphenols. Neurosci Biobehav Rev 2017; 73: 39-47.
[http://dx.doi.org/10.1016/j.neubiorev.2016.11.022] [PMID: 27914941]

[187] Koizumi M, Tatebe J, Watanabe I, Yamazaki J, Ikeda T, Morita T. Aryl hydrocarbon receptor mediates indoxyl sulfate-induced cellular senescence in human umbilical vein endothelial cells. J Atheroscler Thromb 2014; 21(9): 904-16.
[http://dx.doi.org/10.5551/jat.23663] [PMID: 24727683]

[188] Ming M, Zhao B, Shea CR, *et al.* Loss of sirtuin 1 (SIRT1) disrupts skin barrier integrity and sensitizes mice to epicutaneous allergen challenge. J Allergy Clin Immunol 2015; 135(4): 936-945.e4.
[http://dx.doi.org/10.1016/j.jaci.2014.09.035] [PMID: 25445829]

[189] Sutter CH, Olesen KM, Bhuju J, Guo Z, Sutter TR. AHR regulates metabolic reprogramming to promote SIRT1-dependent keratinocyte differentiation. J Invest Dermatol 2019; 139(4): 818-26.
[http://dx.doi.org/10.1016/j.jid.2018.10.019] [PMID: 30393078]

[190] Senft AP, Dalton TP, Nebert DW, *et al.* Mitochondrial reactive oxygen production is dependent on the aromatic hydrocarbon receptor. Free Radic Biol Med 2002; 33(9): 1268-78.
[http://dx.doi.org/10.1016/S0891-5849(02)01014-6] [PMID: 12398935]

[191] Carreira VS, Fan Y, Wang Q, *et al.* Ah receptor signaling controls the expression of cardiac development and homeostasis genes. Toxicol Sci 2015; 147(2): 425-35.
[http://dx.doi.org/10.1093/toxsci/kfv138] [PMID: 26139165]

[192] Tappenden DM, Lynn SG, Crawford RB, *et al.* The aryl hydrocarbon receptor interacts with ATP5α1, a subunit of the ATP synthase complex, and modulates mitochondrial function. Toxicol Appl Pharmacol 2011; 254(3): 299-310.
[http://dx.doi.org/10.1016/j.taap.2011.05.004] [PMID: 21616089]

[193] Hwang HJ, Dornbos P, Steidemann M, Dunivin TK, Rizzo M, LaPres JJ. Mitochondrial-targeted aryl hydrocarbon receptor and the impact of 2,3,7,8-tetrachlorodibenzo-p-dioxin on cellular respiration and the mitochondrial proteome. Toxicol Appl Pharmacol 2016; 304: 121-32.
[http://dx.doi.org/10.1016/j.taap.2016.04.005] [PMID: 27105554]

[194]   Yano M, Terada K, Mori M. AIP is a mitochondrial import mediator that binds to both import receptor Tom20 and preproteins. J Cell Biol 2003; 163(1): 45-56.
[http://dx.doi.org/10.1083/jcb.200305051] [PMID: 14557246]

[195]   Cristina D, Cary M, Lunceford A, Clarke C, Kenyon C. A regulated response to impaired respiration slows behavioral rates and increases lifespan in Caenorhabditis elegans. PLoS Genet 2009; 5(4): e1000450.
[http://dx.doi.org/10.1371/journal.pgen.1000450] [PMID: 19360127]

[196]   Liu Y, Samuel BS, Breen PC, Ruvkun G. Caenorhabditis elegans pathways that surveil and defend mitochondria. Nature 2014; 508(7496): 406-10.
[http://dx.doi.org/10.1038/nature13204] [PMID: 24695221]

[197]   Mao K, Ji F, Breen P, *et al.* Mitochondrial dysfunction in C. elegans activates mitochondrial relocalization and nuclear hormone receptor-dependent detoxification genes. Cell Metab 2019; 29(5): 1182-91.
[http://dx.doi.org/10.1016/j.cmet.2019.01.022] [PMID: 30799287]

CHAPTER 7

Taurine and Skeletal Muscle Disorders: Highlighting the Mitochondria-dependent Mechanisms

Abstract: Skeletal muscle tissue contains a massive taurine (TAU) in millimolar concentrations. Several studies mentioned the importance of TAU in normal skeletal muscle function. It has been found that this amino acid plays a wide range of functions, ranging from osmoregulatory properties to the regulation of cytoplasmic Ca^{2+} homeostasis. Recent findings mentioned that TAU deficiency in the skeletal muscle leads to decreased exercise capacity, severe weakness, and muscle waste. On the other hand, it has been repeatedly shown that TAU supplementation could increase skeletal muscle performance in many disorders. These data mention the essential role of TAU in the skeletal muscle. Interestingly, it has been found that the effect of TAU on cellular mitochondria is an important feature of this amino acid in skeletal muscles. The current chapter highlights the physiological roles of TAU in muscle and its importance in the pathophysiology of skeletal muscle disorders. Then, the essential role of TAU in cellular mitochondria and its importance in muscle function is described. And the relevance of this amino acid in managing skeletal muscle pathologies is discussed.

Keywords: Amino acid, ATP, Bioenergetics, Cell death, Exercise, Muscle waste, Oxidative stress.

INTRODUCTION

Skeletal muscle is one of the most taurine (TAU)-containing tissues [1 - 3]. Physiologically, several functions, including the osmoregulatory properties, calcium (Ca^{2+}) ion regulation, and the phospholipids bio membranes, are attributed to TAU in the skeletal muscle [5 - 7]. Nowadays, it is well-known that TAU plays many other essential roles in the skeletal muscle. TAU plays a vital role in mitochondrial function and energy metabolism in skeletal muscles.

Many investigations revealed that TAU depletion had deleterious consequences on skeletal muscle function [4 - 6]. TAU depletion led to significant mitochondrial abnormalities (morphological and functional). Dissipation of the mitochondrial membrane potential ($\Delta\Psi_m$), mitochondrial permeabilization, enhan-

Reza Heidari and M. Mehdi Ommati

ced mitochondria-mediated ROS formation, mitochondria-mediated cell death, and impaired energy metabolism are consequences of TAU depletion in the skeletal muscle [4 - 11]. It has also been found that skeletal muscle TAU depletion could enhance muscle senescence and atrophy [12]. These two later disorders could also be mitochondria-related mechanisms.

Another exciting feature of TAU is its use in energy drinks as well as by athletes to increase their stamina [13 - 15]. In this regard, it has been found that TAU could significantly enhance energy metabolism in the skeletal muscle. Moreover, TAU prevents muscle injury and efficiently enhances muscle recovery after heavy exercise [13 - 15].

Enhancement of protein catabolism, increased sarcoplasmic Ca^{2+}, oxidative stress, and inflammatory response are cellular processes that seem to be involved in the onset of muscle dysfunction [4, 16 - 18]. More importantly, there are robust clues about the significant role of mitochondrial function and cellular energy metabolism in skeletal muscle disorders with different etiologies [19 - 24]. Hence, it is essential to find pharmacological options against these disorders.

In the current chapter, a review of the physiological roles of TAU in skeletal muscle is provided. Then, the effects of this amino acid on mitochondrial function and its associated pathologies are highlighted. Finally, the application of TAU as a therapeutic agent against skeletal muscle disorders is discussed in detail. The data collected here might provide clues for developing effective therapeutic options against a wide range of skeletal muscle-related disorders or finding strategies to enhance human skeletal muscle strength for various purposes.

MECHANISMS OF TAURINE ACTION IN THE SKELETAL MUSCLE

Skeletal muscle is contained a considerable amount of TAU [1, 2, 25 - 27]. The TAU transporter TauT is highly expressed in the skeletal muscle and could primarily concentrate TAU in this tissue (>100 fold higher than plasma TAU concentration) [1, 2, 4, 25 - 27]. Due to the massive concentration of TAU in this tissue, this amino acid seems to play a crucial role in the skeletal muscle. The observation that skeletal muscle function is significantly impaired in experimental models of TAU deficiency highlights the vital role of this amino acid in muscle function [12, 28]. Significant muscle senescence and energy crisis occurred in TAU deficiency models [12]. Membrane stabilization and the action of TAU as an osmolyte are well-investigated physiological roles of this amino acid in the skeletal muscle [4]. Moreover, crucial functions such as regulating intracellular Ca^{2+} homeostasis are also attributed to TAU [26, 29 - 31]. Other actions of TAU in skeletal muscle include anti-inflammatory effects, antioxidant properties, and regulation of ion channels [4].

As mentioned, a good body of evidence indicates the crucial role of TAU in regulating mitochondrial function and enhancing organ performance in the skeletal muscle and many other organs [4, 32 - 41]. In this context, investigations of TAU deficient models revealed significant mitochondrial impairment, mitochondria-mediated cell death, and severe tissue atrophy in skeletal muscle [12, 28]. These studies revealed that TAU deficiency leads to the dissipation of mitochondrial membrane potential ($\Delta\Psi_m$), impaired mitochondrial respiratory chain complexes activity, decreased mitochondrial energy metabolism, increased mitochondrial permeabilization, and the release of cell death mediators from this organelle [12, 28]. On the other hand, several studies indicate the positive role of TAU supplementation in skeletal muscle mitochondrial indices in various experimental models [42 - 46]. The effects of TAU on many skeletal diseases also seem to be mediated through a mitochondria-dependent mechanism (Fig. **1**) [4, 16, 32].

TAURINE REGULATES ION CHANNELS IN THE SKELETAL MUSCLE

The regulation of skeletal muscle ion channels is a crucial mechanism for TAU in this tissue [4]. In this regard, the voltage-gated chloride channel, CLC-1, seems to be a significant target for TAU in skeletal muscles [4] (Fig. **2**). The Cl$^-$ ion plays a key role in the sarcolemma's electrical stability and muscle relaxation [4]. Several genetic defects in CLC-1 have been identified. These mutations are directly related to myotonia-related muscle disorders [4]. Myotonia is a muscle disorder related to decreased Cl$^-$ ion influx to the muscle fiber. This situation leads to delayed muscle relaxation, severe spasms, and muscle stiffness [4, 47 - 49]. Fortunately, a good body of evidence indicates the activation role of TAU on CLC-1 and myofibers Cl$^-$ ion influx [4, 50 - 52] (Fig. **2**). Hence, TAU is able to decrease skeletal muscle excitability and spasms significantly. Interestingly, it has been found that long-term administration of TAU significantly diminished myotonic symptoms [4, 53 - 55]. Based on these data, the effects of TAU on CLC-1 and Cl$^-$ ion current could have positive effects in muscular disorders such as myotonia. However, more clinical studies, especially with large sample sizes, are needed to confirm this effect of TAU and finally its application in clinical settings.

TAU also regulates the activity of voltage-gated sodium channels (NaV1.4) in skeletal muscles [4] (Fig. **2**). It has been found that high concentrations of TAU (*e.g.*, 10 mM) can significantly reduce sodium (Na$^+$) current in the muscle fiber [4, 16, 56]. The role of TAU in blocking Na$^+$ channels could provide beneficial effects in muscular disorders such as myotonia, especially myotonic disorders associated with mutations in Na$^+$ channels (*e.g.*, paramyotonia congenita) [4].

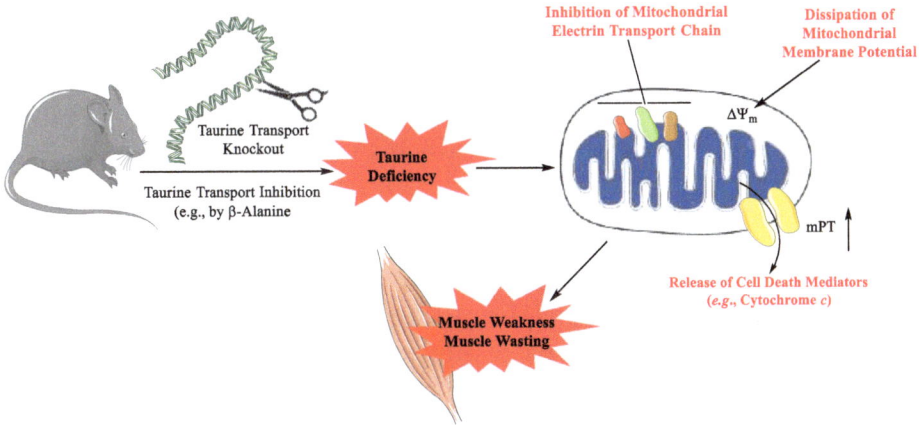

Fig. (1). It is well known that the stimulation of taurine deficiency by taurine transporter inhibitors (*e.g.*, β-alanine) or knocking out taurine transporters causes severe mitochondrial impairment. Taurine deficiency and mitochondrial dysfunction in the skeletal muscle could lead to muscle weakness and skeletal muscle waste.

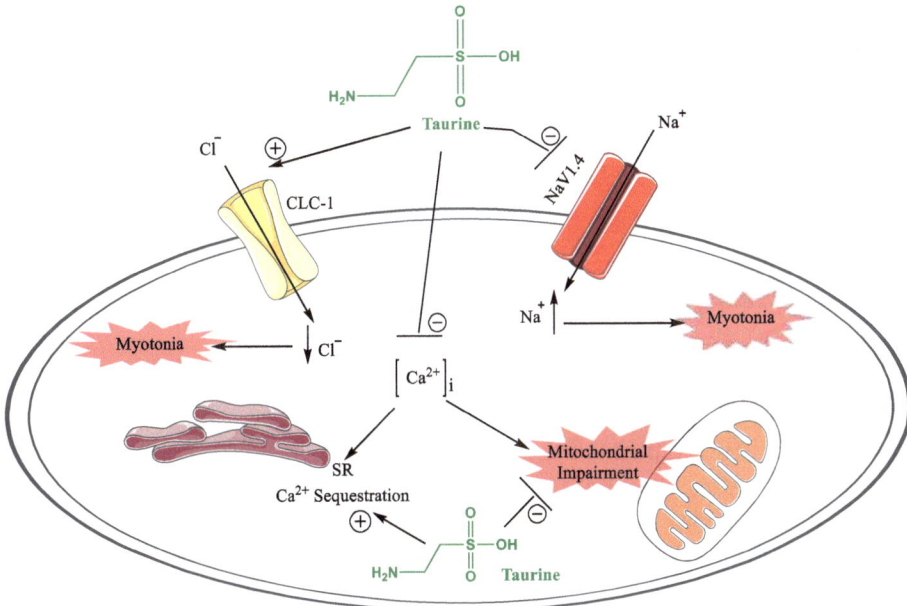

Fig. (2). A schematic representation of the action of taurine on the levels of essential ions in skeletal muscle fiber. Decreased Cl$^-$ ion levels or increased Na$^+$ content are associated with muscle disorders such as myotonia. Disturbances in cytoplasmic Ca^{2+} ions are also well-known factors linked with muscular dystrophy and myopathy. It has been found that TAU could significantly protect against muscular disorders by regulating the myofibers levels of the mentioned ions. SR: Sarcoplasmic reticulum.

Calcium (Ca^{2+}) is another vital ion whose role in the pathophysiology of skeletal muscle disorders has been widely investigated [57 - 60] (Fig. **2**). Ca^{2+} ion dyshomeostasis plays a crucial role in many skeletal muscle disorders, such as muscle degeneration and dystrophy [61 - 63]. For instance, the crucial role of cytoplasmic Ca^{2+} overload has been repeatedly mentioned in aging-related muscle dystrophy, cachexia, hypoxia-induced muscle injury, Duchenne muscular dystrophy, and related myopathies [61 - 65].

Disturbances in cellular Ca^{2+} homeostasis could directly affect skeletal muscle mitochondrial function and energy metabolism (Fig. **2**). Decreased mitochondrial membrane potential, the suppressed activity of the mitochondrial respiratory chain, mitochondria-facilitated reactive oxygen species (ROS) formation, and depletion of skeletal muscle ATP levels have been reported in cases of Ca^{2+} ion dyshomeostasis [22, 65, 66]. As repeatedly mentioned in the current book, the effects of TAU on Ca^{2+} sequestration (by mitochondria or endoplasmic reticulum) is an exciting feature of this amino acid [26, 29 - 31, 67, 68] (Fig. **2**). The role of TAU in modulating Ca^{2+} levels could significantly prevent mitochondrial injury, inhibit the activation of cytotoxic enzymes (*e.g.*, proteases), and prevent mitochondria-mediated cell death [69, 70]. All these data highlight the effects of TAU on Ca^{2+} ion homeostasis as a crucial mechanism for its cytoprotective properties in skeletal muscle disorders.

TAURINE IS ACTIVELY INCORPORATED IN THE SYNTHESIS OF SKELETAL MUSCLE MITOCHONDRIAL COMPONENTS

The incorporation of TAU in mitochondrial tRNA and its role in protein synthesis in this organelle is another key mechanism of its function in the skeletal muscle [33, 71 - 74]. Proper modification of mitochondrial tRNA by TAU guarantees the synthesis of proteins (*e.g.*, respiratory chain complexes) and, consequently, ATP metabolism [33, 71, 73, 74]. Meanwhile, impaired mitochondrial function due to the lack of tRNA modification by TAU could significantly enhance mitochondria-originated ROS formation and oxidative stress [75 - 77]. Interestingly, it has been found that some muscular disorders, such as several forms of myopathic states or chronic fatigue syndrome, are linked with a lack of mitochondrial tRNA modification by TAU [71]. Decreased ATP levels and a significant increase in oxidative stress are biomarkers in these situations [7, 71]. The incorporation of TAU in basic mitochondrial structures such as tRNA mentions that chronic supplementation of this amino acid could be helpful in athletes' performance or military personals stamina and preserve their optimum function.

EVIDENCE OF THE POSITIVE EFFECT OF TAURINE O MUSCULAR DISORDERS LINKED WITH MITOCHONDRIAL IMPAIRMENT

Many investigations indicate that several skeletal muscle disorders benefit from TAU supplementation. Mitochondrial impairment and oxidative stress are basic mechanisms involved in the pathogenesis of these muscle disorders. The following parts highlight the effects of TAU on skeletal muscle disorders with a focus on mitochondrial function and oxidative stress markers.

A wide range of skeletal muscle disorders has been identified in humans. Muscle wasting (sarcopenia, cachexia) and atrophy, myotonia, impaired protein catabolism in skeletal muscles, and different kinds of myopathies have been described in the literature. Aging, malnutrition, prolonged inactivity, and diseases such as cancer, cirrhosis, and chronic kidney disease are associated with muscle atrophy and mass loss [78]. Muscle atrophy and weakness severely affect the quality of life. On the other hand, there is no specific pharmacological approach for treating or preventing muscle atrophy. Regular exercise is the only accepted intervention to slow or prevent muscle atrophy [78]. Therefore, finding new therapeutic options for muscle atrophy has significant clinical value. Many studies suggest a crucial role for mitochondrial-dependent mechanisms in the pathogenesis of skeletal muscle disorders such as impaired proteins catabolism, muscle wasting, atrophy, exercise intolerance, and different kinds of myopathies [24, 79 - 84]. Hence, it is important to find effective pharmacological options against these disorders. In this regard, the effects of TAU on several common skeletal muscle disorders are described here, focusing on the effects of this amino acid on mitochondria-related mechanisms.

Impaired protein catabolism and protein breakdown are major causes of muscle wasting in different forms of muscle atrophy [85]. Sarcopenia, aging-related muscle atrophy, cachexia, and immobility-related atrophy are different forms of muscle wasting that severely debilitate patients and influence their quality of life. In this complication, protein degradation exceeds protein synthesis, and muscle atrophy will occur. Two major protein degradation mechanisms, including the autophagy-lysosome system and ubiquitin-proteasome, are involved in the mechanism of muscle atrophy [85] (Fig. **3**).

Muscle mass in a person depends on many factors, including physical activity and hormonal status. In adults, a process named "protein turnover" means the formation and degradation of proteins control skeletal muscle mass and fiber size [85, 86]. On the other hand, many factors could lead to muscle shrinkage, atrophy, and loss of myofibers' cytoplasm and organelles [85]. Actually, muscle atrophy could be a physiological process, for example, during aging [85]. However, severe muscle atrophy is a pathologic condition that needs medical intervention.

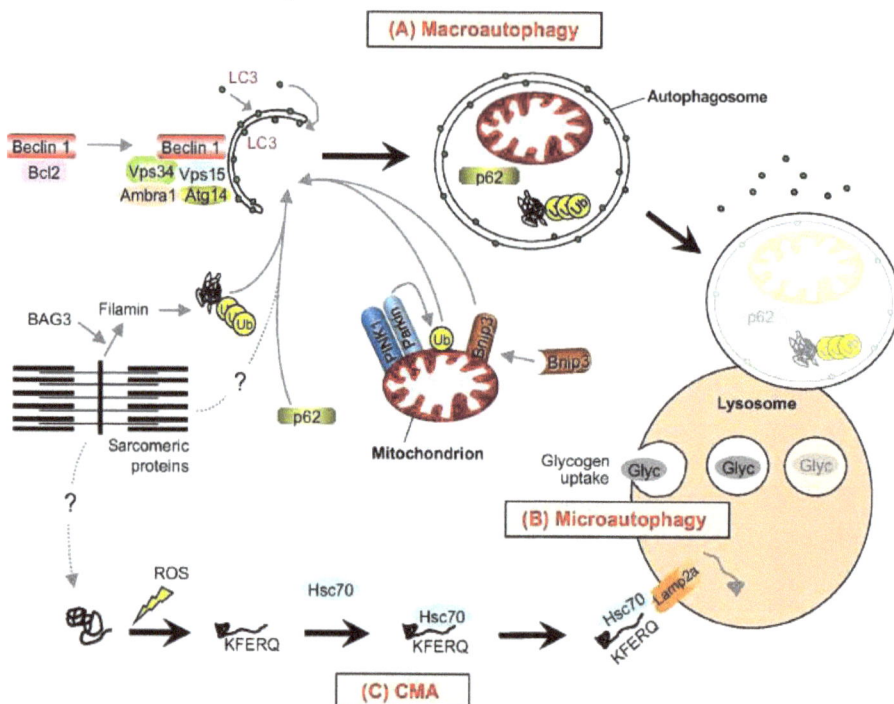

Fig. (3). Macroautophagy, microautophagy, and chaperone-mediated autophagy (CMA) contribute to protein degradation and organelle removal in skeletal muscles. **(A)** Macroautophagy is triggered by activating a regulatory complex (containing Vps34, Beclin 1, Vps15, Ambra1, and Atg14) that induces LC3 recruitment to the nascent autophagosome (isolation membrane). Selective removal of mitochondria (mitophagy; a specific form of macroautophagy) requires the PINK1-parkin complex and Bnip3 factors. Proteins committed to lysosomal degradation (including BAG3 and filamin, shown here) are labeled by polyubiquitin chains and delivered to the autophagosome by the p62 scaffold protein. **(B)** Microautophagy involves the direct engulfment of small portions of cytoplasm into lysosomes. Glycogen (Glyc) is reportedly taken up and broken down by microautophagy in skeletal muscles. **(C)** In CMA, proteins that different agents damage, such as reactive oxygen species (ROS), expose a specific amino acid sequence (the KFERQ motif) recognized by the Hsc70 chaperone, which in turn delivers them to the lysosome *via* interaction with Lamp2a receptors. Dotted lines depict pathways whose molecular mechanisms and roles in adult skeletal muscle have not yet been fully defined. Note: This figure and its caption were adapted from [86] with the kind permission of The Company of Biologists (CC-BY license).

As mentioned, the autophagy/lysosomal process is involved in the mechanism of severe atrophy. In the following parts, first, this mechanism is described. Then, the effects of amino acid TAU as a potential therapeutic target in this disorder are highlighted.

THE ROLE OF THE AUTOPHAGY-LYSOSOME SYSTEM IN MUSCLE ATROPHY

Nowadays, it is well-established that autophagy is involved in various pathological muscle wasting conditions [87 - 89]. A brief review of multiple forms of autophagy, their regulation, and their role in muscle homeostasis is shown in Fig. (3). In summary, autophagy is a homeostatic mechanism for degrading long-lived proteins and organelles through the lysosomal machinery [90] (Fig. 3).

The autophagy process plays an essential role in muscle catabolism [91]. Nowadays, it has been found that a plethora of diseases could activate autophagy in the skeletal muscle [85]. Conditions such as cancer, sepsis, severe fasting, aging, chemotherapeutic pharmaceuticals, muscle disuse, and denervation could activate autophagy in the skeletal muscle [91, 92]. Interestingly, it has also been detected that autophagy could have physiological roles. For instance, autophagy could regulate muscle glucose in exercise [85]. Autophagy in exercise is believed to be essential for remodeling damaged proteins and organelles and replacing them with more functional ones [85].

As mentioned in various parts of this chapter, mitochondria are vital organelles involved in many regulatory mechanisms to preserve muscle function [93, 94]. Processes such as mitochondrial dynamics (Fusion/Fission) and remodeling of mitochondria with processes such as autophagy (mitophagy in this case) continuously occur in the skeletal muscle (Fig. 3).

Several proteins, namely Parkin, PIMK1, Binp3, and Binp3L, are involved in the regulation of mitophagy (Fig. 3). Any abnormality in the action of these proteins could lead to mitochondrial impairment [95, 96]. It has been found that proteins involved in mitophagy, such as PINK1, usually are absent in the mitochondria because they are degraded by mitochondrial protease enzymes [95, 96]. On the other hand, in damaged mitochondria, PINK1 is not degraded and accumulates in this organelle (Fig. 3). PINK1 could induce the recruitment of the Parkin protein to mitochondria. This last event activates mitophagy through the ubiquitination of the mitochondrial outer membrane proteins (Fig. 3). Afterward, a protein named p62 recognizes ubiquitylated proteins and brings autophagic vesicles to marked mitochondria [97, 98]. As shown in Fig. 3, Binp3 and Binp3L are BH3-only proteins located on the mitochondrial membrane and bind to LC3 after stress (Fig. 3). Therefore, these proteins recruit autophagosomes to damage mitochondria [85] (Fig. 3).

It is essential to mention that mitochondrial impairment is a typical process in atrophying muscle, and the mitochondrial network is dramatically remodeled.

Therefore, all mentioned mechanisms remove these damaged proteins and organelles. The net result of such events is muscle atrophy. Despite the mechanisms involved in the mitochondrial impairment in skeletal muscle and autophagy, it appears that preserving its functionality with robust and safe pharmaceuticals could have therapeutic capability.

Interestingly, several experiments revealed that TAU could robustly blunt autophagy and skeletal muscle waste [99]. TAU could also inhibit autophagy and its consequences in other organs [100, 101]. These data provide clues for using TAU as an option against several skeletal muscle disorders.

There is a good body of data indicating the potential of TAU to restore muscle function in many other pathological conditions associated with muscle wasting. In this regard, the effects of TAU on different forms of muscle atrophy, senescence-associated muscle dysfunction, and sarcopenia have been explored [4, 27, 54, 102 - 104]. It should be mentioned that rather than the pivotal role of the autophagy-lysosomal system in muscle atrophy, more simple mechanisms could also be involved in impaired mitochondrial function, depleted myofibers energy, and skeletal muscle disorders.

Several forms of muscular dystrophy have been identified in humans. Duchenne muscular dystrophy (DMD) is one of the best-investigated forms of muscle disorder [105 - 111]. The lack of a protein named "dystrophin" is believed to be involved in the etiology of muscle dysfunction in DMD [112 - 114]. Dystrophin is an essential protein responsible for sarcolemma integrity and Ca^{2+} homeostasis in skeletal muscle tissue [61, 115, 116]. Ca^{2+} ion dyshomeostasis is common in many skeletal muscle disorders [117 - 119]. Impaired sarcolemma integrity could lead to deleterious consequences, such as impaired muscle excitation-contraction coupling disturbances in Ca^{2+} ion homeostasis [61]. These pathologic events could lead to vast muscular dysfunction [61]. The dyshomeostasis of Ca^{2+} levels also significantly impairs mitochondrial dysfunction and energy metabolism [61, 120] (Fig. **1**). Hence, DMD is connected with mitochondrial abnormalities. On the other hand, TAU is a promising compound for regulating cytoplasmic Ca^{2+} homeostasis and preventing this ion's deleterious effects on mitochondrial function.

The connection between Ca^{2+} dyshomeostasis and mitochondrial impairment is a well-known phenomenon [121, 122]. Therefore, Ca^{2+} overload could cause mitochondrial dysfunction in skeletal muscle disorders. In this regard, several studies revealed the connection between mitochondrial impairment and Ca^{2+} dyshomeostasis in complications such as muscle atrophy, extensive exercise/overload-induced muscle injury, or aging-related skeletal muscle complications [122 - 125]. Significant disturbances in mitochondrial membrane potential ($\Delta\Psi_m$), decreased ATP metabolism, and mitochondrial permeability have been reported in connection with Ca^{2+} overload in skeletal muscle diseases [122 - 125]. As repeatedly mentioned, the effect of TAU in regulating cytoplasmic Ca^{2+} overload and preventing its deleterious effects on cell function is an important feature of this amino acid [26, 29 - 31]. Several studies revealed that TAU could significantly preserve mitochondrial function against Ca^{2+} overload and cytotoxicity [126 - 133]. Interestingly, it has also been found that TAU significantly increased the level of calsequestrin 1 in the muscle [26]. Calsequestrin 1 is a Ca^{2+}-binding protein responsible for preserving high levels of Ca^{2+} in the sarcoplasmic reticulum [26]. This event will provide enough Ca^{2+} needed for muscle contraction [27]. On the other hand, this protein prevents cytoplasmic Ca^{2+} dyshomeostasis as a deleterious event that could lead to cell death and organ damage.

The upregulation of apoptosis-inducing factors and mitochondria-mediated cell death is also mentioned in experimental models of muscle diseases [134]. It has been found that mitochondria-mediated cell death plays a vital role in muscle wasting [62, 66, 71, 79, 82, 107, 109, 123]. Namely, apoptosis-inducing factors (AIF) and cytochrome c are cell death mediators involved in muscle damage and atrophy [135]. Several investigations reported that the induction of mitochondrial permeability and release of cell death mediators from this organelle also play a crucial role in the pathogenesis of various skeletal muscle complications (*e.g.*, different forms of muscle atrophy) [134, 136 - 138]. Cytochrome c and apoptosis-inducing factor (AIF) are well-known mitochondria-originated cell death mediators involved in the pathogenesis of skeletal muscle injury [134, 136 - 138]. TAU is an excellent mPT sealing agent, a part of its mechanism against muscle disorders and atrophy could be mediated through this path [9, 10, 31, 44, 51, 73, 77, 139 - 169].

Another interesting finding related to the effects of TAU on muscle atrophy and muscle regeneration is associated with the effects of this amino acid on satellite cells and other myoblasts [14, 170 - 173]. Excitingly, it has been found that TAU is significantly localized in satellite cells [174]. Satellite cells are skeletal muscle stem cells that differentiate to mature skeletal muscle cells [170]. Satellite cells are involved in muscle regeneration in response to injury or physiological conditions (*e.g.*, aging) [170, 172]. Several studies revealed that satellite cells' mitochondria become dysfunctional in various pathological conditions [175 - 177]. On the other hand, it has been found that TAU stimulates protein synthesis and proliferation of myoblasts through mitochondrial-dependent mechanisms [178]. Based on these data, the effect of TAU on protein anabolism in muscle, *via* a mitochondria-dependent mechanism, could play a key role in muscle regeneration and growth. Hence, TAU supplementation in various clinical conditions associated with muscle injury and atrophy, as well as administration in athletes as a stimulator of protein synthesis and muscle growth, could be beneficial.

Increased free radicals and oxidative stress are joint events in most skeletal muscle disorders [179 - 182]. Oxidative stress could damage several intracellular targets in the skeletal muscle. Mitochondria seem to be critical sources of ROS and oxidative stress in muscle disease [180, 182 - 184]. In this regard, several antioxidant molecules, especially mitochondria-targeted antioxidants, have been applied to minimize the adverse effects of oxidative stress in the muscle [181, 182, 185 - 189]. Several molecules, such as MitoQ, SkQ1, SS-31, and XJB-5-131, have been designed for this purpose [186, 188, 189]. On the other hand, the antioxidative stress properties of TAU have been repeatedly mentioned in previous studies [34, 35, 140, 190 - 196]. In the field of investigation on skeletal muscle disorders, it has also been found that TAU protects skeletal muscle against oxidative stress [26, 164, 197]. It is well-known that TAU primarily provides its antioxidant properties through a mitochondria-dependent mechanism [198]. As mentioned, TAU incorporates mitochondrial tRNA and regulates the synthesis of respiratory chain complexes [92, 199]. As mitochondrial DNA (mtDNA) encodes many proteins (*e.g.,* electron transport chain complexes) independently from the nuclear DNA, any defect in the mitochondrial tRNA structure could influence protein synthesis and, consequently, mitochondrial function [92, 199]. The lack of TAU modification of mitochondrial tRNA could lead to significant ROS formation due to the inappropriate function of electron transport chain components [199, 200]. Moreover, it has been found that the inhibition of cellular trafficking of TAU caused a significant increase in mitochondria-facilitated ROS formation and oxidative stress (*e.g.,* excessive superoxide anion, $O_2^{\cdot-}$, generation) [77, 153, 201]. On the other hand, it has been found that TAU supplementation blunted these adverse effects [77, 153].

All the data collected in this chapter provided clues that high TAU concentrations in skeletal muscle play a crucial physiological role and could be employed as a pharmacological option to alleviate and/or treat a variety of skeletal muscle disorders. Based on these data, at least four significant mechanisms could be delineated for the protective properties of TAU in the skeletal muscle. First, as an essential and primary mechanism, TAU could prevent protein catabolism to avoid muscle waste by blocking the autophagy/lysosomal system. Obviously, this mechanism needs much research to be fully proved. The second important mechanism of cytoprotection provided by TAU in the skeletal muscle is its effects on Ca^{2+} ion concentration. Clearly, Ca^{2+} plays a pivotal role in activating many cytotoxic enzymes, such as different proteases. More importantly, Ca^{2+} could adversely damage mitochondria and impair energy metabolism in the skeletal muscle. The effects of TAU on Ca^{2+} sequestration play a pivotal role in its positive effect on skeletal muscle disorders. The third important mechanism for the positive effects of TAU in skeletal muscle is the alleviation of mitochondria-facilitated ROS formation. As severely mentioned in this chapter, TAU could regulate the synthesis of mitochondrial proteins (*e.g.*, electron transport chain component) and prevent their malfunction. Hence, this amino acid can decrease mitochondria-mediated ROS formation and oxidative stress. Finally, it should be noted that a plethora of studies indicate that TAU could significantly inhibit mitochondrial permeabilization. This effect of TAU substantially prevents the release of cell death mediators, protects skeletal muscle, and improves its performance.

CONCLUSION

Although further research is needed to fill the gap between experimental and human studies, it seems that TAU is an excellent candidate for alleviating skeletal muscle damage with different etiologies. Unfortunately, despite a huge body of evidence on the positive effects of TAU in skeletal muscle disorders in animal models, there is no comprehensive clinical investigation in this field. Hence, designing investigations on patients with skeletal muscle disorders deserve further research and could have tremendous clinical value. Finally, it should be mentioned that TAU is used in humans at very high doses (*e.g.*, 12 g/day) with no significant adverse effects. Therefore, this amino acid could be readily applied in human cases of skeletal muscle disorders.

REFERENCES

[1]   Lambert IH, Kristensen DM, Holm JB, Mortensen OH. Physiological role of taurine - from organism to organelle. Acta Physiol (Oxf) 2015; 213(1): 191-212.
        [http://dx.doi.org/10.1111/apha.12365] [PMID: 25142161]

[2]   Hansen SH, Andersen ML, Birkedal H, Cornett C, Wibrand F. The important role of taurine in oxidative metabolism Taurine 6. Springer 2006; pp. 129-35.

[3]   Iwata H, Obara T, Kim BK, Baba A. Regulation of taurine transport in rat skeletal muscle. J Neurochem 1986; 47(1): 158-63.
        [http://dx.doi.org/10.1111/j.1471-4159.1986.tb02844.x] [PMID: 3711895]

[4]   De Luca A, Pierno S, Camerino DC. Taurine: the appeal of a safe amino acid for skeletal muscle disorders. J Transl Med 2015; 13(1): 243.
        [http://dx.doi.org/10.1186/s12967-015-0610-1] [PMID: 26208967]

[5]   Hamilton EJ, Berg HM, Easton CJ, Bakker AJ. The effect of taurine depletion on the contractile properties and fatigue in fast-twitch skeletal muscle of the mouse. Amino Acids 2006; 31(3): 273-8.
        [http://dx.doi.org/10.1007/s00726-006-0291-4] [PMID: 16583307]

[6]   De Luca A, Pierno S, Camerino DC. Effect of taurine depletion on excitation-contraction coupling and Cl− conductance of rat skeletal muscle. Eur J Pharmacol 1996; 296(2): 215-22.
        [http://dx.doi.org/10.1016/0014-2999(95)00702-4] [PMID: 8838459]

[7]   Tsutomu S, Asuteka N, Takeo S. Human mitochondrial diseases caused by lack of taurine modification in mitochondrial tRNAs. Wiley Interdiscip Rev RNA 2011; 2(3): 376-86.
        [http://dx.doi.org/10.1002/wrna.65] [PMID: 21957023]

[8]   Hansen S, Andersen M, Cornett C, Gradinaru R, Grunnet N. A role for taurine in mitochondrial function. J Biomed Sci 2010; 17(1): S23.
        [http://dx.doi.org/10.1186/1423-0127-17-S1-S23] [PMID: 20804598]

[9]   Schaffer SW, Jong CJ, Ito T, Azuma J. Role of taurine in the pathologies of MELAS and MERRF. Amino Acids 2014; 46(1): 47-56.
        [http://dx.doi.org/10.1007/s00726-012-1414-8] [PMID: 23179085]

[10]   Schaffer S, Ito T, Azuma J, Jong C, Kramer J. Mechanisms underlying development of taurine-deficient cardiomyopathy. Hearts 2020; 1(2): 86-98.
        [http://dx.doi.org/10.3390/hearts1020010]

[11]   Jong C, Ito T, Mozaffari M, Azuma J, Schaffer S. Effect of β-alanine treatment on mitochondrial taurine level and 5-taurinomethyluridine content. J Biomed Sci 2010; 17(1): S25.
        [http://dx.doi.org/10.1186/1423-0127-17-S1-S25] [PMID: 20804600]

[12]   Ito T, Yoshikawa N, Inui T, Miyazaki N, Schaffer SW, Azuma J. Tissue depletion of taurine accelerates skeletal muscle senescence and leads to early death in mice. PLoS One 2014; 9(9): e107409.
        [http://dx.doi.org/10.1371/journal.pone.0107409] [PMID: 25229346]

[13]   Gutiérrez-Hellín J, Varillas-Delgado D. Energy drinks and sports performance, cardiovascular risk, and genetic associations; future prospects. Nutrients 2021; 13(3): 715.
        [http://dx.doi.org/10.3390/nu13030715] [PMID: 33668219]

[14]   Kurtz JA, VanDusseldorp TA, Doyle JA, Otis JS. Taurine in sports and exercise. J Int Soc Sports Nutr 2021; 18(1): 39.
        [http://dx.doi.org/10.1186/s12970-021-00438-0] [PMID: 34039357]

[15]   Imagawa TF, Hirano I, Utsuki K, *et al.* Caffeine and taurine enhance endurance performance. Int J Sports Med 2009; 30(7): 485-8.
        [http://dx.doi.org/10.1055/s-0028-1104574] [PMID: 19455480]

[16]   Camerino DC, Tricarico D, Pierno S, *et al.* Taurine and skeletal muscle disorders. Neurochem Res 2004; 29(1): 135-42.
        [http://dx.doi.org/10.1023/B:NERE.0000010442.89826.9c] [PMID: 14992272]

[17]   Ito T, Oishi S, Takai M, *et al.* Cardiac and skeletal muscle abnormality in taurine transporter-knockout mice. J Biomed Sci 2010; 17(1): S20.
        [http://dx.doi.org/10.1186/1423-0127-17-S1-S20] [PMID: 20804595]

[18]   Scicchitano BM, Sica G. The beneficial effects of taurine to counteract sarcopenia. Curr Protein Pept Sci 2018; 19(7): 673-80.
        [http://dx.doi.org/10.2174/1389203718666161122113609] [PMID: 27875962]

[19]   Lodi R, Schapira AHV, Manners D, *et al.* Abnormal in vivo skeletal muscle energy metabolism in Huntington's disease and dentatorubropallidoluysian atrophy. Ann Neurol 2000; 48(1): 72-6.
        [http://dx.doi.org/10.1002/1531-8249(200007)48:1<72::AID-ANA11>3.0.CO;2-I] [PMID: 10894218]

[20]   Kelley DE, He J, Menshikova EV, Ritov VB. Dysfunction of mitochondria in human skeletal muscle in type 2 diabetes. Diabetes 2002; 51(10): 2944-50.
        [http://dx.doi.org/10.2337/diabetes.51.10.2944] [PMID: 12351431]

[21]   Chabi B, Ljubicic V, Menzies KJ, Huang JH, Saleem A, Hood DA. Mitochondrial function and apoptotic susceptibility in aging skeletal muscle. Aging Cell 2008; 7(1): 2-12.
        [http://dx.doi.org/10.1111/j.1474-9726.2007.00347.x] [PMID: 18028258]

[22]   Calvani R, Joseph AM, Adhihetty PJ, *et al.* Mitochondrial pathways in sarcopenia of aging and disuse

muscle atrophy. Biol Chem 2013; 394(3): 393-414.
[http://dx.doi.org/10.1515/hsz-2012-0247] [PMID: 23154422]

[23] Hepple RT. Mitochondrial involvement and impact in aging skeletal muscle. Front Aging Neurosci 2014; 6: 211.
[http://dx.doi.org/10.3389/fnagi.2014.00211] [PMID: 25309422]

[24] Ripolone M, Ronchi D, Violano R, *et al.* Impaired muscle mitochondrial biogenesis and myogenesis in spinal muscular atrophy. JAMA Neurol 2015; 72(6): 666-75.
[http://dx.doi.org/10.1001/jamaneurol.2015.0178] [PMID: 25844556]

[25] Jacobsen JG, Smith LH. Biochemistry and physiology of taurine and taurine derivatives. Physiol Rev 1968; 48(2): 424-511.
[http://dx.doi.org/10.1152/physrev.1968.48.2.424] [PMID: 4297098]

[26] Goodman CA, Horvath D, Stathis C, Mori T, Croft K, Murphy RM, *et al.* Taurine supplementation increases skeletal muscle force production and protects muscle function during and after high-frequency *in vitro* stimulation. Journal of Applied Physiology (Bethesda, Md: 1985). 2009;107(1):144-54.
[http://dx.doi.org/10.1152/japplphysiol.00040.2009]

[27] De Carvalho FG, Galan BSM, Santos PC, *et al.* Taurine: A potential ergogenic aid for preventing muscle damage and protein catabolism and decreasing oxidative stress produced by endurance exercise. Front Physiol 2017; 8: 710.
[http://dx.doi.org/10.3389/fphys.2017.00710] [PMID: 28979213]

[28] Warskulat U, Flögel U, Jacoby C, *et al.* Taurine transporter knockout depletes muscle taurine levels and results in severe skeletal muscle impairment but leaves cardiac function uncompromised. FASEB J 2004; 18(3): 577-9.
[http://dx.doi.org/10.1096/fj.03-0496fje] [PMID: 14734644]

[29] El Idrissi A. Taurine increases mitochondrial buffering of calcium: role in neuroprotection. Amino Acids 2008; 34(2): 321-8.
[http://dx.doi.org/10.1007/s00726-006-0396-9] [PMID: 16955229]

[30] Palmi M, Youmbi GT, Fusi F, *et al.* Potentiation of mitochondrial Ca^{2+} sequestration by taurine. Biochem Pharmacol 1999; 58(7): 1123-31.
[http://dx.doi.org/10.1016/S0006-2952(99)00183-5] [PMID: 10484070]

[31] Palmi M, Youmbi GT, Sgaragli G, Meini A, Benocci A, Fusi F, *et al.* The mitochondrial permeability transition and taurine.Taurine 4: Taurine and Excitable Tissues Advances in Experimental Medicine and Biology. Boston, MA: Springer US 2002; pp. 87-96.
[http://dx.doi.org/10.1007/0-306-46838-7_8]

[32] Ommati MM, Farshad O, Jamshidzadeh A, Heidari R. Taurine enhances skeletal muscle mitochondrial function in a rat model of resistance training. PharmaNutrition 2019; 9: 100161.
[http://dx.doi.org/10.1016/j.phanu.2019.100161]

[33] Jong CJ, Sandal P, Schaffer SW. The role of taurine in mitochondria health: More than just an antioxidant. Molecules 2021; 26(16): 4913.
[http://dx.doi.org/10.3390/molecules26164913] [PMID: 34443494]

[34] Heidari R, Behnamrad S, Khodami Z, Ommati MM, Azarpira N, Vazin A. The nephroprotective properties of taurine in colistin-treated mice is mediated through the regulation of mitochondrial function and mitigation of oxidative stress. Biomed Pharmacother 2019; 109: 103-11.
[http://dx.doi.org/10.1016/j.biopha.2018.10.093] [PMID: 30396066]

[35] Jamshidzadeh A, Heidari R, Abasvali M, *et al.* Taurine treatment preserves brain and liver mitochondrial function in a rat model of fulminant hepatic failure and hyperammonemia. Biomed Pharmacother 2017; 86: 514-20.
[http://dx.doi.org/10.1016/j.biopha.2016.11.095] [PMID: 28024286]

[36] Ahmadi N, Ghanbarinejad V, Ommati MM, Jamshidzadeh A, Heidari R. Taurine prevents mitochondrial membrane permeabilization and swelling upon interaction with manganese: Implication in the treatment of cirrhosis-associated central nervous system complications. J Biochem Mol Toxicol 2018; 32(11): e22216.
[http://dx.doi.org/10.1002/jbt.22216] [PMID: 30152904]

[37] Rutherford JA, Spriet LL, Stellingwerff T. The effect of acute taurine ingestion on endurance performance and metabolism in well-trained cyclists. Int J Sport Nutr Exerc Metab 2010; 20(4): 322-9.
[http://dx.doi.org/10.1123/ijsnem.20.4.322] [PMID: 20739720]

[38] Liu Z, Qi B, Zhang M, *et al.* Role of taurine supplementation to prevent exercise-induced oxidative stress in healthy young men. Amino Acids 2004; 26(2): 203-7.
[http://dx.doi.org/10.1007/s00726-003-0002-3] [PMID: 15042451]

[39] Lee HM, Paik IY, Park TS. Effects of dietary supplementation of taurine, carnitine or glutamine on endurance exercise performance and fatigue parameters in athletes. Korean Journal of Nutrition 2016; 36(7): 711-9.

[40] Abdoli N, Sadeghian I, Azarpira N, Ommati MM, Heidari R. Taurine mitigates bile duct obstruction-associated cholemic nephropathy: effect on oxidative stress and mitochondrial parameters. Clin Exp Hepatol 2021; 7(1): 30-40.
[http://dx.doi.org/10.5114/ceh.2021.104675] [PMID: 34027113]

[41] Heidari R, Ghanbarinejad V, Ommati MM, Jamshidzadeh A, Niknahad H. Mitochondria protecting amino acids: Application against a wide range of mitochondria-linked complications. PharmaNutrition 2018; 6(4): 180-90.
[http://dx.doi.org/10.1016/j.phanu.2018.09.001]

[42] Mortensen O, Olsen H, Frandsen L, *et al.* A maternal low protein diet has pronounced effects on mitochondrial gene expression in offspring liver and skeletal muscle; protective effect of taurine. J Biomed Sci. 2010; 17(1): S38.
[http://dx.doi.org/10.1186/1423-0127-17-S1-S38] [PMID: 20804614]

[43] Mortensen OH, Olsen HL, Frandsen L, *et al.* Gestational protein restriction in mice has pronounced effects on gene expression in newborn offspring's liver and skeletal muscle; protective effect of taurine. Pediatr Res 2010; 67(1): 47-53.
[http://dx.doi.org/10.1203/PDR.0b013e3181c4735c] [PMID: 19823102]

[44] Ma Y, Maruta H, Sun B, Wang C, Isono C, Yamashita H. Effects of long-term taurine supplementation on age-related changes in skeletal muscle function of Sprague–Dawley rats. Amino Acids 2021; 53(2): 159-70.
[http://dx.doi.org/10.1007/s00726-020-02934-0] [PMID: 33398526]

[45] Wen C, Li F, Zhang L, *et al.* Taurine is involved in energy metabolism in muscles, adipose tissue, and the liver. Mol Nutr Food Res 2019; 63(2): 1800536.
[http://dx.doi.org/10.1002/mnfr.201800536] [PMID: 30251429]

[46] Silva LA, Silveira PCL, Ronsani MM, *et al.* Taurine supplementation decreases oxidative stress in skeletal muscle after eccentric exercise. Cell Biochem Funct 2011; 29(1): 43-9.
[http://dx.doi.org/10.1002/cbf.1716] [PMID: 21264889]

[47] Adrian RH, Bryant SH. On the repetitive discharge in myotonic muscle fibres. J Physiol 1974; 240(2): 505-15.
[http://dx.doi.org/10.1113/jphysiol.1974.sp010620] [PMID: 4420758]

[48] Camerino DC, Tricarico D, Desaphy JF. Ion channel pharmacology. Neurotherapeutics 2007; 4(2): 184-98.
[http://dx.doi.org/10.1016/j.nurt.2007.01.013] [PMID: 17395128]

[49] Jentsch TJ. CLC chloride channels and transporters: from genes to protein structure, pathology and physiology. Crit Rev Biochem Mol Biol 2008; 43(1): 3-36.

[http://dx.doi.org/10.1080/10409230701829110] [PMID: 18307107]

[50]   Conte-Camerino D, Franconi F, Mambrini M, *et al.* The action of taurine on chloride conductance and excitability characteristics of rat striated muscle fibers. Pharmacol Res Commun 1987; 19(10): 685-701.
[http://dx.doi.org/10.1016/0031-6989(87)90099-3] [PMID: 2450378]

[51]   Pierno S, Tricarico D, De Luca A, *et al.* Effects of taurine analogues on chloride channel conductance of rat skeletal muscle fibers: a structure-activity relationship investigation. Naunyn Schmiedebergs Arch Pharmacol 1994; 349(4): 416-21.
[http://dx.doi.org/10.1007/BF00170889] [PMID: 8058113]

[52]   Camerino DC, De Luca A, Mambrini M, *et al.* The effects of taurine on pharmacologically induced myotonia. Muscle Nerve 1989; 12(11): 898-904.
[http://dx.doi.org/10.1002/mus.880121105] [PMID: 2608084]

[53]   Durelli L, Mutani R, Fassio F, Satta A, Bartoli E. Taurine and hyperexcitable human muscle: Effects of taurine on potassium-induced hyperexcitability of dystrophic myotonic and normal muscles. Ann Neurol 1982; 11(3): 258-65.
[http://dx.doi.org/10.1002/ana.410110305] [PMID: 7092178]

[54]   Durelli L, Mutani R, Fassio F. The treatment of myotonia: Evaluation of chronic oral taurine therapy. Neurology. 1983;33(5):599.

[55]   Trip J, Drost G, van Engelen BG, Faber CG. Drug treatment for myotonia. Cochrane Database Syst Rev 2006; 2006(1): CD004762.
[PMID: 16437496]

[56]   De Luca A, Pierno S, Tricarico D, Desaphy J-F, Liantonio A, Barbieri M, *et al.* Taurine and Skeletal Muscle Ion Channels.Taurine 4: Taurine and Excitable Tissues Advances in Experimental Medicine and Biology. Boston, MA: Springer US 2002; pp. 45-56.
[http://dx.doi.org/10.1007/0-306-46838-7_5]

[57]   Berchtold MW, Brinkmeier H, Müntener M. Calcium ion in skeletal muscle: its crucial role for muscle function, plasticity, and disease. Physiol Rev 2000; 80(3): 1215-65.
[http://dx.doi.org/10.1152/physrev.2000.80.3.1215] [PMID: 10893434]

[58]   Agrawal A, Suryakumar G, Rathor R. Role of defective Ca^{2+} signaling in skeletal muscle weakness: Pharmacological implications. J Cell Commun Signal 2018; 12(4): 645-59.
[http://dx.doi.org/10.1007/s12079-018-0477-z] [PMID: 29982883]

[59]   Wirth KJ, Scheibenbogen C. Pathophysiology of skeletal muscle disturbances in Myalgic Encephalomyelitis/Chronic Fatigue Syndrome (ME/CFS). J Transl Med 2021; 19(1): 162.
[http://dx.doi.org/10.1186/s12967-021-02833-2] [PMID: 33882940]

[60]   MacLennan DH, Zvaritch E. Mechanistic models for muscle diseases and disorders originating in the sarcoplasmic reticulum. Biochim Biophys Acta Mol Cell Res 2011; 1813(5): 948-64.
[http://dx.doi.org/10.1016/j.bbamcr.2010.11.009] [PMID: 21118704]

[61]   Zabłocka B, Górecki DC, Zabłocki K. Disrupted calcium homeostasis in Duchenne muscular dystrophy: A common mechanism behind diverse consequences. Int J Mol Sci 2021; 22(20): 11040.
[http://dx.doi.org/10.3390/ijms222011040] [PMID: 34681707]

[62]   Mareedu S, Million ED, Duan D, Babu GJ. Abnormal calcium handling in Duchenne muscular dystrophy: Mechanisms and potential therapies. Front Physiol 2021; 12: 647010.
[http://dx.doi.org/10.3389/fphys.2021.647010] [PMID: 33897454]

[63]   Hopf FW, Turner PR, Steinhardt RA. Calcium misregulation and the pathogenesis of muscular dystrophy. Subcell Biochem 2007; 45: 429-64.
[http://dx.doi.org/10.1007/978-1-4020-6191-2_16] [PMID: 18193647]

[64]   Costelli P, Reffo P, Penna F, Autelli R, Bonelli G, Baccino FM. Ca2$^+$-dependent proteolysis in muscle wasting. Int J Biochem Cell Biol 2005; 37(10): 2134-46.

[http://dx.doi.org/10.1016/j.biocel.2005.03.010] [PMID: 15893952]

[65]   Clanton TL. Hypoxia-induced reactive oxygen species formation in skeletal muscle. J Appl Physiol 2007; 102(6): 2379-88.
[http://dx.doi.org/10.1152/japplphysiol.01298.2006] [PMID: 17289907]

[66]   Hyatt HW, Powers SK. Disturbances in calcium homeostasis promotes skeletal muscle atrophy: Lessons from ventilator-induced diaphragm wasting. Front Physiol 2020; 11: 615351.
[http://dx.doi.org/10.3389/fphys.2020.615351] [PMID: 33391032]

[67]   Ye HB, Shi HB, Yin SK. Mechanisms underlying taurine protection against glutamate-induced neurotoxicity. Can J Neurol Sci 2013; 40(5): 628-34.
[http://dx.doi.org/10.1017/S0317167100014840] [PMID: 23968934]

[68]   Mohammadi H, Ommati MM, Farshad O, Jamshidzadeh A, Nikbakht MR, Niknahad H, *et al.* Taurine and isolated mitochondria: A concentration-response study. Trends Pharmacol Sci 2019; 5(4): 197-206.

[69]   Yang Y, Zhang Y, Liu X, *et al.* Exogenous taurine attenuates mitochondrial oxidative stress and endoplasmic reticulum stress in rat cardiomyocytes. Acta Biochim Biophys Sin (Shanghai) 2013; 45(5): 359-67.
[http://dx.doi.org/10.1093/abbs/gmt034] [PMID: 23619568]

[70]   Jong C, Ito T, Prentice H, Wu JY, Schaffer S. Role of mitochondria and endoplasmic reticulum in taurine-deficiency-mediated apoptosis. Nutrients 2017; 9(8): 795.
[http://dx.doi.org/10.3390/nu9080795] [PMID: 28757580]

[71]   Ito T, Yoshikawa N, Schaffer SW, Azuma J. Tissue taurine depletion alters metabolic response to exercise and reduces running capacity in mice. J Amino Acids 2014; 2014: 1-10.
[http://dx.doi.org/10.1155/2014/964680] [PMID: 25478210]

[72]   Kirino Y, Yasukawa T, Ohta S, *et al.* Codon-specific translational defect caused by a wobble modification deficiency in mutant tRNA from a human mitochondrial disease. Proc Natl Acad Sci USA 2004; 101(42): 15070-5.
[http://dx.doi.org/10.1073/pnas.0405173101] [PMID: 15477592]

[73]   Schaffer SW, Jong CJ, Warner D, Ito T, Azuma J. Taurine deficiency and MELAS are closely related syndromes. Adv Exp Med Biol 2013; 776: 153-65.
[http://dx.doi.org/10.1007/978-1-4614-6093-0_16] [PMID: 23392880]

[74]   Asano K, Suzuki T, Saito A, *et al.* Metabolic and chemical regulation of tRNA modification associated with taurine deficiency and human disease. Nucleic Acids Res 2018; 46(4): 1565-83.
[http://dx.doi.org/10.1093/nar/gky068] [PMID: 29390138]

[75]   Jong CJ, Azuma J, Schaffer SW. Role of mitochondrial permeability transition in taurine deficiency-induced apoptosis. Exp Clin Cardiol 2011; 16(4): 125-8.
[PMID: 22131855]

[76]   Suzuki T, Suzuki T, Wada T, Saigo K, Watanabe K. Novel taurine-containing uridine derivatives and mitochondrial human diseases. Nucleic Acids Symp Ser 2001; 1(1): 257-8.
[http://dx.doi.org/10.1093/nass/1.1.257] [PMID: 12836362]

[77]   Jong CJ, Azuma J, Schaffer S. Mechanism underlying the antioxidant activity of taurine: prevention of mitochondrial oxidant production. Amino Acids 2012; 42(6): 2223-32.
[http://dx.doi.org/10.1007/s00726-011-0962-7] [PMID: 21691752]

[78]   Cohen S, Nathan JA, Goldberg AL. Muscle wasting in disease: molecular mechanisms and promising therapies. Nat Rev Drug Discov 2015; 14(1): 58-74.
[http://dx.doi.org/10.1038/nrd4467] [PMID: 25549588]

[79]   Picca A, Calvani R, Bossola M, *et al.* Update on mitochondria and muscle aging: all wrong roads lead to sarcopenia. Biol Chem 2018; 399(5): 421-36.
[http://dx.doi.org/10.1515/hsz-2017-0331] [PMID: 29384724]

[80]　VanderVeen BN, Fix DK, Carson JA. Disrupted skeletal muscle mitochondrial dynamics, mitophagy, and biogenesis during cancer cachexia: A role for inflammation. Oxid Med Cell Longev 2017; 2017: 1-13.
[http://dx.doi.org/10.1155/2017/3292087] [PMID: 28785374]

[81]　Bellanti F, Lo Buglio A, Vendemiale G. Mitochondrial impairment in sarcopenia. Biology (Basel) 2021; 10(1): 31.
[http://dx.doi.org/10.3390/biology10010031] [PMID: 33418869]

[82]　Hyatt H, Deminice R, Yoshihara T, Powers SK. Mitochondrial dysfunction induces muscle atrophy during prolonged inactivity: A review of the causes and effects. Arch Biochem Biophys 2019; 662: 49-60.
[http://dx.doi.org/10.1016/j.abb.2018.11.005] [PMID: 30452895]

[83]　Trevino MB, Zhang X, Standley RA, *et al.* Loss of mitochondrial energetics is associated with poor recovery of muscle function but not mass following disuse atrophy. Am J Physiol Endocrinol Metab 2019; 317(5): E899-910.
[http://dx.doi.org/10.1152/ajpendo.00161.2019] [PMID: 31479303]

[84]　Romanello V, Sandri M. Mitochondrial quality control and muscle mass maintenance. Front Physiol 2016; 6: 422.
[http://dx.doi.org/10.3389/fphys.2015.00422] [PMID: 26793123]

[85]　Sandri M. Protein breakdown in muscle wasting: Role of autophagy-lysosome and ubiquitin-proteasome. Int J Biochem Cell Biol 2013; 45(10): 2121-9.
[http://dx.doi.org/10.1016/j.biocel.2013.04.023] [PMID: 23665154]

[86]　Bonaldo P, Sandri M. Cellular and molecular mechanisms of muscle atrophy. Dis Model Mech 2013; 6(1): 25-39.
[http://dx.doi.org/10.1242/dmm.010389] [PMID: 23268536]

[87]　Xia Q, Huang X, Huang J, *et al.* The role of autophagy in skeletal muscle diseases. Front Physiol 2021; 12: 638983.
[http://dx.doi.org/10.3389/fphys.2021.638983] [PMID: 33841177]

[88]　Park SS, Seo YK, Kwon KS. Sarcopenia targeting with autophagy mechanism by exercise. BMB Rep 2019; 52(1): 64-9.
[http://dx.doi.org/10.5483/BMBRep.2019.52.1.292] [PMID: 30526769]

[89]　Franco-Romero A, Sandri M. Role of autophagy in muscle disease. Mol Aspects Med 2021; 82: 101041.
[http://dx.doi.org/10.1016/j.mam.2021.101041] [PMID: 34625292]

[90]　Mizushima N, Yamamoto A, Matsui M, Yoshimori T, Ohsumi Y. *In vivo* analysis of autophagy in response to nutrient starvation using transgenic mice expressing a fluorescent autophagosome marker. Mol Biol Cell 2004; 15(3): 1101-11.
[http://dx.doi.org/10.1091/mbc.e03-09-0704] [PMID: 14699058]

[91]　Bechet D, Tassa A, Taillandier D, Combaret L, Attaix D. Lysosomal proteolysis in skeletal muscle. Int J Biochem Cell Biol 2005; 37(10): 2098-114.
[http://dx.doi.org/10.1016/j.biocel.2005.02.029] [PMID: 16125113]

[92]　Schaffer SW, Azuma J, Mozaffari M. Role of antioxidant activity of taurine in diabetesThis article is one of a selection of papers from the NATO Advanced Research Workshop on Translational Knowledge for Heart Health (published in part 1 of a 2-part Special Issue). Can J Physiol Pharmacol 2009; 87(2): 91-9.
[http://dx.doi.org/10.1139/Y08-110] [PMID: 19234572]

[93]　De Mario A, Gherardi G, Rizzuto R, Mammucari C. Skeletal muscle mitochondria in health and disease. Cell Calcium 2021; 94: 102357.
[http://dx.doi.org/10.1016/j.ceca.2021.102357] [PMID: 33550207]

[94]   Johannsen DL, Ravussin E. The role of mitochondria in health and disease. Curr Opin Pharmacol 2009; 9(6): 780-6.
[http://dx.doi.org/10.1016/j.coph.2009.09.002] [PMID: 19796990]

[95]   Zhang T, Xue L, Li L, *et al.* BNIP3 protein suppresses PINK1 kinase proteolytic cleavage to promote mitophagy. J Biol Chem 2016; 291(41): 21616-29.
[http://dx.doi.org/10.1074/jbc.M116.733410] [PMID: 27528605]

[96]   Choubey V, Zeb A, Kaasik A. Molecular mechanisms and regulation of mammalian mitophagy. Cells 2021; 11(1): 38.
[http://dx.doi.org/10.3390/cells11010038] [PMID: 35011599]

[97]   Narendra DP, Youle RJ. Targeting mitochondrial dysfunction: role for PINK1 and Parkin in mitochondrial quality control. Antioxid Redox Signal 2011; 14(10): 1929-38.
[http://dx.doi.org/10.1089/ars.2010.3799] [PMID: 21194381]

[98]   Kitagishi Y, Nakano N, Ogino M, Ichimura M, Minami A, Matsuda S. PINK1 signaling in mitochondrial homeostasis and in aging (Review). Int J Mol Med 2017; 39(1): 3-8.
[http://dx.doi.org/10.3892/ijmm.2016.2827] [PMID: 27959386]

[99]   Barbiera A, Sorrentino S, Lepore E, *et al.* Taurine attenuates catabolic processes related to the onset of sarcopenia. Int J Mol Sci 2020; 21(22): 8865.
[http://dx.doi.org/10.3390/ijms21228865] [PMID: 33238549]

[100]   Li Y, Hu Z, Chen B, *et al.* Taurine attenuates methamphetamine-induced autophagy and apoptosis in PC12 cells through mTOR signaling pathway. Toxicol Lett 2012; 215(1): 1-7.
[http://dx.doi.org/10.1016/j.toxlet.2012.09.019] [PMID: 23041169]

[101]   Luo Y, Tian Y, Zhao C. Taurine attenuates liver autophagy and injury of offspring in gestational diabetic mellitus rats. Life Sci 2020; 257: 117889.
[http://dx.doi.org/10.1016/j.lfs.2020.117889] [PMID: 32502541]

[102]   Schaffer S, Kim HW. Effects and mechanisms of taurine as a therapeutic agent. Biomol Ther (Seoul) 2018; 26(3): 225-41.
[http://dx.doi.org/10.4062/biomolther.2017.251] [PMID: 29631391]

[103]   Goodman CA, Horvath D, Stathis C, *et al.* Taurine supplementation increases skeletal muscle force production and protects muscle function during and after high-frequency *in vitro* stimulation. J Appl Physiol 2009; 107(1): 144-54.
[http://dx.doi.org/10.1152/japplphysiol.00040.2009] [PMID: 19423840]

[104]   McLeay Y, Stannard S, Barnes M. The effect of taurine on the recovery from eccentric exercise-induced muscle damage in males. Antioxidants 2017; 6(4): 79.
[http://dx.doi.org/10.3390/antiox6040079] [PMID: 29039798]

[105]   Petrillo S, Pelosi L, Piemonte F, *et al.* Oxidative stress in Duchenne muscular dystrophy: focus on the NRF2 redox pathway. Hum Mol Genet 2017; 26(14): 2781-90.
[http://dx.doi.org/10.1093/hmg/ddx173] [PMID: 28472288]

[106]   Ragusa RJ, Chow CK, Porter JD. Oxidative stress as a potential pathogenic mechanism in an animal model of Duchenne muscular dystrophy. Neuromuscul Disord 1997; 7(6-7): 379-86.
[http://dx.doi.org/10.1016/S0960-8966(97)00096-5] [PMID: 9327402]

[107]   Kelly-Worden M, Thomas E. Mitochondrial dysfunction in Duchenne muscular dystrophy. Open Journal of Endocrine and Metabolic Diseases. 2014.
[http://dx.doi.org/10.4236/ojemd.2014.48020]

[108]   Ramadasan-Nair R, Gayathri N, Mishra S, *et al.* Mitochondrial alterations and oxidative stress in an acute transient mouse model of muscle degeneration: implications for muscular dystrophy and related muscle pathologies. J Biol Chem 2014; 289(1): 485-509.
[http://dx.doi.org/10.1074/jbc.M113.493270] [PMID: 24220031]

[109]   Canton M, Menazza S, Di Lisa F. Oxidative stress in muscular dystrophy: from generic evidence to specific sources and targets. J Muscle Res Cell Motil 2014; 35(1): 23-36.
[http://dx.doi.org/10.1007/s10974-014-9380-2] [PMID: 24619215]

[110]   Kourakis S, Timpani CA, de Haan JB, Gueven N, Fischer D, Rybalka E. Targeting Nrf2 for the treatment of Duchenne muscular dystrophy. Redox Biol 2021; 38: 101803.
[http://dx.doi.org/10.1016/j.redox.2020.101803] [PMID: 33246292]

[111]   Lawler JM. Exacerbation of pathology by oxidative stress in respiratory and locomotor muscles with Duchenne muscular dystrophy. J Physiol 2011; 589(9): 2161-70.
[http://dx.doi.org/10.1113/jphysiol.2011.207456] [PMID: 21486793]

[112]   Berger J, Berger S, Hall TE, Lieschke GJ, Currie PD. Dystrophin-deficient zebrafish feature aspects of the Duchenne muscular dystrophy pathology. Neuromuscul Disord 2010; 20(12): 826-32.
[http://dx.doi.org/10.1016/j.nmd.2010.08.004] [PMID: 20850317]

[113]   Nakamura A, Takeda S. Mammalian models of Duchenne Muscular Dystrophy: pathological characteristics and therapeutic applications. J Biomed Biotechnol 2011; 2011: 1-8.
[http://dx.doi.org/10.1155/2011/184393] [PMID: 21274260]

[114]   Deconinck AE, Rafael JA, Skinner JA, *et al.* Utrophin-dystrophin-deficient mice as a model for Duchenne muscular dystrophy. Cell 1997; 90(4): 717-27.
[http://dx.doi.org/10.1016/S0092-8674(00)80532-2] [PMID: 9288751]

[115]   Nowak KJ, Davies KE. Duchenne muscular dystrophy and dystrophin: pathogenesis and opportunities for treatment. EMBO Rep 2004; 5(9): 872-6.
[http://dx.doi.org/10.1038/sj.embor.7400221] [PMID: 15470384]

[116]   Gao QQ, McNally EM. The dystrophin complex: structure, function and implications for therapy. Compr Physiol 2015; 5(3): 1223-39.
[http://dx.doi.org/10.1002/cphy.c140048] [PMID: 26140716]

[117]   Vallejo-Illarramendi A, Toral-Ojeda I, Aldanondo G, López de Munain A. Dysregulation of calcium homeostasis in muscular dystrophies. Expert Rev Mol Med 2014; 16: e16.
[http://dx.doi.org/10.1017/erm.2014.17] [PMID: 25293420]

[118]   Lee JM, Noguchi S. Calcium dyshomeostasis in tubular aggregate myopathy. Int J Mol Sci 2016; 17(11): 1952.
[http://dx.doi.org/10.3390/ijms17111952] [PMID: 27879676]

[119]   Amici DR, Pinal-Fernandez I, Mázala DAG, *et al.* Calcium dysregulation, functional calpainopathy, and endoplasmic reticulum stress in sporadic inclusion body myositis. Acta Neuropathol Commun 2017; 5(1): 24.
[http://dx.doi.org/10.1186/s40478-017-0427-7] [PMID: 28330496]

[120]   Rugowska A, Starosta A, Konieczny P. Epigenetic modifications in muscle regeneration and progression of Duchenne muscular dystrophy. Clin Epigenetics 2021; 13(1): 13.
[http://dx.doi.org/10.1186/s13148-021-01001-z] [PMID: 33468200]

[121]   Brookes PS, Yoon Y, Robotham JL, Anders MW, Sheu SS. Calcium, ATP, and ROS: a mitochondrial love-hate triangle. Am J Physiol Cell Physiol 2004; 287(4): C817-33.
[http://dx.doi.org/10.1152/ajpcell.00139.2004] [PMID: 15355853]

[122]   Finkel T, Menazza S, Holmström KM, *et al.* The ins and outs of mitochondrial calcium. Circ Res 2015; 116(11): 1810-9.
[http://dx.doi.org/10.1161/CIRCRESAHA.116.305484] [PMID: 25999421]

[123]   Debattisti V, Horn A, Singh R, *et al.* Dysregulation of mitochondrial Ca^{2+} uptake and sarcolemma repair underlie muscle weakness and wasting in patients and mice lacking MICU1. Cell Rep 2019; 29(5): 1274-1286.e6.
[http://dx.doi.org/10.1016/j.celrep.2019.09.063] [PMID: 31665639]

[124] Zhou J, Dhakal K, Yi J. Mitochondrial Ca^{2+} uptake in skeletal muscle health and disease. Sci China Life Sci 2016; 59(8): 770-6.
[http://dx.doi.org/10.1007/s11427-016-5089-3] [PMID: 27430885]

[125] Michelucci A, Liang C, Protasi F, Dirksen RT. Altered Ca^{2+} handling and oxidative stress underlie mitochondrial damage and skeletal muscle dysfunction in aging and disease. Metabolites 2021; 11(7): 424.
[http://dx.doi.org/10.3390/metabo11070424] [PMID: 34203260]

[126] Timbrell JA, Seabra V, Waterfield CJ. The *in vivo* and *in vitro* protective properties of taurine. Gen Pharmacol 1995; 26(3): 453-62.
[http://dx.doi.org/10.1016/0306-3623(94)00203-Y] [PMID: 7789717]

[127] Ohta H, Azuma J, Awata N, *et al.* Mechanism of the protective action of taurine against isoprenaline induced myocardial damage. Cardiovasc Res 1988; 22(6): 407-13.
[http://dx.doi.org/10.1093/cvr/22.6.407] [PMID: 3224353]

[128] Schaffer S, Azuma J, Takahashi K, Mozaffari M. Why is taurine cytoprotective?Taurine 5: Beginning the 21st Century. Advances in Experimental Medicine and Biology.. Boston, MA: Springer US 2003; pp. 307-21.
[http://dx.doi.org/10.1007/978-1-4615-0077-3_39]

[129] Yang YJ, Han YY, Chen K, Zhang Y, Liu X, Li S, *et al.* TonEBP modulates the protective effect of taurine in ischemia-induced cytotoxicity in cardiomyocytes. Cell Death Dis. 2015;6(12):e2025-e.
[http://dx.doi.org/10.1038/cddis.2015.372]

[130] Hanna J, Chahine R, Aftimos G, *et al.* Protective effect of taurine against free radicals damage in the rat myocardium. Exp Toxicol Pathol 2004; 56(3): 189-94.
[http://dx.doi.org/10.1016/j.etp.2004.08.004] [PMID: 15625788]

[131] Azuma J, Hamaguchi T, Ohta H, Takihara K, Awata N, Sawamura A, *et al.* Calcium overload-induced myocardial damage caused by isoproterenol and by adriamycin: Possible role of taurine in its prevention.The Biology of Taurine: Methods and Mechanisms Advances in Experimental Medicine and Biology. Boston, MA: Springer US 1987; pp. 167-79.
[http://dx.doi.org/10.1007/978-1-4899-0405-8_18]

[132] Roysommuti S, Azuma J, Takahashi K, Schaffer S. Taurine cytoprotection: From cell to system. Journal of Physiological and Biomedical Sciences 2003; 16(2): 17-27.

[133] Leon R, Wu H, Jin Y, *et al.* Protective function of taurine in glutamate-induced apoptosis in cultured neurons. J Neurosci Res 2009; 87(5): 1185-94.
[http://dx.doi.org/10.1002/jnr.21926] [PMID: 18951478]

[134] Bano D, Prehn JHM. Apoptosis-inducing factor (AIF) in physiology and disease: The tale of a repented natural born killer. EBioMedicine 2018; 30: 29-37.
[http://dx.doi.org/10.1016/j.ebiom.2018.03.016] [PMID: 29605508]

[135] Joza N, Oudit GY, Brown D, *et al.* Muscle-specific loss of apoptosis-inducing factor leads to mitochondrial dysfunction, skeletal muscle atrophy, and dilated cardiomyopathy. Mol Cell Biol 2005; 25(23): 10261-72.
[http://dx.doi.org/10.1128/MCB.25.23.10261-10272.2005] [PMID: 16287843]

[136] Memme JM, Slavin M, Moradi N, Hood DA. Mitochondrial bioenergetics and turnover during chronic muscle disuse. Int J Mol Sci 2021; 22(10): 5179.
[http://dx.doi.org/10.3390/ijms22105179] [PMID: 34068411]

[137] Schwartz LM. Atrophy and programmed cell death of skeletal muscle. Cell Death Differ 2008; 15(7): 1163-9.
[http://dx.doi.org/10.1038/cdd.2008.68] [PMID: 18483492]

[138] Marzetti E, Hwang JCY, Lees HA, *et al.* Mitochondrial death effectors: Relevance to sarcopenia and disuse muscle atrophy. Biochim Biophys Acta, Gen Subj 2010; 1800(3): 235-44.

[http://dx.doi.org/10.1016/j.bbagen.2009.05.007] [PMID: 19450666]

[139] Heidari R, Babaei H, Eghbal MA. Ameliorative effects of taurine against methimazole-induced cytotoxicity in isolated rat hepatocytes. Sci Pharm 2012; 80(4): 987-99.
[http://dx.doi.org/10.3797/scipharm.1205-16] [PMID: 23264945]

[140] Heidari R, Babaei H, Eghbal MA. Amodiaquine-induced toxicity in isolated rat hepatocytes and the cytoprotective effects of taurine and/or N-acetyl cysteine. Res Pharm Sci 2014; 9(2): 97-105.
[PMID: 25657778]

[141] Kim KS, Jang MJ, Fang S, *et al.* Anti-obesity effect of taurine through inhibition of adipogenesis in white fat tissue but not in brown fat tissue in a high-fat diet-induced obese mouse model. Amino Acids 2019; 51(2): 245-54.
[http://dx.doi.org/10.1007/s00726-018-2659-7] [PMID: 30255260]

[142] Acharya M, Lau-Cam CA. Comparison of the protective actions of N-acetylcysteine, hypotaurine and taurine against acetaminophen-induced hepatotoxicity in the rat. J Biomed Sci 2010; 17(Suppl 1): S35.
[http://dx.doi.org/10.1186/1423-0127-17-S1-S35] [PMID: 20804611]

[143] Schaffer SW, Jong CJ, Ito T, Azuma J. Effect of taurine on ischemia–reperfusion injury. Amino Acids 2014; 46(1): 21-30.
[http://dx.doi.org/10.1007/s00726-012-1378-8] [PMID: 22936072]

[144] Takahashi Y, Kanagawa H. Effects of glutamine, glycine and taurine on the development of *in vitro* fertilized bovine zygotes in a chemically defined medium. J Vet Med Sci 1998; 60(4): 433-7.
[http://dx.doi.org/10.1292/jvms.60.433] [PMID: 9592714]

[145] Shim K, Park G, Kim S-B. Effects of taurine supplementation on mitochondrial function in chronic ethanol administered rats. J Community Nutr 2005; 7(3): 163-8.

[146] Eby G, Halcomb WW. Elimination of cardiac arrhythmias using oral taurine with l-arginine with case histories: Hypothesis for nitric oxide stabilization of the sinus node. Med Hypotheses 2006; 67(5): 1200-4.
[http://dx.doi.org/10.1016/j.mehy.2006.04.055] [PMID: 16797868]

[147] Albrecht J, Wegrzynowicz M. Endogenous neuro-protectants in ammonia toxicity in the central nervous system: facts and hypotheses. Metab Brain Dis 2005; 20(4): 253-63.
[http://dx.doi.org/10.1007/s11011-005-7904-6] [PMID: 16382336]

[148] Bhat MA, Ahmad K, Khan MSA, *et al.* Expedition into taurine biology: Structural insights and therapeutic perspective of taurine in neurodegenerative diseases. Biomolecules 2020; 10(6): 863.
[http://dx.doi.org/10.3390/biom10060863] [PMID: 32516961]

[149] El Idrissi A, Trenkner E. Growth factors and taurine protect against excitotoxicity by stabilizing calcium homeostasis and energy metabolism. J Neurosci 1999; 19(21): 9459-68.
[http://dx.doi.org/10.1523/JNEUROSCI.19-21-09459.1999] [PMID: 10531449]

[150] Jagadeesan G, Sankarsami Pillai S. Hepatoprotective effects of taurine against mercury induced toxicity in rats. J Environ Biol 2007; 28(4): 753-6.
[PMID: 18405108]

[151] Wu G. Important roles of dietary taurine, creatine, carnosine, anserine and 4-hydroxyproline in human nutrition and health. Amino Acids 2020; 52(3): 329-60.
[http://dx.doi.org/10.1007/s00726-020-02823-6] [PMID: 32072297]

[152] Jong CJ, Schaffer S. Mechanism underlying the antioxidant activity of taurine. The FASEB Journal. 2013;27(S1):1086.1-1.
[http://dx.doi.org/10.1096/fasebj.27.1_supplement.1086.1]

[153] Shetewy A, Shimada-Takaura K, Warner D, *et al.* Mitochondrial defects associated with β-alanine toxicity: relevance to hyper-beta-alaninemia. Mol Cell Biochem 2016; 416(1-2): 11-22.
[http://dx.doi.org/10.1007/s11010-016-2688-z] [PMID: 27023909]

[154] Curtis L, Epstein P. Nutritional treatment for acute and chronic traumatic brain injury patients. J Neurosurg Sci 2014; 58(3): 151-60.
[PMID: 24844176]

[155] Triebel S, Sproll C, Reusch H, Godelmann R, Lachenmeier DW. Rapid analysis of taurine in energy drinks using amino acid analyzer and Fourier transform infrared (FTIR) spectroscopy as basis for toxicological evaluation. Amino Acids 2007; 33(3): 451-7.
[http://dx.doi.org/10.1007/s00726-006-0449-0] [PMID: 17051421]

[156] Kerai MDJ, Waterfield CJ, Kenyon SH, Asker DS, Timbrell JA. Reversal of ethanol-induced hepatic steatosis and lipid peroxidation by taurine: a study in rats. Alcohol Alcohol 1999; 34(4): 529-41.
[http://dx.doi.org/10.1093/alcalc/34.4.529] [PMID: 10456581]

[157] Schaffer S, Takahashi K, Azuma J. Role of osmoregulation in the actions of taurine. Amino Acids 2000; 19(3-4): 527-46.
[http://dx.doi.org/10.1007/s007260070004] [PMID: 11140357]

[158] Kirino Y, Goto Y, Campos Y, Arenas J, Suzuki T. Specific correlation between the wobble modification deficiency in mutant tRNAs and the clinical features of a human mitochondrial disease. Proc Natl Acad Sci USA 2005; 102(20): 7127-32.
[http://dx.doi.org/10.1073/pnas.0500563102] [PMID: 15870203]

[159] Nielsen BS, Larsen EH, Ladefoged O, Lam HR. Subchronic, Low-Level Intraperitoneal Injections of Manganese (IV) Oxide and Manganese (II) Chloride Affect Rat Brain Neurochemistry. Int J Toxicol 2017; 36(3): 239-51.
[http://dx.doi.org/10.1177/1091581817704378] [PMID: 28460583]

[160] Fang YJ, Chiu CH, Chang YY, *et al.* Taurine ameliorates alcoholic steatohepatitis *via* enhancing self-antioxidant capacity and alcohol metabolism. Food Res Int 2011; 44(9): 3105-10.
[http://dx.doi.org/10.1016/j.foodres.2011.08.004]

[161] Rikimaru M, Ohsawa Y, Wolf AM, *et al.* Taurine ameliorates impaired the mitochondrial function and prevents stroke-like episodes in patients with MELAS. Intern Med 2012; 51(24): 3351-7.
[http://dx.doi.org/10.2169/internalmedicine.51.7529] [PMID: 23257519]

[162] Chen B, Abaydula Y, Li D, Tan H, Ma X. Taurine ameliorates oxidative stress by regulating PI3K/Akt/GLUT4 pathway in HepG2 cells and diabetic rats. J Funct Foods 2021; 85: 104629.
[http://dx.doi.org/10.1016/j.jff.2021.104629]

[163] Oja SS, Saransaari P. Taurine and epilepsy. Epilepsy Res 2013; 104(3): 187-94.
[http://dx.doi.org/10.1016/j.eplepsyres.2013.01.010] [PMID: 23410665]

[164] Spriet LL, Whitfield J. Taurine and skeletal muscle function. Curr Opin Clin Nutr Metab Care 2015; 18(1): 96-101.
[http://dx.doi.org/10.1097/MCO.0000000000000135] [PMID: 25415270]

[165] Oja SS, Saransaari P. Taurine as osmoregulator and neuromodulator in the brain. Metab Brain Dis 1996; 11(2): 153-64.
[http://dx.doi.org/10.1007/BF02069502] [PMID: 8776717]

[166] Lin CJ, Chiu CC, Chen YC, Chen ML, Hsu TC, Tzang BS. Taurine attenuates hepatic inflammation in chronic alcohol-fed rats through inhibition of TLR4/MyD88 signaling. J Med Food 2015; 18(12): 1291-8.
[http://dx.doi.org/10.1089/jmf.2014.3408] [PMID: 26090712]

[167] Kim C, Cha YN. Taurine chloramine produced from taurine under inflammation provides anti-inflammatory and cytoprotective effects. Amino Acids 2014; 46(1): 89-100.
[http://dx.doi.org/10.1007/s00726-013-1545-6] [PMID: 23933994]

[168] Kaplan JL, Stern JA, Fascetti AJ, *et al.* Taurine deficiency and dilated cardiomyopathy in golden retrievers fed commercial diets. PLoS One 2018; 13(12): e0209112.
[http://dx.doi.org/10.1371/journal.pone.0209112] [PMID: 30543707]

[169] Kim HY, Kim HV, Yoon JH, *et al.* Taurine in drinking water recovers learning and memory in the adult APP/PS1 mouse model of Alzheimer's disease. Sci Rep 2014; 4(1): 7467.
[http://dx.doi.org/10.1038/srep07467] [PMID: 25502280]

[170] Pessemesse L, Tintignac L, Blanchet E, *et al.* Regulation of mitochondrial activity controls the duration of skeletal muscle regeneration in response to injury. Sci Rep 2019; 9(1): 12249.
[http://dx.doi.org/10.1038/s41598-019-48703-2] [PMID: 31439911]

[171] Seidel U, Huebbe P, Rimbach G. Taurine: A Regulator of Cellular Redox Homeostasis and Skeletal Muscle Function. Mol Nutr Food Res 2019; 63(16): 1800569.
[http://dx.doi.org/10.1002/mnfr.201800569] [PMID: 30211983]

[172] Barbiera A, Sorrentino S, Fard D, *et al.* Taurine administration counteracts aging-associated impingement of skeletal muscle regeneration by reducing inflammation and oxidative stress. Antioxidants 2022; 11(5): 1016.
[http://dx.doi.org/10.3390/antiox11051016] [PMID: 35624880]

[173] McIntosh LM, Garrett KL, Megeney L, Rudnicki MA, Anderson JE. Regeneration and myogenic cell proliferation correlate with taurine levels in dystrophin- and MyoD-Deficient muscles. Anat Rec 1998; 252(2): 311-24.
[http://dx.doi.org/10.1002/(SICI)1097-0185(199810)252:2<311::AID-AR17>3.0.CO;2-Q] [PMID: 9776086]

[174] Lobo MVT, Alonso FJM, del Río RM. Immunocytochemical localization of taurine in different muscle cell types of the dog and rat. Histochem J 2000; 32(1): 53-61.
[http://dx.doi.org/10.1023/A:1003910429346] [PMID: 10805385]

[175] Tsitkanou S, Della Gatta PA, Russell AP. Skeletal muscle satellite cells, mitochondria, and microRNAs: Their involvement in the pathogenesis of ALS. Front Physiol 2016; 7: 403.
[http://dx.doi.org/10.3389/fphys.2016.00403] [PMID: 27679581]

[176] Joseph J, Doles JD. Disease-associated metabolic alterations that impact satellite cells and muscle regeneration: perspectives and therapeutic outlook. Nutr Metab (Lond) 2021; 18(1): 33.
[http://dx.doi.org/10.1186/s12986-021-00565-0] [PMID: 33766031]

[177] Chatre L, Verdonk F, Rocheteau P, Crochemore C, Chrétien F, Ricchetti M. A novel paradigm links mitochondrial dysfunction with muscle stem cell impairment in sepsis. Biochim Biophys Acta Mol Basis Dis 2017; 1863(10) (10, Part B): 2546-53.
[http://dx.doi.org/10.1016/j.bbadis.2017.04.019] [PMID: 28456665]

[178] Hao Q, Wang L, Zhang M, Wang Z, Li M, Gao X. Taurine stimulates protein synthesis and proliferation of C2C12 myoblast cells through the PI3K-ARID4B-mTOR pathway. Br J Nutr 2022; 128(10): 1875-86.
[PMID: 34881695]

[179] Serra AJ, Prokić MD, Vasconsuelo A, Pinto JR. Oxidative stress in muscle diseases: Current and future therapy. Oxid Med Cell Longev 2018; 2018: 1-4.
[http://dx.doi.org/10.1155/2018/6439138] [PMID: 29854088]

[180] Kozakowska M, Pietraszek-Gremplewicz K, Jozkowicz A, Dulak J. The role of oxidative stress in skeletal muscle injury and regeneration: focus on antioxidant enzymes. J Muscle Res Cell Motil 2015; 36(6): 377-93.
[http://dx.doi.org/10.1007/s10974-015-9438-9] [PMID: 26728750]

[181] Ghiasvand R, Hariri M. Muscle and oxidative stress Oxidative Stress and Antioxidant Protection. John Wiley & Sons, Ltd 2016; pp. 205-20.
[http://dx.doi.org/10.1002/9781118832431.ch14]

[182] Mosca N, Petrillo S, Bortolani S, *et al.* Redox homeostasis in muscular dystrophies. Cells 2021; 10(6): 1364.
[http://dx.doi.org/10.3390/cells10061364] [PMID: 34205993]

[183] Chandwaney R, Leichtweis S, Leeuwenburgh C, Ji LL. Oxidative stress and mitochondrial function in skeletal muscle: Effects of aging and exercise training. Age (Omaha) 1998; 21(3): 109-17.
[http://dx.doi.org/10.1007/s11357-998-0017-5] [PMID: 23604368]

[184] Ahn B, Ranjit R, Premkumar P, *et al.* Mitochondrial oxidative stress impairs contractile function but paradoxically increases muscle mass *via* fibre branching. J Cachexia Sarcopenia Muscle 2019; 10(2): 411-28.
[http://dx.doi.org/10.1002/jcsm.12375] [PMID: 30706998]

[185] Bhatti JS, Bhatti GK, Reddy PH. Mitochondrial dysfunction and oxidative stress in metabolic disorders — A step towards mitochondria based therapeutic strategies. Biochim Biophys Acta Mol Basis Dis 2017; 1863(5): 1066-77.
[http://dx.doi.org/10.1016/j.bbadis.2016.11.010] [PMID: 27836629]

[186] Broome SC, Woodhead JST, Merry TL. Mitochondria-targeted antioxidants and skeletal muscle function. Antioxidants 2018; 7(8): 107.
[http://dx.doi.org/10.3390/antiox7080107] [PMID: 30096848]

[187] Min K, Smuder AJ, Kwon O, Kavazis AN, Szeto HH, Powers SK. Mitochondrial-targeted antioxidants protect skeletal muscle against immobilization-induced muscle atrophy. J Appl Physiol 2011; 111(5): 1459-66.
[http://dx.doi.org/10.1152/japplphysiol.00591.2011] [PMID: 21817113]

[188] Broome SC, Braakhuis AJ, Mitchell CJ, Merry TL. Mitochondria-targeted antioxidant supplementation improves 8 km time trial performance in middle-aged trained male cyclists. J Int Soc Sports Nutr 2021; 18(1): 58.
[http://dx.doi.org/10.1186/s12970-021-00454-0] [PMID: 34419082]

[189] Williamson J, Hughes CM, Cobley JN, Davison GW. The mitochondria-targeted antioxidant MitoQ, attenuates exercise-induced mitochondrial DNA damage. Redox Biol 2020; 36: 101673.
[http://dx.doi.org/10.1016/j.redox.2020.101673] [PMID: 32810739]

[190] Niknahad H, Jamshidzadeh A, Heidari R, Zarei M, Ommati MM. Ammonia-induced mitochondrial dysfunction and energy metabolism disturbances in isolated brain and liver mitochondria, and the effect of taurine administration: relevance to hepatic encephalopathy treatment. Clin Exp Hepatol 2017; 3(3): 141-51.
[http://dx.doi.org/10.5114/ceh.2017.68833] [PMID: 29062904]

[191] Heidari R, Babaei H, Eghbal MA. Cytoprotective effects of taurine against toxicity induced by isoniazid and hydrazine in isolated rat hepatocytes. Arh Hig Rada Toksikol 2013; 64(2): 201-10.
[http://dx.doi.org/10.2478/10004-1254-64-2013-2297] [PMID: 23819928]

[192] Heidari R, Abdoli N, Ommati MM, Jamshidzadeh A, Niknahad H. Mitochondrial impairment induced by chenodeoxycholic acid: The protective effect of taurine and carnosine supplementation. Trends in Pharmaceutical Sciences. 2018;4(2).

[193] Jamshidzadeh A, Abdoli N, Niknahad H, Azarpira N, Mardani E, Mousavi S, *et al.* Taurine alleviates brain tissue markers of oxidative stress in a rat model of hepatic encephalopathy. Trends Pharmacol Sci 2017; 3(3): 181-92.

[194] Mousavi K, Niknahad H, Ghalamfarsa A, *et al.* Taurine mitigates cirrhosis-associated heart injury through mitochondrial-dependent and antioxidative mechanisms. Clin Exp Hepatol 2020; 6(3): 207-19.
[http://dx.doi.org/10.5114/ceh.2020.99513] [PMID: 33145427]

[195] Heidari R, Jamshidzadeh A, Ghanbarinejad V, Ommati MM, Niknahad H. Taurine supplementation abates cirrhosis-associated locomotor dysfunction. Clin Exp Hepatol 2018; 4(2): 72-82.
[http://dx.doi.org/10.5114/ceh.2018.75956] [PMID: 29904723]

[196] Ommati MM, Heidari R, Ghanbarinejad V, Abdoli N, Niknahad H. Taurine treatment provides neuroprotection in a mouse model of manganism. Biol Trace Elem Res 2019; 190(2): 384-95.

[http://dx.doi.org/10.1007/s12011-018-1552-2] [PMID: 30357569]

[197]   Thirupathi A, Pinho RA, Baker JS, István B, Gu Y. Taurine reverses oxidative damages and restores the muscle function in overuse of exercised muscle. Front Physiol 2020; 11: 582449.
[http://dx.doi.org/10.3389/fphys.2020.582449] [PMID: 33192592]

[198]   Jong CJ, Sandal P, Schaffer SW. The role of taurine in mitochondria health: More than just an antioxidant. Molecules 2021; 26(16): 4913.
[http://dx.doi.org/10.3390/molecules26164913] [PMID: 34443494]

[199]   Suzuki T, Suzuki T, Wada T, Saigo K, Watanabe K. Taurine as a constituent of mitochondrial tRNAs: new insights into the functions of taurine and human mitochondrial diseases. EMBO J 2002; 21(23): 6581-9.
[http://dx.doi.org/10.1093/emboj/cdf656] [PMID: 12456664]

[200]   Yasukawa T, Kirino Y, Ishii N, *et al.* Wobble modification deficiency in mutant tRNAs in patients with mitochondrial diseases. FEBS Lett 2005; 579(13): 2948-52.
[http://dx.doi.org/10.1016/j.febslet.2005.04.038] [PMID: 15893315]

[201]   Baliou S, Adamaki M, Ioannou P, *et al.* Protective role of taurine against oxidative stress (Review). Mol Med Rep 2021; 24(2): 605.
[http://dx.doi.org/10.3892/mmr.2021.12242] [PMID: 34184084]

CHAPTER 8

Taurine and the Renal System: Effects on Mitochondrial Function and Energy Metabolism

Abstract: Renal tissue is the main organ responsible for regulating the human taurine (TAU) pools. A large amount of intact (un-metabolized) TAU is excreted through the urine daily. On the other hand, it has been found that TAU plays a fundamental role in renal function. Several physiological roles, including regulating the blood flow, acting as an osmolyte, and controlling ions transport, are attributed to TAU in the kidneys. Besides, many investigations revealed that TAU could provide several pharmacological roles in renal disorders. It has been found that the antioxidant properties of TAU, its effects on processes such as the renin-angiotensin system, nitric oxide synthesis, and, most importantly, the regulation of mitochondrial function in the kidney could play a fundamental role in the pharmacological effects of this amino acid in the kidney. The current chapter provides a brief review of TAU's fundamental role in renal function. Then, the beneficial effects of TAU administration in renal disease are highlighted, focusing on the impact of this compound on mitochondria-related mechanisms. The data collected in this chapter might shed light on the potential clinical application of TAU as a safe drug candidate against a wide range of renal diseases.

Keywords: Chronic renal damage, Energy metabolism, Kidney disease, Renal injury.

INTRODUCTION

Taurine is mainly excreted in urine as an intact molecule [1, 2]. Actually, the kidney regulates the body's TAU pool. On the other hand, several vital processes are also regulated by TAU in the kidney [1, 3 - 7]. Some examples of TAU's action in the kidneys are regulating the blood flow, acting as an osmolyte, and controlling ions transport [1]. Kidneys profoundly regulate TAU homeostasis [1]. There are a plethora of investigations on the identification of transporters responsible for renal TAU excretion/reabsorption [1]. On the other hand, several physiological roles have been identified for TAU in the kidney [1, 4, 8 - 10]. The osmoregulatory properties of TAU are the best-known physiological role of this compound in the kidney [1].

Reza Heidari and M. Mehdi Ommati

There are a plethora of investigations regarding the renoprotective properties of TAU [5, 11 - 15].

The antioxidant properties of TAU are another exciting feature of this amino acid in renal disease [11, 12, 14 - 18]. These studies noted robust effects of TAU in mitigating biomarkers of oxidative stress in the renal tissue [11 - 18].

The direct effect of TAU on reactive species is also an old concept believed to be responsible for the protective properties of this amino acid [19]. However, more studies revealed that TAU is a weak radical scavenger and practically reacts with no primary ROS forms [20].

An exciting and widely acceptable mechanism for the antioxidant properties of TAU in the kidney and many other organs is supposed to be mediated through the effects of this amino acid on mitochondrial function [21]. In this regard, a plethora of investigations mentioned that TAU supplementation improved mitochondrial indices of functionality and, more importantly, decreased mitochondria-facilitated ROS formation and oxidative stress. An essential part of the current chapter is devoted to the effects of TAU on renal mitochondria and its relevance to managing human renal disease.

THE CRITICAL ROLE OF CELLULAR MITOCHONDRIA AND ENERGY METABOLISM IN THE KIDNEY

Renal tissue consumes a tremendous amount of energy daily. Most of the ATP consumed by the kidney is used for the reabsorption of infiltrated chemicals through glomeruli [22]. Many chemicals, including glucose, amino acids, phosphine, vitamins, minerals, and several ions, are reabsorbed in an energy-dependent manner [23 - 26]. Renal tissue contains numerous mitochondria whose proper function guarantees appropriate ATP metabolism and renal function. Na^+/K^+ ATPase pump is an essential component of chemical reabsorption in the kidney [26, 27]. Actually, the Na^+/K^+ ATPase pump produces an electrochemical sodium gradient used for the reabsorption process of other chemicals in the kidney (Fig. **1**). As shown in Fig. (**1**), Na^+/K^+ ATPase pumps Na^+ out of the tubular cells and simultaneously imports K^+ ions into the cell. Both of these pumping gradients are against the concentration gradient of these ions and are energy (ATP) dependent processes (Fig. **1**). In renal cells, the Na^+ electrochemical gradient is used for reabsorption of many chemicals into the bloodstream (Fig. **1**).

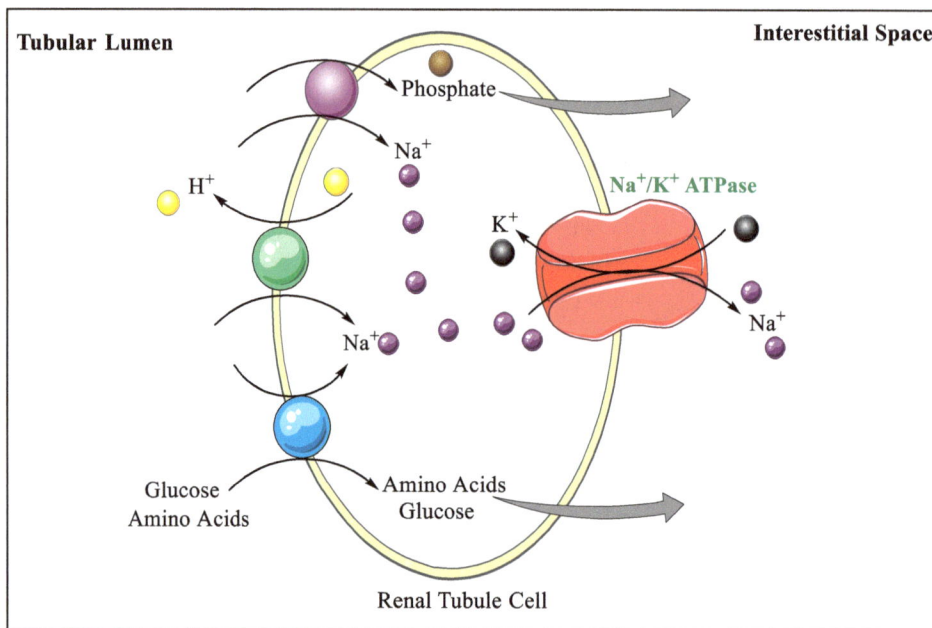

Fig. (1). Schematic representation of the pivotal role of enough ATP level and proper Na^+/K^+ ATPase pump for the reabsorption of chemicals from glomeruli. Any mitochondrial impairment and energy crisis could disrupt this process and lead to deleterious evenest such as essential molecules waste through urine and endangering organisms' life. Renal tissue contains numerous mitochondria that guarantee enough level of ATP required for these processes. Several diseases or xenobiotics could impair mitochondrial function and impair this restorative procedure.

As mentioned, ATP plays a critical role in renal function. In this regard, diseases or xenobiotics that could damage mitochondria could influence renal function and cause deleterious consequences such as body electrolyte disturbances [23, 28 - 33]. Therefore, targeting mitochondria could be a viable therapeutic intervention for many renal disorders.

Since its introduction as a safe and effective therapeutic agent, TAU has positively affected renal function. Most importantly, it has been found that TAU has tremendous effects on renal mitochondrial indices. Hence, this amino acid could be an excellent candidate for managing kidney diseases in clinical stages. In the forthcoming arts, the effects of TAU on renal disorders with a focus on the effects of this amino acid on mitochondrial function are provided.

EFFECT OF TAURINE ON THE KIDNEY: FOCUS ON MITOCHONDRIAL-RELATED PATHOLOGIES

The kidney regulates the whole body's TAU through its excretion [1]. The effects of TAU against several renal diseases and xenobiotics-induced nephrotoxicity are mentioned in previous studies. It seems that the positive impact of TAU on cellular mitochondria in the kidneys is mediated through a mitochondria-dependent mechanism. Several investigations revealed that TAU exerts cytoprotective properties against xenobiotics-induced kidney injury or renal diseases [1, 14, 34 - 39]. Several studies mentioned that TAU provides antioxidative stress in the renal tissue through a mitochondrial-linked pathway [35] (Fig. **2**).

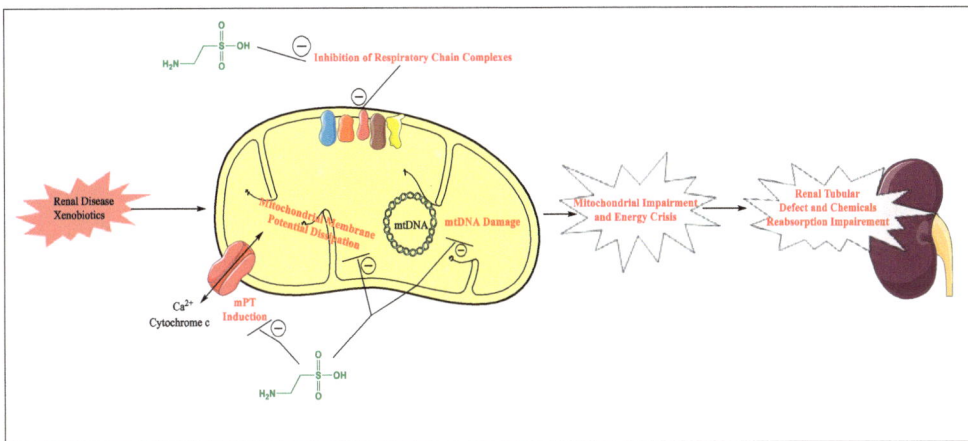

Fig. (2). The renoprotective properties of taurine and its relevance to the effects of this amino acid on cellular mitochondria. Several renal diseases, as well as xenobiotics, could affect the kidney. It appears that mitochondrial injury and its associated complications lay a pivotal role in the disease/xenobiotics-induced kidney injury. Therefore, protecting this organelle could serve as a possible therapeutic intervention point. As a safe amino acid that could tremendously influence many mitochondrial indices, TAU could be an excellent candidate in this field. These data mention the effects of TAU on cellular mitochondria as a critical mechanism by which this amino acid exerts its positive effects on kidney function.

Many pharmaceuticals and toxicants have been identified to have adverse effects on renal function [40 - 44]. Several mechanisms, including changes in the renal blood flow, induction of severe oxidative stress, and cell necrosis, have been proposed for the mechanisms of xenobiotics-induced renal injury [24, 45 - 53]. On the other hand, mitochondrial impairment and related events are the most plausible mechanisms for xenobiotics-induced nephrotoxicity [54 - 56].

Numerous xenobiotics, including many pharmaceuticals, could induce renal injury. As mentioned, the mechanisms of renal injury caused by a high percentage of these chemicals are mediated through their adverse effects on renal mitochondria. Several cases of renal damage are reported in association with antibiotics [53, 57 - 65], anticonvulsants [66 - 68], anticancer drugs [69 - 71], antimetabolites and immunosuppressant drugs [72 - 79], natural toxicants [80, 81], and many other xenobiotics. All these data could indicate the crucial role of mitochondrial impairment in the pathogenesis of xenobiotics-induced renal injury. Hence, it is essential to target this vital organelle and protect the kidney tissue from the adverse effects of pharmaceuticals and a wide range of other xenobiotics.

The forthcoming sections review the evidence of mitochondrial impairment in the pathogenesis of xenobiotics-induced renal injury, focusing on the role of these agents on mitochondrial function. In each section, the positive roles of TAU in these complications are also discussed.

TAURINE AND XENOBIOTICS-INDUCED RENAL INJURY: RELEVANCE TO MITOCHONDRIAL IMPAIRMENT

The effects of TAU on renal injury induced by a wide range of xenobiotics, including natural toxins, heavy metals, and drugs, have been tested. Generally, the main mechanisms of cytoprotection of TAU in the kidney could be divided into three categories. Obviously, these classifications are based on our current knowledge and could change with further research in this field.

Firstly, many studies mentioned that TAU essentially ameliorates oxidative stress markers in xenobiotics-induced renal injury. For example, in renal injury induced by toxicants such as carbon tetrachloride, acetaminophen, thioacetamide, or other drugs such as tamoxifen, TAU significantly decreased ROS formation and lipid peroxidation, probably by stabilizing biomembranes [11, 18, 82]. This amino acid also significantly enhanced kidney tissue antioxidant capacity and its ability to deal with toxic insults [11, 18, 83 - 85]. Although the exact mechanisms of antioxidant properties of TAU in these cases were largely unknown, it appeared that this amino acid could boost cellular enzymatic and non-enzymatic antioxidant capacity.

Secondly, it is well-investigated that the role of TAU on mitochondrial function could be pivotal in its protective properties [21, 86 - 92]. Mitochondria are the primary sources of ROS [93]. Many studies revealed the nephrotoxic agents mentioned in previous sections (*e.g.*, antibiotics, anticonvulsants, anticancer drugs, antimetabolites, and immunosuppressant drugs, natural toxicants) have severe adverse effects on mitochondrial function [94 - 96]. These agents could severely dissipate mitochondrial membrane potential ($\Psi\Delta_m$), induce mitochondrial permeabilization, cause mitochondria-mediated cell death, and, most importantly, increase mitochondria-facilitated ROS formation and oxidative stress [28].

Finally, it should be mentioned that another interesting mechanism for TAU in the renal system (like the mechanism mentioned for the effect of this amino acid in the liver) is mediated through the inhibition of the enzyme CYP2E1 in this organ [14]. As previously mentioned (See chapter TAU and liver), TAU is a potent inhibitor of CYP2E1 [14, 97 - 101]. In the investigation of the renoprotective properties of TAU, Joydeep *et al.* reported that an acute dose of acetaminophen (which is metabolized by CYP2E1) in mice caused a tremendous increase in plasma level of blood urea nitrogen (BUN), creatinine, and uric acid [14]. Moreover, TNF-α, nitric oxide, urinary γ-glutamyl transpeptidase (γ-GT) activity, and most importantly, the urinary excretion of proteins and glucose were also observed [14]. Interestingly, these researchers found a significant decrease in Na^+/K^+–ATPase pump activity [14]. Joydeep *et al.* reported that biomarkers of oxidative stress were considerably increased in the renal tissue of acetaminophen–treated rats. They found that TAU significantly blunted these adverse effects and protected the kidney. However, the impact of TAU on Na^+/K^+–ATPase pump activity is an essential point that should be bolded here. The effect of TAU on this pump could prevent harmful events such as serum electrolyte balance. Another more critical mechanism for TAU found in the current study is its positive effects on mitochondrial function [14]. It was found that TAU prevented acetaminophen-induced mitochondrial injury and ATP depletion in the kidney of mice. This could provide enough energy for processes like the Na^+/K^+-ATPase pump's activity and significantly prevent mitochondria-mediated cell death and renal damage. These data suggest that TAU could act as a potent protective agent against renal damage with different etiologies.

The effects of TAU on renal blood flow is an essential feature of this amino acid [1]. It has been found that TAU could significantly influence renal vascular resistance [102 - 104]. It is supposed that TAU could control arterial renal blood pressure through the autonomic nervous system [105, 106]. Long-term TAU consumption could significantly regulate renal blood pressure, improve renal health, and enhance functionality [1]. Another mechanism for the effects of TAU on renal vasculature and blood flow is mediated through nitric oxide (NO) synthesis [104]. It has been found that TAU significantly increases the serum level of NO and the tissue level of NO synthetase enzyme [104]. The effect of TAU on the renin-angiotensin system is another mechanism for increasing renal blood flow in various pathologies [106]. Although the mentioned mechanism may not be directly related to renal mitochondrial function, enhanced blood flow could provide more oxygen for the mitochondrial oxidative phosphorylation process.

EFFECTS OF TAURINE ON MITOCHONDRIA-CONNECTED PATHOLOGIES IN SOME COMMON RENAL DISORDERS

The amino acid TAU could protect the kidney against xenobiotics and their toxic effects (mainly by modulating oxidative stress and mitochondrial function). It has been found that this amino acid has profound protective effects against several common human renal function disorders. In the next part, some examples of the two most common renal diseases are provided to describe the potential protective properties of TAU for these complications.

RENAL ISCHEMIA-REPERFUSION INJURY

Renal ischemia/reperfusion injury is one of the most investigated fields for assessing the renoprotective properties of TAU [5, 107, 108]. Ischemia/reperfusion (I/R) injury is a condition that includes sudden and complete impairment of blood flow to a particular organ [109, 110]. (I/R) injury is mechanistically related to severe oxidative stress and inflammatory response [109, 110]. It is well known that I/R could lead to acute kidney injury (AKI) and renal failure [109]. These events could be a big issue in situations such as organ transplantation [109].

Several well-investigated routes could mediate the inflammatory response and severe oxidative stress mechanisms. The following parts describe the role of inflammatory response and oxidative stress in the mechanisms of renal injury in I/R. Finally, it should be mentioned that mitochondrial impairment also plays a crucial role in renal I/R. This part describes the connection between inflammatory response, oxidative stress, and mitochondrial injury in renal I/R.

The infiltration of inflammatory cells and inflammation is an essential feature of I/R injury [109]. Infiltrated cells secrete different cytokines that could profoundly affect intracellular components [109]. It has been found that cytokines such as interleukin 6 (IL6) and TNFα play a crucial role in renal dysfunction of renal I/R injury [109]. Interestingly, it has been found that cytokines could adversely affect mitochondrial function [111]. Doll *et al.* reported that TNFα caused a rapid and profound reduction in mitochondrial function in HT-22 cells [111]. Other adverse effects of TNFα, such as severe mitochondrial membrane potential dissipation, have also been reported in their investigation [111].

Hence preventing the adverse effects of cytokines on vital organelles such as mitochondria could serve as a therapeutic point of intervention in renal I/R injury. Interestingly, it has been found that TAU could significantly decrease inflammatory response in renal I/R injury and mitigate the inflammatory response [35, 112, 113]. The protective effects of TAU on mitochondria and preventing the adverse effects of harmful molecules such as cytokines could serve as a mechanism for its protection against renal I/R injury.

The xanthine oxidase enzyme is another important pathway for the induction of oxidative stress in I/R injury [114]. In normal conditions, the enzyme xanthine oxidase is required to produce uric acid by breaking purine nucleotides [114]. Physiologically, xanthine oxidase activity is associated with a small production of ROS [114]. In normal cells, when hypoxanthine is oxidized to xanthine, there is a simultaneous reduction of NAD^+ or oxygen and NADH production by xanthine dehydrogenase [114]. In an ischemic situation, xanthine dehydrogenase is stereochemically converted into xanthine oxidoreductase due to lower oxygen and, consequently, lower ATP metabolism. When blood flow is restored to normal, the enzyme xanthine oxidase reacts with oxygen to induce hypoxanthine, forming xanthine and uric acid using O_2. Finally, a massive amount of ROS is formed in the tissue [114]. Several parts of this chapter mention that excess ROS could significantly damage mitochondria [14]. For example, ROS are well-known inducers of mPT and could cause the release of cell death mediators from this organelle [115]. As mitochondria are potential targets for TAU to induce their cytoprotective mechanisms, the effects of TAU against I/R oxidative stress-induced mitochondrial injury might play a role in its renoprotective properties.

Interestingly, the positive effects of TAU against renal I/R injury have been repeatedly mentioned. In these studies, TAU could significantly decrease oxidative stress, protect mitochondria, and preserve its functionality [116 - 118]. Based on these data, TAU could be readily used as a protecting agent against renal I/R injury. This application of TAU could have a profound biomedical application in fields such as organ transplantation. Finally, the effects of TAU on oxidative stress markers and mitochondrial indices could significantly preserve kidneys in the I/R model. Obviously, large-scale clinical studies are needed to confirm these data and use TAU as a safe amino acid for this purpose.

NEPHROLITHIASIS

The formation of calcium oxalate (CaOx) stones is a common feature in large populations [119]. Several studies tried to describe the mechanisms of CaOx stones formation and the mechanisms of renal epithelial cell injury induced by these compounds [120 - 122]. Many of these investigations mentioned that the cellular damage promoted by these stones could further promote crystal retention in the renal tubule. These cascades of events are believed to lead to a situation termed "nephrolithiasis" [123 - 126].

Two significant sources of ROS have been identified in nephrolithiasis. First, it has been found that the enzyme NADPH oxidase is involved in the overproduction of ROS and the induction of severe damage to renal epithelial cells [127] (Fig. **3**). A key mechanism for the damage of renal epithelial cells by CaOx is mediated by severe oxidative stress and its associated complications [128 - 131].

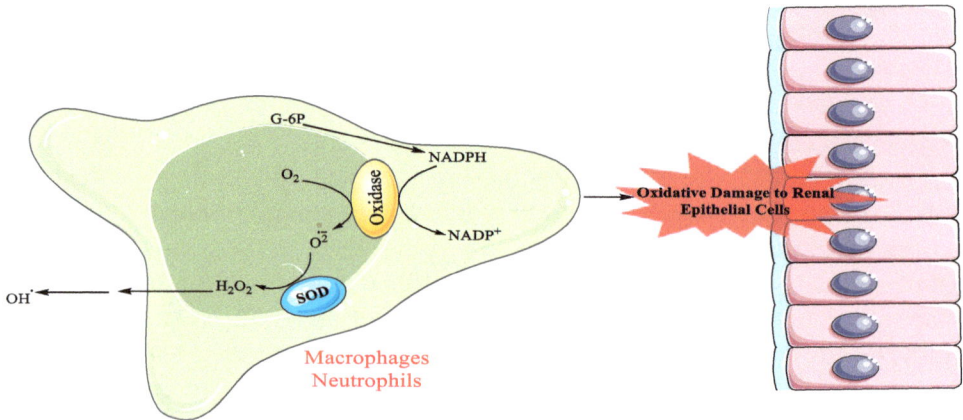

Fig. (3). The enzyme NADPH oxidase is involved in overproducing ROS, inducing severe damage to renal epithelial cells. NADPH oxidase is present in infiltrated cells such as macrophages and neutrophils, which migrate to the renal epithelium during nephrolithiasis. Safe antioxidants or inhibitors of NADPH oxidase enzymes might have ameliorative effects against renal injury during nephrolithiasis. G-6P: Glucose-6-phosphate. SOD: Superoxide dismutase.

NADPH oxidase is an inflammatory cell enzyme that produces a large superoxide anion (O_2^-). Hence, its hyperactivation could lead to severe oxidative stress. It has been found that NADPH oxidase could be a significant source of ROS in the kidney [132, 133]. NADPH oxidase converts O2 into reactive species such as $O_2^{\cdot -}$ which consequently converts them into more dangerous species such as hydroxyl radical (OH^-) (Fig. **3**).

Interestingly, the development of oxidative stress associated with NADPH oxidase is also connected with changes in renal tubule mitochondria. These data mention that these two events are interconnected. Based on the data mentioned in this part, several studies tried to inhibit NADPH oxidase activity by reducing the symptoms of nephrolithiasis [134 - 138]. However, these agents may not suit *in vivo* situations or might develop severe adverse effects. Hence, these days, antioxidant molecules (discussed in the following sections) are the best candidates for alleviating the signs and preventing tissue damage induced by nephrolithiasis [139, 140].

As oxidative stress and its associated events play a crucial role in the pathogenesis of renal injury in urolithiasis, many antioxidant agents have been applied to alleviate oxidative stress and mitochondrial damage in nephrolithiasis [139, 141 - 145]. Most of these agents are not pure compounds, must be used in substantial diseases, and could develop adverse effects in patients. Moreover, no ideal agent has been developed for this purpose to date. An important point that should be mentioned here is the significant decrease in renal tissue's enzymatic and non-enzymatic defense mechanisms in nephrolithiasis [131, 146 - 152]. On the other hand, it has been found that administering some of these antioxidant molecules, such as vitamin E, methionine, and flavonoids, has just partially alleviated the signs and symptoms of nephrotoxicity. On the other hand, it has been found that TAU could significantly activate cellular signaling (*e.g.*, Nrf2) involved in the expression and activation of antioxidant enzymes [153 - 156]. Therefore, a part of the antioxidant properties of TAU in the renal tissue could be mediated through this mechanism.

Mitochondria are crucial sources identified for ROS formation and oxidative stress in nephrolithiasis [157 - 159]. Other events such as severe mitochondrial dysfunction, the release of mitochondrial cell death mediators, dissipation of mitochondrial membrane potential, and significance in the ATP level of patients with nephrolithiasis have been reported [157 - 159].

Physiologically, mitochondria produce an amount of ROS during the oxidative phosphorylation process. However, mitochondria-mediated ROS formation is dramatically elevated in physiological conditions (*e.g.*, genetic defects [160 - 162]. A reason for enhanced mitochondria-mediated ROS formation in nephrolithiasis could be due to the toxic effects of CaOx on different parts of mitochondria, such as permeability transition, mitochondrial membrane complexes activity, morphological changes of mitochondria, and the dissipation of mitochondrial membrane potential [157 - 159, 163 - 165]. Despite the reason for the toxicity of CaOx on renal tubule mitochondria, it seems that targeting this organelle could serve as a viable therapeutic target of intervention in this organelle.

As repeatedly mentioned, mitochondria are significant targets for TAU function. Hence, the action of TAU on mitochondrial function could play a pivotal role in its protective properties against nephrolithiasis as a painful and debilitating disorder that influences patients' quality of life, and in some severe cases, it could even entail renal failure. In many parts of this book, it has been mentioned that TAU plays a pivotal role in mitochondrial function. These functions could vary from participating in essential mitochondrial components such as mitochondrial tRNA to sealing mitochondrial transition pores and enhancing the activity of mitochondrial respiratory chain complexes and ATP metabolism. These effects could protect renal tubule mitochondria and prevent kidney damage in nephrolithiasis.

Interestingly, some studies investigated the effects of TAU in experimental models of urolithiasis and tried to evaluate the effects of this amino acid on the mitochondria [35, 166]. An exciting study by Sun *et al.* revealed that TAU could act by the signaling mechanism of Akt/mTOR to suppress oxidative stress and autophagy in an experimental model of urolithiasis [166]. This study indicates that the effects of TAU in ameliorating ROS (by any origin, *e.g.*, mitochondria and NADPH oxidase) could play a pivotal role in its protective properties in nephrolithiasis [166]. Sun *et al.* also revealed that TAU could significantly decrease cell apoptosis, an event that could be related to the effects of this amino acid on mitochondria [166]. More interestingly, Sun *et al.* revealed that TAU could significantly mitigate mitochondria-originated oxidative stress [166]. This point is important because a crucial part of the antioxidant properties of TAU in many disorders is mediated through regulating mitochondria-mediated oxidative stress. Another exciting finding by Sun *et al.* revealed that mitochondrial morphology in the TAU-treated group was near normal compared to the CaOx-treated group when electron microscope micrographs were compared [166]. This data could also give an excellent clue on the protective effects of TAU on mitochondria in nephrolithiasis.

All the data in this section robustly indicate a therapeutic potential for TAU in renal diseases such as nephrolithiasis. More epidemiologic studies and clinical trials could reveal the importance of this amino acid in such disorders.

CHOLESTASIS/CIRRHOSIS-INDUCED RENAL INJURY

Cholestasis/cirrhosis is a severe complication that could lead to fulminant renal failure and the need for organ transplantation [167 - 171]. Several factors are involved in the pathogenesis of renal injury in cholestasis/cirrhosis. First, it is believed that the renal vasculature is disrupted, and blood flow in the kidney is impaired. Hence, renal tissue suffers from ischemia, and insufficient oxygen is available for vital processes such as oxidative phosphorylation [172 - 174]. Fortunately, as mentioned before, regulating renal blood flow is an exciting feature of TAU [102 - 106]. It has been found that TAU could act on the renin-angiotensin system and nitric oxide synthesis and consequently provide more blood and oxygen for the kidney tissue [102 - 106].

Besides the mentioned mechanisms, several cytotoxic molecules accumulated in the body during cholestasis/cirrhosis are believed to be nephrotoxic. Bile acids are physiologically produced from the cholesterol molecule in the liver. Generally, bile acids (most of them very hydrophobic chemicals) have severe cytotoxic properties. It has been found that these molecules' elevated serum and tissue levels (*e.g.*, in cholestasis/cirrhosis) could be toxic to various organs [43, 175 - 179]. Different organs, including the liver and kidneys, are severely affected by cytotoxic bile acids [167 - 169, 171]. Cholestasis/cirrhosis-induced renal injury (primarily by bile acids) is known as "cholemic nephropathy" [167 - 169, 171].

Hydrophobic cytotoxic bile acids are well-known for their oxidative stress-inducing properties [43, 167, 180 - 182]. Severe oxidative stress and its consequences induced by these agents could lead to severe renal tubule injury [183 - 186]. Most importantly, cytotoxic bile acids are deleterious mitochondrial toxicants [115, 187 - 195]. Hydrophobic bile could robustly induce mitochondrial permeability transition (mPT) [187, 196 - 199]. Consequently, releasing cell death mediators (*e.g.*, Cytochrome *c* and apoptosis-inducing factor) from mitochondria facilitates kidney tissue toxicity [200]. Interestingly, it has been found that mitochondrial impairment could play a central role in the pathogenesis of bile acids-induced renal injury and the waste of essential electrolytes in bile duct ligated rats [185]. Therefore, targeting mitochondria with robust protective agents might be a potential therapeutic point of intervention against bile acids-induced renal damage (*e.g.*, in clinical settings).

CONCLUSION

TAU plays a pivotal role in the renal system as an osmolyte, regulator of ions homeostasis, and adjustment of renal blood flow. However, many studies mentioned that TAU could protect against renal disorders and xenobiotics-induced renal injury. The effects of TAU on oxidative stress biomarkers and its role in modulating kidney tissue mitochondrial function appear to be the most prominent mechanism of action of this amino acid in the kidney. Interestingly, some clinical studies mentioned that TAU could significantly improve renal function in clinical settings. As repeatedly mentioned in the current chapter of this book, TAU could have tremendous effects on renal mitochondria as a critical target for many nephrotoxic xenobiotics as well as in several renal disorders. Hence, the protective properties of taurine could be mediated through the positive effects of this amino acid on cellular mitochondria. Risk assessment studies approved taurine safety in humans, even at very high doses [201]. Therefore, this amino acid could be an appropriate agent to prevent drug-induced renal injury. All these data mention TAU as a good candidate for managing renal diseases.

REFERENCES

[1]   Chesney RW, Han X, Patters AB. Taurine and the renal system. J Biomed Sci 2010; 17(1): S4.
       [http://dx.doi.org/10.1186/1423-0127-17-S1-S4] [PMID: 20804616]

[2] Jacobsen JG, Smith LH. Biochemistry and physiology of taurine and taurine derivatives. Physiol Rev 1968; 48(2): 424-511.
[http://dx.doi.org/10.1152/physrev.1968.48.2.424] [PMID: 4297098]

[3] Hansen SH. The role of taurine in diabetes and the development of diabetic complications. Diabetes Metab Res Rev 2001; 17(5): 330-46.
[http://dx.doi.org/10.1002/dmrr.229] [PMID: 11747139]

[4] Lambert IH, Kristensen DM, Holm JB, Mortensen OH. Physiological role of taurine - from organism to organelle. Acta Physiol (Oxf) 2015; 213(1): 191-212.
[http://dx.doi.org/10.1111/apha.12365] [PMID: 25142161]

[5] Guz G, Oz E, Lortlar N, *et al.* The effect of taurine on renal ischemia/reperfusion injury. Amino Acids 2007; 32(3): 405-11.
[http://dx.doi.org/10.1007/s00726-006-0383-1] [PMID: 17006602]

[6] Han X, Chesney RW. The role of taurine in renal disorders. Amino Acids 2012; 43(6): 2249-63.
[http://dx.doi.org/10.1007/s00726-012-1314-y] [PMID: 22580723]

[7] Huxtable RJ. Physiological actions of taurine. Physiol Rev 1992; 72(1): 101-63.
[http://dx.doi.org/10.1152/physrev.1992.72.1.101] [PMID: 1731369]

[8] Graham LA, Dominiczak AF, Ferreri NR. Role of renal transporters and novel regulatory interactions in the TAL that control blood pressure. Physiol Genomics 2017; 49(5): 261-76.
[http://dx.doi.org/10.1152/physiolgenomics.00017.2017] [PMID: 28389525]

[9] Baliou S, Adamaki M, Ioannou P, *et al.* Ameliorative effect of taurine against diabetes and renal□associated disorders (Review). Med Int 2021; 1(2): 3.
[http://dx.doi.org/10.3892/mi.2021.3] [PMID: 36699147]

[10] Lerdweeraphon W, Wyss JM, Boonmars T, Roysommuti S. Perinatal taurine exposure affects adult oxidative stress. Am J Physiol Regul Integr Comp Physiol 2013; 305(2): R95-7.
[http://dx.doi.org/10.1152/ajpregu.00142.2013] [PMID: 23616107]

[11] Ozden S, Catalgol B, Gezginci-Oktayoglu S, Arda-Pirincci P, Bolkent S, Alpertunga B. Methiocarb-induced oxidative damage following subacute exposure and the protective effects of vitamin E and taurine in rats. Food Chem Toxicol 2009; 47(7): 1676-84.
[http://dx.doi.org/10.1016/j.fct.2009.04.018] [PMID: 19394395]

[12] Tabassum H, Parvez S, Rehman H, Dev Banerjee B, Siemen D, Raisuddin S. Nephrotoxicity and its prevention by taurine in tamoxifen induced oxidative stress in mice. Hum Exp Toxicol 2007; 26(6): 509-18.
[http://dx.doi.org/10.1177/0960327107072392] [PMID: 17698946]

[13] Heidari R, Rasti M, Shirazi Yeganeh B, Niknahad H, Saeedi A, Najibi A. Sulfasalazine-induced renal and hepatic injury in rats and the protective role of taurine. Bioimpacts 2016; 6(1): 3-8.
[http://dx.doi.org/10.15171/bi.2016.01] [PMID: 27340618]

[14] Das J, Ghosh J, Manna P, Sil PC. Taurine protects acetaminophen-induced oxidative damage in mice kidney through APAP urinary excretion and CYP2E1 inactivation. Toxicology 2010; 269(1): 24-34.
[http://dx.doi.org/10.1016/j.tox.2010.01.003] [PMID: 20067817]

[15] Trachtman H, Sturman JA. Taurine: A therapeutic agent in experimental kidney disease. Amino Acids 1996; 11(1): 1-13.
[http://dx.doi.org/10.1007/BF00805717] [PMID: 24178634]

[16] Odetti P, Pesce C, Traverso N, *et al.* Comparative trial of N-acetyl-cysteine, taurine, and oxerutin on skin and kidney damage in long-term experimental diabetes. Diabetes 2003; 52(2): 499-505.
[http://dx.doi.org/10.2337/diabetes.52.2.499] [PMID: 12540627]

[17] Ha H, Yu MR, Kim KH. Melatonin and taurine reduce early glomerulopathy in diabetic rats. Free Radic Biol Med 1999; 26(7-8): 944-50.

[http://dx.doi.org/10.1016/S0891-5849(98)00276-7] [PMID: 10232838]

[18]   Boşgelmez II, Güvendik G. Effects of taurine on oxidative stress parameters and chromium levels altered by acute hexavalent chromium exposure in mice kidney tissue. Biol Trace Elem Res 2004; 102(1-3): 209-26.
[http://dx.doi.org/10.1385/BTER:102:1-3:209] [PMID: 15621940]

[19]   Shi X, Flynn DC, Porter DW, Leonard SS, Vallyathan V, Castranova V. Efficacy of taurine based compounds as hydroxyl radical scavengers in silica induced peroxidation. Ann Clin Lab Sci 1997; 27(5): 365-74.
[PMID: 9303176]

[20]   Mehta TR, Dawson R Jr. Taurine is a weak scavenger of peroxynitrite and does not attenuate sodium nitroprusside toxicity to cells in culture. Amino Acids 2001; 20(4): 419-33.
[http://dx.doi.org/10.1007/s007260170038] [PMID: 11452985]

[21]   Schaffer S, Kim HW. Effects and mechanisms of taurine as a therapeutic agent. Biomol Ther (Seoul) 2018; 26(3): 225-41.
[http://dx.doi.org/10.4062/biomolther.2017.251] [PMID: 29631391]

[22]   Bhargava P, Schnellmann RG. Mitochondrial energetics in the kidney. Nat Rev Nephrol 2017; 13(10): 629-46.
[http://dx.doi.org/10.1038/nrneph.2017.107] [PMID: 28804120]

[23]   Hall AM, Bass P, Unwin RJ. Drug-induced renal Fanconi syndrome. QJM 2014; 107(4): 261-9.
[http://dx.doi.org/10.1093/qjmed/hct258] [PMID: 24368854]

[24]   Bergeron M, Gougoux A. Renal Fanconi syndrome eLS. John Wiley & Sons, Ltd 2001.

[25]   Berman E, Nicolaides M, Maki RG, *et al.* Altered bone and mineral metabolism in patients receiving imatinib mesylate. N Engl J Med 2006; 354(19): 2006-13.
[http://dx.doi.org/10.1056/NEJMoa051140] [PMID: 16687713]

[26]   Chakraborti S, Rahaman SM, Alam MN, Mandal A, Ghosh B, Dey K, et al. Na+/K+-ATPase: A Perspective. In: Chakraborti S, Dhalla NS, editors. Regulation of Membrane Na+-K+ ATPase. Advances in Biochemistry in Health and Disease: Springer International Publishing; 2016. p. 3-30.

[27]   Lote C. Principles of renal physiology: Springer Science & Business Media; 2012.

[28]   Heidari R. The footprints of mitochondrial impairment and cellular energy crisis in the pathogenesis of xenobiotics-induced nephrotoxicity, serum electrolytes imbalance, and Fanconi's syndrome: A comprehensive review. Toxicology 2019; 423: 1-31.
[http://dx.doi.org/10.1016/j.tox.2019.05.002] [PMID: 31095988]

[29]   Heidari R, Jafari F, Khodaei F, Shirazi Yeganeh B, Niknahad H. Mechanism of valproic acid-induced Fanconi syndrome involves mitochondrial dysfunction and oxidative stress in rat kidney. Nephrology (Carlton) 2018; 23(4): 351-61.
[http://dx.doi.org/10.1111/nep.13012] [PMID: 28141910]

[30]   Ommati MM, Farshad O, Ghanbarinejad V, Mohammadi HR, Khadijeh M, Negar A, *et al.* The nephroprotective role of carnosine against ifosfamide-induced renal injury and electrolytes imbalance is mediated *via* the regulation of mitochondrial Function and Alleviation of Oxidative Stress. Drug Res (Stuttg) 2019.
[PMID: 31671464]

[31]   Emadi E, Abdoli N, Ghanbarinejad V, *et al.* The potential role of mitochondrial impairment in the pathogenesis of imatinib-induced renal injury. Heliyon 2019; 5(6): e01996.
[http://dx.doi.org/10.1016/j.heliyon.2019.e01996] [PMID: 31294126]

[32]   Lin Y, Pan F, Wang Y, *et al.* Adefovir dipivoxil-induced Fanconi syndrome and its predictive factors: A study of 28 cases. Oncol Lett 2017; 13(1): 307-14.
[http://dx.doi.org/10.3892/ol.2016.5393] [PMID: 28123560]

[33] Pan F, Wang Y, Zhang X, *et al.* Long-term adefovir therapy may induce Fanconi syndrome: A report of four cases. Exp Ther Med 2017; 14(1): 424-30.
[http://dx.doi.org/10.3892/etm.2017.4483] [PMID: 28672949]

[34] Das J, Sil PC. Taurine ameliorates alloxan-induced diabetic renal injury, oxidative stress-related signaling pathways and apoptosis in rats. Amino Acids 2012; 43(4): 1509-23.
[http://dx.doi.org/10.1007/s00726-012-1225-y] [PMID: 22302365]

[35] Li CY, Deng YL, Sun BH. Taurine protected kidney from oxidative injury through mitochondrial-linked pathway in a rat model of nephrolithiasis. Urol Res 2009; 37(4): 211-20.
[http://dx.doi.org/10.1007/s00240-009-0197-1] [PMID: 19513707]

[36] Heidari R, Behnamrad S, Khodami Z, Ommati MM, Azarpira N, Vazin A. The nephroprotective properties of taurine in colistin-treated mice is mediated through the regulation of mitochondrial function and mitigation of oxidative stress. Biomed Pharmacother 2019; 109: 103-11.
[http://dx.doi.org/10.1016/j.biopha.2018.10.093] [PMID: 30396066]

[37] Pushpakiran G, Mahalakshmi K, Anuradha CV. Taurine restores ethanol-induced depletion of antioxidants and attenuates oxidative stress in rat tissues. Amino Acids 2004; 27(1): 91-6.
[http://dx.doi.org/10.1007/s00726-004-0066-8] [PMID: 15309576]

[38] Shalby AB, Assaf N, Ahmed HH. Possible mechanisms for N-acetyl cysteine and taurine in ameliorating acute renal failure induced by cisplatin in rats. Toxicol Mech Methods 2011; 21(7): 538-46.
[http://dx.doi.org/10.3109/15376516.2011.568985] [PMID: 21470069]

[39] Tsunekawa M, Wang S, Kato T, Yamashita T, Ma N. Taurine administration mitigates cisplatin induced acute nephrotoxicity by decreasing DNA damage and inflammation: An immunocytochemical study Taurine 10 Advances in Experimental Medicine and Biology. Dordrecht: Springer 2017; pp. 703-16.
[http://dx.doi.org/10.1007/978-94-024-1079-2_55]

[40] George B, You D, Joy MS, Aleksunes LM. Xenobiotic transporters and kidney injury. Adv Drug Deliv Rev 2017; 116: 73-91.
[http://dx.doi.org/10.1016/j.addr.2017.01.005] [PMID: 28111348]

[41] Mohammadi A, Ahmadizadeh M. Effects of antioxidants on xenobiotics-induced nephrotoxicity. J Renal Inj Prev 2018; 7(2): 56-7.
[http://dx.doi.org/10.15171/jrip.2018.14]

[42] Radi ZA. Kidney pathophysiology, toxicology, and drug-induced injury in drug development. Int J Toxicol 2019; 38(3): 215-27.
[http://dx.doi.org/10.1177/1091581819831701] [PMID: 30845865]

[43] Heidari R, Ghanbarinejad V, Mohammadi H, *et al.* Dithiothreitol supplementation mitigates hepatic and renal injury in bile duct ligated mice: Potential application in the treatment of cholestasis-associated complications. Biomed Pharmacother 2018; 99: 1022-32.
[http://dx.doi.org/10.1016/j.biopha.2018.01.018] [PMID: 29307496]

[44] Dixon J, Lane K, MacPhee I, Philips B. Xenobiotic metabolism: the effect of acute kidney injury on non-renal drug clearance and hepatic drug metabolism. Int J Mol Sci 2014; 15(2): 2538-53.
[http://dx.doi.org/10.3390/ijms15022538] [PMID: 24531139]

[45] Gracey DM, Snelling P, McKenzie P, Strasser SI. Tenofovir-associated Fanconi syndrome in patients with chronic hepatitis B monoinfection. Antivir Ther 2013; 18(7): 945-8.
[http://dx.doi.org/10.3851/IMP2649] [PMID: 23839869]

[46] Heidari R, Ahmadi A, Mohammadi H, Ommati MM, Azarpira N, Niknahad H. Mitochondrial dysfunction and oxidative stress are involved in the mechanism of methotrexate-induced renal injury and electrolytes imbalance. Biomed Pharmacother 2018; 107: 834-40.
[http://dx.doi.org/10.1016/j.biopha.2018.08.050] [PMID: 30142545]

[47]   Niknahad AM, Ommati MM, Farshad O, Moezi L, Heidari R. Manganese-induced nephrotoxicity Is mediated through oxidative stress and mitochondrial impairment. Journal of Renal and Hepatic Disorders 2020; 4(2): 1-10.
[http://dx.doi.org/10.15586/jrenhep.2020.66]

[48]   Ommati MM, Farshad O, Mousavi K, *et al.* Agmatine alleviates hepatic and renal injury in a rat model of obstructive jaundice. PharmaNutrition 2020; 13: 100212.
[http://dx.doi.org/10.1016/j.phanu.2020.100212]

[49]   Ahmadian E. Mitochondrial damages in drug-induced nephrotoxicity. Journal of Advanced Chemical and Pharmaceutical Materials 2019; 2(2): 116-8.

[50]   Heidari R, Ghanbarinejad V, Ommati MM, Jamshidzadeh A, Niknahad H. Mitochondria protecting amino acids: Application against a wide range of mitochondria-linked complications. PharmaNutrition 2018; 6(4): 180-90.
[http://dx.doi.org/10.1016/j.phanu.2018.09.001]

[51]   Ahmadi A, Niknahad H, Li H, *et al.* The inhibition of NFκB signaling and inflammatory response as a strategy for blunting bile acid-induced hepatic and renal toxicity. Toxicol Lett 2021; 349: 12-29.
[http://dx.doi.org/10.1016/j.toxlet.2021.05.012] [PMID: 34089816]

[52]   Ommati MM, Mohammadi H, Mousavi K, *et al.* Metformin alleviates cholestasis-associated nephropathy through regulating oxidative stress and mitochondrial function. Liver Res 2021; 5(3): 171-80.
[http://dx.doi.org/10.1016/j.livres.2020.12.001]

[53]   Mousavi K, Niknahad H, Li H, *et al.* The activation of nuclear factor-E2-related factor 2 (Nrf2)/heme oxygenase-1 (HO-1) signaling blunts cholestasis-induced liver and kidney injury. Toxicol Res (Camb) 2021; 10(4): 911-27.
[http://dx.doi.org/10.1093/toxres/tfab073] [PMID: 34484683]

[54]   Porter GA, Bennett WM. Nephrotoxic acute renal failure due to common drugs. Am J Physiol 1981; 241(1): F1-8.
[PMID: 7018267]

[55]   Dykens JA, Will Y. Drug-induced mitochondrial dysfunction: John Wiley & Sons; 2008.

[56]   Ralto KM, Parikh SM, editors. Mitochondria in acute kidney injury. 2016: Elsevier.

[57]   Waugh CD. Amphotericin B xPharm: The Comprehensive Pharmacology Reference. New York: Elsevier 2007; pp. 1-5.

[58]   Herlitz LC, Mohan S, Stokes MB, Radhakrishnan J, D'Agati VD, Markowitz GS. Tenofovir nephrotoxicity: acute tubular necrosis with distinctive clinical, pathological, and mitochondrial abnormalities. Kidney Int 2010; 78(11): 1171-7.
[http://dx.doi.org/10.1038/ki.2010.318] [PMID: 20811330]

[59]   Taneja OP, Grover NK, Thakur LC, Bhatia VN. Effects of blood levels of tetracycline and oxytetracycline on hepatic and renal functions in normal subjects. Chemotherapy 1974; 20(4): 201-11.
[http://dx.doi.org/10.1159/000221809] [PMID: 4413117]

[60]   Cox M. Tetracycline nephrotoxicity. In: M.D GAP, editor. Nephrotoxic Mechanisms of Drugs and Environmental Toxins: Springer US; 1982. p. 165-77.
[http://dx.doi.org/10.1007/978-1-4684-4214-4_15]

[61]   Bihorac A, Özener Ç, Akoglu E, Kullu S. Tetracycline-induced acute interstitial nephritis as a cause of acute renal failure. Nephron J 1999; 81(1): 72-5.
[http://dx.doi.org/10.1159/000045249] [PMID: 9884423]

[62]   Miller CS, McGarity GJ. Tetracycline-induced renal failure after dental treatment. J Am Dent Assoc 2009; 140(1): 56-60.
[http://dx.doi.org/10.14219/jada.archive.2009.0018] [PMID: 19119167]

[63]   Kirst HA, Allen NE. Aminoglycoside Antibiotics- Reference Module in Chemistry, Molecular Sciences and Chemical Engineering. Elsevier 2013.

[64]   Martínez-Salgado C, López-Hernández FJ, López-Novoa JM. Glomerular nephrotoxicity of aminoglycosides. Toxicol Appl Pharmacol 2007; 223(1): 86-98.
[http://dx.doi.org/10.1016/j.taap.2007.05.004] [PMID: 17602717]

[65]   Lopez-Novoa JM, Quiros Y, Vicente L, Morales AI, Lopez-Hernandez FJ. New insights into the mechanism of aminoglycoside nephrotoxicity: an integrative point of view. Kidney Int 2011; 79(1): 33-45.
[http://dx.doi.org/10.1038/ki.2010.337] [PMID: 20861826]

[66]   Nanau RM, Neuman MG. Adverse drug reactions induced by valproic acid. Clin Biochem 2013; 46(15): 1323-38.
[http://dx.doi.org/10.1016/j.clinbiochem.2013.06.012] [PMID: 23792104]

[67]   Feldkamp J, Becker A, Witte OW, Scharff D, Scherbaum WA. Long-term anticonvulsant therapy leads to low bone mineral density--evidence for direct drug effects of phenytoin and carbamazepine on human osteoblast-like cells. Exp Clin Endocrinol Diabetes 2000; 108(1): 37-43.
[PMID: 10768830]

[68]   Knorr M, Schaper J, Harjes M, Mayatepek E, Rosenbaum T. Fanconi syndrome caused by antiepileptic therapy with valproic Acid. Epilepsia 2004; 45(7): 868-71.
[http://dx.doi.org/10.1111/j.0013-9580.2004.05504.x] [PMID: 15230715]

[69]   Liamis G, Filippatos TD, Elisaf MS. Electrolyte disorders associated with the use of anticancer drugs. Eur J Pharmacol 2016; 777: 78-87.
[http://dx.doi.org/10.1016/j.ejphar.2016.02.064] [PMID: 26939882]

[70]   Jungsuwadee P, Vore M, Clair DKS. Chemotherapy-induced oxidative stress in nontargeted normal tissues.Oxidative stress in cancer biology and therapy oxidative stress in applied basic research and clinical practice. Humana Press 2012; pp. 97-129.
[http://dx.doi.org/10.1007/978-1-61779-397-4_6]

[71]   Kintzel PE. Anticancer drug-induced kidney disorders. Drug Saf 2001; 24(1): 19-38.
[http://dx.doi.org/10.2165/00002018-200124010-00003] [PMID: 11219485]

[72]   Oikonomou KA, Kapsoritakis AN, Stefanidis I, Potamianos SP. Drug-induced nephrotoxicity in inflammatory bowel disease. Nephron Clin Pract 2011; 119(2): c89-96.
[http://dx.doi.org/10.1159/000326682] [PMID: 21677443]

[73]   Mchenry PM, Allan JG, Rodger RSC, Lever RS. Nephrotoxicity due to azathioprine. Br J Dermatol 1993; 128(1): 106.
[http://dx.doi.org/10.1111/j.1365-2133.1993.tb00161.x] [PMID: 8427817]

[74]   Jahovic N, Çevik H, Şehirli AÖ, Yeğen BÇ, Şener G. Melatonin prevents methotrexate-induced hepatorenal oxidative injury in rats. J Pineal Res 2003; 34(4): 282-7.
[http://dx.doi.org/10.1034/j.1600-079X.2003.00043.x] [PMID: 12662351]

[75]   Kepka L, Lassence AD, Ribrag V, *et al.* Successful rescue in a patient with high dose methotrexate-induced nephrotoxicity and acute renal failure. Leuk Lymphoma 1998; 29(1-2): 205-9.
[http://dx.doi.org/10.3109/10428199809058397] [PMID: 9638991]

[76]   Widemann BC, Adamson PC. Understanding and managing methotrexate nephrotoxicity. Oncologist 2006; 11(6): 694-703.
[http://dx.doi.org/10.1634/theoncologist.11-6-694] [PMID: 16794248]

[77]   Campbell GA, Hu D, Okusa MD. Acute kidney injury in the cancer patient. Adv Chronic Kidney Dis 2014; 21(1): 64-71.
[http://dx.doi.org/10.1053/j.ackd.2013.08.002] [PMID: 24359988]

[78]   Çetiner M, Şener G, Şehirli AÖ, *et al.* Taurine protects against methotrexate-induced toxicity and

inhibits leukocyte death. Toxicol Appl Pharmacol 2005; 209(1): 39-50.
[http://dx.doi.org/10.1016/j.taap.2005.03.009] [PMID: 15890378]

[79]   el-Badawi MG, Abdalla MA, Bahakim HM, Fadel RA. Nephrotoxicity of low-dose methotrexate in guinea pigs: an ultrastructural study. Nephron J 1996; 73(3): 462-6.
[http://dx.doi.org/10.1159/000189111] [PMID: 8832608]

[80]   Grollman AP, Shibutani S, Moriya M, *et al.* Aristolochic acid and the etiology of endemic (Balkan) nephropathy. Proc Natl Acad Sci USA 2007; 104(29): 12129-34.
[http://dx.doi.org/10.1073/pnas.0701248104] [PMID: 17620607]

[81]   Debelle FD, Vanherweghem JL, Nortier JL. Aristolochic acid nephropathy: A worldwide problem. Kidney Int 2008; 74(2): 158-69.
[http://dx.doi.org/10.1038/ki.2008.129] [PMID: 18418355]

[82]   Surai PF, Earle-Payne K, Kidd MT. Taurine as a natural antioxidant: From direct antioxidant effects to protective action in various toxicological models. Antioxidants 2021; 10(12): 1876.
[http://dx.doi.org/10.3390/antiox10121876] [PMID: 34942978]

[83]   Mapuskar KA, Steinbach EJ, Zaher A, *et al.* Mitochondrial superoxide dismutase in cisplatin-induced kidney injury. Antioxidants 2021; 10(9): 1329.
[http://dx.doi.org/10.3390/antiox10091329] [PMID: 34572961]

[84]   Manna P, Sinha M, Sil PC. Taurine plays a beneficial role against cadmium-induced oxidative renal dysfunction. Amino Acids 2009; 36(3): 417-28.
[http://dx.doi.org/10.1007/s00726-008-0094-x] [PMID: 18414974]

[85]   Ali SN, Arif A, Ansari FA, Mahmood R. Cytoprotective effect of taurine against sodium chlorate-induced oxidative damage in human red blood cells: an *ex vivo* study. Amino Acids 2022; 54(1): 33-46.
[http://dx.doi.org/10.1007/s00726-021-03121-5] [PMID: 34993628]

[86]   Chang L, Zhao J, Xu J, Jiang W, Tang CS, Qi YF. Effects of taurine and homocysteine on calcium homeostasis and hydrogen peroxide and superoxide anions in rat myocardial mitochondria. Clin Exp Pharmacol Physiol 2004; 31(4): 237-43.
[http://dx.doi.org/10.1111/j.1440-1681.2004.03983.x] [PMID: 15053820]

[87]   Menzie J, Prentice H, Wu JY. Neuroprotective mechanisms of taurine against ischemic stroke. Brain Sci 2013; 3(4): 877-907.
[http://dx.doi.org/10.3390/brainsci3020877] [PMID: 24961429]

[88]   Palmi M, Youmbi GT, Fusi F, *et al.* Potentiation of mitochondrial Ca^{2+} sequestration by taurine. Biochem Pharmacol 1999; 58(7): 1123-31.
[http://dx.doi.org/10.1016/S0006-2952(99)00183-5] [PMID: 10484070]

[89]   Schaffer SW, Azuma J, Mozaffari M. Role of antioxidant activity of taurine in diabetesThis article is one of a selection of papers from the NATO Advanced Research Workshop on Translational Knowledge for Heart Health (published in part 1 of a 2-part Special Issue). Can J Physiol Pharmacol 2009; 87(2): 91-9.
[http://dx.doi.org/10.1139/Y08-110] [PMID: 19234572]

[90]   Shimada K, Jong CJ, Takahashi K, Schaffer SW, Eds. Role of ROS production and turnover in the antioxidant activity of taurine. Cham: Springer International Publishing 2015.

[91]   Takatani T, Takahashi K, Uozumi Y, *et al.* Taurine inhibits apoptosis by preventing formation of the Apaf-1/caspase-9 apoptosome. Am J Physiol Cell Physiol 2004; 287(4): C949-53.
[http://dx.doi.org/10.1152/ajpcell.00042.2004] [PMID: 15253891]

[92]   Schuller-Levis GB, Park E. Taurine: new implications for an old amino acid. FEMS Microbiol Lett 2003; 226(2): 195-202.
[http://dx.doi.org/10.1016/S0378-1097(03)00611-6] [PMID: 14553911]

[93]   Brookes PS, Yoon Y, Robotham JL, Anders MW, Sheu SS. Calcium, ATP, and ROS: a mitochondrial

love-hate triangle. Am J Physiol Cell Physiol 2004; 287(4): C817-33.
[http://dx.doi.org/10.1152/ajpcell.00139.2004] [PMID: 15355853]

[94] Hamed SA. The effect of antiepileptic drugs on the kidney function and structure. Expert Rev Clin Pharmacol 2017; 10(9): 993-1006.
[http://dx.doi.org/10.1080/17512433.2017.1353418] [PMID: 28689437]

[95] Özlem Hergüner M, Altunbaşak Ş, Doğan A, *et al.* Effects of sodium valproate on renal functions in rats. Ren Fail 2006; 28(7): 593-7.
[http://dx.doi.org/10.1080/08860220600843821] [PMID: 17050243]

[96] Gai Z, Gui T, Kullak-Ublick GA, Li Y, Visentin M. The role of mitochondria in drug-induced kidney injury. Front Physiol 2020; 11: 1079.
[http://dx.doi.org/10.3389/fphys.2020.01079] [PMID: 33013462]

[97] Heidari R, Jamshidzadeh A, Niknahad H, *et al.* Effect of taurine on chronic and acute liver injury: Focus on blood and brain ammonia. Toxicol Rep 2016; 3: 870-9.
[http://dx.doi.org/10.1016/j.toxrep.2016.04.002] [PMID: 28959615]

[98] Kerai MDJ, Waterfield CJ, Kenyon SH, Asker DS, Timbrell JA. Taurine: Protective properties against ethanol-induced hepatic steatosis and lipid peroxidation during chronic ethanol consumption in rats. Amino Acids 1998; 15(1-2): 53-76.
[http://dx.doi.org/10.1007/BF01345280] [PMID: 9871487]

[99] Yao HT, Lin P, Chang YW, *et al.* Effect of taurine supplementation on cytochrome P450 2E1 and oxidative stress in the liver and kidneys of rats with streptozotocin-induced diabetes. Food Chem Toxicol 2009; 47(7): 1703-9.
[http://dx.doi.org/10.1016/j.fct.2009.04.030] [PMID: 19406192]

[100] Das J, Ghosh J, Manna P, Sil PC. Acetaminophen induced acute liver failure *via* oxidative stress and JNK activation: Protective role of taurine by the suppression of cytochrome P450 2E1. Free Radic Res 2010; 44(3): 340-55.
[http://dx.doi.org/10.3109/10715760903513017] [PMID: 20166895]

[101] Miyazaki T, Matsuzaki Y. Taurine and liver diseases: a focus on the heterogeneous protective properties of taurine. Amino Acids 2014; 46(1): 101-10.
[http://dx.doi.org/10.1007/s00726-012-1381-0] [PMID: 22918604]

[102] Roysommuti S, Lerdweeraphon W, Malila P, Jirakulsomchok D, Wyss JM. Perinatal taurine alters arterial pressure control and renal function in adult offspring. Adv Exp Med Biol 2009; 643: 145-56.
[http://dx.doi.org/10.1007/978-0-387-75681-3_15] [PMID: 19239145]

[103] Satoh H, Kang J. Modulation by taurine of human arterial stiffness and wave reflection. Adv Exp Med Biol 2009; 643: 47-55.
[http://dx.doi.org/10.1007/978-0-387-75681-3_5] [PMID: 19239135]

[104] Hu J, Xu X, Yang J, Wu G, Sun C, Lv Q. Antihypertensive effect of taurine in rat. Adv Exp Med Biol 2009; 643: 75-84.
[http://dx.doi.org/10.1007/978-0-387-75681-3_8] [PMID: 19239138]

[105] Roysommuti S, Suwanich A, Jirakulsomchok D, Wyss JM. Perinatal taurine depletion increases susceptibility to adult sugar-induced hypertension in rats. Adv Exp Med Biol 2009; 643: 123-33.
[http://dx.doi.org/10.1007/978-0-387-75681-3_13] [PMID: 19239143]

[106] Yasuo N, Yukio Y, Lovenberg W. Effect of dietary taurine on blood pressure in spontaneously hypertensive rats. Biochem Pharmacol 1978; 27(23): 2689-92.
[http://dx.doi.org/10.1016/0006-2952(78)90043-6] [PMID: 728224]

[107] Cavdar Z, Ural C, Celik A, *et al.* Protective effects of taurine against renal ischemia/reperfusion injury in rats by inhibition of gelatinases, MMP-2 and MMP-9, and p38 mitogen-activated protein kinase signaling. Biotech Histochem 2017; 92(7): 524-35.
[http://dx.doi.org/10.1080/10520295.2017.1367033] [PMID: 28895768]

[108] Wang J, Yan LI, Zhang L, *et al.* Taurine inhibits ischemia/reperfusion-induced compartment syndrome in rabbits1. Acta Pharmacol Sin 2005; 26(7): 821-7.
[http://dx.doi.org/10.1111/j.1745-7254.2005.00128.x] [PMID: 15960888]

[109] Malek M, Nematbakhsh M. Renal ischemia/reperfusion injury; from pathophysiology to treatment. J Renal Inj Prev 2015; 4(2): 20-7.
[PMID: 26060833]

[110] Najafi H, Abolmaali SS, Heidari R, *et al.* Nitric oxide releasing nanofibrous Fmoc-dipeptide hydrogels for amelioration of renal ischemia/reperfusion injury. J Control Release 2021; 337: 1-13.
[http://dx.doi.org/10.1016/j.jconrel.2021.07.016] [PMID: 34271033]

[111] Doll DN, Rellick SL, Barr TL, Ren X, Simpkins JW. Rapid mitochondrial dysfunction mediates TNF-alpha-induced neurotoxicity. J Neurochem 2015; 132(4): 443-51.
[http://dx.doi.org/10.1111/jnc.13008] [PMID: 25492727]

[112] Schaffer SW, Jong CJ, Ito T, Azuma J. Effect of taurine on ischemia–reperfusion injury. Amino Acids 2014; 46(1): 21-30.
[http://dx.doi.org/10.1007/s00726-012-1378-8] [PMID: 22936072]

[113] Xu Y, Niu Y, Li H, Pan G. Downregulation of lncRNA TUG1 attenuates inflammation and apoptosis of renal tubular epithelial cell induced by ischemia-reperfusion by sponging miR-449b-5p *via* targeting HMGB1 and MMP2. Inflammation 2020; 43(4): 1362-74.
[http://dx.doi.org/10.1007/s10753-020-01214-z] [PMID: 32206944]

[114] Wu MY, Yiang GT, Liao WT, *et al.* Current mechanistic concepts in ischemia and reperfusion injury. Cell Physiol Biochem 2018; 46(4): 1650-67.
[http://dx.doi.org/10.1159/000489241] [PMID: 29694958]

[115] Paumgartner G, Beuers U. Ursodeoxycholic acid in cholestatic liver disease: Mechanisms of action and therapeutic use revisited. Hepatology 2002; 36(3): 525-31.
[http://dx.doi.org/10.1053/jhep.2002.36088] [PMID: 12198643]

[116] Mozaffari MS, Abdelsayed R, Patel C, Wimborne H, Liu J, Schaffer SW. Differential effects of taurine treatment and taurine deficiency on the outcome of renal ischemia reperfusion injury. J Biomed Sci. 2010; 17(1): S32.
[http://dx.doi.org/10.1186/1423-0127-17-S1-S32] [PMID: 20804608]

[117] Kingston R. The therapeutic role of taurine in ischaemia-reperfusion injury.Apoptosome: An up-an--coming therapeutical tool. Dordrecht: Springer Netherlands 2010; pp. 283-304.
[http://dx.doi.org/10.1007/978-90-481-3415-1_15]

[118] Rojas-Morales P, León-Contreras JC, Aparicio-Trejo OE, *et al.* Fasting reduces oxidative stress, mitochondrial dysfunction and fibrosis induced by renal ischemia-reperfusion injury. Free Radic Biol Med 2019; 135: 60-7.
[http://dx.doi.org/10.1016/j.freeradbiomed.2019.02.018] [PMID: 30818054]

[119] Asplin JR. Hyperoxaluric calcium nephrolithiasis. Endocrinol Metab Clin North Am 2002; 31(4): 927-49.
[http://dx.doi.org/10.1016/S0889-8529(02)00030-0] [PMID: 12474639]

[120] Scheid C, Koul H, Hill WA, *et al.* Oxalate toxicity in LLC-PK1 cells, a line of renal epithelial cells. J Urol 1996; 155(3): 1112-6.
[http://dx.doi.org/10.1016/S0022-5347(01)66402-4] [PMID: 8583575]

[121] Tsujihata M. Mechanism of calcium oxalate renal stone formation and renal tubular cell injury. Int J Urol 2008; 15(2): 115-20.
[http://dx.doi.org/10.1111/j.1442-2042.2007.01953.x] [PMID: 18269444]

[122] Khan SR. Role of renal epithelial cells in the initiation of calcium oxalate stones. Nephron, Exp Nephrol 2004; 98(2): e55-60.
[http://dx.doi.org/10.1159/000080257] [PMID: 15499208]

[123] Lingeman JE. Pathogenesis of Nephrolithiasis. J Urol 2013; 189(2): 417-8.
       [http://dx.doi.org/10.1016/j.juro.2012.11.069] [PMID: 23159272]

[124] Aggarwal KP, Narula S, Kakkar M, Tandon C. Nephrolithiasis: molecular mechanism of renal stone
       formation and the critical role played by modulators. BioMed Res Int 2013; 2013: 1-21.
       [http://dx.doi.org/10.1155/2013/292953] [PMID: 24151593]

[125] Paliouras C, Tsampikaki E, Alivanis P, Aperis G. Pathophysiology of Nephrolithiasis. Nephrology
       Research & Reviews 2012; 4(2): 58-65.
       [http://dx.doi.org/10.4081/nr.2012.e14]

[126] Sakhaee K. Recent advances in the pathophysiology of nephrolithiasis. Kidney Int 2009; 75(6): 585-
       95.
       [http://dx.doi.org/10.1038/ki.2008.626] [PMID: 19078968]

[127] Thamilselvan V, Menon M, Thamilselvan S. Oxalate-induced activation of PKC-α and -δ regulates
       NADPH oxidase-mediated oxidative injury in renal tubular epithelial cells. Am J Physiol Renal
       Physiol 2009; 297(5): F1399-410.
       [http://dx.doi.org/10.1152/ajprenal.00051.2009] [PMID: 19692488]

[128] Thamilselvan S, Byer KJ, Hackett RL, Khan SR. Free radical scavengers, catalase and superoxide
       dismutase provide protection from oxalate-associated injury to LLC-PK1 and MDCK cells. J Urol
       2000; 164(1): 224-9.
       [http://dx.doi.org/10.1016/S0022-5347(05)67499-X] [PMID: 10840464]

[129] Thamilselvan S, Hackett RL, Khan SR. Lipid peroxidation in ethylene glycol induced hyperoxaluria
       and calcium oxalate nephrolithiasis. J Urol 1997; 157(3): 1059-63.
       [http://dx.doi.org/10.1016/S0022-5347(01)65141-3] [PMID: 9072543]

[130] Rashed T, Menon M, Thamilselvan S. Molecular mechanism of oxalate-induced free radical
       production and glutathione redox imbalance in renal epithelial cells: effect of antioxidants. Am J
       Nephrol 2004; 24(5): 557-68.
       [http://dx.doi.org/10.1159/000082043] [PMID: 15539792]

[131] Thamilselvan S, Khan SR, Menon M. Oxalate and calcium oxalate mediated free radical toxicity in
       renal epithelial cells: effect of antioxidants. Urol Res 2003; 31(1): 3-9.
       [http://dx.doi.org/10.1007/s00240-002-0286-x] [PMID: 12624656]

[132] Hanna IR, Taniyama Y, Szöcs K, Rocic P, Griendling KK. NAD(P)H oxidase-derived reactive oxygen
       species as mediators of angiotensin II signaling. Antioxid Redox Signal 2002; 4(6): 899-914.
       [http://dx.doi.org/10.1089/152308602762197443] [PMID: 12573139]

[133] Shiose A, Kuroda J, Tsuruya K, *et al.* A novel superoxide-producing NAD(P)H oxidase in kidney. J
       Biol Chem 2001; 276(2): 1417-23.
       [http://dx.doi.org/10.1074/jbc.M007597200] [PMID: 11032835]

[134] Zuo J, Khan A, Glenton PA, Khan SR. Effect of NADPH oxidase inhibition on the expression of
       kidney injury molecule and calcium oxalate crystal deposition in hydroxy-L-proline-induced
       hyperoxaluria in the male Sprague-Dawley rats. Nephrol Dial Transplant 2011; 26(6): 1785-96.
       [http://dx.doi.org/10.1093/ndt/gfr035] [PMID: 21378157]

[135] Joshi S, Peck AB, Khan SR. NADPH oxidase as a therapeutic target for oxalate induced injury in
       kidneys. Oxid Med Cell Longev 2013; 2013: 1-18.
       [http://dx.doi.org/10.1155/2013/462361] [PMID: 23840917]

[136] Joshi S, Khan SR. NADPH oxidase: a therapeutic target for hyperoxaluria-induced oxidative stress –
       an update. Future Med Chem 2019; 11(23): 2975-8.
       [http://dx.doi.org/10.4155/fmc-2019-0275] [PMID: 31659918]

[137] Altenhöfer S, Radermacher KA, Kleikers PWM, Wingler K, Schmidt HHHW. Evolution of NADPH
       Oxidase Iinhibitors: selectivity and mechanisms for target engagement. Antioxid Redox Signal 2015;
       23(5): 406-27.

[http://dx.doi.org/10.1089/ars.2013.5814] [PMID: 24383718]

[138] Qin B, Wang Q, Lu Y, *et al.* Losartan ameliorates calcium oxalate-induced elevation of stone-related proteins in renal tubular vells by inhibiting NADPH oxidase and oxidative stress. Oxid Med Cell Longev 2018; 2018: 1-12.
[http://dx.doi.org/10.1155/2018/1271864] [PMID: 29849862]

[139] Kizivat T, Smolić M, Marić I, *et al.* Antioxidant pre-treatment reduces the toxic effects of oxalate on renal epithelial cells in a cell culture codel of urolithiasis. Int J Environ Res Public Health 2017; 14(1): 109.
[http://dx.doi.org/10.3390/ijerph14010109] [PMID: 28125004]

[140] Zhu J, Wang Q, Li C, *et al.* Inhibiting inflammation and modulating oxidative stress in oxalate-induced nephrolithiasis with the Nrf2 activator dimethyl fumarate. Free Radic Biol Med 2019; 134: 9-22.
[http://dx.doi.org/10.1016/j.freeradbiomed.2018.12.033] [PMID: 30599261]

[141] Ceban E, Banov P, Galescu A, Botnari V. Oxidative stress and antioxidant status in patients with complicated urolithiasis. J Med Life 2016; 9(3): 259-62.
[PMID: 27974930]

[142] Göknar N, Oktem F, Arı E, Demir AD, Torun E. Is oxidative stress related to childhood urolithiasis? Pediatr Nephrol 2014; 29(8): 1381-6.
[http://dx.doi.org/10.1007/s00467-014-2773-z] [PMID: 24526098]

[143] Ashok P, Koti B, Vishwanathswamy AHM. Antiurolithiatic and antioxidant activity of Mimusops elengi on ethylene glycol-induced urolithiasis in rats. Indian J Pharmacol 2010; 42(6): 380-3.
[http://dx.doi.org/10.4103/0253-7613.71925] [PMID: 21189910]

[144] Marhoume FZ, Aboufatima R, Zaid Y, *et al.* Antioxidant and polyphenol-rich ethanolic extract of Rubia tinctorum L. prevents urolithiasis in an ethylene glycol experimental model in rats. Molecules 2021; 26(4): 1005.
[http://dx.doi.org/10.3390/molecules26041005] [PMID: 33672875]

[145] Zeng X, Xi Y, Jiang W. Protective roles of flavonoids and flavonoid-rich plant extracts against urolithiasis: A review. Crit Rev Food Sci Nutr 2019; 59(13): 2125-35.
[http://dx.doi.org/10.1080/10408398.2018.1439880] [PMID: 29432040]

[146] P S, P F, C Y, P T. Renal tubular cell damage and oxidative stress in renal stone patients and the effect of potassium citrate treatment. Urol Res 2005; 33(1).

[147] A M, R S. Role of glutathione on renal mitochondrial status in hyperoxaluria. Mol Cell Biochem 1998; 185(1-2): 77-84.

[148] Itoh Y, Yasui T, Okada A, Tozawa K, Hayashi Y, Kohri K. Preventive effects of green tea on renal stone formation and the role of oxidative stress in nephrolithiasis. J Urol 2005; 173(1): 271-5.
[http://dx.doi.org/10.1097/01.ju.0000141311.51003.87] [PMID: 15592095]

[149] Khan SR. Hyperoxaluria-induced oxidative stress and antioxidants for renal protection. Urol Res 2005; 33(5): 349-57.
[http://dx.doi.org/10.1007/s00240-005-0492-4] [PMID: 16292585]

[150] Selvam R. Calcium oxalate stone disease: role of lipid peroxidation and antioxidants. Urol Res 2002; 30(1): 35-47.
[http://dx.doi.org/10.1007/s00240-001-0228-z] [PMID: 11942324]

[151] Selvam R, Ravichandran V. Restoration of tissue antioxidants and prevention of renal stone deposition in vitamin B6 deficient rats fed with vitamin E or methionine. Indian J Exp Biol 1993; 31(11): 882-7.
[PMID: 8112761]

[152] Thamilselvan S, Menon M. Vitamin E therapy prevents hyperoxaluria-induced calcium oxalate crystal deposition in the kidney by improving renal tissue antioxidant status. BJU Int 2005; 96(1): 117-26.
[http://dx.doi.org/10.1111/j.1464-410X.2005.05579.x] [PMID: 15963133]

[153] Yang W, Huang J, Xiao B, *et al.* Taurine protects pouse ppermatocytes from ionizing radiation-induced damage through activation of Nrf2/HO-1 signaling. Cell Physiol Biochem 2017; 44(4): 1629-39.
[http://dx.doi.org/10.1159/000485762] [PMID: 29216642]

[154] Sun Q, Jia N, Yang J, Chen G. Nrf2 signaling pathway mediates the antioxidative effects of taurine against corticosterone-induced cell death in HUMAN SK-N-SH cells. Neurochem Res 2018; 43(2): 276-86.
[http://dx.doi.org/10.1007/s11064-017-2419-1] [PMID: 29063347]

[155] Ghanim A, Farag M, Anwar M, Ali N, Hawas M, Elsallab H, *et al.* Taurine alleviates kidney injury in a thioacetamide rat model by mediating Nrf2/HO-1, NQO-1 and MAPK/NF-κB signaling pathways. Can J Physiol Pharmacol 2022; 100(4): 352-60.

[156] Cheong SH, Lee D-S. Taurine chloramine prevents neuronal HT22 cell damage through nrf2-related heme oxygenase-1 Taurine 10. Springer 2017; pp. 145-57.

[157] Patel M, Yarlagadda V, Adedoyin O, *et al.* Oxalate induces mitochondrial dysfunction and disrupts redox homeostasis in a human monocyte derived cell line. Redox Biol 2018; 15: 207-15.
[http://dx.doi.org/10.1016/j.redox.2017.12.003] [PMID: 29272854]

[158] Khan SR. Reactive oxygen species, inflammation and calcium oxalate nephrolithiasis. Transl Androl Urol 2014; 3(3): 256-76.
[PMID: 25383321]

[159] Wang Z, Zhang Y, Zhang J, Deng Q, Liang H. Recent advances on the mechanisms of kidney stone formation (Review). Int J Mol Med 2021; 48(2): 149.
[http://dx.doi.org/10.3892/ijmm.2021.4982] [PMID: 34132361]

[160] Supinski GS, Schroder EA, Callahan LA. Mitochondria and critical illness. Chest 2020; 157(2): 310-22.
[http://dx.doi.org/10.1016/j.chest.2019.08.2182] [PMID: 31494084]

[161] He Z, Ning N, Zhou Q, Khoshnam SE, Farzaneh M. Mitochondria as a therapeutic target for ischemic stroke. Free Radic Biol Med 2020; 146: 45-58.
[http://dx.doi.org/10.1016/j.freeradbiomed.2019.11.005] [PMID: 31704373]

[162] Nishikawa T, Araki E. Impact of mitochondrial ROS production in the pathogenesis of diabetes mellitus and its complications. Antioxid Redox Signal 2007; 9(3): 343-53.
[http://dx.doi.org/10.1089/ars.2006.1458] [PMID: 17184177]

[163] Chaiyarit S, Thongboonkerd V. Mitochondrial dysfunction and kidney stone disease. Front Physiol 2020; 11: 566506.
[http://dx.doi.org/10.3389/fphys.2020.566506] [PMID: 33192563]

[164] Cao LC, Honeyman TW, Cooney R, Kennington L, Scheid CR, Jonassen JA. Mitochondrial dysfunction is a primary event in renal cell oxalate toxicity. Kidney Int 2004; 66(5): 1890-900.
[http://dx.doi.org/10.1111/j.1523-1755.2004.00963.x] [PMID: 15496160]

[165] Wigner P, Grębowski R, Bijak M, Szemraj J, Saluk-Bijak J. The molecular aspect of nephrolithiasis development. Cells 2021; 10(8): 1926.
[http://dx.doi.org/10.3390/cells10081926] [PMID: 34440695]

[166] Sun Y, Dai S, Tao J, *et al.* Taurine suppresses ROS-dependent autophagy *via* activating Akt/mTOR signaling pathway in calcium oxalate crystals-induced renal tubular epithelial cell injury. Aging (Albany NY) 2020; 12(17): 17353-66.
[http://dx.doi.org/10.18632/aging.103730] [PMID: 32931452]

[167] Holt S, Marley R, Fernando B, *et al.* Acute cholestasis-induced renal failure: Effects of antioxidants and ligands for the thromboxane A2 receptor. Kidney Int 1999; 55(1): 271-7.
[http://dx.doi.org/10.1046/j.1523-1755.1999.00252.x] [PMID: 9893136]

[168] Kaler B, Karram T, Morgan WA, Bach PH, Yousef IM, Bomzon A. Are bile acids involved in the renal dysfunction of obstructive jaundice? An experimental study in bile duct ligated rats. Ren Fail 2004; 26(5): 507-16.
[http://dx.doi.org/10.1081/JDI-200031753] [PMID: 15526908]

[169] Krones E, Eller K, Pollheimer MJ, *et al.* NorUrsodeoxycholic acid ameliorates cholemic nephropathy in bile duct ligated mice. J Hepatol 2017; 67(1): 110-9.
[http://dx.doi.org/10.1016/j.jhep.2017.02.019] [PMID: 28242240]

[170] Krones E, Wagner M, Eller K, Rosenkranz AR, Trauner M, Fickert P. Bile acid-induced cholemic nephropathy. Dig Dis 2015; 33(3): 367-75.
[http://dx.doi.org/10.1159/000371689] [PMID: 26045271]

[171] Wardle EN. Renal failure in obstructive jaundice--pathogenic factors. Postgrad Med J 1975; 51(598): 512-4.
[http://dx.doi.org/10.1136/pgmj.51.598.512] [PMID: 1234333]

[172] Tinti F, Umbro I, D'Alessandro M, *et al.* Cholemic nephropathy as cause of acute and chronic kidney disease. update on an under-diagnosed disease. Life (Basel) 2021; 11(11): 1200.
[http://dx.doi.org/10.3390/life11111200] [PMID: 34833076]

[173] Liu J, Qu J, Chen H, *et al.* The pathogenesis of renal injury in obstructive jaundice: A review of underlying mechanisms, inducible agents and therapeutic strategies. Pharmacol Res 2021; 163: 105311.
[http://dx.doi.org/10.1016/j.phrs.2020.105311] [PMID: 33246170]

[174] Krones E, Pollheimer MJ, Rosenkranz AR, Fickert P. Cholemic nephropathy – Historical notes and novel perspectives. Biochim Biophys Acta Mol Basis Dis 2018; 1864(4) (4, Part B): 1356-66.
[http://dx.doi.org/10.1016/j.bbadis.2017.08.028] [PMID: 28851656]

[175] Fickert P, Krones E, Pollheimer MJ, *et al.* Bile acids trigger cholemic nephropathy in common bile-duct-ligated mice. Hepatology 2013; 58(6): 2056-69.
[http://dx.doi.org/10.1002/hep.26599] [PMID: 23813550]

[176] Green J, Better OS. Systemic hypotension and renal failure in obstructive jaundice-mechanistic and therapeutic aspects. J Am Soc Nephrol 1995; 5(11): 1853-71.
[http://dx.doi.org/10.1681/ASN.V5111853] [PMID: 7620083]

[177] Heidari R. Brain mitochondria as potential therapeutic targets for managing hepatic encephalopathy. Life Sci 2019; 218: 65-80.
[http://dx.doi.org/10.1016/j.lfs.2018.12.030] [PMID: 30578865]

[178] Heidari R, Abdoli N, Ommati MM, Jamshidzadeh A, Niknahad H. Mitochondrial impairment induced by chenodeoxycholic acid: The protective effect of taurine and carnosine supplementation. Trends in Pharmaceutical Sciences. 2018;4(2).

[179] Abdoli N, Sadeghian I, Mousavi K, Azarpira N, Ommati MM, Heidari R. Suppression of cirrhosis-related renal injury by N-acetyl cysteine. Current Research in Pharmacology and Drug Discovery 2020; 1: 30-8.
[http://dx.doi.org/10.1016/j.crphar.2020.100006] [PMID: 34909640]

[180] Sastre J, Serviddio G, Tormos AM, Monsalve M, Sastre J. Mitochondrial dysfunction in cholestatic liver diseases. Front Biosci (Elite Ed) 2012; E4(6): 2233-52.
[http://dx.doi.org/10.2741/e539] [PMID: 22202034]

[181] Copple B, Jaeschke H, Klaassen C. Oxidative stress and the pathogenesis of cholestasis. Semin Liver Dis 2010; 30(2): 195-204.
[http://dx.doi.org/10.1055/s-0030-1253228] [PMID: 20422501]

[182] Krähenbühl S, Talos C, Lauterburg BH, Reichen J. Reduced antioxidative capacity in liver mitochondria from bile duct ligated rats*1. Hepatology 1995; 22(2): 607-12.
[http://dx.doi.org/10.1016/0270-9139(95)90586-3] [PMID: 7635430]

[183]   Ljubuncic P, Tanne Z, Bomzon A. Evidence of a systemic phenomenon for oxidative stress in cholestatic liver disease. Gut 2000; 47(5): 710-6.
[http://dx.doi.org/10.1136/gut.47.5.710] [PMID: 11034590]

[184]   Bomzon A, Holt S, Moore K. Bile acids, oxidative stress, and renal function in biliary obstruction. Semin Nephrol 1997; 17(6): 549-62.
[PMID: 9353865]

[185]   Heidari R, Mandegani L, Ghanbarinejad V, *et al.* Mitochondrial dysfunction as a mechanism involved in the pathogenesis of cirrhosis-associated cholemic nephropathy. Biomed Pharmacother 2019; 109: 271-80.
[http://dx.doi.org/10.1016/j.biopha.2018.10.104] [PMID: 30396085]

[186]   Martínez-Cecilia D, Reyes-Díaz M, Ruiz-Rabelo J, *et al.* Oxidative stress influence on renal dysfunction in patients with obstructive jaundice: A case and control prospective study. Redox Biol 2016; 8: 160-4.
[http://dx.doi.org/10.1016/j.redox.2015.12.009] [PMID: 26774750]

[187]   Krähenbühl S, Talos C, Fischer S, Reichen J. Toxicity of bile acids on the electron transport chain of isolated rat liver mitochondria*1. Hepatology 1994; 19(2): 471-9.
[http://dx.doi.org/10.1016/0270-9139(94)90027-2] [PMID: 7904981]

[188]   Sokol RJ, McKim JM Jr, Goff MC, *et al.* Vitamin E reduces oxidant injury to mitochondria and the hepatotoxicity of taurochenodeoxycholic acid in the rat. Gastroenterology 1998; 114(1): 164-74.
[http://dx.doi.org/10.1016/S0016-5085(98)70644-4] [PMID: 9428230]

[189]   Rolo AP, Palmeira CM, Wallace KB. Mitochondrially mediated synergistic cell killing by bile acids. Biochim Biophys Acta Mol Basis Dis 2003; 1637(1): 127-32.
[http://dx.doi.org/10.1016/S0925-4439(02)00224-7] [PMID: 12527417]

[190]   Palmeira CM, Rolo AP. Mitochondrially-mediated toxicity of bile acids. Toxicology 2004; 203(1-3): 1-15.
[http://dx.doi.org/10.1016/j.tox.2004.06.001] [PMID: 15363577]

[191]   Perez MJ, Briz O. Bile-acid-induced cell injury and protection. World J Gastroenterol 2009; 15(14): 1677-89.
[http://dx.doi.org/10.3748/wjg.15.1677] [PMID: 19360911]

[192]   Heidari R, Ghanbarinejad V, Mohammadi H, *et al.* Mitochondria protection as a mechanism underlying the hepatoprotective effects of glycine in cholestatic mice. Biomed Pharmacother 2018; 97: 1086-95.
[http://dx.doi.org/10.1016/j.biopha.2017.10.166] [PMID: 29136945]

[193]   Heidari R, Niknahad H. The role and study of mitochondrial impairment and oxidative stress in cholestasis. Experimental Cholestasis Research Methods in Molecular Biology. New York, NY: Springer 2019; pp. 117-32.
[http://dx.doi.org/10.1007/978-1-4939-9420-5_8]

[194]   Ommati MM, Farshad O, Niknahad H, *et al.* Cholestasis-associated reproductive toxicity in male and female rats: The fundamental role of mitochondrial impairment and oxidative stress. Toxicol Lett 2019; 316: 60-72.
[http://dx.doi.org/10.1016/j.toxlet.2019.09.009] [PMID: 31520699]

[195]   Siavashpour A, Khalvati B, Azarpira N, Mohammadi H, Niknahad H, Heidari R. Poly (ADP-Ribose) polymerase-1 (PARP-1) overactivity plays a pathogenic role in bile acids-induced nephrotoxicity in cholestatic rats. Toxicol Lett 2020; 330: 144-58.
[http://dx.doi.org/10.1016/j.toxlet.2020.05.012] [PMID: 32422328]

[196]   Attili AF, Angelico M, Cantafora A, Alvaro D, Capocaccia L. Bile acid-induced liver toxicity: Relation to the hydrophobic-hydrophilic balance of bile acids. Med Hypotheses 1986; 19(1): 57-69.
[http://dx.doi.org/10.1016/0306-9877(86)90137-4] [PMID: 2871479]

[197] Guicciardi ME, Gores GJ. Bile acid-mediated hepatocyte apoptosis and cholestatic liver disease. Dig Liver Dis 2002; 34(6): 387-92.
[http://dx.doi.org/10.1016/S1590-8658(02)80033-0] [PMID: 12132783]

[198] Rolo AP, Oliveira PJ, Moreno AJM, Palmeira CM. Bile acids affect liver mitochondrial bioenergetics: possible relevance for cholestasis therapy. Toxicol Sci 2000; 57(1): 177-85.
[http://dx.doi.org/10.1093/toxsci/57.1.177] [PMID: 10966524]

[199] Yerushalmi B, Dahl R, Devereaux MW, Gumpricht E, Sokol RJ. Bile acid-induced rat hepatocyte apoptosis is inhibited by antioxidants and blockers of the mitochondrial permeability transition. Hepatology 2001; 33(3): 616-26.
[http://dx.doi.org/10.1053/jhep.2001.22702] [PMID: 11230742]

[200] Rodrigues CM, Fan G, Ma X, Kren BT, Steer CJ. A novel role for ursodeoxycholic acid in inhibiting apoptosis by modulating mitochondrial membrane perturbation. J Clin Invest 1998; 101(12): 2790-9.
[http://dx.doi.org/10.1172/JCI1325] [PMID: 9637713]

[201] Schwarzer R, Kivaranovic D, Mandorfer M, *et al.* Randomised clinical study: the effects of oral taurine 6g/day vs placebo on portal hypertension. Aliment Pharmacol Ther 2018; 47(1): 86-94.
[http://dx.doi.org/10.1111/apt.14377] [PMID: 29105115]

CHAPTER 9

The Mechanism of Action of Taurine in the Digestive System

Abstract: Several transporters have been identified for taurine (TAU) absorption from the gastrointestinal (GI) tract. The Na^+/Cl^--dependent taurine transporter (TauT) and PAT1 (SLC36A1) are well-known TAU transporters in the GI. These transporters efficiently deliver TAU from GI to the bloodstream. On the other hand, no metabolic pathway has been identified for TAU in the human body. But, it has been found that GI-resident bacteria are able to metabolize TAU to sulfur-containing chemicals (*e.g.,* H_2S). Hence, GI is the primary place for TAU metabolism. TAU-conjugated compounds such as bile acids are also excreted through GI. Compounds such as H_2S could be re-absorbed from GI and have a tremendous physiological effect on other organs (*e.g.,* heart and vessels). Finally, it should be noted that several studies mentioned that TAU could protect GI in various pathological conditions (*e.g.,* xenobiotics-induced GI damage). In the current chapter, a brief review of the absorption, metabolism, and excretion of TAU is provided. Then, the importance of TAU metabolites in the GI and other organs is highlighted. Finally, the effects of TAU on GI complications are discussed, focusing on the effects of this amino acid on oxidative stress biomarkers and mitochondrial impairment. These data could give a new concept of the physiological roles of TAU as well as its effects on GI complications.

Keywords: Absorption, Gastrointestinal disease, Peptic ulcer, Sulfur-containing chemicals, Taurine metabolism.

INTRODUCTION

Taurine (TAU) is readily synthesized from the amino acids methionine and cysteine in the liver of many species (*e.g.,* dogs and rats) [1 - 4]. However, many other species, including humans, depends on the dietary sources of TAU [5 - 8]. TAU is readily absorbed from our gastrointestinal (GI) tract [1]. Some TAU transporters have been identified for TAU in our GI. The SLC35A1 and Na^+/Cl^--dependent transporters are the most investigated TAU transporters in the human intestine [1, 9]. The affinity and capacity of these transporters for TAU are different, but they efficiently transport TAU from the intestine to the bloodstream [1, 9, 10]

Reza Heidari and M. Mehdi Ommati

An exciting feature of the connection between TAU and the GI is the metabolism of this amino acid. Actually, no metabolic pathway (enzyme) has been identified for TAU in the human body to date. On the other hand, it is well-known that several GI-resident bacteria are able to metabolize TAU and convert this amino acid into sulfur-containing chemicals [11]. Most interestingly, some of these TAU metabolites, such as H_2S could have profound biological activities in the GI and may be absorbed into the bloodstream and affect other vital organs [11]. Interestingly, some investigations mentioned that long-term TAU supplementation could change the gut microbiome favoring beneficial microbes and improving GI function [12]. The role of gut bacteria in TAU metabolism and its relevance to human diseases are discussed in the current chapter.

Several studies tested the protective properties of TAU against GI disorders and/or xenobiotics-induced GI injury [13 - 15]. In some cases, it seems that the effects of TAU on mitochondrial function and oxidative stress biomarkers play a role in its positive effects on these disorders. The impacts of TAU on GI disease and xenobiotics-induced GI disturbances are also discussed herein.

TAURINE IN THE DIGESTIVE SYSTEM: ABSORPTION, METABOLISM, AND EXCRETION

As mentioned in previous chapters (refer to chapter one for more information), the capacity of the human liver for TAU synthesis is negligible, and we receive a considerable amount of our body TAU from exogenous sources [3, 5 - 8, 16]. Several transporting systems have been identified in the gastrointestinal (GI) tract for taurine (TAU) absorption. Among these transporters, the Na^+/Cl^--dependent taurine transporter (TauT) and PAT1 (SLC36A1) are well-known transporters identified for TAU absorption from GI [10]. It has been found that TauT has a low capacity but a high affinity for TAU uptake and transport from the small intestine brush border [9]. On the other hand, another TAU transport system has been identified in GI. This transport system has a very high capacity for TAU transport from the GI [9, 17]. Therefore, these transporters, such as TauT and PAT1, are expressed in the intestinal brush border and abundantly found in organs such as the brain, heart, skeletal muscle, reproductive organs, and the liver [9, 18 - 20]. Actually, when TAU reaches the bloodstream by intestinal TauT and PAT1, it is rapidly uptaken by different organs [21, 22]. It has been found that some organs, such as skeletal muscle, express a very high level of TAU transporters [23 - 28]. Thus, it is unsurprising that this tissue contains a massive amount of this amino acid [1, 26, 29, 30]. Other tissues, such as the heart, also express a high level of TAU transporters [27, 31, 32]. Tissues such as the liver have a relatively low level of TAU transporter [2, 33]. As mentioned in Chapter 1, when TAU enters an organ through transporters such as TauT, it compartmentalizes in various organelles (*e.g.*, mitochondria) and induces physiological/pharmaco-logical actions.

Pharmacokinetic studies have also been conducted on TAU in humans. In a study by Ghandforoush-Sattari *et al.,* the pharmacokinetics of TAU in healthy volunteers was evaluated [34]. They found that the administration of 4 g of TAU solution to fasting volunteers (in the morning) gave a peak plasma of the amino acid, C_{max}) of 86.1 ± 19.0 mg/L after 1.5 ± 0.6 h after TAU administration [34]. They also found that the plasma elimination half-life ($T_{1/2}$) of TAU was 1 ± 0.3h and its clearance/bioavailability was 21.1 ± 7.8 L/h [34]. These pharmacokinetic data are precious for drug development studies and TAU application for therapeutic purposes. In another study by Rodella *et al.*, they claimed that TAU is well absorbed in its crystal solution [35]. All these studies give vital clues about TAU formulation for future therapeutic purposes.

An exciting finding of the TAU and GI system relates to TAU metabolism. There is no TAU metabolizing enzyme in human cells. However, TAU is metabolized by gut bacteria to sulfur-containing compounds (Fig. **1**) [11, 36]. TAU acts as an organic sulfonate substrate in the gut [11]. Some gut bacteria have been identified using TAU as a substrate to produce sulfite [11, 36]. Sulfite acts as an electron donor for the anaerobic bacteria to respirate and produce energy [11, 36]. Sulfite respiration (Fig. **1**) is a phenomenon in anaerobic bacteria that finally leads to the release of H_2S [11, 36]. Sulfite is reduced to H_2S by the bacterial sulfite reductase enzyme [11, 36]. The produced H_2S might also be oxidized to bio-sulfur compounds by other sulfide-oxidizing bacteria [11, 36]. Acetaldehyde is another product made by TAU metabolism by gut bacteria (Fig. **1**). It is believed that acetaldehyde is further metabolized to acetyl-CoA by bacterial dehydrogenase enzymes [11, 36] (Fig. **1**).

Interestingly, recent studies identified some bacteria in the human intestine responsible for TAU metabolism [11]. *Bilophila wadsworthia* is an opportunistic pathogen in the human GI [37]. *B. wadsworthia* presents a very low abundance in the healthy human colonic microbiota [37]. The abundance of *B. wadsworthia* is less than 0.01% of whole gut microbiota in healthy subjects [37]. Some investigations revealed that a high level of *B. wadsworthia* in the GI is associated with several human diseases such as appendicitis and colorectal cancer [38, 39]. The conditions such as hypoxia might also increase *B. wadsworthia* population because of the death of other normal flora [37 - 39]. Other microorganisms have also been identified for TAU metabolism and the production of sulfite and H_2S in GI [36]. *Clostridium butyricum* and *Anaerostipes hadrus* are also TAU metabolizing bacteria in the human GI tract [36].

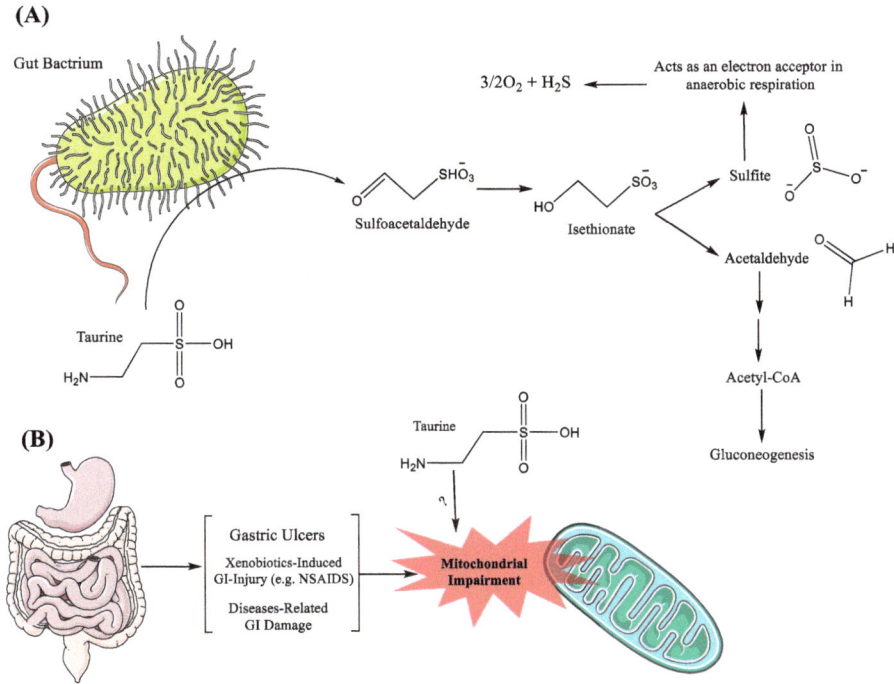

Fig. (1). Effects of taurine in the digestive system. Anaerobic gut bacteria degrade taurine to different chemicals needed for respiration and energy metabolism in these microorganisms (A). H_2S is an essential metabolite of TAU in the GI. The balance between production and the removal of H_2S after TAU digestion depends on multiple factors, including gut microbiota. Therefore, the abundance of H_2S production in the GI might vary between populations based on their GI microbiota.

The role of H_2S produced in GI and its effects on human health and diseases has also been widely investigated [40 - 42]. Several studies mentioned the link between high H_2S levels in GI and complications such as colon cancer, GI barrier disintegrity, GI bacterial antibiotic resistance, and inflammatory bowel disease (IBD) [43 - 47]. On the other hand, many investigations mentioned the GI-original H_2S as a signaling molecule responsible for some health benefits in the GI tract and even other organs (*e.g.*, the heart) [42, 48]. The role of H_2S in antioxidant and redox signaling is also an exciting field of investigation [40, 49]. Hence, there are controversial results about GI-derived H_2S on host health and diseases [41].

H_2S is a well-known inhibitor of mitochondrial respiration in eukaryotic cells [50, 51]. On the other hand, surprisingly, it has been found that H_2S could promote mitochondrial respiration and energy production under exceptional circumstances [52]. Fu *et al.* found that a protein called cystathionine lyase (CSE) is translocated to the mitochondria [52]. CSE is able to produce H_2S in mitochondria [52]. They found that NaHS as an H_2S donor stimulated ATP production under hypoxic conditions [52].

Several studies mentioned the role of TAU in IBD and colitis [53 - 56]. It has also been found that TAU has anti-inflammatory properties in GI [53, 57]. On the other hand, there is no report on the high TAU consumption and GI disorders in humans to date. All these findings mention the controversial results about the role of TAU metabolites in the GI. More investigations of TAU metabolism and its relation to health and disease could answer questions about the exact role of this amino acid in the human GI. On the other hand, there is no clear evidence of the amount of H_2S produced in the gut or reaching the systemic circulation in different individuals after TAU consumption.

Another interesting finding of the effect of TAU on gut microbe is mentioned in a study by Yu *et al.* [12]. They found that TAU could influence gut microbes and metabolism [12]. It has been found that TAU supplementation could significantly decrease the abundance of pathogenic bacteria such as Helicobacter [12]. More importantly, the serum level of toxic molecules such as lipopolysaccharide (LPS) was significantly decreased in TAU-treated animals [12]. Yu *et al.* concluded that TAU is able to regulate gut microbiology and prevent the growth of harmful microbes [12].

As repeatedly mentioned in the current book, the conjugation of bile acids with TAU is an essential physiological role for this amino acid. Bile acids conjugation by TAU occurs in the liver, and the conjugates are excreted in the bile's GI tract. TAU-conjugated bile acids are finally excreted in the feces. However, it should be mentioned that a large amount of TAU is excreted by kidneys as an intact TAU molecule.

TAURINE AND GI DISORDERS

The protective properties of TAU and its derivatives on GI complications, such as gastric ulcers, have been repeatedly investigated [13, 15]. Enhancing the secretion of bicarbonate and mucus, decreasing the release of NO, and the antioxidant effects of TAU have been proposed to be involved in its effects against gastric ulcers [13, 15]. On the other hand, several GI disorders have been identified in which mitochondrial impairment is involved in their pathogenesis [58, 59]. As repeatedly mentioned in this book, TAU provides its cytoprotective properties by regulating mitochondrial function in various organs [60 - 71]. The following parts describe the effects of TAU on GI with a focus on some of the most GI toxic agents. In each case, it has also been tried to explain the potential mechanisms of action of TAU.

Annual ethanol consumption is a significant cause of many gastrointestinal diseases globally, including multiple mucosal ulcers. Therefore, finding therapeutic options to reduce this complication can be helpful. Yu *et al.* reported that TAU could significantly protect gastric mucosa by a tremendous decrease in gastric ulcer index in absolute ethanol-fed animals [13]. In their study, TAU formulation decreased nitric oxide, enhanced mucosal superoxide dismutase (SOD) activity, improved the level of gastric prostaglandin E2 (PGE2) production, decreased malondialdehyde (MDA) level, and enhanced glutathione (GSH) content in the gastric mucosal of ethanol-treated animals [13]. The effects of TAU on MDA and GSH and its role in decreasing NO production could significantly blunt oxidative stress and its associated contents in this model. NO could also interact with other reactive oxygen species and produce molecules such as peroxynitrite ($ONOO\bullet^-$). The $ONOO\bullet^-$ is a very cytotoxic species that could cause apoptosis or necrosis of gastric mucosal cells [13]. Therefore, TAU prevents the formation of this deleterious species and protects the gastric mucosa. Moreover, PEGE2 is a chemical responsible for mucus secretion, thus providing a physical barrier to gastric ulcers and protecting from GI acid. Finally, it should be mentioned that in the study by Yu *et al.*, they used a TAU-zinc complex.

Alendronate is widely used to manage bone disorders [72]. However, severe gastrointestinal disturbances, including erosive esophagitis, gastritis, and gastric ulcer, have been reported in association with its administration [73 - 75]. However, the exact mechanism induced by alendronate is not fully cleared yet. Sener *et al.* reported that the alendronate damage to gastric mucosa could be associated with oxidative stress-dependent mechanisms [14]. In the investigation conducted by Sener *et al.*, they found that the ulcer index caused by alendronate significantly decreased when animals received TAU [14]. On the other hand, the acidity of mucosa was significantly decreased in TAU-treated animals compared with the alendronate group. Moreover, TAU treatment significantly improved biomarkers of oxidative stress (increased MDA and depletion of GSH) in the alendronate-treated groups [14]. Another interesting finding in the study by Sener *et al.* was the effect of TAU on myeloperoxidase (MPO) activity. The decrease in MPO activity could indicate the decrease in the infiltration of inflammatory cells (*e.g.*, neutrophils) and suppression of the inflammatory response in the gastric mucosa induced by alendronate. Actually, TAU provides potent anti-inflammatory properties, and its effects, at least a partial part, against the alendronate-induced GI damage could be mediated through this mechanism [76, 77].

Another case reporting the gastroprotective properties of TAU is carried out by Motawi *et al.* [15]. Non-steroidal anti-inflammatory drugs (NSAIDs), including indomethacin, could severely damage gastric mucosa and cause gastric ulcers

[15]. The study conducted by Motawi *et al.* found that TAU could significantly blunt indomethacin-induced gastric damage. Like the previous two reported cases in the current chapter, mitigation of oxidative stress and protecting mucosa by enhancing PGE2 and mucus secretion were involved in the gastroprotective properties of TAU [15]. Moreover, the effects of TAU on inflammatory biomarkers appear to be also involved in its gastroprotective properties in the study by Motawi *et al.* [15]. In an earlier study by Son *et al.*, they focused on the role of TAU in modulating gastric mucosa action of inflammatory cells and the effects of this amino acid in its gastroprotective [78]. Although the study of Son *et al.* was conducted earlier, the doses of indomethacin and TAU, as well as the biomarkers assessed in these investigations, are different [15, 78].

In another study by Ainad-Tabet *et al.*, they found that TAU provided robust anti-inflammatory activity in an animal model of intestinal damage [79]. They found that the levels of immunoglobulins (IgG and IgM) and cytokines (TNF-α and IL6) were significantly decreased in TAU-treated groups [79]. TAU also alleviated intestinal histopathological alterations induced by β- Lactoglobulin sensitization [79]. They concluded that the effects of TAU on inflammatory markers might play a pivotal role in the positive impact of TAU in their study [79]. Although Ainad-Tabet *et al.* did not assess, as inflammatory response, oxidative stress, and mitochondrial function are mechanistically related events, the effects of TAU on these parameters also may be involved in its protective effect in their study. Obviously, this issue needs further research to be cleared.

CONCLUSION

All the mentioned studies above were instances of the gastroprotective effects of TAU. As mentioned in all the above cases, oxidative stress and its associated complications were involved in those disorders. As it is well-known that oxidative stress and mitochondrial function are firmly connected, mitochondrial impairment might also be involved in the pathogenesis of such disorders. Therefore, more future investigations on the role of mitochondria in GI disorders could shed light on the protective properties of TAU in this system and finally find safe therapeutic options in this field.

REFERENCES

[1]   Lambert IH, Kristensen DM, Holm JB, Mortensen OH. Physiological role of taurine - from organism to organelle. Acta Physiol (Oxf) 2015; 213(1): 191-212.
        [http://dx.doi.org/10.1111/apha.12365] [PMID: 25142161]

[2]   Bella DL, Hirschberger LL, Kwon YH, Stipanuk MH. Cysteine metabolism in periportal and perivenous hepatocytes: perivenous cells have greater capacity for glutathione production and taurine synthesis but not for cysteine catabolism. Amino Acids 2002; 23(4): 453-8.
        [http://dx.doi.org/10.1007/s00726-002-0213-z] [PMID: 12436215]

[3]　　Stipanuk MH. Role of the liver in regulation of body cysteine and taurine levels: a brief review. Neurochem Res 2004; 29(1): 105-10.
[http://dx.doi.org/10.1023/B:NERE.0000010438.40376.c9] [PMID: 14992268]

[4]　　Bouckenooghe T, Remacle C, Reusens B. Is taurine a functional nutrient? Curr Opin Clin Nutr Metab Care 2006; 9(6): 728-33.
[http://dx.doi.org/10.1097/01.mco.0000247469.26414.55] [PMID: 17053427]

[5]　　Hansen SH, Grunnet N. Taurine, Glutathione and Bioenergetics.Taurine 8 Advances in Experimental Medicine and Biology: Springer New York. 2013; pp. 3-12.

[6]　　Huxtable RJ. Taurine in nutrition and neurology: Springer Science & Business Media; 2013.

[7]　　Laidlaw SA, Grosvenor M, Kopple JD. The taurine content of common foodstuffs. JPEN J Parenter Enteral Nutr 1990; 14(2): 183-8.
[http://dx.doi.org/10.1177/0148607190014002183] [PMID: 2352336]

[8]　　Xu Y-J, Arneja AS, Tappia PS, Dhalla NS. The potential health benefits of taurine in cardiovascular disease. Exp Clin Cardiol 2008; 13(2): 57-65.
[PMID: 19343117]

[9]　　Baliou S, Kyriakopoulos A, Goulielmaki M, Panayiotidis M, Spandidos D, Zoumpourlis V. Significance of taurine transporter (TauT) in homeostasis and its layers of regulation (Review). Mol Med Rep 2020; 22(3): 2163-73.
[http://dx.doi.org/10.3892/mmr.2020.11321] [PMID: 32705197]

[10]　Anderson CMH, Howard A, Walters JRF, Ganapathy V, Thwaites DT. Taurine uptake across the human intestinal brush-border membrane is *via* two transporters: H⁺-coupled PAT1 (SLC36A1) and Na⁺- and Cl⁻-dependent TauT (SLC6A6). J Physiol 2009; 587(4): 731-44.
[http://dx.doi.org/10.1113/jphysiol.2008.164228] [PMID: 19074966]

[11]　Peck SC, Denger K, Burrichter A, Irwin SM, Balskus EP, Schleheck D. A glycyl radical enzyme enables hydrogen sulfide production by the human intestinal bacterium *Bilophila wadsworthia*. Proc Natl Acad Sci USA 2019; 116(8): 3171-6.
[http://dx.doi.org/10.1073/pnas.1815661116] [PMID: 30718429]

[12]　Yu H, Guo Z, Shen S, Shan W. Effects of taurine on gut microbiota and metabolism in mice. Amino Acids 2016; 48(7): 1601-17.
[http://dx.doi.org/10.1007/s00726-016-2219-y] [PMID: 27026373]

[13]　Yu C, Mei XT, Zheng YP, Xu DH. Gastroprotective effect of taurine zinc solid dispersions against absolute ethanol-induced gastric lesions is mediated by enhancement of antioxidant activity and endogenous PGE2 production and attenuation of NO production. Eur J Pharmacol 2014; 740: 329-36.
[http://dx.doi.org/10.1016/j.ejphar.2014.07.014] [PMID: 25041839]

[14]　Sener G, Sehirli O, Cetinel S, Midillioğlu S, Gedik N, Ayanoğlu-Dülger G. Protective effect of taurine against alendronate-induced gastric damage in rats. Fundam Clin Pharmacol 2005; 19(1): 93-100.
[http://dx.doi.org/10.1111/j.1472-8206.2004.00310.x] [PMID: 15660965]

[15]　Motawi TK, Abd Elgawad HM, Shahin NN. Modulation of indomethacin-induced gastric injury by spermine and taurine in rats. J Biochem Mol Toxicol 2007; 21(5): 280-8.
[http://dx.doi.org/10.1002/jbt.20194] [PMID: 17912696]

[16]　Schuller-Levis GB, Park E. Taurine: new implications for an old amino acid. FEMS Microbiol Lett 2003; 226(2): 195-202.
[http://dx.doi.org/10.1016/S0378-1097(03)00611-6] [PMID: 14553911]

[17]　Lichter-Konecki U. Hypothermia Treatment in Hyperammonemia and Encephalopathy. Clinical trial registration. clinicaltrials.gov; 2015. Report No.: NCT01624311.

[18]　Han X, Patters AB, Jones DP, Zelikovic I, Chesney RW. The taurine transporter: mechanisms of regulation. Acta Physiol (Oxf) 2006; 187(1-2): 61-73.

[http://dx.doi.org/10.1111/j.1748-1716.2006.01573.x] [PMID: 16734743]

[19]   Bröer S. Amino acid transport across mammalian intestinal and renal epithelia. Physiol Rev 2008; 88(1): 249-86.
        [http://dx.doi.org/10.1152/physrev.00018.2006] [PMID: 18195088]

[20]   Desforges M, Parsons L, Westwood M, Sibley CP, Greenwood SL. 2013. Taurine transport in human placental trophoblast is important for regulation of cell differentiation and survival. Cell Death Dis. 2013;4(3):e559-e.
        [http://dx.doi.org/10.1038/cddis.2013.81]

[21]   Schaffer SW, Ju Jong C, Kc R, Azuma J. Physiological roles of taurine in heart and muscle. J Biomed Sci 2010; 17(Suppl 1): S2.
        [http://dx.doi.org/10.1186/1423-0127-17-S1-S2] [PMID: 20804594]

[22]   Ito T, Kimura Y, Uozumi Y, *et al.* Taurine depletion caused by knocking out the taurine transporter gene leads to cardiomyopathy with cardiac atrophy. J Mol Cell Cardiol 2008; 44(5): 927-37.
        [http://dx.doi.org/10.1016/j.yjmcc.2008.03.001] [PMID: 18407290]

[23]   Miyazaki T, Honda A, Ikegami T, Matsuzaki Y, Eds. The role of taurine on skeletal muscle cell differentiation 2013. New York, NY: Springer 2013.

[24]   De Luca A, Pierno S, Camerino DC. Effect of taurine depletion on excitation-contraction coupling and Cl− conductance of rat skeletal muscle. Eur J Pharmacol 1996; 296(2): 215-22.
        [http://dx.doi.org/10.1016/0014-2999(95)00702-4] [PMID: 8838459]

[25]   Horvath DM, Murphy RM, Mollica JP, Hayes A, Goodman CA. The effect of taurine and β-alanine supplementation on taurine transporter protein and fatigue resistance in skeletal muscle from mdx mice. Amino Acids 2016; 48(11): 2635-45.
        [http://dx.doi.org/10.1007/s00726-016-2292-2] [PMID: 27444300]

[26]   Spriet LL, Whitfield J. Taurine and skeletal muscle function. Curr Opin Clin Nutr Metab Care 2015; 18(1): 96-101.
        [http://dx.doi.org/10.1097/MCO.0000000000000135] [PMID: 25415270]

[27]   Ito T, Oishi S, Takai M, *et al.* Cardiac and skeletal muscle abnormality in taurine transporter-knockout mice. J Biomed Sci 2010; 17(1): S20.
        [http://dx.doi.org/10.1186/1423-0127-17-S1-S20] [PMID: 20804595]

[28]   Warskulat U, Flögel U, Jacoby C, *et al.* Taurine transporter knockout depletes muscle taurine levels and results in severe skeletal muscle impairment but leaves cardiac function uncompromised. FASEB J 2004; 18(3): 577-9.
        [http://dx.doi.org/10.1096/fj.03-0496fje] [PMID: 14734644]

[29]   Hansen SH, Andersen ML, Birkedal H, Cornett C, Wibrand F. The important role of taurine in oxidative metabolism Taurine 6. Springer 2006; pp. 129-35.

[30]   Iwata H, Obara T, Kim BK, Baba A. Regulation of taurine transport in rat skeletal muscle. J Neurochem 1986; 47(1): 158-63.
        [http://dx.doi.org/10.1111/j.1471-4159.1986.tb02844.x] [PMID: 3711895]

[31]   Schaffer SW, Shimada-Takaura K, Jong CJ, Ito T, Takahashi K. Impaired energy metabolism of the taurine-deficient heart. Amino Acids 2016; 48(2): 549-58.
        [http://dx.doi.org/10.1007/s00726-015-2110-2] [PMID: 26475290]

[32]   Wójcik OP, Koenig KL, Zeleniuch-Jacquotte A, Costa M, Chen Y. The potential protective effects of taurine on coronary heart disease. Atherosclerosis 2010; 208(1): 19-25.
        [http://dx.doi.org/10.1016/j.atherosclerosis.2009.06.002] [PMID: 19592001]

[33]   Miyazaki T, Matsuzaki Y. Taurine and liver diseases: a focus on the heterogeneous protective properties of taurine. Amino Acids 2014; 46(1): 101-10.
        [http://dx.doi.org/10.1007/s00726-012-1381-0] [PMID: 22918604]

[34]   Ghandforoush-Sattari M, Mashayekhi S, Krishna CV, Thompson JP, Routledge PA. Pharmacokinetics of oral taurine in healthy volunteers. J Amino Acids 2010; 2010: 346237.
[PMID: 22331997]

[35]   Rodella P, Takase L, Santos J, Scarim C, de Oliveira Vizioli E, Chung M. The effect of taurine on hepatic disorders. Current Updates in Hepatology and Gastroenterology 2017; 1(1): 1-12.

[36]   Xing M, Wei Y, Hua G, *et al.* A gene cluster for taurine sulfur assimilation in an anaerobic human gut bacterium. Biochem J 2019; 476(15): 2271-9.
[http://dx.doi.org/10.1042/BCJ20190486] [PMID: 31350331]

[37]   Baron EJ. Bilophila wadsworthia: a unique Gram-negative anaerobic rod. Anaerobe 1997; 3(2-3): 83-6.
[http://dx.doi.org/10.1006/anae.1997.0075] [PMID: 16887567]

[38]   Baron EJ, Curren M, Henderson G, *et al.* Bilophila wadsworthia isolates from clinical specimens. J Clin Microbiol 1992; 30(7): 1882-4.
[http://dx.doi.org/10.1128/jcm.30.7.1882-1884.1992] [PMID: 1629348]

[39]   Yazici C, Wolf PG, Kim H, *et al.* Race-dependent association of sulfidogenic bacteria with colorectal cancer. Gut 2017; 66(11): 1983-94.
[http://dx.doi.org/10.1136/gutjnl-2016-313321] [PMID: 28153960]

[40]   Linden DR. Hydrogen sulfide signaling in the gastrointestinal tract. Antioxid Redox Signal 2014; 20(5): 818-30.
[http://dx.doi.org/10.1089/ars.2013.5312] [PMID: 23582008]

[41]   Wallace JL. Physiological and pathophysiological roles of hydrogen sulfide in the gastrointestinal tract. Antioxid Redox Signal 2010; 12(9): 1125-33.
[http://dx.doi.org/10.1089/ars.2009.2900] [PMID: 19769457]

[42]   Singh S, Lin H. Hydrogen sulfide in physiology and diseases of the digestive tract. Microorganisms 2015; 3(4): 866-89.
[http://dx.doi.org/10.3390/microorganisms3040866] [PMID: 27682122]

[43]   Attene-Ramos MS, Nava GM, Muellner MG, Wagner ED, Plewa MJ, Gaskins HR. DNA damage and toxicogenomic analyses of hydrogen sulfide in human intestinal epithelial FHs 74 Int cells. Enviro Mol Mutagen 2010; 51(4): 304-14.
[http://dx.doi.org/10.1002/em.20546] [PMID: 20120018]

[44]   Blachier F, Beaumont M, Kim E. Cysteine-derived hydrogen sulfide and gut health. Curr Opin Clin Nutr Metab Care 2019; 22(1): 68-75.
[http://dx.doi.org/10.1097/MCO.0000000000000526] [PMID: 30461448]

[45]   Ijssennagger N, van der Meer R, van Mil SWC. Sulfide as a mucus barrier-breaker in inflammatory bowel disease? Trends Mol Med 2016; 22(3): 190-9.
[http://dx.doi.org/10.1016/j.molmed.2016.01.002] [PMID: 26852376]

[46]   Shatalin K, Shatalina E, Mironov A, Nudler E. H2S: a universal defense against antibiotics in bacteria. Science 2011; 334(6058): 986-90.
[http://dx.doi.org/10.1126/science.1209855] [PMID: 22096201]

[47]   Luhachack L, Nudler EH. ₂S as a bacterial defense against antibiotics. Hydrogen Sulfide and Its Therapeutic Applications.. Springer 2013; pp. 173-80.

[48]   Wallace JL, Dicay M, McKnight W, Martin GR. Hydrogen sulfide enhances ulcer healing in rats. FASEB J 2007; 21(14): 4070-6.
[http://dx.doi.org/10.1096/fj.07-8669com] [PMID: 17634391]

[49]   Wang R. Hydrogen sulfide: the third gasotransmitter in biology and medicine. Antioxid Redox Signal 2010; 12(9): 1061-4.
[http://dx.doi.org/10.1089/ars.2009.2938] [PMID: 19845469]

[50]   Eghbal MA, Pennefather PS, O'Brien PJ. H2S cytotoxicity mechanism involves reactive oxygen species formation and mitochondrial depolarisation. Toxicology 2004; 203(1-3): 69-76.
[http://dx.doi.org/10.1016/j.tox.2004.05.020] [PMID: 15363583]

[51]   Truong DH, Eghbal MA, Hindmarsh W, Roth SH, O'Brien PJ. Molecular mechanisms of hydrogen sulfide toxicity. Drug Metab Rev 2006; 38(4): 733-44.
[http://dx.doi.org/10.1080/03602530600959607] [PMID: 17145698]

[52]   Fu M, Zhang W, Wu L, Yang G, Li H, Wang R. Hydrogen sulfide (H_2S) metabolism in mitochondria and its regulatory role in energy production. Proc Natl Acad Sci USA 2012; 109(8): 2943-8.
[http://dx.doi.org/10.1073/pnas.1115634109] [PMID: 22323590]

[53]   Son MW, Ko JI, Doh HM, *et al.* Protective effect of taurine on TNBS-induced inflammatory bowel disease in rats. Arch Pharm Res 1998; 21(5): 531-6.
[http://dx.doi.org/10.1007/BF02975370] [PMID: 9875490]

[54]   Giriş M, Depboylu B, Doğru-Abbasoğlu S, *et al.* Effect of taurine on oxidative stress and apoptosis-related protein expression in trinitrobenzene sulphonic acid-induced colitis. Clin Exp Immunol 2008; 152(1): 102-10.
[http://dx.doi.org/10.1111/j.1365-2249.2008.03599.x] [PMID: 18241224]

[55]   Son M, Ko JI, Kim WB, Kang HK, Kim BK. Taurine can ameliorate inflammatory bowel disease in rats Taurine 3. Springer 1998; pp. 291-8.
[http://dx.doi.org/10.1007/978-1-4899-0117-0_37]

[56]   Zhao Z, Satsu H, Fujisawa M, *et al.* Attenuation by dietary taurine of dextran sulfate sodium-induced colitis in mice and of THP-1-induced damage to intestinal Caco-2 cell monolayers. Amino Acids 2008; 35(1): 217-24.
[http://dx.doi.org/10.1007/s00726-007-0562-8] [PMID: 17619120]

[57]   Shimizu M, Zhao Z, Ishimoto Y, Satsu H. Dietary taurine attenuates dextran sulfate sodium (DSS)-induced experimental colitis in mice Taurine 7. Springer 2009; pp. 265-71.
[http://dx.doi.org/10.1007/978-0-387-75681-3_27]

[58]   Somasundaram S, Sigthorsson G, Simpson RJ, *et al.* Uncoupling of intestinal mitochondrial oxidative phosphorylation and inhibition of cyclooxygenase are required for the development of NSAID-enteropathy in the rat. Aliment Pharmacol Ther 2000; 14(5): 639-50.
[http://dx.doi.org/10.1046/j.1365-2036.2000.00723.x] [PMID: 10792129]

[59]   Maity P, Bindu S, Dey S, *et al.* Indomethacin, a non-steroidal anti-inflammatory drug, develops gastropathy by inducing reactive oxygen species-mediated mitochondrial pathology and associated apoptosis in gastric mucosa: a novel role of mitochondrial aconitase oxidation. J Biol Chem 2009; 284(5): 3058-68.
[http://dx.doi.org/10.1074/jbc.M805329200] [PMID: 19049974]

[60]   De Luca A, Pierno S, Camerino DC. Taurine: the appeal of a safe amino acid for skeletal muscle disorders. J Transl Med 2015; 13(1): 243.
[http://dx.doi.org/10.1186/s12967-015-0610-1] [PMID: 26208967]

[61]   Ommati MM, Farshad O, Jamshidzadeh A, Heidari R. Taurine enhances skeletal muscle mitochondrial function in a rat model of resistance training. PharmaNutrition 2019; 9: 100161.
[http://dx.doi.org/10.1016/j.phanu.2019.100161]

[62]   Jong CJ, Sandal P, Schaffer SW. The role of taurine in mitochondria health: More than just an antioxidant. Molecules 2021; 26(16): 4913.
[http://dx.doi.org/10.3390/molecules26164913] [PMID: 34443494]

[63]   Heidari R, Behnamrad S, Khodami Z, Ommati MM, Azarpira N, Vazin A. The nephroprotective properties of taurine in colistin-treated mice is mediated through the regulation of mitochondrial function and mitigation of oxidative stress. Biomed Pharmacother 2019; 109: 103-11.
[http://dx.doi.org/10.1016/j.biopha.2018.10.093] [PMID: 30396066]

[64]   Jamshidzadeh A, Heidari R, Abasvali M, *et al.* Taurine treatment preserves brain and liver mitochondrial function in a rat model of fulminant hepatic failure and hyperammonemia. Biomed Pharmacother 2017; 86: 514-20.
[http://dx.doi.org/10.1016/j.biopha.2016.11.095] [PMID: 28024286]

[65]   Ahmadi N, Ghanbarinejad V, Ommati MM, Jamshidzadeh A, Heidari R. Taurine prevents mitochondrial membrane permeabilization and swelling upon interaction with manganese: Implication in the treatment of cirrhosis-associated central nervous system complications. J Biochem Mol Toxicol 2018; 32(11): e22216.
[http://dx.doi.org/10.1002/jbt.22216] [PMID: 30152904]

[66]   Hansen S, Andersen M, Cornett C, Gradinaru R, Grunnet N. A role for taurine in mitochondrial function. J Biomed Sci 2010; 17(Suppl 1): S23.
[http://dx.doi.org/10.1186/1423-0127-17-S1-S23] [PMID: 20804598]

[67]   Rutherford JA, Spriet LL, Stellingwerff T. The effect of acute taurine ingestion on endurance performance and metabolism in well-trained cyclists. Int J Sport Nutr Exerc Metab 2010; 20(4): 322-9.
[http://dx.doi.org/10.1123/ijsnem.20.4.322] [PMID: 20739720]

[68]   Liu Z, Qi B, Zhang M, *et al.* Role of taurine supplementation to prevent exercise-induced oxidative stress in healthy young men. Amino Acids 2004; 26(2): 203-7.
[http://dx.doi.org/10.1007/s00726-003-0002-3] [PMID: 15042451]

[69]   Lee HM, Paik IY, Park TS. Effects of dietary supplementation of taurine, carnitine or glutamine on endurance exercise performance and fatigue parameters in athletes. Korean Journal of Nutrition 2016; 36(7): 711-9.

[70]   Abdoli N, Sadeghian I, Azarpira N, Ommati MM, Heidari R. Taurine mitigates bile duct obstruction-associated cholemic nephropathy: effect on oxidative stress and mitochondrial parameters. Clin Exp Hepatol 2021; 7(1): 30-40.
[http://dx.doi.org/10.5114/ceh.2021.104675] [PMID: 34027113]

[71]   Heidari R, Ghanbarinejad V, Ommati MM, Jamshidzadeh A, Niknahad H. Mitochondria protecting amino acids: Application against a wide range of mitochondria-linked complications. PharmaNutrition 2018; 6(4): 180-90.
[http://dx.doi.org/10.1016/j.phanu.2018.09.001]

[72]   Kanis JA, Gertz BJ, Singer F, Ortolani S. Rationale for the use of alendronate in osteoporosis. Osteoporos Int 1995; 5(1): 1-13.
[http://dx.doi.org/10.1007/BF01623652] [PMID: 7703618]

[73]   Zhou M, Zheng Y, Li J, *et al.* Upper gastrointestinal safety and tolerability of oral alendronate: A meta-analysis. Exp Ther Med 2016; 11(1): 289-96.
[http://dx.doi.org/10.3892/etm.2015.2848] [PMID: 26889256]

[74]   Bauer DC, Black D, Ensrud K, *et al.* Upper gastrointestinal tract safety profile of alendronate: the fracture intervention trial. Arch Intern Med 2000; 160(4): 517-25.
[http://dx.doi.org/10.1001/archinte.160.4.517] [PMID: 10695692]

[75]   de Groen PC, Lubbe DF, Hirsch LJ, *et al.* Esophagitis associated with the use of alendronate. N Engl J Med 1996; 335(14): 1016-21.
[http://dx.doi.org/10.1056/NEJM199610033351403] [PMID: 8793925]

[76]   Zaki HF, Salem HA, El-Yamany MF. Taurine: A promising agent of therapeutic potential in experimentally-induced arthritis. Egypt Rheumatol 2011; 33(3): 131-7.
[http://dx.doi.org/10.1016/j.ejr.2011.05.002]

[77]   Marcinkiewicz J, Kontny E. Taurine and inflammatory diseases. Amino Acids 2014; 46(1): 7-20.
[http://dx.doi.org/10.1007/s00726-012-1361-4] [PMID: 22810731]

[78]   Son M, Kim HK, Kim WB, Yang J, Kim BK. Protective effect of taurine on indomethacin-induced gastric mucosal injury. Adv Exp Med Biol 1996; 403(2): 147-55.

[http://dx.doi.org/10.1007/978-1-4899-0182-8_17] [PMID: 8915352]

[79]   Aïnad-Tabet S, Grar H, Haddi A, *et al.* Taurine administration prevents the intestine from the damage induced by beta-lactoglobulin sensitization in a murine model of food allergy. Allergol Immunopathol (Madr) 2019; 47(3): 214-20.
[http://dx.doi.org/10.1016/j.aller.2018.07.010] [PMID: 30270100]

CHAPTER 10

The Role of Taurine in the Reproductive System: A Focus on Mitochondria-related Mechanisms

Abstract: The cytoprotective features of taurine (TAU), including anti-programmed cell death, membrane stabilization, antioxidant, anti-inflammation, osmoregulation, and intracellular calcium homeostasis regulation, have been well addressed in the literature. TAU has also been considered a potent agent for diminishing various xenobiotics-caused by physiological and pathophysiological alterations through its antioxidant action in reproductive and non-reproductive organs. Hence, exogenous TAU administration is the topic of many in-depth investigations. Several studies revealed that the antioxidative effect, anti-cellular death, and anti-inflammatory effects of TAU are involved in inhibiting xenobiotics-induced reproductive toxicity. Hence, the exact targets of TAU during the intracellular routes related to mitochondrial functionality (such as mitochondria-mediated oxidative stress and cell death) triggered by xenobiotics are discussed in this chapter. The data collected in this chapter suggest that TAU could be highly protective against various kinds of xenobiotics-induced gonadotoxicity, spermatotoxicity, and steroidogenotoxicity (hormonal steroids' genotoxicity) *via* its antioxidative, anti-inflammatory, and anti-cell death features. Furthermore, this amino acid also acts as an anti-apoptotic and anti-autophagic molecule by modifying the regulation of some related genes and proteins and inflammatory and mitochondrial-dependent signaling molecules.

Keywords: Antioxidant, Apoptosis, Autophagy, Fertility, Inflammatory response, Oxidative stress.

INTRODUCTION

Having a healthy and efficient reproductive system guarantees the survival of generations of different species. This is also vital in humans. Defects in the reproductive system's function and cumulative damage to the reproductive indices could lead to the birth of babies with various abnormalities. This issue also imposes many social and psychological burdens on families and society. Therefore, identifying the mechanisms of injury of reproductive systems (*e.g.*, induced by diseases or xenobiotics) and using substances that effectively protect the reproductive attributes in both males and females could have tremendous clinical value. Also, finding such materials could be of great importance to developing biological banks for specimens for future applications.

Reza Heidari and M. Mehdi Ommati

Mitochondria are vital organelles that control the normal, forward movement of sperm by producing large amounts of energy (ATP). This ensures that sperm reaches the egg cell easily and can fertilize it. On the other hand, humans receive all the mitochondria of their cells (also the sperm mitochondria) from the egg (mother). Therefore, protecting this vital cell could play an essential role in the generation's survival and prevent various abnormalities in human generations.

Taurine (TAU) is a sulfur-containing amino acid that has been extensively researched for its biological effects. In the field of research on the impacts of TAU on the reproductive system, it has been found that this amino acid could robustly protect sperm and eggs against a wide range of xenobiotics or diseases and protect them in both *in vitro* and/or *in vivo* models. It has also been observed that the level of ATP in TAU-exposed sperm is higher than that of control groups. This point could confirm that these sperms could be more efficient in fertilizing eggs. Numerous studies revealed the protective effects of TAU on damage caused by xenobiotics to sperm, eggs, and various components of the male and female reproductive systems. It has also been shown that the administration of TAU could alleviate the damage caused by multiple human diseases.

This chapter discusses the effects of TAU on fertility parameters, sperm and egg health, and finally, the use of this safe substance in treating human fertility disorders. Attempts have been made in different sections to pay special attention to the effect of this amino acid on other mitochondrial functions and their application as potential therapeutic points of intervention.

THE HISTORY OF TAURINE/HYPOTAURINE ON REPRODUCTIVE PARAMETERS

There are two kinds of antioxidants in the reproductive system, including enzymatic and non-enzymatic antioxidants. **A:** Enzymatic antioxidants (natural antioxidants) include glutathione reductase, glutathione peroxidase, catalase, and superoxide dismutase. **B:** Non-enzymatic antioxidants (synthetic antioxidants or dietary supplements) consist of reduced glutathione (GSH), α-tocopherol (vitamin E), β-carotene (carotenoids), urate, ubiquinone, ascorbic acid (vitamin C), selenium, zinc, hypo taurine (hTAU), and taurine (TAU).

The last non-enzymatic antioxidant, TAU (2-aminoethanesulfonic acid; as the most critical intracellular free beta-amino acid), is present in most tissues of mammals. It has been shown that male motile and immotile gametes might contain various intercellular levels of TAU and hTAU. These chemicals' biological and physiological roles through their antioxidant activities have been assessed in the last century [1 - 4]. However, there is a considerable contradiction among these observations. This chapter aims to cover all those discrepancies.

In-depth investigations have recommended that these vital compounds (TAU and hTAU) play a crucial role in spermatozoa physiology, probably through osmoregulation, neurotransmission, and/or ion modulation [5 - 7]. About fifty years ago, considerable concentrations of both TAU and hTAU have been frequently recorded in male and female reproductive-related organs, gametes, and fluids of various species [1, 8 - 14]. However, as mentioned earlier, there are contradictions about their concentrations in these tissues and cells; for instance, the levels of these elements were equal in the gametes extracted from hamsters and guinea pigs [8]. Holmes *et al.* (1992) highlighted the crucial roles of TAU and hTAU in sperm motility and fertility.

They have also shown that male gametes TAU ranged from 17 to 348 nmol/mg DNA, and hTAU was in the range of 0 to 251 nmol/mg DNA, whereas seminal fluid encompassed 319 to 1590 µmol/L TAU, but no detectable hTAU [4]. They also reported that the average level of hTAU in fertile men (n = 8) was higher, four times that of the gametes from infertile men (n = 9), 149 ± 92 nmol/mg DNA as compared with 35 ± 19 nmol/mg, respectively. In their study, the sperm values for TAU were significantly lower in fertile men (83 ± 33 nmol/mg DNA) than in infertile men (168 ± 119 nmol/mg DNA) [4]. In view of seminal fluid TAU levels, the concentrations were identical in both trial studied groups.

On the other hand, a good body of literature demonstrates that among various mammalian tissues, the reproductive-related organs are unique in containing high levels of hTAU [1, 4, 8, 11 - 14]. Finally, Holmes *et al.* (1992) claimed a close and positive relationship between the concentration of hTAU with some sperm parameters, including sperm morphology, motility, and attention [4]. In contrary to the recent popular belief, they claimed these indices were negatively correlated with the sperm concentration of TAU. Fascinatingly, the high levels of hTAU, which varied in a hormone-dependent manner, were also recorded in the oviducts of the ewe [11] and the reproductive fluids of the rodents, monkeys, and cow [8]; which implies the crucial role of hTAU in the reproductive tissues of females as well. To sum up, it sounds that hTAU, a well-known antioxidant, can play a vital role in mitigating oxidative stress action by inhibiting reactive oxygen species (ROS) formation in the male gametes. On the other hand, the higher observed levels of TAU in the infertile men's gametes in their study were interpreted that the recorded abnormalities in sperm parameters might be induced by accelerated oxidation of hTAU to TAU. Several studies have mentioned that hTAU oxidation is involved in the generation of TAU [1 - 3]. This hypothesis is contrary to the views of modern research indicating the high protective role of TAU on reproductive-related parameters [15, 16].

In the next step, the question arises about where these crucial compounds (hTAU and TAU) come from. The following research can be indicated to answer this question. Although the exact origin of hTAU in the human gamete is not well understood; however, animal experiments proposed an epididymal source. Johnson and colleagues (1972) reported a high concentration of hTAU (45 mmol/L) in epididymal plasma compared to seminal fluids and other accessory sex organs' fluids in boars. In line with the observation by Johnson *et al.* (1972) in porcine, the origin of hTAU is supported by the studies in rats and mice male gonad, epididymis, and seminal vesicle; where the high hTAU level was obtained only in the epididymis [13]. These high obtained epididymal concentrations of hTAU in various studies might indicate that epididymis is probably the leading endogenous site for this crucial compound that is eventually secreted into the epididymal plasma.

On the other hand, other low-molecular-weight non-essential amino acids containing thiol, such as L-cysteine (L-Cys), can pass through the cells and metabolize to TAU. Furthermore, this intracellular free beta-amino acid (TAU) is transformed into acyl-taurine upon combination with sperm plasma membrane fatty acids, which ultimately improves osmoregulation and plasma membrane integrity of the sperm [17]. In male gonads, TAU has been identified in interstitial cells (Leydig cells, LCs), vascular endothelial cells, and other interstitial cells [18]. Furthermore, male gametes are rich in TAU [19], and subsequently, seminal fluid will be rich. Altogether, there are two crucial sources of TAU for the intracellular levels of this amino acid considered as follows: a biosynthetic path from cysteine (as mentioned above) and/or the selective uptake from the extracellular environment; for instance, it can come from dietary bases and/or from some tissues (*e.g.*, it can be synthesized in liver) and released into circulatory system [20].

As mentioned earlier, a considerable hTAU level in male gametes plays a crucial role in the antioxidant system, osmoregulation, and ion modulation. There are important reasons for the presence of the antioxidant system in male gametes, including A) long-term maturation and storage time of sperm [4]; B) the high concentrations of polyunsaturated fatty acids (PUFA) [21]; C) post-ejaculated spermatozoa exposed to air; and D) inactivation of intracellular ROS generated by seminal leucocytes [22 - 26]. In addition to high concentrations of hTAU in male gametes, the defense mechanisms of sperm against ROS may consist of superoxide dismutase, the ratio of GSH to oxidized form (GSSG), and glutathione peroxidase [27 - 29]. Aitken *et al.* (1989) reported that sperm from patients with oligozoospermia could produce high levels of ROS as compared with those in normal fertile men with average sperm count [30]; hence, Holmes *et al.* (1992) concluded that gametes under any kind of stress might generate high levels of

ROS, which can trigger the conversion of hTAU to TAU. Hereafter, based on the earlier reports, the low hTAU level might be considered a marker for sperm stress rather than a fundamental reason for anomalies in sperm.

In contrast with the literature published in the last century, the past decade has witnessed a steady accumulation of observations that TAU is a fertility stimulant in different species [15, 16]. Perhaps some of the reasons for these discrepancies are mentioned in the last section of the article conducted by Holmes *et al.* (1992); where the authors frankly pointed out that "whereas we observed that exogenous and endogenous hTAU was stable in a fertile individual with normal semen parameters, including a high hTAU content, we cannot conclude from our studies whether differences in sperm hTAU content between fertile and infertile individuals occur before or after ejaculation" and or in the last paragraph, they highlighted that "the correlation coefficient of sperm hTAU content with various sperm and semen parameters was about 0.5 ($r2_{det}$ = 0.25). This coefficient of determination indicates that most of the variation in these parameters is controlled by factors other than hTAU. Therefore, perhaps the alterations observed in the reproductive indices in their work were related to the post-ejaculatory periods and other co-variants that were not considered in their studies. Hence, it can be assumed that a typical content of hTAU does not necessarily protect the gametes against the adverse effects of various xenobiotics; in other words, not all harsh situations lead to a decrease in gametes' hTAU concentration. In the following sections, TAU's ameliorative role and biological function in reproductive parameters through improving mitochondrial function and their concentrations in reproductive tissues will be further addressed.

AMELIORATIVE ROLE OF TAU ON XENOBIOTICS-INDUCED GONADOTOXICITY, SPERMATOTOXICITY, AND STEROIDOGENOTOXICITY

Various well-known xenobiotics, including environmental toxicants, drugs, physical injuries, disruptors of endocrine and neuroendocrine systems, immunosuppression, hypoxia, smoking, irradiation, and malnutrition, could adversely affect males' and females' reproductive systems [22]. During the past decade, the authors have frequently reported that various kinds of xenobiotics [31], including drugs (*i.e.*, sulfasalazine) [32], anomalies in the functionality of endogenous organs and their secretions (*i.e.*, liver, bile acids, and thymus) [27], heavy metals and other toxic elements (*i.e.*, arsenic, lead, lithium, fluoride) [22 - 25, 28, 29, 33 - 35], and nanoparticles (*i.e.*, single-walled and multi-walled carbon nanotubes) [26] in rodents could impair the functionality of male and female reproductive system through impairment in spermatogenesis and steroidogenesis, as well as reduction of the weight of the male and female sex organs possibly *via* triggering oxidative stress and consequent intracellular routes, such as mitochondrial impairment that will be discussed in following sections.

The crucial testicular histological properties (*i.e.*, LCs and Sertoli cells presence, centrally localized male gametes, and well-organized germinal epithelium) [36] are interrupted by xenobiotics resulting in gonadotoxicity. However, histopathological investigations have revealed that TAU could considerably recover the testicular pathology pointing toward its strength in improving xenobiotics-induced gonadotoxicity.

Remarkable Point

It is getting progressively clear that any significant decrement in the male gonad's weight upon xenobiotics exposure indicates toxicity. There is a close relation between male gonad weight and the quantity of differentiated spermatogenic cells. Hence, a considerable reduction in the testis weight can be a valid index of gonadotoxicity (except in the condition of inflammation that testicular mass and weight will be increased). Subsequently, it might be expected that this anomaly may be because of the considerable decrement in the steroidogenesis function (through decrement in the expression of the related genes and proteins, as described below, and subsequent decrement in testosterone level) and marked decrease in spermatogenesis [26, 32, 37, 38]. Pre-treatment of TAU protected the exposed animals from retardation in testicular growth [39].

Seminal testosterone content impacts the metabolism, maturation, and spermatozoa performance [21, 40]. However, the authors have not observed a significant correlation between plasma testosterone content and semen characteristics in roosters [41]. Because of the considerable contradictions in this issue that we have also highlighted frequently [21, 41], it needs to be discussed more carefully in the field of endocrinology (*i.e.*, steroidogenesis) and its relationship with reproductive parameters and fertility. For instance, in 1986 and 1988, Cecil and Bakst reported that there is no association between seminal plasma and blood testosterone content with sperm quality indices in turkey [42, 43]; while it has been shown that seminal testosterone content was associated with sperm count in Leghorn cockerels [44]. Furthermore, neither negative [45] nor positive correlation [42] was obtained between blood and seminal testosterone concentrations. Blood testosterone content was not correlated with the male gametes' parameters in bovines [46]; however, positively associated with fertility [47]. However, a positive association was observed by Meeker and colleagues (2007) between blood testosterone levels and sperm motility in men [48]. In contrast and interestingly, Sundqvist *et al.* (1984) observed a negative correlation between blood testosterone content and male gametes quality in mink [49]. Based on the above literature, more scholarly investigations are needed before an association between the lower serum testosterone content and reproductive indices (*i.e.*, seminal characteristics) and/or spermatotoxicity-related indices in xenobiotics-exposed animals is established.

On the other hand, it has been well illustrated that TAU can act as a capacitating agent [8, 50], sperm motility factor [51, 52], enhancer of sperm membrane integrity, the regulator of calcium transport, and modifier of protein phosphorylation [53]. However, a good body of literature shows that TAU can considerably mitigate these adverse effects of xenobiotics-induced toxicity in male and female gonads. For instance, Wei *et al.* (2007) reported that TAU significantly improved testicular ischemia-reperfusion injury, the primary pathophysiology of testicular torsion-detorsion [15].

It is getting progressively clear that over-biosynthesis of ROS (*i.e.*, hypochlorous acid, hydrogen peroxide, superoxide anion, and hydroxyl radicals) and reactive nitrogen species play an essential role in losing ipsilateral testicular spermatogenesis [54, 55]. These reactive species could induce testicular injury *via* DNA damage, lipid peroxidation of the membrane, and denaturation of its protein [54, 56]. In addition, it is well established that neutrophils are one of the crucial sources of ROS biosynthesis [57]. Therefore, it can be assumed that the observed ameliorative effects of TAU in their studies might be relatively the consequence of a reduction in the biogenesis of ROS through diminishing neutrophil recruitment to the testis. One of the potent oxidants that can induce remarkable destruction in host tissues is HClO [58]. The activation of neutrophils results in the generation of HClO from H_2O_2 [58, 59]. As mentioned earlier, TAU is well-known as a highly potent antioxidant. Hence, TAU can interact with this acid to generate TAU- chloramine, ultimately reducing its cytotoxicity [60].

Moreover, more scholarly reports have documented that in addition to this acid, TAU can also quench and detoxify other ROS, including superoxide anion, nitric oxide, and hydrogen peroxide in the liver [61] and hydroxyl radicals in the heart [62]. Hence, TAU prevents lipid peroxidation through its antioxidative properties and has a crucial impact on osmoregulation, spermatozoa motility, capacitation, and acrosome reaction [19]. Altogether, it can be assumed that TAU consumption can be suggested as a new approach to the therapy of xenobiotics-induced gonadotoxicity and spermatotoxicity through steroidogenotoxicity (Fig. **1**). In this view, Wei *et al.* (2007) reported that the administration of TAU (100mg/kg body weight for five consecutive days, orally) caused a considerable rescue of testicular spermatogenesis upon 120 min of testicular torsion. In another study, pre-treatment with TAU could considerably prevent the heavy metals-induced gonadotoxicity and keep the male gonad's architecture [63]. The survey conducted by Aly and Khafagy (2014) has also shown that pre-exposure (24 h before the administration of endosulfan) to 100 mg/kg/day of TAU could considerably mitigate the observed reduction in the testicular weight, sperm count, motility, viability, and daily sperm production in the rats challenged with 5 mg/kg/day of endosulfan for 15 consecutive days by oral gavage [39]. They have shown that the decreased epididymal sperm chromatin integrity, epididymal L-carnitine, level of serum testosterone, and testicular 3ß-HSD, 17ß-HSD, G6PDH (a crucial testicular enzyme involved in providing reducing equivalents for the steroids hydroxylation), and LDH-X (a specific isoenzyme of lactate dehydrogenase distinguishing as a well-known indicator for normal metabolism of male gametes locating in the inner mitochondrial membrane of these germ cells) were considerably mitigated in the endosulfan-treated rats pre-exposed to TAU [39] (Fig. **1**).

Many investigations have focused on the parallel relationship between L-carnitine content and mitochondrial functionality [64]. However, this compound is also introduced as a valid biochemical marker for the functionality of epididymis [65], and its positive correlation with sperm count, motility, and maturation is discussed [66]. The presence of L-carnitine in male gametes has been proven; hence, any decrement in the content of epididymal L-carnitine might indicate a decrease in sperm concentration in the epididymis or a reduction of L-carnitine concentration in the gamete itself. On the other hand, except for the spermatozoa L-carnitine content, epididymal tissue fluid has a higher amount of this element than sperms [67]. Hence, it can be assumed that most of the decrease in L-carnitine concentration indicates a reduction in epididymal fluid content and consequently reflects a detrimental effect on the functionality of epididymis to transport and/or concentrate L-carnitine. In this regard, Aly *et al.* (2014) have reported that the recorded decrement in epididymal male gametes concentration and epididymal L-carnitine level seems to be in the same line. However, they reported that these changes returned to a normal condition by pre-treatment of TAU (Fig. **1**). The effects of TAU on the reproductive system could be mediated through different mechanisms, some of which are addressed in the following sections.

TAURINE AND APOPTOSIS THROUGH MITOCHONDRIAL FUNCTION AND INFLAMMATORY RESPONSES

Under non-stress situations, mitochondria are the primary site for generating oxygen-derived oxidants, commonly known as ROS, swiftly trapped by cellular antioxidants. Oxidative injury triggered by ROS is a crucial factor in infertility in males and females [22, 24 - 29, 33] (Fig. **1**). There is a good collection of information on xenobiotics illustrating the unquestionable role of ROS in performing its deleterious effects (Fig. **1**). One of the well-known detrimental effects is called apoptosis, an active cellular process of self-destruction managed by related genes. The activated cells die in a precise route either in reaction to different environmental stimuli and chemicals (various kinds of xenobiotics) or spontaneously.

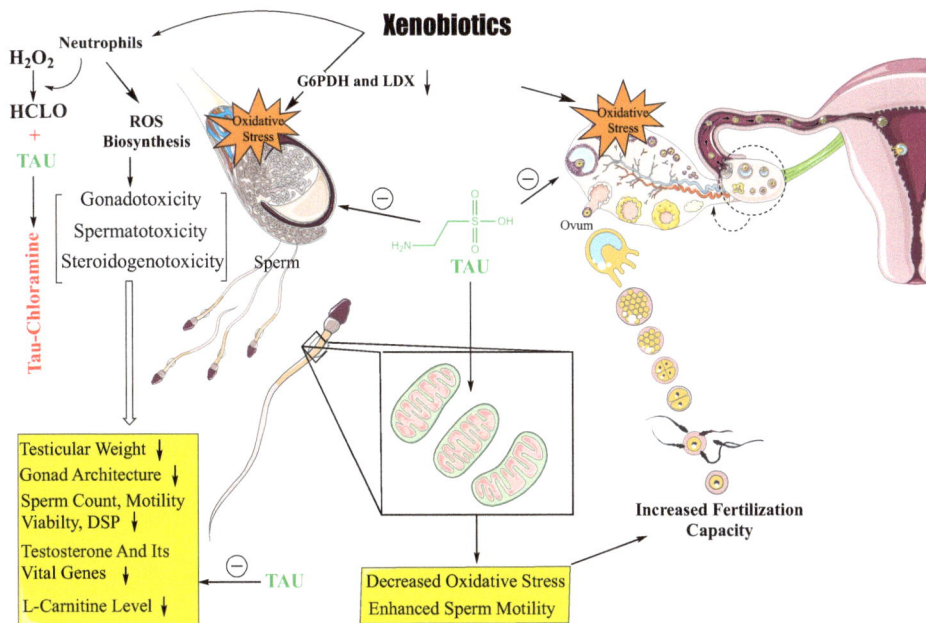

Fig. (1). Mitochondria-mediated effects of taurine (TAU) in the reproductive system. A significant part of the positive effects of taurine in the reproductive system, especially in males, is mediated through the results of this amino acid on cellular mitochondria. H_2O_2: hydrogen peroxide; HCLO: hypochlorous acid; ROS: reactive oxygen species; G6PDH: glucose-6-P-dehydrogenase; LDX: lactate dehydrogenase-X; DSP: daily sperm production.

Meanwhile, xenobiotics can induce adverse effects on mitochondrial function, such as mitochondrial membrane polarization, causing further ROS biosynthesis. In various types of spermatogenic cells and reproductive-related organs, there is an acceptable correlation exists between oxidative stress and subsequent ROS formation with apoptosis [63, 68]. Hence, it can be assumed that these reactive species-induced decreased mitochondrial membrane potential ($\Delta\Psi_m$) operates as an indispensable mediator of apoptosis [69]. More scholarly reports have documented that xenobiotics induced ROS formation and decreased $\Delta\Psi_m$, which ultimately endorsed the apoptosis mitochondria-mediated route.

The mitochondrion has been described as a well-known sensor for oxidative stress. Consequently, oxidative stress-induced $\Delta\Psi_m$ loss or dysfunction and damage can cause cellular death by releasing proapoptotic factors and cytochrome *c* into the cytosol (Figs. **2** and **3**). Upon cytochrome *c* translocation into the cytosol, important cascade events in mitochondrial routes are activated that ultimately cause apoptosome generation and caspase cascade activation [70]. Many in-depth investigations have reviewed the crucial roles of the Bcl-2 family of proteins in incrementing mitochondrial permeability *via* selective outer membrane permeabilization or through the PTPC (permeability transition pore complex).

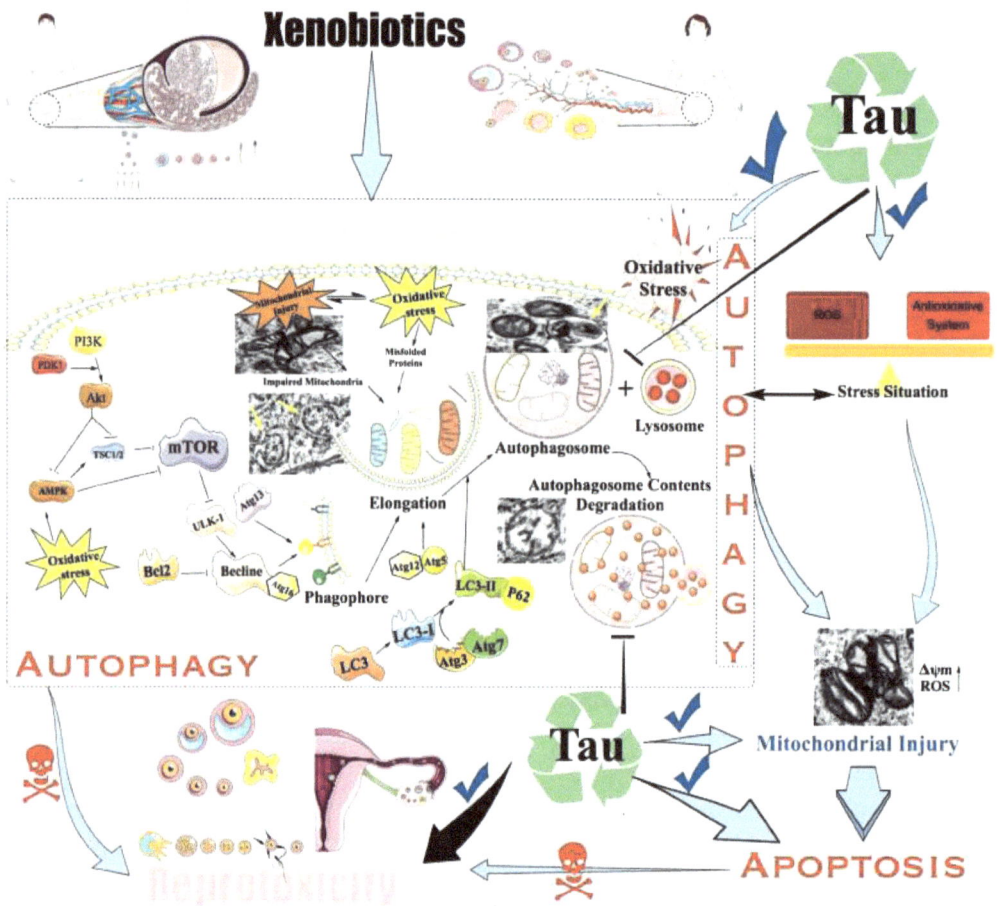

Fig. (2). A flow diagram of the most involved genes in the autophagy cascade route and its interconnection with oxidative stress, mitochondrial impairment, and apoptosis. Taurine (TAU) can mitigate the adverse effects induced by xenobiotics through mitochondrial and non-mitochondrial-related routes. ROS: reactive oxygen species; $\Delta\Psi_m$: mitochondrial membrane potential. The above schematic illustration of autophagy-related genes and proteins is redesigned by a recent publication by authors (DOI: 10.1016/j.ecoenv.2020.110973) [25].

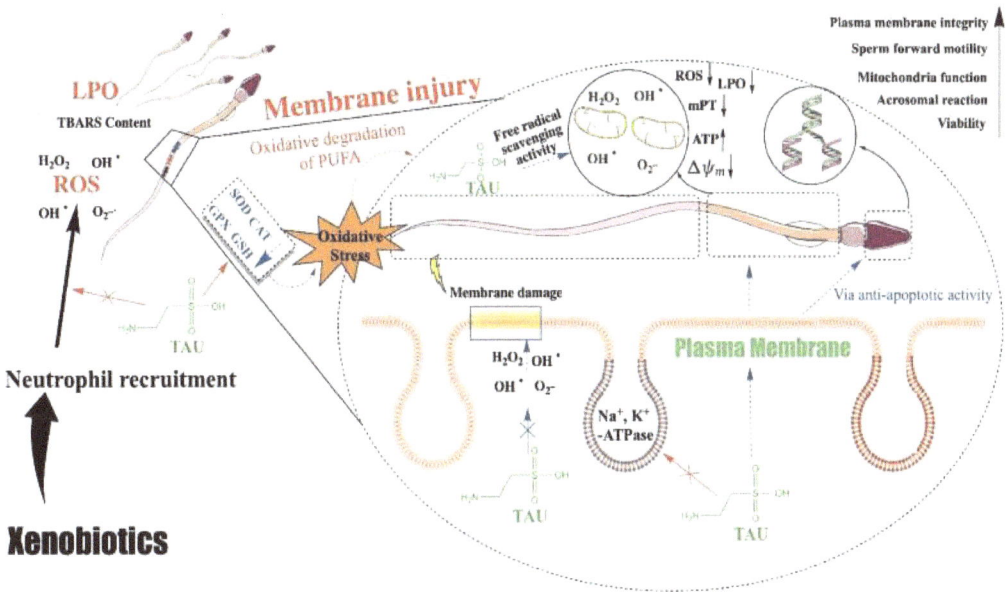

Fig. (3). TAU mitigates xenobiotics-induced oxidative stress *via* mitochondrial-dependent and independent pathways. ROS: reactive oxygen species; LPO: lipid peroxidation; TBARS: thiobarbituric acid-reactive substances; mPT: mitochondrial permeability transition; $\Delta\Psi_m$: mitochondrial membrane potential; ATP: adenosine triphosphate; SOD: superoxide dismutase; CAT: catalase; GPX: glutathione peroxidase; GSH: reduced glutathione.

Two vital anti-apoptotic members of the Bcl-2 family, including Bcl-2 and Bcl-X, can tangibly retard cytochrome c release. In this regard, it has been shown that oxidative stress-mediated alterations in blood biochemical attributes, such as hyperglycemia, considerably instigated apoptosis that may follow the intrinsic mitochondrial routes with the interruption in the balance between pro-apoptotic Bax and antiapoptotic Bcl-2 proteins. This disruption can dramatically reduce the loss of $\Delta\Psi_m$ and subsequently cytochrome c release into the cytosol. This releasement triggers caspase-9 and caspase-3 activation, where caspase-3 instigates apoptosis through activating DNases and cleaving PARP [71 - 73]. In contracts, some important pro-apoptotic members of the Bcl-2 family, including Bid, Bad, and Bik, counteract the cytoprotective effect of Bcl-2 and Bcl- X *via* triggering cytochrome c release [74, 75]. However, Das *et al.* (2009) have reported that heavy metals, such as arsenic, significantly upregulated the Bad expression level and concomitantly downregulated the Bcl-2 expression level, which subsequently led to a reduction in the $\Delta\Psi_m$ and an increment in cytochrome c release, as well as the activation of caspase-3. Finally, they claimed pre-exposure with TAU could effectively mitigate the caspase-3 activation, cytochrome c release, and improved $\Delta\Psi_m$ through the reciprocal regulation of

Bcl-2/Bad. In this regard, Aly and Khafagy (2014) have reported that the spermatozoa $\Delta\Psi_m$ and mitochondrial cytochrome c content were considerably improved in the endosulfan-treated rodents pre-exposed to TAU [39]. Meanwhile, they have also reported that testicular caspases-3, -8, and -9 activities were significantly increased in the male gonads of the treated animals, while TAU imposed considerable protection from endosulfan-induced apoptosis. Hence, it can be concluded that $\Delta\Psi_m$ occurs continually after mitochondrial cytochrome c is released into the cytosol.

This releasement triggers the activation of caspase-8 and then 9. After the activation of caspase-9, caspase-3 is up-regulated, leading to the induction of apoptotic processes [76] (Fig. **4**). Upon exposure to xenobiotics (*i.e.*, endosulfan), it has been shown that caspases- 3 and 9 activities were considerably increased. A cascade-related route should be initiated to activate caspase-8, which triggers caspase-9 activation [77]. Eventually, caspase-3 is stimulated by caspase-8 and 9 activations, inducing apoptosis [78, 79]. Hence, it is primarily expected that these xenobiotics trigger apoptosis in the male gonad through the activation of caspase-8 and 9 (Fig. **4**). However, it has been shown that pre-treatment with TAU could significantly suppress the adverse effects of xenobiotics, leading to the activation of caspases- 3, increased $\Delta\Psi_m$ and the cytochrome c releasement [39] (Fig. **4**).

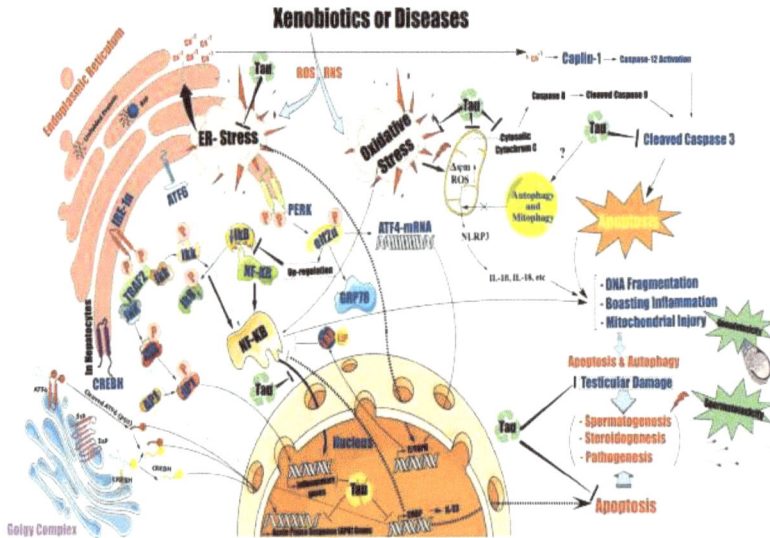

Fig. (4). Schematic representation of the ameliorative effects of taurine (TAU) against xenobiotics or diseases-induced gonadotoxicity and spermatotoxicity through ER-stress-induced acute-phase response and UPR pathways initiating inflammation intermediated by NF-κB or AP-1 and/or *via* the oxidative stress-induced cytochrome c releasement and NF-κB activation. The three UPR signaling arms were investigated, including PERK, IRE1, and ATF6, by ER stress. ROS: reactive oxygen species; RNS: reactive nitrogen species.

In the animals exposed to xenobiotics, it has also been shown that the activities of glucose-6-P-dehydrogenase (G6PDH) and lactate dehydrogenase-X (LDH- X) were notably decreased, causing oxidative stress induction and, consequently, cell death (Fig. **1**). As mentioned earlier, testicular G6PDH is one of the well-known testicular enzymes involved in the hydroxylation of steroidogenesis-related steroids [80] and has a close relationship with the metabolism of GSH; hence, any abnormality in its content and activity can cause oxidative stress in tissue and ultimately may lead to cellular death [81]. However, another good marker for normal metabolism of spermatozoa, LDH-X (located in the inner mitochondrial membrane of spermatogenic cells of developing and mature gonads), has a crucial role in the transportation of cytoplasmic hydrogen to mitochondria with the help of redox coupling α-hydroxy acid/ α-keto acid associated with the metabolism of spermatozoa [69, 82]. Any alteration in their expression is associated with decreased male gametes count, and motility in the animals challenged with toxicants; meanwhile, TAU has been shown to considerably mitigate these decrements in their gene expressions and activations induced by xenobiotics [39].

However, there is a close correlation between immune responses-mediated inflammatory activation routes and apoptosis, as it has been shown that the tumor necrosis factor (TNF)- α /TNF type-I receptor (TNFRI) and Fas ligand (FasL)/Fas receptor (Fas) apoptotic pathways are two well-known and crucial mechanisms controlling the apoptosis initiation in various tissues. Chen *et al.* (2002) have highlighted that one of the critical factors in the host immune response to infection is TNF-α. This vital component can trigger apoptosis by its type-I receptor (p55, TNFRI) [83]. In this regard, it has been shown that serum TNF- α concentration was notably decreased in the arsenic-exposed rats who were pre-treated with TAU.

To investigate the molecular mechanism of the protective effect of TAU against testicular apoptosis caused by toxic metals, such as arsenic, signaling pathways of MAPKs have been investigated. This heavy metal has increased phospho-ERK1/2 and phospho-p38 gene expression, although no significant differences were detected in the total ERK1/2 and p38 gene expression. Literature data reporting a bilateral role, either pro-apoptotic or anti-apoptotic, of NF-kB (as a well-known transcription factor and foremost regulator of stress responses) in male gamete response to xenobiotics-induced injuries [84, 85] (Fig. **4**). Meanwhile, Das *et al.* (2009) have also reported that NF-kB (p65) was significantly upregulated upon exposure to arsenic, emphasizing its pro-apoptotic role in testicular response to this metalloid. Under normal physiological conditions, IκB family inhibitors (*i.e.*, such as IκB- α) maintain NF-kB in an inactive form. IκB- α, by its ankyrin motifs, interacts with NF-kB, covering nuclear localization signals on NF-kB subunits. In pathophysiology anomalies induced by various types of stress, it is reported that upon IκB-α degradation or dissociation caused by phosphorylation, the release of transcriptionally competent NF-kB dimers is hastened. However, it has also been reported that the expressions of IκB-α and NF-kB were significantly downregulated and upregulated after exposure to xenobiotics [63] (Fig. **4**). Another well-characterized kinase promoting cellular survival is Akt. In stress situations induced by toxicants, the phospho-Akt level was significantly decreased. At the same time, TAU could tangibly mitigate the downregulation of phosphor-Akt and up-regulation of phospho-ERK 1/2, phospho-p38, and NF-B (p65).

Based on the above literature, we can conclude that this crucial amino acid improves xenobiotics-induced gonadotoxicity by preventing oxidative- and ER-stress- intermediated inflammatory responses (for more details, see section 10. 6) and apoptotic pathways.

TAURINE AND AUTOPHAGY IN THE REPRODUCTIVE SYSTEM

There are a considerable number of intracellular routes involved in moderating the adverse effects induced by different kinds of stress, including modifications in antioxidant enzymes, metallothioneins formation, heat shock proteins, apoptosis, and autophagy (a bulk degradation event), which are distinguished as crucial defense mechanisms in the cellular adaptation against various types of stress [24, 25]. However, it has been well shown that this evolutionarily conserved catabolic process, autophagy, would also be instigated independently as a unique cell death pathway through numerous xenobiotics, such as environmental stress conditions and diseases.

As a well-known physiological process, autophagy is involved in numerous intracellular and physiological events (*i.e.*, cell death, protein and organelle turnover, and autophagosomal/lysosomal degradation through the lysosomal pathway), among which, more than a few intracellular stimulators can instigate this crucial route, including oxidative and endoplasmic reticulum (ER)-stress, starvation, intracellular injured organelles, and misfolded proteins accumulation, bacterial and viral infections, hypoxia, hyperthermia, aging, cellular energy crisis, mitochondrial impairment, growth factor deficiency, toxic elements, and so on [29]. Some physiologically continuous steps, such as cargo selection and covering, vesicle production, a fusion of vacuole autophagosome, and cargo degradation, are involved in autophagy (Fig. **2**). These steps regulate *via* various autophagy-related (Atg) genes and protein complexes; some of the important ones are evaluated in recent publications of authors, including mammalian target of rapamycin (mTOR), Atg8 (microtubule-associated protein one light-chain, the mammalian homolog of LC3), TSC2, Atg6 (also known as Beclin1), ULK1, Atg

3/ 5/ 12/ 13, PDK1, phosphatidylinositol 3-kinase (PI3K), P62, AKT, and AMPK. A schematic illustration of the autophagy process with a focus on the data published in our current investigations has been presented in Fig. **2**.

Meanwhile, we have just reported the crucial role of this pathway on heavy metals (such as arsenic trioxide (As_2O_3) -induced reproductive toxicity [24, 25, 29] and blood-brain barrier injury [86, 87]. As we have frequently highlighted in recent years, oxidative stress, apoptosis, autophagy, and mitochondrial impairment are closely interconnected [24, 25, 29, 88 - 90]. For this purpose, the detrimental effects of As_2O_3 on vital intracellular mechanisms, such as oxidative stress, mitochondrial impairment, and autophagy in the HPG axis of the F1-male and female generation, have been evaluated by authors [24, 25, 29]. The importance of autophagy in germ cell death, spermatogenesis, and functionality of Sertoli and Leydig cells has been reported [24, 91]. Meanwhile, specific autophagic-related proteins, such as Beclin1, p62, Atg5, Atg16, LC3, PINK1, mTOR, and AMPKα 1/2, present in human male gametes, have been reported [92].

Polycystic ovary syndrome (PCOS) is well-known for connecting the endocrine system and metabolic disorders in females. This syndrome has become incalculably predominant among females of fertile age. The female gonad is the primary organ affected by PCOS. It has been shown that any anomalies or dysfunctionality in this vital organ induced by this syndrome can cause irreparable damage to the female reproductive system. The past decade has authenticated observations that macroautophagy/autophagy has a crucial responsibility in the female gonads from the beginning of the formation of oocytes until the time of the final Graafian follicle's ovulation and fertilization. However, progress in the field has revealed a considerable role of autophagy in PCOS-induced pathogenesis. Meanwhile, defective autophagy in the female gametes during foliculogenesis is recorded in the PCOS ovary. Hence, we can assume that surveying various cascade events of the autophagy route can prepare a platform for forecasting the possible reason for changed ovarian physiology in patients suffering from PCOS [93].

However, it should be highlighted that depending on the different stress conditions (*i.e.*, chronic or acute phases, doses, or concentrations of xenobiotics), the dual role of autophagy as a double-edged sword is well reported. For example, Yahyavy *et al.* (2020) have reported that the expressions of autophagy-related genes and the percentage of LC3-II-positive cells were considerably increased in the TM3 cells exposed to TAU (100 μg/mL) and consequently decreased oxidative stress [94]. Their results also showed that TAU, in the presence of an autophagy inhibitor (3-Methyladenine), tangibly increased oxidative stress and consequently reduced the concentration of testosterone [94]. Hence, they concluded that this bulk degradation event could be involved in the increment of testosterone level of the mice Leydig TM3 cells exposed to TAU through the decrement of oxidative stress.

In recent years, the growing use of TAU (a wide-distributed cytoprotective amino acid with high potential antioxidant properties) raises many important questions regarding its possible therapeutic role in organs, tissues, and cells through mitigating factors such as the autophagy-induced adverse effect on the reproductive system. A great body of literature has demonstrated that numerous xenobiotics can considerably induce adverse effects on the reproductive system through autophagy. For instance, the reprotoxic, embryotoxic, neurotoxic, carcinogenic, nephrotoxic, teratogenic, hepatotoxic, and immunotoxic effects of ochratoxin A (OTA; one of the most harmful mycotoxins) in laboratory and farm animals, as well as in humans, has been well reported. Meanwhile, the endocrine disruptor role of OTS (a biologically probable cause of male gonad cancer in humans), with reducing capabilities of male gametes quality and gonadotoxicity, has been shown. However, it has also been reported that OTA (4.0–8.0 μM) can instigate autophagy through the upregulation of LC3-II protein expression and fluorescence intensity of GFP-LC3 dots. They have also said that upon exposure to TAU, OTA-induced autophagy was mitigated through the decrement of LC3-II expression and fluorescence intensity of GFP-LC3 dots, resulting in the maintenance of cellular homeostasis. In another study, Li *et al.* (2019) reported that Di-(2-Ethylhexyl) phthalate (DEHP; as an environmental endocrine disruptor) could cause reprotoxicity [95]. They have also shown that this toxic element can trigger apoptosis in INS-1 cells through autophagy and oxidative stress. Meanwhile, they reported that TAU could considerably decrease DEHP-mediated excessive autophagy.

TAURINE MITIGATES OXIDATIVE STRESS *VIA* MITOCHONDRIAL-DEPENDENT AND INDEPENDENT PATHWAYS: WITH AN EYE TO STEROIDOGENESIS AND SPERMATOGENESIS

Xenobiotics are well-known reprotoxicity inducers. It is shown that oxidative stress induced by xenobiotics is a potential causative factor in interpreting male and female reproductive failure [22 - 25, 33, 96, 97]. We have frequently presented that male gametes can be susceptible to oxidative stress and subsequent adverse cellular events due to the high amount of PUFA and low antioxidant capacity [21, 29, 32, 33, 98]. Based on the above literature, over-generated ROS is associated with impaired spermatogenesis and steroidogenesis. Various forms of ROS, including oxygen free radicals (*i.e.*, hydroxyl, superoxide, alkoxyl, peroxyl, and hydro-peroxyl radicals), cause testicular injury through multiple mechanisms, such as depletion of thiols groups, peroxidation of lipids, oxidation of proteins, and DNA injury. Peroxidation of lipids (a kind of oxidative degradation of PUFA) which is indicated by thiobarbituric acid-reactive substances (TBARS) content, has been interconnected with alterations in spermatozoa membrane integrity, enzyme inactivation [21, 32, 99] (Fig. **3**). As evident from many investigations, alterations in lipid peroxidation are complemented by either decrement in the antioxidant enzymes activities (*i.e.*, superoxide dismutase (SOD), catalase (CAT), and glutathione peroxidase (GPX)) or the reduced glutathione (GSH) levels. CAT and GPX are protected by SOD against superoxide anion. SOD protects CAT and GPX against superoxide anion. The equilibrium of this enzyme system is crucial to dispose of the peroxides and superoxide anion produced in the male gonad [100]. Hence, any reduction in the mentioned enzyme activities, concomitant with an increment in lipid peroxidation rate, could reflect the detrimental effects of various xenobiotics on the testicular and ovarian antioxidant systems (Fig. **3**).

Furthermore, GSH content positively correlates with xenobiotics' detoxification and the cellular antioxidant power against ROS and other free radicals. However, this crucial compound is vital in cellular redox state regulation, and any decrement in its cellular content can be indicated by oxidative stress [88, 101 - 105] (Fig. **3**). Interestingly, recent studies have delineated that TAU can considerably reverse all these deleterious effects and consequent oxidative stress-correlated alterations induced by xenobiotics (Fig. **3**). Cozzi *et al.* (1995) reported that these ameliorative effects of TAU as a potent antioxidant in organ injuries had been related to its specific features by scavenging ROS and stabilizing biological membranes [106]. However, many investigations have shown that TAU can present its protective role through its direct or indirect antioxidative activities as follow:

Direct Antioxidant: TAU can quench and detoxify several reactive intermediates, including hydroxyl radical ($\cdot$OH) [3], H_2O_2 [106], and nitric oxide [61]. However, many recent studies questioned the direct radical scavenging properties of TAU.

Indirect Antioxidant: TAU can prevent the alterations in mitochondrial indices such as membrane permeabilization and dissipation of $\Delta\Psi_m$ induced by oxidative stress [107 - 117].

Literature data demonstrated that xenobiotics can trigger apoptosis in gonads of the various species through the activation of caspase-3 and regulation of Bcl-2/Bad along with the reduction of mitochondrial functionality and subsequent increased level of cytosolic cytochrome *c*. They can alter the activation of LC3-I and II, Beclin1, Atg3, Atg5, Atg12, Atg13, mTOR, AMPK, PI3K, AKT, PDK1, TSC2, ULK1, P62, and NF-B (p65) in male and female gonads [24, 25, 29, 63].

Furthermore, we have recently observed oxidative stress and mitochondrial impairment fingerprints in xenobiotics-induced (heavy and toxic metals) testosterone release suppression in pubertal and mature mice through the downregulation of 3β-HSD, StAR, 17β-HSD, and CYP11a expression. Similar to our observations, Das *et al.* (2009) have also reported that heavy metals (*i.e.*, $NaAsO_2$) can considerably decrease testicular Δ^5-3ß-HSD and 17ß-HSD activities and subsequently decrease the plasma testosterone, testicular sperm count, and sperm motility through the increased level of ROS, serum TNF-α, TBARS content, and reduced activities of the antioxidant enzymes and glutathione in male gonads. However, as mentioned earlier by the authors, oxidative stress and subsequent events, such as mitochondrial impairments, seem to be crucial routes involved in the pathogenesis of male and female reprotoxicity with different etiologies [22 - 25, 27]. Until the recent decade, there have been relatively reasonable investigations on the influence of crucial antioxidants as promising preventive or curative elements that can be applied as therapeutic tools in testicular anomalies. Among the various available antioxidants, this free ß-amino acid, TAU, might be considered an influential candidate in this regard. Murugesan and colleagues (2008) have shown that a marked decrease in the activity of testicular androgenic enzymes and, subsequently, decrement in serum testosterone might be due to the increased contents of ROS and TBARS [118]. Additionally, it mentioned that the poor steroidogenesis might be due to a degeneration of the gonad and or activation of apoptosis in the LCs of animals exposed to xenobiotics [119]. Although, it showed that pre-exposure to TAU could considerably normalize the activities of testicular steroidogenic enzymes and consequent blood testosterone level [39].

Furthermore, this conditional amino acid has been recognized as the major free amino acid in the male reproductive system [18]. It has also been well shown that TAU can act as an antioxidant in mitigating gametes lipid peroxidation [120], as a capacitating agent [8, 50], maintaining sperm chromatin integrity (through directly scavenging ROS and ultimately inhibiting DNA damage) [39], and or as a potent factor stimulating sperm motility (Fraser, 1986; Boatman *et al.*, 1990) (Fig. **3**). However, it has been proved that TAU exposure proficiently restored DNA from oxidative damage *via* its anti-apoptotic activity [121] (Fig. **3**).

It has also been reported that TAU can alter the activity of phospholipid methyl transferase in golden hamster spermatozoa [122]. The crucial role of TAU and hTAU as potent inhibitors for plasma membrane Na^+, K^+-ATPase in membrane homogenates of epididymal sperm cells has also been reported by Mrsny and Meizel (1985). They concluded that these compounds could considerably sustain sperm motility and fertility in hamsters [123] (Fig. **3**). Previous investigations have also mentioned the effects of TAU on mitochondrial-dependent apoptosis and its relevance to reproductive toxicity. For instance, Das *et al.* (2009) claimed that TAU significantly improved the decreased testicular weight, sperm concentration, motility, activity of 3β-HSD and 17β-HSD, as well as plasma testosterone level in arsenic-treated rats. Meanwhile, they have illustrated that this amino acid, concomitant with an increase in antioxidant enzyme activities, the ratio of GSH/GSSG, and intracellular total antioxidant capacity, considerably mitigates the generation of ROS, protein carbonylation, and TBARS content in these challenged rats. Finally, they presented that TAU had an ameliorative role in male gametes through oxidative stress-associated alterations, mitochondrial-dependent, and independent apoptosis in the rats exposed to $NaAsO_2$. As previously referred to, neutrophils are well-known cells involved in the generation of ROS [57], and different testicular generation of these free radicals is accountable for testicular damage (*i.e.*, after testicular torsion-detorsion) [54]. Hence, it is assumed that TAU probably presents an extra valuable effect by reducing neutrophil recruitment and ROS generation (Fig. **3**). Meanwhile, a significant part of the positive effects of TAU on the male and/or female reproductive system could be mediated through the results of this amino acid on cellular mitochondria (Figs. **1** - **4**).

It has been shown that TAU tangibly mitigated ROS formation, oxidative stress, and the malondialdehyde level (TBARS content) in the testis tissue [15]. Similar to these observations, it has been reported that TAU effectively mitigated the oxidative stress induction stimulated by endosulfan as evidenced by a decrement in H_2O_2 level and TBARS content and increment in the antioxidant enzymes, such as CAT, SOD, and GPX activities and GSH content [39]. Hence, it can be assumed that TAU can mitigate oxidative stress and apoptosis through vital mechanisms of both mitochondria and non-mitochondrial pathways. Based on the above literature, the highlighted points provide insight into the mode of action of the xenobiotics-induced reprotoxicity and, concomitantly, the beneficial effects provided by TAU to counteract xenobiotics-induced oxidative stress, autophagy, and apoptosis in the male and female gonads and also to restore the suppressed spermatogenesis and steroidogenesis, so verifying to be a highly potent cytoprotective agent.

Xenobiotics-induced ER Stress and Mitochondrial Dysfunctionality Instigates Inflammation: The Ameliorative Role of Taurine

As mentioned in the previous sections, any reduction in antioxidant levels and/or anomalous increase in ROS levels can cause severe cellular damage in reproductive and non-reproductive tissues through activating ER-stress, devastating normal mitochondrial function, interrupting the DNA, and boosting inflammation *via* triggering of NF-κB, and other vital inflammatory-related indices. Mapping the relations between mitochondria, metabolism, and inflammation has been an exciting topic for many researchers, as a failure of this network is correlated to numerous chronic inflammatory disorders. Dysfunctional mitochondria produce ROS, necessitating inflammasome activation through NLRP3 inflammasome [124].

The injured organelles trigger unique signals to stimulate the apoptotic and autophagic signaling-related routes as an outcome of oxidative- and ER-stress [24, 25, 29, 72, 125 - 127]. For instance, it has been shown that the NLRP3 inflammasome is adversely regulated by autophagy (a catabolic cascade that eliminates injured or dysfunctional organelles, such as mitochondria (called mitophagy) [124]. In this regard, Tschopp (2011) has reported that rotenone could significantly trigger mitochondrial ROS formation, NLRP3 inflammasome activation, and IL-1β and IL-18 secretion (Fig. **4**). Therefore, ROS-producing mitochondria are regularly eliminated through mitophagy to prevent cellular damage. To the best of the authors, no comprehensive investigation of TAU's ameliorative role on the male and female reproductive system through mitophagy activation has been performed. Hence, a new research window is felt in future investigations (Fig. **4**).

However, the past decade has witnessed many interpretations deciphering the role of oxidative-, ER- stress, NF-κB, and crucial inflammatory cytokines facilitating inflammation, apoptosis, and autophagy in the induction of testicular damage (by evaluating spermatogenesis, steroidogenesis, and pathogenesis) through mitochondrial and non-mitochondrial related routes [24, 25, 29, 36, 128]. Various xenobiotics could considerably lead to the formation of ROS [23, 26, 32, 33, 88, 97, 129 - 135] and reactive nitrogen species [RNS] in reproductive organs that hasten cellular oxidative- and ER-stress [121].

A review of the published literature showed that stress in the ER could activate some crucial routes depending on the intensity of the pressure (for instance, the activation of various inflammatory processes [including the acute-phase response (APR) and the process initiated by transcriptional factors (*i.e.*, NF-kB and activator protein-1 (AP-1))] and unfolded protein response [UPR] signaling routes), ultimately affecting the cell fate. However, as mentioned, inflammatory responses initiated by ER stress are correlated with several xenobiotics and diseases. Therefore, therapeutic targeting of ER-mediated inflammation is challenging; and could be considered for medicinal purposes. On the other hand, the importance of immune cells in ER stress is well understood [136 - 138]. Therefore, it is not astonishing that in the tissues exposed to ER stress, communication between the stressed cells and other cells (*i.e.*, immune cells) in that tissue does not occur rapidly. The ER stress-instigated communication mainly causes inflammatory responses contributing to the control of tissue injuries and/or in the recovery of tissues. Nevertheless, ER stress-induced inflammation could lead to the pathological condition's progression under particular circumstances, such as gonadotoxicity (Fig. **4**).

In the past decade, investigations have documented that ER stress-induced UPR signaling routes are interconnected with the biosynthesis of numerous pro-inflammatory molecules (*i.e.*, MCP-1, IL-6, IL 8, and TNF-α) [139]. Recent investigations have reported that all three vital branches of the UPR, including those deriving from ATF6, IRE1α, and PERK, can mediate related signaling routes which eventually trigger a pro-inflammatory transcriptional program that in numerous cases is controlled by the transcription factors, such as NF-κB and AP-1 (Fig. **4**) [140 - 142]. Meanwhile, it has also shown that all three UPR branches can govern the activation of NF-κB; however, they claimed that the same is not valid for AP-1. Furthermore, they also presented that apart from pro-inflammatory programs based on individual transcription factors, UPR-related routes might cause the highly intricate inflammatory process identified as APR [143]. Hence, there are several mechanisms through which UPR signaling induced by ER stress leads to the activation of NF-κB, AP-1, and APR [136] (Fig. **4**).

Over the years, more scholarly reports have explained that all these three UPR signaling branches deriving from the UPR sensors (such as PERK, IRE1α, and ATF6) can be considerably upregulated and then activated NF-κB [140, 141] (Fig. **4**). Furthermore, except for the UPR, other routes are involved in triggering ER-stress (including oxidative stress) concomitant with a promotion in the NF-κB activation, resulting in the collection of misfolded proteins and/or leakage of ER-Ca^{+2} into the cytosol [141]. However, as illustrated in Fig. (**4**), there is an inhibitory effect on the expression of IκB by the activation of the PERK-eIF2α arm of the UPR, resulting in an increment of the NF-κB to IκB ratio and the subsequent release of the NF-κB protein to carry out its transcriptional role in the nucleus (Fig. **4**) [144].

There is a relation between the UPR signaling pathway and activation of the pro-inflammatory cytokine, like IL-23; where it has been shown that except for NF-κB activation (through ATF4 route), another PERK-eIF2α arm of the UPR-activated transcription factor (*e.g.*, CHOP) can instigate the activation of IL-23 (Fig. **4**) [145]. However, there is a piece of contradictory evidence demonstrating that ER-stress-activated CHOP can adversely regulate inflammatory-related responses through alteration in the expression and activation of NF-κB and JNK (applicable to AP-1) (Fig. **4**) [146]. Hence, it can be assumed that the PERK branch of UPR is dichotomous in regulating inflammation; for instance, it can activate, suppress, and control the inflammatory process.

However, there is an affinity for IRE1α to bind with tumor-necrosis factor-α (TNF-α)-receptor-associated factor 2 (TRAF2). Ultimately this new complex, IRE1α-TRAF2, can recruit IκB kinase (IKK) (Fig. **4**). Afterward, IκB could be degraded by the activation of IKK, freeing NF-κB [147, 148]. Ultimately, another branch of UPR, called ATF6, can be involved in the activation of NF-κB (Fig. **4**) [140, 149]. A solid body of evidence supports that xenobiotics-induced ER-stress can activate NF-κB through the ATF6 branch [149]. To sum up, upon exposure to xenobiotics, all three UPR branches can instigate the activation of NF-κB in different routes. However, xenobiotics-triggered ER-stress caused a transient up-regulation of the transcription factor C/EBPβ, resulting in a constant accumulation of its translational products (*i.e.*, liver activating protein (LAP) and liver-enriched inhibitory protein (LIP)) (Fig. **4**) [149]. Consequently, these two mentioned translational products (LAP-LIP) could act as an automatic brake on the path of inflammation by decreasing the functionality of NF-κB (Fig. **4**) [150].

The APR is a cluster of physiological routes occurring upon the instigation of inflammation, trauma, infection, and other malignant circumstances- induced innate immune response (through the activation of numerous pro-inflammatory elements, such as IL-1, IL-6, and TNF-α). Two crucial molecules are involved in the signaling-induced ER-stress-intermediated APR named ATF6 and cyclic-AMP-responsive-element-binding protein H (CREBH). However, it should be highlighted that CREBH is only expressed in hepatocytes [141]. Under ER-stress circumstances, ATF6 and CREBH instigate a new route titled regulated intramembrane proteolysis (RIP) (Fig. **4**), where transcription factors (ATF6 and CREBH) move from the ER to the Golgi complex and then cleave into their functional isoforms, mainly by S_1P and S_2P proteases (Fig. **4**) [141, 151]. The stimulated fragments of ATF6 and CREBH, their active isoforms, translocate into the nucleus to form APR-associated genes' transcription (Fig. **4**). Once again, the authors are going to highlight that CREBH-mediated APR derives principally from liver cells. However, due to the importance of the issue and the crucial role of this path in this process, it is mentioned in this section.

Emerging evidence from the literature supports the promising therapeutic role of natural antioxidants, such as carnosine, Kombucha, *Phyllanthus niruri* protein, melatonin, curcumin, mangiferin, genistein, *Terminalia arjuna*, morin, and TAU, against a broad spectrum of anomalies induced by xenobiotics through cellular-related routes (such as inflammatory signaling cascades, as described in details above([72, 152 - 164]. Taurine exerts its ameliorative effects primarily *via* its antioxidative and anti-inflammatory features [165]. Meanwhile, the ameliorative role of TAU on xenobiotics-triggered inflammatory responses through the activation of NF-κB has been well reported in the literature and presented briefly below [121, 166].

It has been shown that TAU significantly facilitated the translocation of the NF-κB into the nucleus, thereby inhibiting NF-κB mediated inflammatory response. Multiple lines of research have revealed that ROS can increase NF-κB-mediated inflammation accompanied by the increment levels of the pro-inflammatory cytokines, chemokines, and adhesion molecules [72]. For instance, Ghosh *et al.* [121] have shown that TAU exposure (100 mg kg^{-1} body weight) for 42 consecutive days after diabetic induction by STZ (50 mg kg^{-1} body weight, i.p., once) significantly improved diabetes-induced adverse effects related to reproductive dysfunction through intricate molecular mechanisms, including decreased ER-stress induction through down-regulation of calpain-1 and caspase-12, as well as CHOP and GRP78 *via* eIF2α signaling, inhibition of NF-κB - translocation in the nucleus (caused a substantial decrement in the levels of the inflammatory cytokines), mitigation of the mitochondria-related apoptotic routes and consequent DNA fragmentation (Fig. **4**). They have reported that the up-regulated genes of TNF- α, IL-1β, IL-6, MCP-1, ICAM-1, and VCAM-1 in the STZ-induced diabetic animals were considerably decreased upon exposure to TAU through its powerful anti-inflammatory features. However, as mentioned earlier, there is a close relation between ER stress and apoptotic death of testicular cells [36, 121, 167]. ER stress triggers PERK activation by its phosphorylation, which triggers the activation of eIF2α. The up-regulation of eIF2α can activate a downstream molecule called CHOP. On the other hand, PERK can increase the releasement of the GRP78 resulting in a UPR activation [167]. It has been shown that the accumulation of intracellular Ca^{2+} can activate calpain-1 resulting in caspase-12 activation (Fig. **4**) [36]. In this regard, it has been shown that diabetic rats showed a considerable up-regulation in p-PERK, p-eIF2α, GRP78, calpain-1, cleaved caspase-12, and CHOP genes expression, where treatment with TAU tangibly mitigated such alterations, thereby preventing oxidative- and ER-stres--mediated testicular apoptotic and autophagic death (Fig. **4**). Hence, this potential therapeutic agent can cause a preventive role in oxidative and ER-stress-related indices mediated xenobiotics-induced testicular complications through the mitochondrial and non-mitochondrial related routes.

To sum up, it can be concluded that TAU has a high potential to present protection against xenobiotics-induced reprotoxicity through oxidative stress (changes in the levels of the antioxidant enzymes), ER-stress (UPR and acute-phase response pathways), and consequently inflammation (NF-κB signaling cascade), as well as apoptosis mediated damage through improving the status of the markers of testicular injury, controlling intracellular redox balance, preventing inflammatory-related responses, and finally oxidative and ER-stress stimulated mitochondrial-dependent apoptotic route (Fig. **4**).

CONCLUSION

The current chapter demonstrated that xenobiotics have a high potential to induce reproductive toxicity by altering the expression levels of some vital autophagic, apoptotic, inflammatory, oxidative/endoplasmic stress-related genes and proteins *via* mitochondrial and non-mitochondrial-associated routes. Furthermore, it has been shown that xenobiotics induced pyroptotic cell death through the activation of the NLRP3 inflammasome. Moreover, we mentioned that xenobiotics-triggered autophagy was implicated in the heavy metals-induced NLRP3 inflammasome activation and pyroptotic cell death. Finally, based on the literature, we claimed that TAU could considerably mitigate xenobiotics-mediated inflammation and pyroptosis *via* the autophagic- inflammasomal pathway. Hence, all mentioned adverse effects could be reversed by TAU. This chapter provides a novel insight into xenobiotics-induced reprotoxicity and the potential molecular mechanism by which TAU causes ameliorative effects. The knowledge of this chapter might be applied to enhance therapeutic strategies by TAU against xenobiotics-mediated reproductive toxicity through mitochondrial-related routes.

REFERENCES

[1]   Van der Horst C. Hypotaurine in the reproductive tract Natural Sulfur Compounds. Springer 1980; pp. 225-34.
[http://dx.doi.org/10.1007/978-1-4613-3045-5_19]

[2]   Fellman JH, Roth ES. The biological oxidation of hypotaurine to taurine: hypotaurine as an antioxidant. Prog Clin Biol Res 1985; 179: 71-82.
[PMID: 2997795]

[3]   Aruoma OI, Halliwell B, Hoey BM, Butler J. The antioxidant action of taurine, hypotaurine and their metabolic precursors. Biochem J 1988; 256(1): 251-5.
[http://dx.doi.org/10.1042/bj2560251] [PMID: 2851980]

[4]   Holmes RP, Goodman HO, Shihabi ZK, Jarow JP. The taurine and hypotaurine content of human semen. J Androl 1992; 13(3): 289-92.
[PMID: 1601750]

[5]   Jacobsen JG, Smith LH. Biochemistry and physiology of taurine and taurine derivatives. Physiol Rev 1968; 48(2): 424-511.
[http://dx.doi.org/10.1152/physrev.1968.48.2.424] [PMID: 4297098]

[6]   Sturman JA, Hayes KC. The biology of taurine in nutrition and development Adv Nutr Res. Springer 1980; pp. 231-99.

[7]   Wright CE, Tallan HH, Lin YY, Gaull GE. Taurine: biological update. Annu Rev Biochem 1986; 55(1): 427-53.
[http://dx.doi.org/10.1146/annurev.bi.55.070186.002235] [PMID: 3527049]

[8]   Meizel S, Lui CW, Working PK, Mrsny RJ. Taurine and hypotaurine: their effects on motility, capacitation and the acrosome reaction of hamster sperm *in vitro* and their presence in sperm and reproductive tract fluids of several mammals. Dev Growth Differ 1980; 22(3): 483-94.
[http://dx.doi.org/10.1111/j.1440-169X.1980.00483.x]

[9]   Velázquez A, Delgado NM, Rosado A. Taurine content and amino acid composition of human acrosome. Life Sci 1986; 38(11): 991-5.

[http://dx.doi.org/10.1016/0024-3205(86)90232-8] [PMID: 3081776]

[10] Casslén BG. Free amino acids in human uterine fluid. Possible role of high taurine concentration. J Reprod Med 1987; 32(3): 181-4.
[PMID: 3572897]

[11] Van Der Horst CJG, Brand A. Occurrence of hypotaurine and inositol in the reproductive tract of the ewe and its regulation by pregnenolone and progesterone. Nature 1969; 223(5201): 67-8.
[http://dx.doi.org/10.1038/223067a0] [PMID: 5792431]

[12] Van der Horst CJG, Grooten HJG. The occurrence of hypotaurine and other sulfur-containing amino acids in seminal plasma and spermatozoa of boar, bull and dog. Biochim Biophys Acta, Gen Subj 1966; 117(2): 495-7.
[http://dx.doi.org/10.1016/0304-4165(66)90107-3] [PMID: 6006677]

[13] Johnson LA, Pursel VG, Gerrits RJ, Thomas CH. Free amino acid composition of porcine seminal, epididymal and seminal vesicle fluids. J Anim Sci 1972; 34(3): 430-4.
[http://dx.doi.org/10.2527/jas1972.343430x] [PMID: 5010631]

[14] Kochakian CD. Free amino acids of sex organs of the mouse: regulation by androgen. Am J Physiol 1975; 228(4): 1231-5.
[http://dx.doi.org/10.1152/ajplegacy.1975.228.4.1231] [PMID: 1169001]

[15] Wei SM, Yan ZZ, Zhou J. Beneficial effect of taurine on testicular ischemia-reperfusion injury in rats. Urology 2007; 70(6): 1237-42.
[http://dx.doi.org/10.1016/j.urology.2007.09.030] [PMID: 18158068]

[16] Devreker F, Van den Bergh M, Biramane J, Winston RL, Englert Y, Hardy K. Effects of taurine on human embryo development *in vitro*. Hum Reprod 1999; 14(9): 2350-6.
[http://dx.doi.org/10.1093/humrep/14.9.2350] [PMID: 10469709]

[17] Amidi F, Pazhohan A, Shabani Nashtaei M, Khodarahmian M, Nekoonam S. The role of antioxidants in sperm freezing: a review. Cell Tissue Bank 2016; 17(4): 745-56.
[http://dx.doi.org/10.1007/s10561-016-9566-5] [PMID: 27342905]

[18] Lobo MVT, Alonso FJM, del Río RM. Immunohistochemical localization of taurine in the male reproductive organs of the rat. J Histochem Cytochem 2000; 48(3): 313-20.
[http://dx.doi.org/10.1177/002215540004800301] [PMID: 10681385]

[19] Li JH, Ling YQ, Fan JJ, Zhang XP, Cui S. Expression of cysteine sulfinate decarboxylase (CSD) in male reproductive organs of mice. Histochem Cell Biol 2006; 125(6): 607-13.
[http://dx.doi.org/10.1007/s00418-005-0095-8] [PMID: 16252094]

[20] Huxtable RJ. Physiological actions of taurine. Physiol Rev 1992; 72(1): 101-63.
[http://dx.doi.org/10.1152/physrev.1992.72.1.101] [PMID: 1731369]

[21] Ommati MM, Zamiri MJ, Akhlaghi A, *et al.* Seminal characteristics, sperm fatty acids, and blood biochemical attributes in breeder roosters orally administered with sage (*Salvia officinalis*) extract. Anim Prod Sci 2013; 53(6): 548-54.
[http://dx.doi.org/10.1071/AN12257]

[22] Ommati MM, Heidari R. Amino acids ameliorate heavy metals-induced oxidative stress in male/female reproductive tissue Toxicology. Elsevier 2021; pp. 371-86.

[23] Ommati MM, Arabnezhad MR, Farshad O, *et al.* The role of mitochondrial impairment and oxidative stress in the pathogenesis of lithium-induced reproductive toxicity in male mice. Front Vet Sci 2021; 8(125): 603262.
[http://dx.doi.org/10.3389/fvets.2021.603262] [PMID: 33842567]

[24] Ommati MM, Manthari RK, Tikka C, *et al.* Arsenic-induced autophagic alterations and mitochondrial impairments in HPG-S axis of mature male mice offspring (F1-generation): A persistent toxicity study. Toxicol Lett 2020; 326: 83-98.
[http://dx.doi.org/10.1016/j.toxlet.2020.02.013] [PMID: 32112876]

[25] Ommati MM, Shi X, Li H, *et al.* The mechanisms of arsenic-induced ovotoxicity, ultrastructural alterations, and autophagic related paths: An enduring developmental study in folliculogenesis of mice. Ecotoxicol Environ Saf 2020; 204: 110973.
[http://dx.doi.org/10.1016/j.ecoenv.2020.110973] [PMID: 32781346]

[26] Farshad O, Heidari R, Zamiri MJ, *et al.* Spermatotoxic Effects of Single-Walled and Multi-Walled Carbon Nanotubes on Male Mice. Front Vet Sci 2020; 7(1007): 591558.
[http://dx.doi.org/10.3389/fvets.2020.591558] [PMID: 33392285]

[27] Ommati MM, Farshad O, Niknahad H, *et al.* Cholestasis-associated reproductive toxicity in male and female rats: The fundamental role of mitochondrial impairment and oxidative stress. Toxicol Lett 2019; 316: 60-72.
[http://dx.doi.org/10.1016/j.toxlet.2019.09.009] [PMID: 31520699]

[28] Ommati MM, Heidari R, Zamiri MJ, Sabouri S, Zaker L, Farshad O, *et al.* The footprints of oxidative stress and mitochondrial impairment in arsenic trioxide-induced testosterone release suppression in pubertal and Mature F1-male Balb/c Mice *via* the Downregulation of 3β-HSD, 17β-HSD, and CYP11a Expression. Biol Trace Elem Res. 2019: 1-10.

[29] Ommati MM, Heidari R, Manthari RK, *et al.* Paternal exposure to arsenic resulted in oxidative stress, autophagy, and mitochondrial impairments in the HPG axis of pubertal male offspring. Chemosphere 2019; 236: 124325.
[http://dx.doi.org/10.1016/j.chemosphere.2019.07.056] [PMID: 31326754]

[30] Aitken RJ, Clarkson JS, Hargreave TB, Irvine DS, Wu FCW. Analysis of the relationship between defective sperm function and the generation of reactive oxygen species in cases of oligozoospermia. J Androl 1989; 10(3): 214-20.
[http://dx.doi.org/10.1002/j.1939-4640.1989.tb00091.x] [PMID: 2501260]

[31] Solano F, Hernández E, Juárez-Rojas L, *et al.* Reproductive disruption in adult female and male rats prenatally exposed to mesquite pod extract or daidzein. Reprod Biol 2022; 22(3): 100683.
[http://dx.doi.org/10.1016/j.repbio.2022.100683] [PMID: 35932513]

[32] Ommati MM, Heidari R, Jamshidzadeh A, *et al.* Dual effects of sulfasalazine on rat sperm characteristics, spermatogenesis, and steroidogenesis in two experimental models. Toxicol Lett 2018; 284: 46-55.
[http://dx.doi.org/10.1016/j.toxlet.2017.11.034] [PMID: 29197623]

[33] Ommati MM, Jamshidzadeh A, Heidari R, *et al.* Carnosine and histidine supplementation blunt lead-induced reproductive toxicity through antioxidative and mitochondria-dependent mechanisms. Biol Trace Elem Res 2019; 187(1): 151-62.
[http://dx.doi.org/10.1007/s12011-018-1358-2] [PMID: 29767280]

[34] Yu Y, Han Y, Niu R, *et al.* Ameliorative effect of VE, IGF-I, and hCG on the fluoride-induced testosterone release suppression in mice Leydig cells. Biol Trace Elem Res 2018; 181(1): 95-103.
[http://dx.doi.org/10.1007/s12011-017-1023-1] [PMID: 28462439]

[35] Sun Z, Li S, Yu Y, *et al.* Alterations in epididymal proteomics and antioxidant activity of mice exposed to fluoride. Arch Toxicol 2018; 92(1): 169-80.
[http://dx.doi.org/10.1007/s00204-017-2054-2] [PMID: 28918527]

[36] Rashid K, Sil PC. Curcumin enhances recovery of pancreatic islets from cellular stress induced inflammation and apoptosis in diabetic rats. Toxicol Appl Pharmacol 2015; 282(3): 297-310.
[http://dx.doi.org/10.1016/j.taap.2014.12.003] [PMID: 25541178]

[37] Katoh C, Kitajima S, Saga Y, Kanno J, Horii I, Inoue T. Assessment of quantitative dual-parameter flow cytometric analysis for the evaluation of testicular toxicity using cyclophosphamide- and ethinylestradiol-treated rats. J Toxicol Sci 2002; 27(2): 87-96.
[http://dx.doi.org/10.2131/jts.27.87] [PMID: 12058451]

[38] Prahalathan C, Selvakumar E, Varalakshmi P. Remedial effect of DL- -lipoic acid against adriamycin

induced testicular lipid peroxidation. Mol Cell Biochem 2004; 267(1/2): 209-14.
[http://dx.doi.org/10.1023/B:MCBI.0000049385.13773.23] [PMID: 15663203]

[39]　Aly HAA, Khafagy RM. Taurine reverses endosulfan-induced oxidative stress and apoptosis in adult rat testis. Food Chem Toxicol 2014; 64: 1-9.
[http://dx.doi.org/10.1016/j.fct.2013.11.007] [PMID: 24262488]

[40]　Sexton TJ. Oxidative metabolism of chicken semen and washed spermatozoa in the presence of various steroid hormones. Comp Biochem Physiol B 1974; 47(4): 799-804.
[http://dx.doi.org/10.1016/0305-0491(74)90025-X] [PMID: 4833557]

[41]　Ommati MM, Heidari R, Zamiri MJ, Shojaee S, Akhlaghi A, Sabouri S. Association of open field behavior with blood and semen characteristics in roosters: an alternative animal model. Rev Int Androl 2018; 16(2): 50-8.
[http://dx.doi.org/10.1016/j.androl.2017.02.002] [PMID: 30300125]

[42]　Cecil HC, Bakst MR. Serum testosterone concentration during two breeding cycles of turkeys with low and high ejaculate volumes. Domest Anim Endocrinol 1986; 3(1): 27-32.
[http://dx.doi.org/10.1016/0739-7240(86)90037-8]

[43]　Cecil HC, Bakst MR. Testosterone concentrations in blood and seminal plasma of turkeys classified as high or low semen producers. Poult Sci 1988; 67(10): 1461-4.
[http://dx.doi.org/10.3382/ps.0671461] [PMID: 3194337]

[44]　Zeman M, Kosutzký J, Bobáková E. Testosterone concentration in the seminal plasma of cocks. Br Poult Sci 1986; 27(2): 261-6.
[http://dx.doi.org/10.1080/00071668608416879] [PMID: 3742262]

[45]　Anderson EM, Navara KJ. Steroid hormone content of seminal plasma influences fertilizing ability of sperm in White Leghorns. Poult Sci 2011; 90(9): 2035-40.
[http://dx.doi.org/10.3382/ps.2010-01299] [PMID: 21844270]

[46]　Gábor G, Mézes M, Tözsér J, Bozó S, Szücs E, Bárány I. Relationship among testosterone response to GnRH administration, testes size and sperm parameters in Holstein-Friesian bulls. Theriogenology 1995; 43(8): 1317-24.
[http://dx.doi.org/10.1016/0093-691X(95)00116-P]

[47]　Andersson M. Relationships between GnRH-induced testosterone maxima, sperm motility and fertility in Ayrshire bulls. Anim Reprod Sci 1992; 27(2-3): 107-11.
[http://dx.doi.org/10.1016/0378-4320(92)90050-N]

[48]　Meeker JD, Godfrey-Bailey L, Hauser R. Relationships between serum hormone levels and semen quality among men from an infertility clinic. J Androl 2006; 28(3): 397-406.
[http://dx.doi.org/10.2164/jandrol.106.001545] [PMID: 17135633]

[49]　Sundqvist C, Lukola A, Valtonen M. Relationship between serum testosterone concentrations and fertility in male mink (Mustela vison). Reproduction 1984; 70(2): 409-12.
[http://dx.doi.org/10.1530/jrf.0.0700409] [PMID: 6699807]

[50]　Meizel S. Molecules that initiate or help stimulate the acrosome reaction by their interaction with the mammalian sperm surface. Am J Anat 1985; 174(3): 285-302.
[http://dx.doi.org/10.1002/aja.1001740309] [PMID: 3934955]

[51]　Fraser LR. Both taurine and albumin support mouse sperm motility and fertilizing ability *in vitro* but there is no obligatory requirement for taurine. Reproduction 1986; 77(1): 271-80.
[http://dx.doi.org/10.1530/jrf.0.0770271] [PMID: 3755176]

[52]　Boatman DE, Bavister BD, Cruz E. Addition of hypotaurine can reactivate immotile golden hamster spermatozoa. J Androl 1990; 11(1): 66-72.
[PMID: 2312401]

[53]　Zhang B, Yang X, Gao X. Taurine protects against bilirubin-induced neurotoxicity *in vitro*. Brain Res 2010; 1320: 159-67.

[http://dx.doi.org/10.1016/j.brainres.2010.01.036] [PMID: 20096270]

[54] Turner TT, Tung KSK, Tomomasa H, Wilson LW. Acute testicular ischemia results in germ cell-specific apoptosis in the rat. Biol Reprod 1997; 57(6): 1267-74.
[http://dx.doi.org/10.1095/biolreprod57.6.1267] [PMID: 9408230]

[55] Filho DW, Torres MA, Bordin ALB, Crezcynski-Pasa TB, Boveris A. Spermatic cord torsion, reactive oxygen and nitrogen species and ischemia–reperfusion injury. Mol Aspects Med 2004; 25(1-2): 199-210.
[http://dx.doi.org/10.1016/j.mam.2004.02.020] [PMID: 15051328]

[56] Prillaman HM, Turner TT. Rescue of testicular function after acute experimental torsion. J Urol 1997; 157(1): 340-5.
[http://dx.doi.org/10.1016/S0022-5347(01)65374-6] [PMID: 8976294]

[57] Babior BM, Peters WA. The O_2^- producing enzyme of human neutrophils. Further properties. J Biol Chem 1981; 256(5): 2321-3.
[http://dx.doi.org/10.1016/S0021-9258(19)69781-4] [PMID: 7462239]

[58] Epstein FH, Weiss SJ. Tissue destruction by neutrophils. N Engl J Med 1989; 320(6): 365-76.
[http://dx.doi.org/10.1056/NEJM198902093200606] [PMID: 2536474]

[59] Babior BM. Oxygen-dependent microbial killing by phagocytes (first of two parts). N Engl J Med 1978; 298(12): 659-68.
[http://dx.doi.org/10.1056/NEJM197803232981205] [PMID: 24176]

[60] Thomas EL. Myeloperoxidase-hydrogen peroxide-chloride antimicrobial system: effect of exogenous amines on antibacterial action against Escherichia coli. Infect Immun 1979; 25(1): 110-6.
[http://dx.doi.org/10.1128/iai.25.1.110-116.1979] [PMID: 39030]

[61] Redmond HP, Wang JH, Bouchier-Hayes D. Taurine attenuates nitric oxide- and reactive oxygen intermediate-dependent hepatocyte injury. Arch Surg 1996; 131(12): 1280-7.
[http://dx.doi.org/10.1001/archsurg.1996.01430240034004] [PMID: 8956769]

[62] Raschke P, Massoudy P, Becker BF. Taurine protects the heart from neutrophil-induced reperfusion injury. Free Radic Biol Med 1995; 19(4): 461-71.
[http://dx.doi.org/10.1016/0891-5849(95)00044-X] [PMID: 7590395]

[63] Das J, Ghosh J, Manna P, Sinha M, Sil PC. Taurine protects rat testes against NaAsO$_2$-induced oxidative stress and apoptosis *via* mitochondrial dependent and independent pathways. Toxicol Lett 2009; 187(3): 201-10.
[http://dx.doi.org/10.1016/j.toxlet.2009.03.001] [PMID: 19429265]

[64] Heidari R, Jafari F, Khodaei F, Shirazi Yeganeh B, Niknahad H. Mechanism of valproic acid-induced Fanconi syndrome involves mitochondrial dysfunction and oxidative stress in rat kidney. Nephrology (Carlton) 2018; 23(4): 351-61.
[http://dx.doi.org/10.1111/nep.13012] [PMID: 28141910]

[65] Hisatomi A, Sakuma S, Fujiwara M, Seki J. Effect of tacrolimus on the cauda epididymis in rats: Analysis of epididymal biochemical markers or antioxidant defense enzymes. Toxicology 2008; 243(1-2): 23-30.
[http://dx.doi.org/10.1016/j.tox.2007.09.017] [PMID: 17988778]

[66] Ng CM, Blackman MR, Wang C, Swerdloff RS. The role of carnitine in the male reproductive system. Ann N Y Acad Sci 2004; 1033(1): 177-88.
[http://dx.doi.org/10.1196/annals.1320.017] [PMID: 15591015]

[67] Cooper TG, Wang XS, Yeung CH, Lewin LM. Successful lowering of epididymal carnitine by administration of pivalate to rats. Int J Androl 1997; 20(3): 180-8.
[http://dx.doi.org/10.1046/j.1365-2605.1997.00059.x] [PMID: 9354188]

[68] Kasahara E, Sato EF, Miyoshi M, *et al.* Role of oxidative stress in germ cell apoptosis induced by di(2-ethylhexyl)phthalate. Biochem J 2002; 365(3): 849-56.

[http://dx.doi.org/10.1042/bj20020254] [PMID: 11982482]

[69]   Khanna S, Lakhera PC, Khandelwal S. Interplay of early biochemical manifestations by cadmium insult in sertoli–germ coculture: An *in vitro* study. Toxicology 2011; 287(1-3): 46-53.
[http://dx.doi.org/10.1016/j.tox.2011.05.013] [PMID: 21664405]

[70]   Gao HB, Tong MH, Hu YQ, *et al.* Mechanisms of glucocorticoid-induced Leydig cell apoptosis. Mol Cell Endocrinol 2003; 199(1-2): 153-63.
[http://dx.doi.org/10.1016/S0303-7207(02)00290-3] [PMID: 12581887]

[71]   Ghosh S, Chowdhury S, Sarkar P, Sil PC. Ameliorative role of ferulic acid against diabetes associated oxidative stress induced spleen damage. Food Chem Toxicol 2018; 118: 272-86.
[http://dx.doi.org/10.1016/j.fct.2018.05.029] [PMID: 29758315]

[72]   Rashid K, Chowdhury S, Ghosh S, Sil PC. Curcumin attenuates oxidative stress induced NFκB mediated inflammation and endoplasmic reticulum dependent apoptosis of splenocytes in diabetes. Biochem Pharmacol 2017; 143: 140-55.
[http://dx.doi.org/10.1016/j.bcp.2017.07.009] [PMID: 28711624]

[73]   Siavashpour A, Khalvati B, Azarpira N, Mohammadi H, Niknahad H, Heidari R. Poly (ADP-Ribose) polymerase-1 (PARP-1) overactivity plays a pathogenic role in bile acids-induced nephrotoxicity in cholestatic rats. Toxicol Lett 2020; 330: 144-58.
[http://dx.doi.org/10.1016/j.toxlet.2020.05.012] [PMID: 32422328]

[74]   Budihardjo I, Oliver H, Lutter M, Luo X, Wang X. Biochemical pathways of caspase activation during apoptosis. Annu Rev Cell Dev Biol 1999; 15(1): 269-90.
[http://dx.doi.org/10.1146/annurev.cellbio.15.1.269] [PMID: 10611963]

[75]   Hengartner MO. The biochemistry of apoptosis. Nature 2000; 407(6805): 770-6.
[http://dx.doi.org/10.1038/35037710] [PMID: 11048727]

[76]   Tang XL, Yang XY, Jung HJ, *et al.* Asiatic acid induces colon cancer cell growth inhibition and apoptosis through mitochondrial death cascade. Biol Pharm Bull 2009; 32(8): 1399-405.
[http://dx.doi.org/10.1248/bpb.32.1399] [PMID: 19652380]

[77]   Li Y, Lim SC. Cadmium-induced apoptosis of hepatocytes is not associated with death receptor-related caspase-dependent pathways in the rat. Environ Toxicol Pharmacol 2007; 24(3): 231-8.
[http://dx.doi.org/10.1016/j.etap.2007.05.010] [PMID: 21783816]

[78]   Denecker G, Vercammen D, Declercq W, Vandenabeele P. Apoptotic and necrotic cell death induced by death domain receptors. Cell Mol Life Sci 2001; 58(3): 356-70.
[http://dx.doi.org/10.1007/PL00000863] [PMID: 11315185]

[79]   Moustapha A, Pérétout PA, Rainey NE, *et al.* Curcumin induces crosstalk between autophagy and apoptosis mediated by calcium release from the endoplasmic reticulum, lysosomal destabilization and mitochondrial events. Cell Death Discov 2015; 1(1): 15017.
[http://dx.doi.org/10.1038/cddiscovery.2015.17] [PMID: 27551451]

[80]   Prasad AK, Pant N, Srivastava SC, Kumar R, Srivastava SP. Effect of dermal application of hexachlorocyclohexane (HCH) on male reproductive system of rat. Hum Exp Toxicol 1995; 14(6): 484-8.
[http://dx.doi.org/10.1177/096032719501400603] [PMID: 8519523]

[81]   Das J, Ghosh J, Manna P, Sil PC. Taurine protects rat testes against doxorubicin-induced oxidative stress as well as p53, Fas and caspase 12-mediated apoptosis. Amino Acids 2012; 42(5): 1839-55.
[http://dx.doi.org/10.1007/s00726-011-0904-4] [PMID: 21476075]

[82]   Gu Y, Davis DR, Lin YC. Developmental changes in lactate dehydrogenase-X activity in young jaundiced male rats. Arch Androl 1989; 22(2): 131-6.
[http://dx.doi.org/10.3109/01485018908986762] [PMID: 2751392]

[83]   Chen G, Goeddel DV. TNF-R1 signaling: a beautiful pathway. Science 2002; 296(5573): 1634-5.
[http://dx.doi.org/10.1126/science.1071924] [PMID: 12040173]

[84] Rasoulpour RJ, Boekelheide K. NF-kappaB is activated in the rat testis following exposure to mono-(2-ethylhexyl) phthalate. Biol Reprod 2005; 72(2): 479-86.
[http://dx.doi.org/10.1095/biolreprod.104.034363] [PMID: 15496515]

[85] Kaur P, Kaur G, Bansal MP. Tertiary-butyl hydroperoxide induced oxidative stress and male reproductive activity in mice: Role of transcription factor NF-κB and testicular antioxidant enzymes. Reprod Toxicol 2006; 22(3): 479-84.
[http://dx.doi.org/10.1016/j.reprotox.2006.03.017] [PMID: 16704919]

[86] Manthari RK, Tikka C, Ommati MM, *et al.* Arsenic-induced autophagy in the developing mouse cerebellum: Involvement of the blood-brain barrier's tight-junction proteins and the PI3K-Akt-mTOR signaling pathway. J Agric Food Chem 2018; 66(32): 8602-14.
[http://dx.doi.org/10.1021/acs.jafc.8b02654] [PMID: 30032600]

[87] Manthari RK, Tikka C, Ommati MM, *et al.* Arsenic induces autophagy in developmental mouse cerebral cortex and hippocampus by inhibiting PI3K/Akt/mTOR signaling pathway: involvement of blood–brain barrier's tight junction proteins. Arch Toxicol 2018; 92(11): 3255-75.
[http://dx.doi.org/10.1007/s00204-018-2304-y] [PMID: 30225639]

[88] Ghanbarinejad V, Jamshidzadeh A, Khalvati B, *et al.* Apoptosis-inducing factor plays a role in the pathogenesis of hepatic and renal injury during cholestasis. Naunyn Schmiedebergs Arch Pharmacol 2021; 394(6): 1191-203.
[http://dx.doi.org/10.1007/s00210-020-02041-7] [PMID: 33527194]

[89] Yuan J, Kong Y, Ommati MM, *et al.* Bisphenol A-induced apoptosis, oxidative stress and DNA damage in cultured rhesus monkey embryo renal epithelial Marc-145 cells. Chemosphere 2019; 234: 682-9.
[http://dx.doi.org/10.1016/j.chemosphere.2019.06.125] [PMID: 31234085]

[90] Ahmadi A, Niknahad H, Li H, *et al.* The inhibition of NFκB signaling and inflammatory response as a strategy for blunting bile acid-induced hepatic and renal toxicity. Toxicol Lett 2021; 349: 12-29.
[http://dx.doi.org/10.1016/j.toxlet.2021.05.012] [PMID: 34089816]

[91] Li WR, Chen L, Chang ZJ, *et al.* Autophagic deficiency is related to steroidogenic decline in aged rat Leydig cells. Asian J Androl 2011; 13(6): 881-8.
[http://dx.doi.org/10.1038/aja.2011.85] [PMID: 21822295]

[92] Sakkas D, El-Fakahany HM. Apoptosis in ejaculated spermatozoa and in the normal and pathological testes: Abortive apoptosis and sperm chromatin damage.A Clinician's Guide to Sperm DNA and Chromatin Damage. Cham: Springer International Publishing 2018; pp. 197-218.
[http://dx.doi.org/10.1007/978-3-319-71815-6_12]

[93] Kumariya S, Ubba V, Jha RK, Gayen JR. Autophagy in ovary and polycystic ovary syndrome: role, dispute and future perspective. Autophagy 2021; 17(10): 2706-33.
[http://dx.doi.org/10.1080/15548627.2021.1938914] [PMID: 34161185]

[94] Yahyavy S, Valizadeh A, Saki G, Khorsandi L. Taurine induces autophagy and inhibits oxidative stress in mice Leydig cells. JBRA Assist Reprod 2020; 24(3): 250-6.
[http://dx.doi.org/10.5935/1518-0557.20190079] [PMID: 32155016]

[95] Li J, Zheng L, Wang X, *et al.* Taurine protects INS-1 cells from apoptosis induced by Di(2-ethylhexyl) phthalate *via* reducing oxidative stress and autophagy. Toxicol Mech Methods 2019; 29(6): 445-56.
[http://dx.doi.org/10.1080/15376516.2019.1588931] [PMID: 30890009]

[96] Kaur P, Bansal MP. Effect of experimental oxidative stress on steroidogenesis and DNA damage in mouse testis. J Biomed Sci 2004; 11(3): 391-7.
[http://dx.doi.org/10.1007/BF02254444] [PMID: 15067223]

[97] Ommati MM, Attari H, Siavashpour A, Shafaghat M, Azarpira N, Ghaffari H, *et al.* Mitigation of cholestasis-associated hepatic and renal injury by edaravone treatment: Evaluation of its effects on oxidative stress and mitochondrial function. Liver Research 2021; 5(3): 181-193.

[98]   Saemi F, Zamiri MJ, Akhlaghi A, Niakousari M, Dadpasand M, Ommati MM. Dietary inclusion of dried tomato pomace improves the seminal characteristics in Iranian native roosters. Poult Sci 2012; 91(9): 2310-5.
       [http://dx.doi.org/10.3382/ps.2012-02304] [PMID: 22912468]

[99]   Vernet P, Aitken RJ, Drevet JR. Antioxidant strategies in the epididymis. Mol Cell Endocrinol 2004; 216(1-2): 31-9.
       [http://dx.doi.org/10.1016/j.mce.2003.10.069] [PMID: 15109742]

[100] Prahalathan C, Selvakumar E, Varalakshmi P. Modulatory role of lipoic acid on adriamycin-induced testicular injury. Chem Biol Interact 2006; 160(2): 108-14.
       [http://dx.doi.org/10.1016/j.cbi.2005.12.007] [PMID: 16434030]

[101] Heidari R, Niknahad H, Sadeghi A, *et al.* Betaine treatment protects liver through regulating mitochondrial function and counteracting oxidative stress in acute and chronic animal models of hepatic injury. Biomed Pharmacother 2018; 103: 75-86.
       [http://dx.doi.org/10.1016/j.biopha.2018.04.010] [PMID: 29635131]

[102] Heidari R, Arabnezhad MR, Ommati MM, Azarpira N, Ghodsimanesh E, Niknahad H. Boldine Supplementation Regulates Mitochondrial Function and Oxidative Stress in a Rat Model of Hepatotoxicity. Ulum-i Daruyi 2019; 25(1): 1-10.
       [http://dx.doi.org/10.15171/PS.2019.1]

[103] Ommati MM, Heidari R. Betaine, heavy metal protection, oxidative stress, and the liver.Toxicology. Academic Press 2021; pp. 387-95.
       [http://dx.doi.org/10.1016/B978-0-12-819092-0.00038-8]

[104] Ommati MM, Mohammadi H, Mousavi K, *et al.* Metformin alleviates cholestasis-associated nephropathy through regulating oxidative stress and mitochondrial function. Liver Res 2021; 5(3): 171-80.
       [http://dx.doi.org/10.1016/j.livres.2020.12.001]

[105] Ghanbarinejad V, Ommati MM, Jia Z, Farshad O, Jamshidzadeh A, Heidari R. Disturbed mitochondrial redox state and tissue energy charge in cholestasis. J Biochem Mol Toxicol 2021; 35(9): e22846.
       [http://dx.doi.org/10.1002/jbt.22846] [PMID: 34250697]

[106] Cozzi R, Ricordy R, Bartolini F, Ramadori L, Perticone P, De Salvia R. Taurine and ellagic acid: Two differently-acting natural antioxidants. Environ Mol Mutagen 1995; 26(3): 248-54.
       [http://dx.doi.org/10.1002/em.2850260310] [PMID: 7588651]

[107] Timbrell JA, Seabra V, Waterfield CJ. The *in vivo* and *in vitro* protective properties of taurine. Gen Pharmacol 1995; 26(3): 453-62.
       [http://dx.doi.org/10.1016/0306-3623(94)00203-Y] [PMID: 7789717]

[108] Gordon RE, Heller RF, Heller RF. Taurine protection of lungs in hamster models of oxidant injury: a morphologic time study of paraquat and bleomycin treatment. Adv Exp Med Biol 1992; 315: 319-28.
       [http://dx.doi.org/10.1007/978-1-4615-3436-5_38] [PMID: 1380761]

[109] Abdoli N, Sadeghian I, Azarpira N, Ommati MM, Heidari R. Taurine mitigates bile duct obstruction-associated cholemic nephropathy: effect on oxidative stress and mitochondrial parameters. Clin Exp Hepatol 2021; 7(1): 30-40.
       [http://dx.doi.org/10.5114/ceh.2021.104675] [PMID: 34027113]

[110] Heidari R, Babaei H, Eghbal MA. Ameliorative effects of taurine against methimazole-induced cytotoxicity in isolated rat hepatocytes. Sci Pharm 2012; 80(4): 987-99.
       [http://dx.doi.org/10.3797/scipharm.1205-16] [PMID: 23264945]

[111] Heidari R, Babaei H, Eghbal MA. Amodiaquine-induced toxicity in isolated rat hepatocytes and the cytoprotective effects of taurine and/or N-acetyl cysteine. Res Pharm Sci 2014; 9(2): 97-105.
       [PMID: 25657778]

[112] Heidari R, Babaei H, Eghbal MA. Cytoprotective effects of taurine against toxicity induced by isoniazid and hydrazine in isolated rat hepatocytes. Arh Hig Rada Toksikol 2013; 64(2): 201-10.
[http://dx.doi.org/10.2478/10004-1254-64-2013-2297] [PMID: 23819928]

[113] Heidari R, Abdoli N, Ommati MM, Jamshidzadeh A, Niknahad H. Mitochondrial impairment induced by chenodeoxycholic acid: The protective effect of taurine and carnosine supplementation. Trends in Pharmaceutical Sciences. 2018;4(2).

[114] Ahmadi N, Ghanbarinejad V, Ommati MM, Jamshidzadeh A, Heidari R. Taurine prevents mitochondrial membrane permeabilization and swelling upon interaction with manganese: Implication in the treatment of cirrhosis-associated central nervous system complications. J Biochem Mol Toxicol 2018; 32(11): e22216.
[http://dx.doi.org/10.1002/jbt.22216] [PMID: 30152904]

[115] Heidari R, Behnamrad S, Khodami Z, Ommati MM, Azarpira N, Vazin A. The nephroprotective properties of taurine in colistin-treated mice is mediated through the regulation of mitochondrial function and mitigation of oxidative stress. Biomed Pharmacother 2019; 109: 103-11.
[http://dx.doi.org/10.1016/j.biopha.2018.10.093] [PMID: 30396066]

[116] Ommati MM, Heidari R, Ghanbarinejad V, Abdoli N, Niknahad H. Taurine treatment provides neuroprotection in a mouse model of manganism. Biol Trace Elem Res 2019; 190(2): 384-95.
[http://dx.doi.org/10.1007/s12011-018-1552-2] [PMID: 30357569]

[117] Ommati MM, Farshad O, Jamshidzadeh A, Heidari R. Taurine enhances skeletal muscle mitochondrial function in a rat model of resistance training. PharmaNutrition 2019; 9: 100161.
[http://dx.doi.org/10.1016/j.phanu.2019.100161]

[118] Murugesan P, Muthusamy T, Balasubramanian K, Arunakaran J. Polychlorinated biphenyl (Aroclor 1254) inhibits testosterone biosynthesis and antioxidant enzymes in cultured rat Leydig cells. Reprod Toxicol 2008; 25(4): 447-54.
[http://dx.doi.org/10.1016/j.reprotox.2008.04.003] [PMID: 18502095]

[119] Ozmen O, Mor F. Apoptosis in adult rabbit testes during subacute endosulfan toxicity. Pestic Biochem Physiol 2012; 102(2): 129-33.
[http://dx.doi.org/10.1016/j.pestbp.2011.12.003]

[120] Alvarez JG, Storey BT. Taurine, hypotaurine, epinephrine and albumin inhibit lipid peroxidation in rabbit spermatozoa and protect against loss of motility. Biol Reprod 1983; 29(3): 548-55.
[http://dx.doi.org/10.1095/biolreprod29.3.548] [PMID: 6626644]

[121] Ghosh S, Chowdhury S, Das AK, Sil PC. Taurine ameliorates oxidative stress induced inflammation and ER stress mediated testicular damage in STZ-induced diabetic Wistar rats. Food Chem Toxicol 2019; 124: 64-80.
[http://dx.doi.org/10.1016/j.fct.2018.11.055] [PMID: 30496779]

[122] Llanos MN, Ronco AM. Sperm phospholipid methyltransferase activity during preparation for exocytosis. Cell Biochem Funct 1994; 12(4): 289-96.
[http://dx.doi.org/10.1002/cbf.290120410] [PMID: 7834819]

[123] Mrsny RJ, Meizel S. Inhibition of hamster sperm Na^+, K^+-ATPase activity by taurine and hypotaurine. Life Sci 1985; 36(3): 271-5.
[http://dx.doi.org/10.1016/0024-3205(85)90069-4] [PMID: 2981386]

[124] Tschopp J. Mitochondria: Sovereign of inflammation? Eur J Immunol 2011; 41(5): 1196-202.
[http://dx.doi.org/10.1002/eji.201141436] [PMID: 21469137]

[125] Chowdhury S, Ghosh S, Rashid K, Sil PC. Deciphering the role of ferulic acid against streptozotocin-induced cellular stress in the cardiac tissue of diabetic rats. Food Chem Toxicol 2016; 97: 187-98.
[http://dx.doi.org/10.1016/j.fct.2016.09.011] [PMID: 27621051]

[126] Liu ZW, Zhu HT, Chen KL, *et al.* Protein kinase RNA- like endoplasmic reticulum kinase (PERK) signaling pathway plays a major role in reactive oxygen species (ROS)- mediated endoplasmic

reticulum stress- induced apoptosis in diabetic cardiomyopathy. Cardiovasc Diabetol 2013; 12(1): 158.
[http://dx.doi.org/10.1186/1475-2840-12-158] [PMID: 24180212]

[127]　Sinha K, Das J, Pal PB, Sil PC. Oxidative stress: the mitochondria-dependent and mitochondria-independent pathways of apoptosis. Arch Toxicol 2013; 87(7): 1157-80.
[http://dx.doi.org/10.1007/s00204-013-1034-4] [PMID: 23543009]

[128]　Guo Y, Sun J, Li T, *et al.* Melatonin ameliorates restraint stress-induced oxidative stress and apoptosis in testicular cells *via* NF-κB/iNOS and Nrf2/ HO-1 signaling pathway. Sci Rep 2017; 7(1): 9599.
[http://dx.doi.org/10.1038/s41598-017-09943-2] [PMID: 28851995]

[129]　Ommati MM, Farshad O, Ghanbarinejad V, *et al.* The nephroprotective role of carnosine against ifosfamide-induced renal injury and electrolytes imbalance is mediated *via* the regulation of mitochondrial function and alleviation of oxidative stress. Drug Res (Stuttg) 2020; 70(1): 49-56.
[http://dx.doi.org/10.1055/a-1017-5085] [PMID: 31671464]

[130]　Ommati MM, Farshad O, Niknahad H, *et al.* Oral administration of thiol-reducing agents mitigates gut barrier disintegrity and bacterial lipopolysaccharide translocation in a rat model of biliary obstruction. Current Research in Pharmacology and Drug Discovery 2020; 1: 10-8.
[http://dx.doi.org/10.1016/j.crphar.2020.06.001] [PMID: 34909638]

[131]　Heidari R, Mandegani L, Ghanbarinejad V, *et al.* Mitochondrial dysfunction as a mechanism involved in the pathogenesis of cirrhosis-associated cholemic nephropathy. Biomed Pharmacother 2019; 109: 271-80.
[http://dx.doi.org/10.1016/j.biopha.2018.10.104] [PMID: 30396085]

[132]　Farshad O, Heidari R, Zare F, *et al.* Effects of cimetidine and N-acetylcysteine on paraquat-induced acute lung injury in rats: a preliminary study. Toxicol Environ Chem 2018; 100(8-10): 785-93.
[http://dx.doi.org/10.1080/02772248.2019.1606225]

[133]　Heidari R, Jamshidzadeh A, Niknahad H, *et al.* Effect of taurine on chronic and acute liver injury: Focus on blood and brain ammonia. Toxicol Rep 2016; 3: 870-9.
[http://dx.doi.org/10.1016/j.toxrep.2016.04.002] [PMID: 28959615]

[134]　Jamshidzadeh A, Heidari R, Abazari F, *et al.* Antimalarial drugs-induced hepatic injury in rats and the protective role of carnosine. Ulum-i Daruyi 2016; 22(3): 170-80.
[http://dx.doi.org/10.15171/PS.2016.27]

[135]　Dalle-Donne I, Rossi R, Giustarini D, Milzani A, Colombo R. Protein carbonyl groups as biomarkers of oxidative stress. Clin Chim Acta 2003; 329(1-2): 23-38.
[http://dx.doi.org/10.1016/S0009-8981(03)00003-2] [PMID: 12589963]

[136]　Garg AD, Kaczmarek A, Krysko DV, Vandenabeele P. ER Stress and Inflammation.Endoplasmic Reticulum Stress in Health and Disease. Dordrecht: Springer Netherlands 2012; pp. 257-79.
[http://dx.doi.org/10.1007/978-94-007-4351-9_11]

[137]　Bettigole SE, Glimcher LH. Endoplasmic reticulum stress in immunity. Annu Rev Immunol 2015; 33(1): 107-38.
[http://dx.doi.org/10.1146/annurev-immunol-032414-112116] [PMID: 25493331]

[138]　Rodvold JJ, Mahadevan NR, Zanetti M. Immune modulation by ER stress and inflammation in the tumor microenvironment. Cancer Lett 2016; 380(1): 227-36.
[http://dx.doi.org/10.1016/j.canlet.2015.09.009] [PMID: 26525580]

[139]　Li Y, Schwabe RF, DeVries-Seimon T, *et al.* Free cholesterol-loaded macrophages are an abundant source of tumor necrosis factor-α and interleukin-6: model of NF-kappaB- and map kinase-dependent inflammation in advanced atherosclerosis. J Biol Chem 2005; 280(23): 21763-72.
[http://dx.doi.org/10.1074/jbc.M501759200] [PMID: 15826936]

[140]　Hotamisligil GS, Erbay E. Nutrient sensing and inflammation in metabolic diseases. Nat Rev Immunol 2008; 8(12): 923-34.
[http://dx.doi.org/10.1038/nri2449] [PMID: 19029988]

[141] Zhang K, Kaufman RJ. From endoplasmic-reticulum stress to the inflammatory response. Nature 2008; 454(7203): 455-62.
[http://dx.doi.org/10.1038/nature07203] [PMID: 18650916]

[142] Verfaillie T, Garg AD, Agostinis P. Targeting ER stress induced apoptosis and inflammation in cancer. Cancer Lett 2013; 332(2): 249-64.
[http://dx.doi.org/10.1016/j.canlet.2010.07.016] [PMID: 20732741]

[143] Austin CA, Umbreit TH, Brown KM, *et al.* Distribution of silver nanoparticles in pregnant mice and developing embryos. Nanotoxicology 2012; 6(8): 912-22.
[http://dx.doi.org/10.3109/17435390.2011.626539] [PMID: 22023110]

[144] Deng J, Lu PD, Zhang Y, *et al.* Translational repression mediates activation of nuclear factor kappa B by phosphorylated translation initiation factor 2. Mol Cell Biol 2004; 24(23): 10161-8.
[http://dx.doi.org/10.1128/MCB.24.23.10161-10168.2004] [PMID: 15542827]

[145] Goodall JC, Wu C, Zhang Y, *et al.* Endoplasmic reticulum stress-induced transcription factor, CHOP, is crucial for dendritic cell IL-23 expression. Proc Natl Acad Sci USA 2010; 107(41): 17698-703.
[http://dx.doi.org/10.1073/pnas.1011736107] [PMID: 20876114]

[146] Jeong M, Cho J, Cho WS, Shin GC, Lee K. The glucosamine-mediated induction of CHOP reduces the expression of inflammatory cytokines by modulating JNK and NF-κB in LPS-stimulated RAW264.7 cells. Genes Genomics 2009; 31(3): 251-60.
[http://dx.doi.org/10.1007/BF03191197]

[147] Urano F, Wang X, Bertolotti A, *et al.* Coupling of stress in the ER to activation of JNK protein kinases by transmembrane protein kinase IRE1. Science 2000; 287(5453): 664-6.
[http://dx.doi.org/10.1126/science.287.5453.664] [PMID: 10650002]

[148] Hu P, Han Z, Couvillon AD, Kaufman RJ, Exton JH. Autocrine tumor necrosis factor alpha links endoplasmic reticulum stress to the membrane death receptor pathway through IRE1alpha-mediated NF-kappaB activation and down-regulation of TRAF2 expression. Mol Cell Biol 2006; 26(8): 3071-84.
[http://dx.doi.org/10.1128/MCB.26.8.3071-3084.2006] [PMID: 16581782]

[149] Yamazaki H, Hiramatsu N, Hayakawa K, Tagawa Y, Okamura M, Ogata R, *et al.* Activation of the Akt-NF-kappaB pathway by subtilase cytotoxin through the ATF6 branch of the unfolded protein response 2009.

[150] Nakajima S, Kato H, Takahashi S, Johno H, Kitamura M. Inhibition of NF-κB by MG132 through ER stress-mediated induction of LAP and LIP. FEBS Lett 2011; 585(14): 2249-54.
[http://dx.doi.org/10.1016/j.febslet.2011.05.047] [PMID: 21627972]

[151] Ye J, Rawson RB, Komuro R, *et al.* ER stress induces cleavage of membrane-bound ATF6 by the same proteases that process SREBPs. Mol Cell 2000; 6(6): 1355-64.
[http://dx.doi.org/10.1016/S1097-2765(00)00133-7] [PMID: 11163209]

[152] Ommati MM, Heidari R, Ghanbarinejad V, Aminian A, Abdoli N, Niknahad H. The neuroprotective properties of carnosine in a mouse model of manganism is mediated *via* mitochondria regulating and antioxidative mechanisms. Nutr Neurosci 2020; 23(9): 731-43.
[http://dx.doi.org/10.1080/1028415X.2018.1552399] [PMID: 30856059]

[153] Banerjee S, Sinha K, Chowdhury S, Sil PC. Unfolding the mechanism of cisplatin induced pathophysiology in spleen and its amelioration by carnosine. Chem Biol Interact 2018; 279: 159-70.
[http://dx.doi.org/10.1016/j.cbi.2017.11.019] [PMID: 29191451]

[154] Bhattacharya S, Gachhui R, Sil PC. Effect of Kombucha, a fermented black tea in attenuating oxidative stress mediated tissue damage in alloxan induced diabetic rats. Food Chem Toxicol 2013; 60: 328-40.
[http://dx.doi.org/10.1016/j.fct.2013.07.051] [PMID: 23907022]

[155] Bhattacharyya S, Banerjee S, Guha C, Ghosh S, Sil PC. A 35 kDa Phyllanthus niruri protein

suppresses indomethacin mediated hepatic impairments: Its role in Hsp70, HO-1, JNKs and Ca $^{2+}$ dependent inflammatory pathways. Food Chem Toxicol 2017; 102: 76-92.
[http://dx.doi.org/10.1016/j.fct.2017.01.028] [PMID: 28159595]

[156]   Mohammadi H, Ommati MM, Farshad O, Jamshidzadeh A, Niknahad H, Heidari R. Taurine and isolated mitochondria: A concentration-response study. Trends Pharmacol Sci 2019; 5(4): 5-6.

[157]   Jamshidzadeh A, Heidari R, Abasvali M, *et al.* Taurine treatment preserves brain and liver mitochondrial function in a rat model of fulminant hepatic failure and hyperammonemia. Biomed Pharmacother 2017; 86: 514-20.
[http://dx.doi.org/10.1016/j.biopha.2016.11.095] [PMID: 28024286]

[158]   Niknahad H, Jamshidzadeh A, Heidari R, Zarei M, Ommati MM. Ammonia-induced mitochondrial dysfunction and energy metabolism disturbances in isolated brain and liver mitochondria, and the effect of taurine administration: relevance to hepatic encephalopathy treatment. Clin Exp Hepatol 2017; 3(3): 141-51.
[http://dx.doi.org/10.5114/ceh.2017.68833] [PMID: 29062904]

[159]   Dutta S, Saha S, Mahalanobish S, Sadhukhan P, Sil PC. Melatonin attenuates arsenic induced nephropathy *via* the regulation of oxidative stress and inflammatory signaling cascades in mice. Food Chem Toxicol 2018; 118: 303-16.
[http://dx.doi.org/10.1016/j.fct.2018.05.032] [PMID: 29763682]

[160]   Pal PB, Sinha K, Sil PC. Mangiferin attenuates diabetic nephropathy by inhibiting oxidative stress mediated signaling cascade, TNFα related and mitochondrial dependent apoptotic pathways in streptozotocin-induced diabetic rats. PLoS One. 2014;9(9):e107220-e.

[161]   Sadhukhan P, Saha S, Sil PC. Antioxidative effect of genistein and mangiferin on sodium fluoride induced oxidative insult of renal cells: A comparative study. Biomarkers Journal. 2016;2(1).

[162]   Vasanthi P, Parameswari CS. Aqueous extract of Terminalia arjuna prevents cyclosporine-induced renal disorders. Comp Clin Pathol 2014; 23(3): 583-8.
[http://dx.doi.org/10.1007/s00580-012-1655-7]

[163]   Sinha K, Sadhukhan P, Saha S, Pal PB, Sil PC. Morin protects gastric mucosa from nonsteroidal anti-inflammatory drug, indomethacin induced inflammatory damage and apoptosis by modulating NF-κB pathway. Biochim Biophys Acta, Gen Subj 2015; 1850(4): 769-83.
[http://dx.doi.org/10.1016/j.bbagen.2015.01.008] [PMID: 25603542]

[164]   Vazin A, Heidari R, Khoddami Z. Curcumin supplementation alleviates polymyxin E-induced nephrotoxicity. J Exp Pharmacol 2020; 12: 129-36.
[http://dx.doi.org/10.2147/JEP.S255861] [PMID: 32581601]

[165]   Sarkar P, Basak P, Ghosh S, Kundu M, Sil PC. Prophylactic role of taurine and its derivatives against diabetes mellitus and its related complications. Food Chem Toxicol 2017; 110: 109-21.
[http://dx.doi.org/10.1016/j.fct.2017.10.022] [PMID: 29050977]

[166]   Nam SY, Kim HM, Jeong HJ. The potential protective role of taurine against experimental allergic inflammation. Life Sci 2017; 184: 18-24.
[http://dx.doi.org/10.1016/j.lfs.2017.07.007] [PMID: 28694089]

[167]   Morishima N, Nakanishi K, Takenouchi H, Shibata T, Yasuhiko Y. An endoplasmic reticulum stress-specific caspase cascade in apoptosis. Cytochrome c-independent activation of caspase-9 by caspase-12. J Biol Chem 2002; 277(37): 34287-94.
[http://dx.doi.org/10.1074/jbc.M204973200] [PMID: 12097332]

CHAPTER 11

Role of Taurine Supplementation in Obesity: Stimulating Fats to Burn in Cellular Power Plants

Abstract: With changes in lifestyle and eating habits, obesity is a significant health issue, especially in developed countries. Obesity could be induced by an imbalance between energy expenditure and energy intake. Obesity harms several body organs' functions by causing impairments in vital intracellular organelles such as mitochondria. Meanwhile, it has been found that chronic inflammation and oxidative stress could induce mitochondrial impairment in various tissues of obese individuals. On the other hand, it has been revealed that there is a negative correlation between obesity and taurine (TAU) biosynthesis. In the current chapter, we tried to present a good body of evidence on the role of mitochondria in various types of fatty tissues, including white adipose tissues (WAT), brown adipose tissues (BAT), and beige/brite/inducible/brown-like adipose tissues (bAT). We also highlighted the effects of TAU on mitochondria related signaling in adipocytes. The data collected in this chapter could help develop new strategies for preventing and treating obesity and its associated complications.

Keywords: Antioxidant, Lipid peroxidation, Mitochondrial impairment, Oxidative stress, Overweight.

INTRODUCTION

Obesity is a significant health issue worldwide that imposes a considerable cost on the healthcare system annually. It is estimated that the annual fee for obesity-related comorbidities exceeds $150 billion annually in the united states [1]. In 2008, approximately 1.5 billion adults were estimated to have a body mass index (BMI) greater than 25 [2]. Changes in dietary habits, especially in developing countries, lead to the obesity crisis. Consuming many fast foods, fructose, and trans fatty acid-rich diets in combination with decreased physical activity have been identified as contributing factors in the obesity crisis [1].

Obesity is a body mass index (BMI) greater than 30 kg/m^2 [3]. Extremely obese patients have a BMI greater than 40 kg/m^2 [1, 3]. It is well-known that obesity is associated with a higher incidence of significant health complications such as metabolic syndrome, diabetes, cardiovascular disease, and cancer [3]. Hence, obesity is considered a major threat to public health, especially in developed

Reza Heidari and M. Mehdi Ommati

countries, and significantly influences people's quality of life [3 - 5]. Based on these data, developing strategies to treat and/or prevent obesity is essential.

Obesity is a chronic condition; thus, managing this complication requires a continuous and integrated approach. The strategies for managing obesity could differ among health care systems worldwide. However, it generally includes changing lifestyle and eating habits and, if necessary, adding medications or even surgical operations [6]. Surgical procedures are often used in morbidly-obese patients [2].

As mentioned, obesity is connected with serious health issues and significantly influences people's quality of life [4, 5]. Several pharmacological interventions have also been developed to manage obesity on overweight. These strategies are usually used as adjuvant therapies when patients' lifestyle changes are insufficient. Most of these medications are centrally-acting agents that affect eating habits (*e.g.*, suppressing appetite). Some other drugs prevent the absorption of food fats. On the other hand, these medications have several adverse effects and low patient compliance. Therefore, finding effective and safe agents to manage obesity is still essential.

Taurine (TAU) is one of the most abundant sulfur-containing free amino acids in various excitable tissues. This amino acid (AA) is evaluated as 0.1% of the total live bodyweight [7], obtained from two sources, including extracellular resources (*i.e.*, active uptake from the diet) and intracellular resources through biosynthetic routes of other sulfur-containing AAs such as cysteine and methionine. Until today, various functions are considered for this vital AA, including membrane stabilizing properties, anti-inflammatory, and anti-oxidative properties. Meanwhile, it has been well shown that TAU can considerably enhance metabolic-related maladies (through improving insulin resistance to control glucose metabolism) [8]. However, it should be highlighted that TAU, as a component of reformed uridine, has a particular function in conjugating mitochondrial tRNAs for two crucial AAs (*e.g.*, leucine and lysine). Meanwhile, the ameliorative role of TAU in the pathologies of mitochondrial myopathy, lactic acidosis, encephalopathy, stroke-like episodes (MELAS), myoclonic epilepsy, and ragged-red fiber syndrome (MERRF) has been well reported. TAU also mitigates plasma and liver cholesterol levels caused by high energy/cholesterol foods, possibly related to bile acid homeostasis [9 - 13].

In the current chapter, the efficacy of the amino acid TAU on several parameters involved in fatty acid metabolism focuses on the effect of this amino acid on mitochondrial function in various forms of fat tissue. Several clinical trials revealed that TAU could control obesity with no significant adverse effects.

TYPES OF ADIPOCYTES AND THEIR RELEVANCE TO ENERGY METABOLISM AND STORAGE

Generally, mammals have two types of adipose tissues with opposite functions, including white adipose tissue (WAT) and brown adipose tissue (BAT). In another classification, three types of fat cells, adipocytes, have been identified in the human body [14, 15]. White, brown, and beige/brite/inducible/brown-like adipocytes form adipose tissue, abbreviated to WAT, BAT, and bAT, respectively [14, 15]. Different adipocytes' morphological and functional activity and their role in the development of obesity and the weight loss process are different [14, 15]. For instance, emerging evidence from the literature demonstrated a close relation between BAT activation and further physiological alterations (*i.e.*, a significant decrease in blood sugar content resulting in an increment of resting energy expenditure and consequently reduced weight).

The WAT is the energy-storing tissue [15] and saves extra energy as a form of triglyceride (TG). This type of adipocyte could go under the "browning" process by different stimuli and produce BAT [15, 16].

As mentioned above, BAT has an opposite function compared to WAT. The BAT is specified in the overindulgence of energy by generating heat to keep the body's temperature and energy consumption. Different stimulations, such as thermal changes, hormones, and cytokines, could cause BAT production [15, 17]. The BAT is a fatty tissue that expends energy and is considered the central place of non-shivering thermogenesis in mammals [15, 17]. Some in-depth animal studies claimed that the thermogenic activity of this type of fatty tissue might protect against obesity. Humans have shown that BAT primarily comprises these inducible adipocytes in adults. However, new studies claimed the classical BAT persistence in certain anatomical spots. Hence, they showed that BAT activity might be negatively related to obesity. The brown-like adipose tissue is formed within WAT after browning and is called bAT (beige/brite/inducible/brown-like adipocytes) [17] and emerges in reaction to particular environmental signals. The bAT has the agonistic functions of BAT and the antagonistic roles of WAT [18]. In general, bAT acts as WAT; nevertheless, as soon as the body receives the signal that heat production is required *via* energy consumption (such as cold stimulation), this type of adipocyte exhibits a function and morphology like those in BAT [19].

WAT contains a large amount of lipid, usually a single droplet, which occupies a large proportion of cell volume [15, 17] (Fig. **1**). However, it should be highlighted that a few numbers mitochondria are found in WAT. On the other hand, the number of mitochondria in BAT is very high, and the size of lipid droplets is minimal [15, 17, 18] (Fig. **1**). Although another fascinating evidence exists about WAT browning resulting in what is identified as BAT, biochemical and ultrastructural analyses showed an increasing number of mitochondrial and uncoupling proteins (UCPs; like the uncoupling protein-1; UCP1) in this type of adipocyte [20]. This mitochondrial inner membrane's protein plays a vital role in the thermogenic activity of BAT and activates bAT through the induction of a proton leak throughout the inner membrane of this organelle; this can produce heat by the electrochemical energy conversion (triggered by fatty acids making *via* lipolysis in some exceptional circumstances, such as cold exposure) [32]. An in-depth study has shown that additional acetyl-CoA oxidation could supply energy to generate heat with the help of UCP1 [21]. However, it should be highlighted that except for UCP1, which is involved in adaptive thermogenesis, other UCPs, such as UCP2 and UCP3, seem to be more involved in mitigating reactive oxygen species (ROS) contents than in adaptive thermogenesis [22]. Meanwhile, along with UCP1-mediated uncoupling, other intracellular pathways, including the creatinine cycling [23] and glycerol-3-phosphate shuttle [24], might also generate heat.

Considering the biological routes involved in managing activity and differentiation of brown fat cells, they might help design BAT-related strategies to increase energy expenditure and fight against obesity, especially in adults and other diseases related to obesity. Some rodent trial investigations have targeted physiological responses; for instance, these studies suggested that diet-generated thermogenesis in BAT might protect against obesity. On the other hand, several pharmaceutical studies have shown dietary agents and/or drugs as the stimulators of BAT and the browning process [20, 25 - 28]. In this regard, resveratrol, metformin, poly-unsaturated fatty acids (PUFA), catechin, and different polyphenol agents have been studied to stimulate WAT browning process [20, 25 - 31]. It has been determined that BAT can act as one of the crucial modulators for thermal homeostasis *via* chemical energy dissipation as a form of heat. The leading site of this process is UCPs located in their mitochondria.

Progress of therapies that target brown fat or WAT browning requires a fundamental knowledge of the fatty tissues' biology and a reasonable interpretation of the effect of changing their activity levels on the metabolism and physiology of the whole body. For this reason, in the following parts, we will try to point out the role of a unique AA, TAU, playing an essential role in the anti-obesity process by regulating some crucial endogenous modulators involved in obesity and improving the functionality of mitochondria in this tissue.

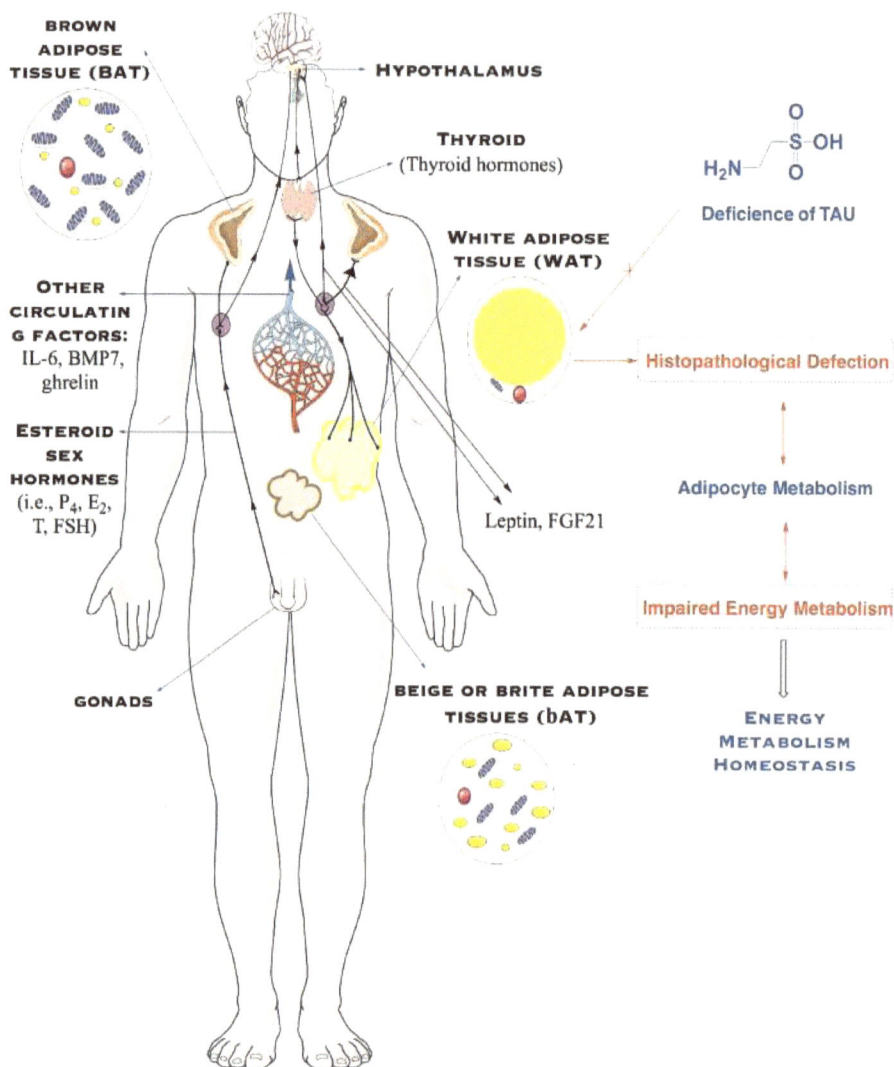

Fig. (1). Morphological characteristics of different adipocytes and their source circulating controllers of fatty tissues. The hypothalamus/ thyroid/ gonad axis plays a crucial role in controlling the activity of fatty tissues. Many of these circulating controllers operate *via* increasing UCP1 expression in mitochondria. White adipocytes contain a sizeable single lipid droplet that occupies a large volume of the cytoplasm. Few mitochondria and a nucleus (brown) are also evident in white adipocytes. Brown adipocytes contain numerous mitochondria, which facilitate the oxidation of fatty acids in these cells. Small droplets of lipids and nuclei (brown) are present in brown adipocytes. Brown-like adipocytes also contain high mitochondria numbers but larger lipid droplets than brown adipocytes. The deficiency of TAU can induce alterations in tissue histology and cause adverse effects on its function, causing compromised energy metabolism and ultimately impairing its homeostasis.

THE CENTRAL MODULATORS IN OBESITY: THE ROLE OF TAURINE

Before starting the main subjects about the crucial parts of TAU and mitochondria in obesity, it is better to refer to some of the well-known endogenous factors (and their relation with TAU) affecting obesity to understand this metabolic disorder better.

Several in-depth studies have comprehensively reported the action and regulatory role of various hormones on the activation of BAT and the browning of WAT. Meanwhile, the past decade has witnessed a steady accumulation of review articles focusing on the regulation of BAT activity and browning by hormonal moderators [32, 33]. In Fig. (**1**), we tried to provide a schematic illustration of the controlling role of some crucial hormones (testosterone (T), estrogen (E), progesterone (P4), follicle-stimulating hormones (FSH)), and some circulating factors (including interleukin-6 (IL-6), bone morphogenic protein-7 (BMP7) and ghrelin, as well as leptin, and fibroblast growth factor-21 (FBS-21)) in the fatty tissues' activity and browning. Except for these mentioned hormones and circulating factors, Dallon and colleagues have shown that daily insulin injection-induced hyperinsulinemia could considerably decrease the respiratory activity of inguinal WAT [IWAT] and interscapular BAT [IBAT] [34].

Leptin not only is one of the crucial hormones released from WAT and discerned for its well-known connection with energy balance regulation through the aryl-hydrocarbon receptor (AHR) and decreasing appetite but it has also been shown that it triggers the sympathetic nervous system (SNS) activity to BAT [35, 36]. Nevertheless, IBAT's SNS activity was not obligatory for the weight loss induced by leptin [37]. However, there is a good body of evidence showing the footprints of some neurons, including Agouti-related protein (AgRP) and proopiomelanocortin (POMC) neurons, in leptin interceded intensified SNS activity to BAT. On the other hand, it is shown that orexigenic peptides, such as neuropeptide Y (NPY) and AgRP secreting from the arcuate nucleus (ARC) of the hypothalamus, were considerably decreased by the high-fat diet (obesity). In this regard, in a laboratory animal model (in mice), Bell and colleagues have reported that AgRP neurons are the key controllers of leptin-induced intensified SNS activity in the inguinal fat [38]. On the other hand, in the leptin-deficient ob/ob (–/–) mice, Martins and coworkers have reported that PGC-1α, ß3-adrenergic receptor, and UCP1 levels were significantly decreased [39]. Meanwhile, Han and colleagues in rat ß-cells have shown that TAU tangibly increased the levels of ATP in UCP2- overexpressing ß-cells, possibly *via* intensifying mitochondrial Ca^{2+} influx through the Ca^{2+} uniporter and triggering mitochondrial metabolic function [40]. It has also been reported that TAU considerably decreased blood glucose levels, insulin resistance, serum content of lipids (*e.g.*, TG, cholesterol, and low and high-density lipoprotein cholesterol), serum leptin (not adiponectin levels) in Otsuka Long-Evans Tokushima fatty rats with a long-term duration of diabetes [41]. In the study, the authors concluded that Tau could improve hyperglycemia and dyslipidemia through improving leptin modulation and insulin sensitivity. In another study, Brazilian authors have shown that although the ameliorative effects of TAU upon feeding behavior control are complex and controlled by various types of genes; however, it preserves hypothalamic leptin action (preventing hypothalamic leptin resistance) in normal and protein-restricted mice fed on a high-fat diet [42].

As evidenced by many investigations, there is a footprint of thyroid hormone activity in WAT browning. Multiple lines of research have revealed that thyroid hormones trigger the mechanism of WAT browning through the central effects of these hormones on energy balance. For instance, Weiner and colleagues reported that both hyperthyroidism and hypothyroidism could trigger the browning process in mice WAT [43]. They said that BAT activity and mass were considerably higher in hyperthyroid mice than in hypothyroid ones. Meanwhile, an in-depth investigation demonstrated that the 3,3′,5-triiodothyronine (T3) form of thyroid hormones could notably increase the activity of BAT by increasing SNS activity to BAT [44]. However, a recent study claimed that 3,3′,5,5′ tetraiodothyronine (T4) treatment and T3 administration to the ventromedial nucleus of the hypothalamus (VMH) were correlated with the WAT browning [45]. These authors also showed that the T3 action-induced BAT activity could be facilitated by declining endoplasmic reticulum stress in the VMH [46]. Meanwhile, it is demonstrated that energy expenditure increment induced by cold stimulation was interconnected with circulating T3 concentration in humans [47]. However, a crucial role for angiotensin type 2 receptor (AT2R) in T3-induced upregulation of browning genes in WAT has been shown [48]; in this case, an agonist of AT2R increased the WAT browning. In contrast, Tsukuda and colleagues have demonstrated that angiotensin II type 1 receptor (AT1R) blockade was interconnected with IWAT browning. Then it could be considered a therapeutic target for treating metabolic disorders [49]. However, it has been reported that bile acids could considerably trigger energy expenditure through increasing intracellular thyroid hormone activation [50]. These authors illustrated that the bile acids administration could tangibly increase energy expenditure in BAT, preventing obesity and resistance to insulin. In this regard, Taş and co-authors have reported that treatment with TAU (1% for five weeks) had an ameliorative role against hypothyroidism-induced intensified oxidative stress [51]. On the other hand, *via* supporting and regulating the healthy generation of bile acids, TAU can inhibit gallstones and help promote the healthy detoxification of estrogen in the liver and bowel. However, further studies are needed to assess the enhancing role of TAU on obesity through thyroid hormone alterations.

A body of literature exists on the role of sex steroid hormones in regulating BAT and WAT function. Frank and co-authors have written that BAT activity in females is significantly higher than in males; hence, they highlighted the crucial role of estrogens in this type of fatty tissue, especially in enhancing thermogenesis [52]. In other two studies, which were conducted by López and Tena-Sempere (2016 and 2017), the minimum level of this ovary-derived hormone (E2) was shown to be associated with decreased activity of BAT [53]; meanwhile, they have also reported that BAT activity was tangibly increased upon treatment with E2 through the activation of hypothalamic AMPK [54]. BAT density and energy expenditure were notably increased by pharmacological activation of estrogen receptor-ß (ER-ß) [55]. In this case, it has also been shown that the effect of TAU is sex-dependent [56], proposing the potential role of sex hormones, chiefly estrogen, in the impact of this AA. Hence, it can be concluded that taking sufficient TAU can be more crucial for women than men due to the biosynthesis of TAU, which is impeded by estrogen.

Another sex steroid hormone involved in gestation, progesterone (P4), was reported to cause a brown-to-white conversion of BAT in rodents [57]. It is established that BAT deletion before pregnancy can cause hyperlipidemia in the mother and fetus, resulting in an increment in body weight and size in the fetus. A polyclonal antibody-induced inhibition in follicle-stimulating hormone (FSH) secretion was reported to trigger beiging, activate BAT and thermogenesis, and decrease WAT, resulting in a decrement of the body fat volume [58]. On the other hand, a considerably high concentration of an FSH-suppressing protein, called Follistatin, is determined in BAT. The highest expression of Follistatin was associated with an increment in BAT density and WAT browning [59]. Based on the above literature, an inhibitory role for FSH inn BAT activity and browning can be assumed. In line with this assumption, Hashimoto and his team have reported that castration could significantly increase IWAT browning in rodents [60]. It has been shown that TAU could considerably alter the gonadotropin hormone levels, FSH and LH, and testosterone content in male rats suffering from hypercholesterolemia [61].

As illustrated in Fig. (**1**), other crucial peptides and hormones also have an essential role in the functionality of these adipose tissues. For instance, a negative correlation is reported for ghrelin with the activity of BAT [62], whereas there was a positive correlation for erythropoietin with thermogenic activity [63]. Brown fat is also a leading source of different kinds of BATokines. These BATokines can affect various endogenous organs. One of the well-known BATokines, secreted by the liver and WAT is fibroblast growth factor-21

(FGF21). A good body of literature demonstrates the impact of FGF21 on BAT and WAT functioning *via* the central nervous system, resulting in an increment of the SNS activity, which ultimately causes body weight loss and enhanced energy expenditure [64 - 66]. On the other hand, it is mentioned that the FGF21 functionality was decreased in obese ladies [67]; therefore, they highlighted a close interconnection between serum levels of FGF21 with insulin resistance and obesity. Finally, they reported the positive effects of TAU *via* the regulation of FGF21 and βklotho co-receptor along with a standard weight-loss diet in obese women [67]. However, there are some contradictions in this area; for instance, Zouhar and colleagues have reported that FGF21 has an independent effect of UCP1 on body temperature that could be attained without any alteration in energy expenditure. Finally, they concluded that body temperature plays a primary role in FGF21 and can be obtained without increasing energy expenditure [68]. The autocrine role of FGF21 has been shown. Furthermore, it has been reported that FGF21 induces WAT browning *via* increased activity of peroxisome proliferator-activated receptor [69, 70] and PPAR-y coactivator α (PGC-1α) activity [71]. PPAR-α regulates the mRNA expression involved in mitochondrial and peroxisome fatty acid oxidation, fatty acid uptake, and TG catabolism (*i.e.*, such carnitine palmitoyltransferase (CPT)-1 α and acyl-CoA oxidase; ACO) [72]. In this regard, these authors have also shown that TAU significantly decreased TG levels in obese rats through enhancing PPAR-α gene expression, which up-regulates ACO and CPT- 1 α gene expressions. In the same vein, Tsuboyama-Kasaoka and colleagues have shown that TAU considerably upregulated the expression levels of transcription factors and cofactors associated with energy expenditure, including PPARα, PPARy, PGC-1, and nuclear respiratory factor 2α in WAT [73]. This activated route can improve hepatic peroxisomal and mitochondrial β-oxidation routes in obese rats supplemented with TAU. Therefore, they showed that TAU has an anti-obesity effect by decreasing TG accumulation by up-regulating the expression of carbohydrate response element-binding protein (ChREBP) and microsomal TG transfer protein (MTP) genes ameliorates hepatic lipid efflux and increases PPAR-α gene expression. Furthermore, TAU considerably increased the mitochondrial and peroxisomal lipid oxidation in the liver through the modulation of the ACO and CPT-1α genes.

A clinical study also reported a considerable decrement in body weight through improvements in metabolisms of lipids in obese human subjects with type 2 diabetes treated with an analog of FGF21, LY2405319 [74]. Hence, they concluded that FGF21-based therapies might be efficient for some metabolic disorders. For more information about BATokines and their roles, see the review by Villarroya and colleagues [75].

MITOCHONDRIA, ADIPOCYTES, AND OBESITY

Mitochondria are considered crucial intracellular organelles for energy metabolism; so there are unique intracellular elements (*i.e.*, specific enzymes and intracellular related pathways) that are able to convert the chemical energy derivative of carbohydrates, lipids, and proteins into adenosine triphosphate (ATP), in the form of accessible energy for cells [76, 77]. Based on the evidence available, numerous crucial functions are determined for this vital organelle, such as cooperation in energy homeostasis, autophagy, apoptosis, and inflammatory-related routes through controlling their quantity or morphology and/or modifying their organization and distribution [78 - 83].

However, accumulated evidence reveals that mitochondria play a pivotal role in adipocytes' differentiation and function by regulating oxidative stress, mitochondrial biogenesis, lipolysis, apoptosis, and efficiency of oxidative phosphorylation [84] and maintaining energy homeostasis in metabolic tissues (*i.e.*, adipose tissues). Hence, adipocyte mitochondria could be a good target for which intervention in its function significantly alters adipogenesis [85] and will help those interested in losing body fat.

In an alive creature, adipose tissue is a well-known organ that manages energy homeostasis. In brief, the fatty tissue can save the overabundant nutrients as a form of TGs in a situation with extra energy. In contrast, this organ can provide nutrients to other tissues by an important intracellular route called lipolysis [84]. Besides their roles in controlling systemic energy homeostasis (*i.e.*, as a supplier of cellular energy), these organelles also have adipocyte-specific functions. For instance, evidence indicates that adipocyte mitochondria participate well in critical adipocyte biology (*i.e.*, adipogenesis, lipid metabolism, and thermogenesis) [85, 86]. Moreover, multiple lines of research have demonstrated that these mitochondria might also play crucial roles in managing whole-body energy homeostasis, regulation of glucose metabolism and insulin sensitivity, and/or crosstalk between muscles and adipose tissues [87, 88].

As illustrated in Table **1**, the WAT is round-shaped cells of various sizes (depending on a single lipid droplet). This single lipid droplet comprises TGs and considers about 90 percent of the whole cell volume. The WAT mitochondria are thin, lengthened, and flexible in quantity (Table **1**). As mentioned in the previous sections, in contradiction to WAT, the BAT has multilocular lipid droplets with mitochondria morphologically different from those in WAT. The mitochondria of BAT are superficially dissimilar from the mitochondria of WAT, where these BAT mitochondria are more abundant, more giant, and encompass packed cristae than those in the WAT (Table **1**) [89]. Many mitochondria in BAT in the images recorded by precise microscopes are detected as brownish elements; because of the iron-containing heme-cofactor in the mitochondrial enzyme (well-known as cytochrome oxidase) [90].

Table 1. Mitochondrial properties of various types of adipocytes.

Mitochondrial Features	WAT	BAT and bAT	DOI
Morphology 1) Size 2) Figure 3) Construction	• Tiny • Ellipsoid • Lengthened	• Bigger than WAT • Sphere-shaped • Packed cristae	10.1152/ajpendo.00183.2009
Content	• Rarity of mitochondria	• BAT: Maximum number • Beige: Minimum to Maximum depends on stimulation	10.2353/ajpath.2009.081155
Development	• Unwell developed	• Well developed	10.2353/ajpath.2009.081155
Key role	• Differentiation • Lipogenesis	• Differentiation • Thermogenesis • Fatty acid oxidation	10.1016/j.cmet.2009.08.014
UCP1 expression	• Minimum	• Maximum	10.2353/ajpath.2009.081155
Tissue-specific mitochondrial genes	• Moscl • Acsm5	• Acss1 • Pdk4	10.1016/j.cmet.2009.08.014
White (WAT); Brown (BAT); Beige (bAT) adipocytes; Molybdenum cofactor sulfurase C-terminal domain containing protein 1 (Moscl); Acyl-coenzymeAsynthase (Acsm5); Acetyl-CoA synthase 2-like (Acss1); Pyruvate dehydrogenase kinase 4 (Pdk4).			

Like other tissues, the mitochondria of WAT also characterize the core source of ATP. Meanwhile, the WAT mitochondria play crucial roles in essential biological routes, including fatty acid oxidation, lipolysis, lipogenesis, and differentiation [86, 91]. However, one of the well-known characteristics of WAT is the minimum number of their mitochondria compared with that of BAT. The minimum fatty acid oxidation-related enzyme expression (*i.e.*, acyl-CoA dehydrogenase) in WAT recommends that fatty acid oxidation activity in these adipocytes is considerably lower than that in BAT (Table **1**) [92 - 95]. An *in-vivo* mitochondrial proteome between WAT and BAT in mice was conducted by Forner and colleagues, who wanted to clarify the tissue-specific functions of mitochondria [96]. Their observations recorded considerable qualitative and quantitative alterations in the mitochondrial proteins of these two adipocyte types. Meanwhile, these researchers also showed that the proteins involved in pathways related to fatty acid metabolism, oxidative phosphorylation (OXPHOS), and the TCA cycle were highly expressed in BAT compared to WAT [96].

The BAT-isolated mitochondria are more similar to those isolated from skeletal muscles. On the other hand, the WAT mitochondria selectively express the relative proteins that modulate lipogenic function. Meanwhile, these mitochondria from WAT could degrade xenobiotics, demonstrating this type of adipocyte's protective role. Notably, two tissue-specific mitochondrial genes, molybdenum cofactor sulfurase C-terminal domain-containing protein 1 (Mosc1, a component of the prodrug-converting complex) and acyl-coenzyme A synthase (Acsm5, with CoA ligase activity), were recorded only in WAT (Table **1**). Whereas acetyl-CoA synthase 2-like (Acss1, which converts acetate to acetyl-CoA), and pyruvate dehydrogenase kinase 4 (Pdk4, which inhibits the pyruvate dehydrogenase complex, thereby reducing the conversion of pyruvate to acetyl-CoA), were exclusively identified in BAT (Table **1**).

As mentioned in previous sections, the prominent role of WAT is to save extra energy, while the crucial one for BAT is energy expenditure through mitochondria-related non-shivering thermogenesis (*via* converting chemical energy into heat in adaptive thermogenesis); hence, BAT, that is produced by the browning of WAT in response to various stimuli (*e.g.*, cold stress situations and ß-adrenergic agonists), is characterized by the massive number of mitochondria. In fact, upon activation of sympathetic stimulation, BAT and bAT release the stored chemical energy (as a form of TGs) through two crucial intracellular routes, lipolysis and fatty acid oxidation. And then, the substrate oxidation-derived energy can be converted to heat [15, 93, 97]; a process called non-shivering thermogenesis of BAT and activated bAT; a critical strategy for small animals and new-borns who require more heat formation due to the large surface-to-volume ratio and hibernation of some unique species [98].

Mitochondria have crucial physiological roles in adipocytes, including adipocyte differentiation, lipid homeostasis, oxidative capacity, glucose utilization and insulin sensitivity, thermogenesis, and WAT browning (Fig. **2**). For more information about the role of various types of mitochondria in adipocytes, see the review article by Lee *et al.* [18] (Fig. **2**). Meanwhile, literature data report a solid relation between the dysfunctionality of mitochondria with metabolic disorders, such as obesity and type 2 diabetes. It has been shown that mitochondrial dysfunction can cause harmful effects on lipid metabolism, adipocyte differentiation, oxidative capacity, insulin sensitivity, and thermogenesis, which ultimately can cause metabolic disorders [18].

Over the years, we frequently reported the improved functionality of mitochondria induced by the administration of some mitochondria-targeted herbal/chemical antioxidants and natural dietary compounds (such as agmatine, silymarin, carnosine, histidine, betaine, boldine, chlorogenic acid, N-acetyl cysteine, methylene blue, Metformin, edaravone, and TAU) [11, 12, 99 - 124], by performing exercise [108, 112]; and by controlling caloric restriction (by probiotic treatment [125]. Meanwhile, it has been shown that these elements can maintain metabolic homeostasis through stimulating adaptive thermogenesis of BAT and browning of WAT [18].

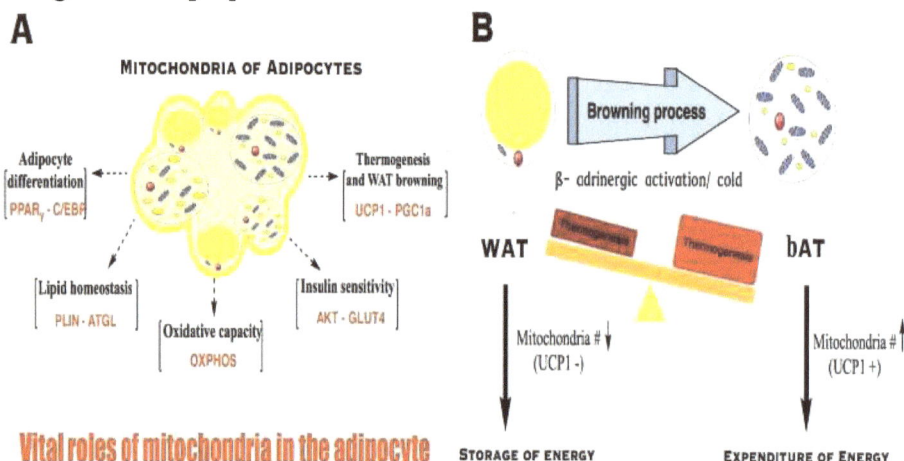

Fig. (2). (A) The critical physiological role of mitochondria in regulating various adipocytes' functions. **(B)** bAT formation by browning process. Like BAT, bAT has an enriched number of mitochondria expressing UCP1 and then induces thermogenesis. Hence, it has been well known that bAT is mainly involved in energy expenditure more than energy storage. PPARy: Peroxisome proliferator-activated receptor; C/EBP: CCAATenhancer-binding protein; PLIN: Perilipin; ATGL: Adipose triglyceride lipase; OXPHOS: Oxidative phosphorylation; GLUT4: Glucose transporter type 4; UCP1: Uncoupling protein-1; PGC1a: PPAR coactivator 1-a. This figure is inspired by a similar figure from DOI:10.3390/ijms20194924.

AMELIORATIVE ROLE OF TAURINE IN ADIPOSE TISSUES' ENERGY METABOLISMS

One of the primary and general processes in the body is energy metabolism (EM). In this way, the body of all organisms can obtain and consume energy to keep its normal function. However, TAU can play a critical role in this physiological event. Therefore, any deficiency of this AA can occur in a feeble EM and EM dysfunction. However, the bio-generation of this AA is limited. Thus, any diet supplementation of TAU can improve EM in various organs, including the functionality of muscle, heart, liver, and adipose tissue. Combining this AA with other high-potential chemicals (like medicines) might facilitate the EM of fatty tissue. In this view, a good body of literature demonstrates that any supplementation of this AA alone or in combination with other high potential chemicals showed a therapeutic role in damaged tissues or acted as a modulator of EM's balance. Due to the importance of this topic, the potential role of TAU in the EM of adipose tissue is discussed in this section.

As mentioned earlier, TAU has a crucial role in maintaining physiological homeostasis; hence, it is not surprising that TAU depletion can cause a disproportion in EM in various tissues, such as adipose tissue, through tissue histological defection and dysfunctionality, which finally results in compromised EM (Fig. **1**).

It is getting progressively clear that any deficiency in TAU can cause abnormality in adipose tissue function by disrupting the metabolism of adipocytes. For instance, Ito and colleagues have shown less abdominal fat mass of TauT-knockout (TauTKO) mice exposed to a typical food [126]. On the other hand, over-exposure to a high-fat diet (60% fat) in these animals caused obesity. Bodyweight was significantly decreased in the TauTKO mice exposed to a regular chow diet, implying nutrition concentrations in the standard chow diet are insufficient for these animals to keep their body weight compared with that in the wild-type [127]. Finally, they concluded that TAU depletion increased glucose disposal, despite decreasing insulin content and lower body weight, suggesting deterioration in tissue EM. In another study, these authors reported that the blood lactate concentration was raised (>3-fold) during treadmill running in TauTKO mice. However, they have not observed a significant difference in the WT mice, recommending an endogenous competition between fatty acids and glucose metabolism [128]. On the other hand, it has been shown that TAU restores the homeostasis of EM in xenobiotics-induced dysfunction of energy expenditure in different organs [129].

Multiple lines of investigation have shown that adipose tissue is considered an energy reservoir and acts as an endocrine organ synthesizing and secreting various types of adipokines (*i.e.*, two critical and well-known ones are leptin and adiponectin). These two adipokines are involved in crucial routes, including food intake, energy expenditure, and glucose homeostasis control [130 - 132], and play essential roles in other endogenous systems, such as the reproductive system [133 - 135]. The functionality of reproduction is closely related to the energy balance. For instance, Dos Santos and colleagues have shown that metabolic abnormalities might cause a dozen complications in pregnancy and ultimately cause alterations in fetal growth [134]. They have also implied that the ratio of leptin to adiponectin might be a clinically valuable marker for identifying various pathologies in pregnancy.

As discussed above, WAT also plays an endocrine function and releases various bioactive elements, including adipokines, tumor necrosis factor-α (TNF-α; the most-assessed cytokine in WAT with the maximum mRNA expression discovered in the adipocyte), the anti-inflammatory interleukin-10 (IL-10), and several other compounds based on the degree of WAT accumulation (Obesity) [127, 130 - 132,

136]. TNF-α is involved in physiological, immunological, and metabolic routes in WAT; meanwhile, its crucial role in the biosynthesis of various cytokines, like IL-10 and other adipokines in WAT (*i.e.*, leptin) is well reported [137, 138]. These compounds have been shown to act locally and distally, with autocrine, paracrine, and endocrine effects [139]. Therefore, we can consider the crucial role of this tissue with other proximal and distal tissues.

Murakami has reviewed the impact and mechanisms of this AA on the development of obesity through the suppression of adipocyte inflammation [131]. However, TAU derivatives (*i.e.*, TAU chloramine (TauCl) and tauroursodeoxycholic acid), synthesized from TAU in the body, also present an anti-obesity effect through a modulatory effect on inflammation and ER stress in adipocytes [131]. Therefore, obesity triggers a slight but chronic inflammation in the fatty tissue, causing several metabolic disorders. In this way, it has been shown that TauCl can prevent nitric oxide (NO) biosynthesis, TNF-α generation, and other pro-inflammatory mediators formation through macrophages [140] and polymorphonuclear leukocytes (PMNs) [141, 142]. Therefore, obesity is a situation of chronic inflammation and oxidative stress. As elucidated in Table **2**, a body of data presented the relation of mitochondrial impairments with metabolic disorders like obesity.

Table 2. The ameliorative roles of Taurine [TAU] on the metabolism of glucose and lipid in obese animals

Study Models	TAU Exposure	Findings	DOI
NAFL-male hamster induced by high-fat/cholesterol dietary	Drinking water containing 0.35 and 0.7% TAU for four weeks	(0.7% TAU): Dec. in weight gain, visceral fat, liver TG and TC. Inc. in energy expenditure.	10.1021/jf103167u
Chronic ethanol feeding induces hepatic steatosis in rats	Drinking water containing 30 g/L TAU for four weeks	Dec. in adiponectin levels and then hepatic steatosis. Inc. in fatty acid oxidation.	10.1002/hep.22811
MSG-caused obesity in male Wistar rats	2.5% TAU in drinking water for 100 d	Dec. in body weight, retroperitoneal and perigonadal fat pad, liver TG. Inc. lipid oxidation.	10.1016/j.lfs.2015.05.019
MSG-caused obesity in male Wistar rats	2.5% TAU in drinking water for 70 d	Dec. in retroperitoneal and periepididymal fat pad, NEFA, and TG.	10.1007/s00726-010-0789-7

Study Models	TAU Exposure	Findings	DOI
MSG-caused obesity in male Wistar rats	2.5% TAU in drinking water for 100 d	Dec. in retroperitoneal and perigonadal fat pad, and insulin level.	10.1007/s00394-015-1114-8
Male Wistar rats	5% TAU of the diet for 14 d	Dec. in cholesteryl ester. Inc. in fatty acid oxidation.	10.3177/jnsv.57.144
Diabetic/obese KK-A(y) mice	Fish oil (7%) + taurine *via* drinking water (4%) for four weeks	Dec. in WAT weight. Inc. in fatty acid oxidation Imp. in hyperglycemia and Hyperinsulinemia.	10.1111/j.1750-3841.2012.02687.x
High-fat diet-induced obese C57BL/6J mice	2.5% TAU in drinking water for 14 weeks	Dec. in subcutaneous, epididymal, mesenteric, and retroperitoneal WAT.	• 10.1002/mnfr.201300150
High-fat diet-induced obese C57BL/6J mice	2.5% TAU in drinking water for 18 weeks	Dec. in body fat, parametrial WAT, adipocyte size. Inc. in resting energy expenditure.	• 10.1210/en.2005-1007
High-fat diet-caused obese weaned male C57BL/6J mice	5% TAU in drinking water for eight weeks	• Dec. in body weight, • retroperitoneal and pre-epididymal fat pad. • Inc. in liver glucose control.	• 10.1002/mnfr.201200345 •
NAFL: Non-alcoholic fatty liver; Inc.: increment; Dec.: decrement; Imp.: improvement; TG: triglyceride; TC: total cholesterol; MSG: monosodium glutamate; NEFA: non-esterified fatty acids.			

The most well-known models to assess anti-obesity effects for various kinds of xenobiotics, including diets, and chemicals, are multiple types of high-fat diet-induced obesity models. TAU improves xenobiotics-induced obesity *via* different physiological and intracellular routes (Table **2**). Progress in the field has revealed that the TAU plasma concentration was considerably lowered in obese humans and animals [73, 143], implying that this metabolic disorder is a TAU-deficient. Tsuboyama-Kasaoka *et al.* (2006) have shown that the protein levels of cysteine dioxygenase and plasma TAU levels were tangibly decreased in WAT (but not in BAT) in the animal exposed to a high-fat diet [73]. Based on their observation, it can be assumed that cysteine dioxygenase in the WAT can control blood TAU levels and that large-scale adipocytes synthesize and release the minimum levels of this AA [73].

Energy expenditure can be considered a popular model to assess the potential anti-obesity effects of TAU. On the other hand, PGC-1α is a potential marker to measure energy expenditure in adipose tissues as a cellular switch from an energy-storage state to an energy-expenditure mood, stimulating mitochondrial biogenesis and fatty acid oxidation, and adaptive thermogenesis [144, 145]. As shown in Table **2**, TAU can mitigate considerably extreme body weight gain and hyperplasia [146]. However, it showed that the diets supplemented with TAU increased the BAT weight and decreased the WAT mass. The mentioned alterations in these two types of adipocytes are related to PGC-1α upregulation [130], implying that TAU triggers energy expenditure. As referred, adipocytes can stimulate the synthesis and release of different molecules (*i.e.*, adiponectin) [134, 135]. The adipokine concentration is decreased in obese humans and rodents [147, 148]; You *et al.* (2013) showed a positive correlation between serum TAU level and adiponectin levels in high-fat diet-induced obese rats. In the same vein, accumulating evidence reveals that the animals exposed to TAU-supplemented diets exhibited a considerable increment in the plasma levels of adiponectin and renovated adiponectin mRNA expression in the adipose tissue compared with those in the obese rats [143, 148, 149].

Moreover, it has been shown that exposure to TAU (3%) for 56 days considerably decreased the total cholesterol (TC) in serum as compared with high-fat diet-induced obese females [148], implying that TAU can essentially reverse obesity by increasing the levels of adiponectin. On the other hand, in different experimental models (*e.g.*, worms), it has also been reported that TAU could decrease fat accumulation by controlling lipid deposition and promoting mobility without any effects on lipid biosynthesis and/or food consumption rate [150]. The anti-obesity roles of TAU were also assessed in obese trained rats [151]. Meanwhile, an in-depth investigation reported that the serum levels of TAU were notably lower in the obese group than the control group and that the adiponectin concentration was increased upon exposure to TAU [143], recommending that TAU can amend lipid peroxidation and insulin sensitivity.

Multiple lines of research have revealed that TAU (0.7%) improved high-fat diet-induced obesity, dose-dependently decreased fat repositories and plasma insulin levels, tangibly limiting the increase in fasting blood glucose content, and increased TAU levels in the WAT, probably standardizing calorie intake and reducing visceral fat in the high-fat diet-induced obese groups [146, 152, 153]. Meanwhile, Chang *et al.* (2011) have shown that the blood concentrations of TC, TG, and non-high-density lipoprotein cholesterol (HDL-C) were considerably mitigated by TAU (0.35% - 0.7%) in the high-fat diet-induced obese groups than the control group [153]. TAU triggers adipocytes lipolysis through two routes [154]:

- By triggering adenosine monophosphate (cAMP)-dependent protein kinase A (PKA) catalytic activity.
- They favor PKA activation *via* the cAMP action and inhibit the H_2O_2 pool increase.

Macrophages- synthesized TauCl might prevent preadipocyte differentiation into adipocytes [155]. Additional investigations presented that TauCl controls the adipokines expression by preventing the signal transducer and activator of the transcription of three signaling routes [156], representing possible applications in obesity-related disorders. Moreover, in the obese rodents induced by monosodium glutamate (MSG), the BAT density in the TAU-exposed rats was considerably higher than in the obese model group. However, the density of WAT was significantly lower than in the model group [157]. They have also shown that the PGC-1α mRNA expression in the WAT and BAT was significantly upregulated in the TAU-supplemented group (notably higher in the BAT). The remarkable point here is the function of PGC-1α switching cells from an energy depository mood to energy expenditure types, including mitochondria's biogenesis and adaptive thermogenesis.

THE ANTI-OBESITY ROLE OF TAU THROUGH MITOCHONDRIAL FUNCTION IMPROVEMENT

There is a close correlation between obesity and mitochondrial impairment, ROS over-biosynthesis, lipoperoxides, and changes in pro-oxidative–antioxidative balance [130]. Multiple lines of research have revealed that mitochondrial functionality can be improved by various xenobiotics (*i.e.*, mitochondria-targeted antioxidants, PPAR agonist thiazolidinedione (TZD), caloric restriction, exercise, and dietary natural and chemical compounds, like TAU). Hence, these factors could be considered novel probable therapeutic approaches for the medication of metabolic disorders. As in the last years, we have frequently reported the ameliorative role of TAU in various organs' injuries by improving the functionality of mitochondria damaged by several types of environmental toxins and drugs-caused multiple organ injuries induced by oxidative stress [10 - 13, 101, 102, 104, 106, 108 - 110, 119]. Therefore, it can be supposed that the improving effects of TAU on mitochondrial biogenesis, morphology, and remodeling might also play a role in the anti-obesity mechanisms of this AA.

In the same vein, it has been frequently shown that TAU stimulates weight loss by encouraging the activity of brown and beige adipocytes through mitochondrial-related routes [129, 158]. Rikimaru and colleagues have shown that challenging mitochondrial myopathy, encephalopathy, lactic acidosis, and stroke (MELAS)-patient-derived cells with TAU improved mitochondrial indices, including mitochondrial membrane potential, mitochondrial oxygen consumption, and the redox status [159]. TAU also can regulate mitochondrial protein synthesis; so, improving the activity of the electron transport chain and keeping the mitochondria against excessive superoxide formation [160]. Moreover, a considerable number of TAU is discovered in the tissues with high oxidative activity implying that this AA can mitigate the leakage of the reactive substances generated in the reactive mitochondrial environment [161]. Based on the above literature, it can be suggested that TAU is vital for maintaining the normal adipocytes' mitochondrial functionality and could normalize mitochondrial impairment stimulated by different types of stresses. Therefore, it can be assumed that TAU can act indirectly as a highly potent antioxidant by presenting adequate pH buffering in the mitochondrial matrix. This AA can also preserve mitochondrial functionality, which results in a considerable decrement in the development of obesity.

β-oxidation of short-chain fatty acids is one of the most crucial functions of cellular mitochondria in adipocytes [162]. On the other hand, lipogenesis is a process in which TGs are formed from fatty acids in WAT [162]. TAU could affect several mitochondria-dependent signaling pathways at molecular levels, leading to BAT formation and fatty acid metabolism [163, 164]. TAU can increase mitochondrial ß-oxidation of fatty acids in the liver and consequently improve the accumulation of plasma and tissue TG [130]. In the same vein, it has been reported that GW3965 (synthetic LXR agonist) increased the activity of mitochondrial β-oxidation in both humans and rodents WAT [165]. LXRs (LXR-α and LXR-β) are well-known as the ligand-activated transcription factors of the nuclear receptor superfamily playing crucial roles in the homeostasis of glucose and lipid and the inflammatory responses [166 - 168]. Hence, this might suggest the vital role of LXR in the control of substrate oxidation and the switch between carbohydrates and lipids as the potential fuels into the cells. There is good murine and human-related literature on the role of LXRs in the WAT. In this regard, Dib *et al.* (2014) have shown that LXRα - knockout mice presented more bodyweight and adipose mass on a high-fat diet than those in the WT control group with the same diet [169]. However, it has been shown that the GW3965- activated LXR ameliorates the glucose tolerance in diet-induced obesity and insulin resistance study [170]. Based on the above literature, it can be proposed that the LXRα activation by TAU might ameliorate the lipids and carbohydrates' metabolisms in adipose tissues, thus improving obesity and insulin resistance.

It has been found that in activated brown-beige adipocytes, a large amount of heat is produced instead of energy after β-oxidation of fatty acids [162]. This process is essential during hibernation in animals and human infants with more thermogenesis demands due to the sizeable surface-to-body ratio [162]. It has also been shown that TAU can express one part of its anti-obesity effects through stimulating thermogenesis (for instance, by triggering the expression of characteristic thermogenic genes) [164]. The thermogenesis in bAT/BAT adipocytes is possible with the help of a group of proteins called UCPs, a BAT marker gene [162]. Interestingly, as mentioned, it has been found that TAU significantly increased the expression of UCP1 in WAT [163]. Similar results were also shown by Tsuboyama-Kasaoka *et al.* (2006). They reported significant increments in the mRNA levels of the ß-subunit of ATP synthetase and uncoupling protein-2 (UCP-2) in WAT, which are crucial for the respiratory activity of mitochondria. Moreover, the expression of their target genes, lipoprotein lipase, acyl-coenzyme A (CoA) oxidase, acyl-CoA synthetase, and medium-chain acyl-CoA dehydrogenase in WAT, enzymes for fatty acid ß-oxidation, were also increased as compared with high-fat-diet- fed mice without TAU.

In this context, one of the well-known inducers for the development of BAT is PGC1α which has been shown to transact the mRNA level of UCP1 and be an effective activator of mitochondrial biogenesis and oxidation of fatty acids [144]. There are some renowned markers to determine mitochondrial biogenesis and oxidation of fatty acids; for instance, mitochondrial cytochrome-*c* (Cyt-*c*) and mitochondrial transcription factor-A (mtTF-A) expression levels indicate the mitochondrial biogenesis activity, whereas medium-chain acyl-CoA dehydrogenase (MCAD) and carnitine palmitoyl-CoA: transferase 1b (Cpt1b) expression levels reflect the fatty acid oxidation level [171]. Guo *et al.* (2019) have reported that in BAT and IWAT (with a more effective in IWAT), the expression of these genes and the protein levels of PGC1α and UCP1 were considerably upregulated upon exposure to TAU. By immunohistochemistry (IHC) staining assays, these researchers have shown that TAU upregulated the expression level of UCP1and decreased the size of adipocytes compared to those in the control PBS group. Moreover, TAU increased the mitochondrial copy number in the IWAT of the mice, proposing improved mitochondrial biogenesis. On the other hand, they have shown that TAU-improved mitochondrial biosynthesis (evaluated by MitoTracker Green (MTG) staining) was blocked by the PGC1α knockdown. Based on their report, it can be concluded that TAU triggers the browning of WAT, particularly in IWAT (subcutaneous fat).

Another high potential regulator for EM and mitochondrial biogenesis is adenosine 5'-monophosphate (AMP)-activated protein kinase (AMPK) [15, 172]. However, the precise intracellular mechanisms by which AMPK regulates energy balance are not comprehensively clarified, although the footprint of PGC1α is traced, claiming that it can either upregulate the mRNA level of PGC1α or directly involved in the phosphorylation of PGC1α [173, 174]. In this regard, Guo *et al.* (2019) have also shown that TAU can phosphorylate the AMPK in adipocytes of high-fat diet-fed mice [163]. The authors have used the siRNA-mediated knockdown of the α1-subunit of AMPK (AMPKα1) in adipocytes to confirm this issue. This AMPK signaling downregulation significantly diminished the positive sign role of TAU in upregulations of PGC1α and UCP1, ameliorating oxygen consumption rate and increasing mitochondrial biosynthesis [163]. Therefore, it can be assumed that AMPK can act as an energy sensor playing a crucial role in controlling complex signaling systems of EM and mitochondrial biogenesis [175, 176]. Furthermore, they also showed that the positive role of TAU in increasing mitochondrial copy number and oxygen consumption rate in IWAT was also diminished by the knockdown of PGC1α. Meanwhile, Tiraby *et al.* (2003) have shown that the PGC1α ectopic expression of WAT caused the acquisition of BAT features, such as mitochondrial, fatty acid oxidation, and thermogenic- related genes up-regulation [145]. Therefore, the anti-obesity role of the TAU/AMPK/PGC1α route through triggering the adipocytes browning was established.

THE EFFECTS OF TAURINE COMBINATION THERAPY IN ADIPOSE TISSUE

W-3 Polyunsaturated fatty acids (PUFAs, such as eicosapentaenoic acid and docosahexaenoic acid) are considered a high potential and functional element rich in seafood. One of the well-known ameliorative effects of these W-3 compounds is their decreasing effects on plasma lipid concentrations. Based on this fact, the combination of fish oil, as a potent component containing a resealable amount of W-3 PUFAs, and TAU is recommended by much in-depth research for preventing obesity through mitochondrial and non-mitochondrial-related routes. In a mice study, it has been shown that WAT gain and blood glucose content was considerably decreased upon challenging type 2 diabetic/obese kk-a(y) mice with a combination of dietary fish oil and TAU (4%) for 28 days [158]. However, they had shown that this reduction effect was considerably higher than when soybean oil was treated alone.

Moreover, the study showed that the mice exposed to a mixture of fish oil and TAU (2%) significantly increased the acyl-CoA oxidase content. Based on their research, we can conclude that combining fish oil (a well-known resource for W-3 PUFA) and TAU can potentially improve adipose metabolism in obese ones by increasing mitochondrial functionality. Moreover, over the years, research has demonstrated that branched-chain amino acids (BCAAs, mainly leucine supplementation) can tangibly change the body fat mass and ameliorate EM, comprising glucose uptake and fatty acid oxidation [177, 178]. However, further studies are needed to assess the ameliorative effects of the BCAA + TAU mixture in preventing and treating obesity. Meanwhile, in the last chapter entitled "Importance of Appropriate TAU Formulation to Target Mitochondria", we comprehensively discussed the newly available techniques for increasing the bio-functionality of TAU through mitochondria-related pathways.

CONCLUSION

Obesity could be induced by an imbalance between energy expenditure and energy intake. Herein, an introduction to different adipocyte types that focus on these cells' mitochondrial function is provided. On the other hand, there is a negative association between obesity and Tau formation. Then, the potential effects of TAU on adipocytes and its role in treating obesity, as one of the significant health challenges worldwide, is highlighted. Even though the intracellular mechanisms involved in the anti-obesity action of TAU remain well-identified, TAU seems to improve obesity through mitochondrial-related and unrelated routes, including triggering energy expenditure, controlling lipid metabolism, anorexic effect, anti-inflammatory, and anti-oxidative effects. Therefore, it can be concluded that TAU, alone and combined with other high potent components, has an anti-obesity impact by improving mitochondria's function. The effects of mitochondria-targeting drugs in fatty tissues are pretty promising; hence, there is a hope to develop effective metabolic disorders therapies. Nevertheless, further investigations are needed to clarify mitochondrial impairments' intracellular mechanisms and their pathogenic influence on developing metabolic complications.

REFERENCES

[1]   Hurt RT, Kulisek C, Buchanan LA, McClave SA. The obesity epidemic: challenges, health initiatives, and implications for gastroenterologists. Gastroenterol Hepatol (N Y) 2010; 6(12): 780-92.
        [PMID: 21301632]

[2]   Finucane MM, Stevens GA, Cowan MJ, *et al.* National, regional, and global trends in body-mass index since 1980: systematic analysis of health examination surveys and epidemiological studies with 960 country-years and 9·1 million participants. Lancet 2011; 377(9765): 557-67.
        [http://dx.doi.org/10.1016/S0140-6736(10)62037-5] [PMID: 21295846]

[3]   Seidell JC, Halberstadt J. The global burden of obesity and the challenges of prevention. Ann Nutr Metab 2015; 66 (Suppl. 2): 7-12.
        [http://dx.doi.org/10.1159/000375143] [PMID: 26045323]

[4]   Visscher TLS, Seidell JC. The public health impact of obesity. Annu Rev Public Health 2001; 22(1): 355-75.
        [http://dx.doi.org/10.1146/annurev.publhealth.22.1.355] [PMID: 11274526]

[5]   Taylor VH, Forhan M, Vigod SN, McIntyre RS, Morrison KM. The impact of obesity on quality of life. Best Pract Res Clin Endocrinol Metab 2013; 27(2): 139-46.
        [http://dx.doi.org/10.1016/j.beem.2013.04.004] [PMID: 23731876]

[6]   Seidell JC, Halberstadt J, Noordam H, Niemer S. An integrated health care standard for the management and prevention of obesity in The Netherlands. Fam Pract 2012; 29 (Suppl. 1): i153-6.
        [http://dx.doi.org/10.1093/fampra/cmr057] [PMID: 22399546]

[7]   Imae M, Asano T, Murakami S. Potential role of taurine in the prevention of diabetes and metabolic syndrome. Amino Acids 2014; 46(1): 81-8.
[http://dx.doi.org/10.1007/s00726-012-1434-4] [PMID: 23224909]

[8]   Chen W, Guo J, Zhang Y, Zhang J. The beneficial effects of taurine in preventing metabolic syndrome. Food Funct 2016; 7(4): 1849-63.
[http://dx.doi.org/10.1039/C5FO01295C] [PMID: 26918249]

[9]   Chen W, Guo JX, Chang P. The effect of taurine on cholesterol metabolism. Mol Nutr Food Res 2012; 56(5): 681-90.
[http://dx.doi.org/10.1002/mnfr.201100799] [PMID: 22648615]

[10]   Heidari R, Jamshidzadeh A, Niknahad H, *et al.* Effect of taurine on chronic and acute liver injury: Focus on blood and brain ammonia. Toxicol Rep 2016; 3: 870-9.
[http://dx.doi.org/10.1016/j.toxrep.2016.04.002] [PMID: 28959615]

[11]   Jamshidzadeh A, Heidari R, Abasvali M, *et al.* Taurine treatment preserves brain and liver mitochondrial function in a rat model of fulminant hepatic failure and hyperammonemia. Biomed Pharmacother 2017; 86: 514-20.
[http://dx.doi.org/10.1016/j.biopha.2016.11.095] [PMID: 28024286]

[12]   Niknahad H, Jamshidzadeh A, Heidari R, Zarei M, Ommati MM. Ammonia-induced mitochondrial dysfunction and energy metabolism disturbances in isolated brain and liver mitochondria, and the effect of taurine administration: relevance to hepatic encephalopathy treatment. Clin Exp Hepatol 2017; 3(3): 141-51.
[http://dx.doi.org/10.5114/ceh.2017.68833] [PMID: 29062904]

[13]   Heidari R, Jamshidzadeh A, Ghanbarinejad V, Ommati MM, Niknahad H. Taurine supplementation abates cirrhosis-associated locomotor dysfunction. Clin Exp Hepatol 2018; 4(2): 72-82.
[http://dx.doi.org/10.5114/ceh.2018.75956] [PMID: 29904723]

[14]   Lafontan M. Adipose tissue and adipocyte dysregulation. Diabetes Metab 2014; 40(1): 16-28.
[http://dx.doi.org/10.1016/j.diabet.2013.08.002] [PMID: 24139247]

[15]   Bartelt A, Heeren J. Adipose tissue browning and metabolic health. Nat Rev Endocrinol 2014; 10(1): 24-36.
[http://dx.doi.org/10.1038/nrendo.2013.204] [PMID: 24146030]

[16]   Jeremic N, Chaturvedi P, Tyagi SC. Browning of white fat: novel insight into factors, mechanisms, and therapeutics. J Cell Physiol 2017; 232(1): 61-8.
[http://dx.doi.org/10.1002/jcp.25450] [PMID: 27279601]

[17]   Giralt M, Villarroya F. White, brown, beige/brite: different adipose cells for different functions? Endocrinology 2013; 154(9): 2992-3000.
[http://dx.doi.org/10.1210/en.2013-1403] [PMID: 23782940]

[18]   Lee JH, Park A, Oh K-J, Lee SC, Kim WK, Bae K-H. The role of adipose tissue mitochondria: Regulation of mitochondrial function for the treatment of metabolic diseases. Int J Mol Sci 2019; 20(19): 4924.
[http://dx.doi.org/10.3390/ijms20194924] [PMID: 31590292]

[19]   Park A, Kim WK, Bae KH. Distinction of white, beige and brown adipocytes derived from mesenchymal stem cells. World J Stem Cells 2014; 6(1): 33-42.
[http://dx.doi.org/10.4252/wjsc.v6.i1.33] [PMID: 24567786]

[20]   Srivastava S, Veech RL. Brown and brite: The fat soldiers in the anti-obesity fight. Front Physiol 2019; 10: 38.
[http://dx.doi.org/10.3389/fphys.2019.00038] [PMID: 30761017]

[21]   Lowell BB, Spiegelman BM. Towards a molecular understanding of adaptive thermogenesis. Nature 2000; 404(6778): 652-60.
[http://dx.doi.org/10.1038/35007527] [PMID: 10766252]

[22]   Bouillaud F, Alves-Guerra MC, Ricquier D. UCPs, at the interface between bioenergetics and metabolism. Biochim Biophys Acta Mol Cell Res 2016; 1863(10): 2443-56.
[http://dx.doi.org/10.1016/j.bbamcr.2016.04.013] [PMID: 27091404]

[23]   Kazak L, Chouchani ET, Jedrychowski MP, *et al.* A creatine-driven substrate cycle enhances energy expenditure and thermogenesis in beige fat. Cell 2015; 163(3): 643-55.
[http://dx.doi.org/10.1016/j.cell.2015.09.035] [PMID: 26496606]

[24]   Anunciado-Koza R, Ukropec J, Koza RA, Kozak LP. Inactivation of UCP1 and the glycerol phosphate cycle synergistically increases energy expenditure to resist diet-induced obesity. J Biol Chem 2008; 283(41): 27688-97.
[http://dx.doi.org/10.1074/jbc.M804268200] [PMID: 18678870]

[25]   Karise I, Bargut TC, del Sol M, Aguila MB, Mandarim-de-Lacerda CA. Metformin enhances mitochondrial biogenesis and thermogenesis in brown adipocytes of mice. Biomed Pharmacother 2019; 111: 1156-65.
[http://dx.doi.org/10.1016/j.biopha.2019.01.021] [PMID: 30841429]

[26]   Yuan T, Li J, Zhao WG, *et al.* Effects of metformin on metabolism of white and brown adipose tissue in obese C57BL/6J mice. Diabetol Metab Syndr 2019; 11(1): 96.
[http://dx.doi.org/10.1186/s13098-019-0490-2] [PMID: 31788033]

[27]   Liao W, Yin X, Li Q, *et al.* Resveratrol-induced white adipose tissue browning in obese mice by remodeling fecal microbiota. Molecules 2018; 23(12): 3356.
[http://dx.doi.org/10.3390/molecules23123356] [PMID: 30567366]

[28]   Silvester AJ, Aseer KR, Yun JW. Dietary polyphenols and their roles in fat browning. J Nutr Biochem 2019; 64: 1-12.
[http://dx.doi.org/10.1016/j.jnutbio.2018.09.028] [PMID: 30414469]

[29]   Seifi K, Rezaei M, Yansari AT, Riazi GH, Zamiri MJ, Heidari R. Saturated fatty acids may ameliorate environmental heat stress in broiler birds by affecting mitochondrial energetics and related genes. J Therm Biol 2018; 78: 1-9.
[http://dx.doi.org/10.1016/j.jtherbio.2018.08.018] [PMID: 30509623]

[30]   Seifi K, Rezaei M, Yansari AT, Zamiri MJ, Riazi GH, Heidari R. Short chain fatty acids may improve hepatic mitochondrial energy efficiency in heat stressed-broilers. J Therm Biol 2020; 89: 102520.
[http://dx.doi.org/10.1016/j.jtherbio.2020.102520] [PMID: 32364974]

[31]   Han Y, Wu JZ, Shen J, *et al.* Pentamethylquercetin induces adipose browning and exerts beneficial effects in 3T3-L1 adipocytes and high-fat diet-fed mice. Sci Rep 2017; 7(1): 1123.
[http://dx.doi.org/10.1038/s41598-017-01206-4] [PMID: 28442748]

[32]   Hu J, Christian M. Hormonal factors in the control of the browning of white adipose tissue. Horm Mol Biol Clin Investig 2017; 31(1): 31.
[http://dx.doi.org/10.1515/hmbci-2017-0017] [PMID: 28731853]

[33]   Ludwig RG, Rocha AL, Mori MA. Circulating molecules that control brown/beige adipocyte differentiation and thermogenic capacity. Cell Biol Int 2018; 42(6): 701-10.
[http://dx.doi.org/10.1002/cbin.10946] [PMID: 29384242]

[34]   Dallon BW, Parker BA, Hodson AE, *et al.* Insulin selectively reduces mitochondrial uncoupling in brown adipose tissue in mice. Biochem J 2018; 475(3): 561-9.
[http://dx.doi.org/10.1042/BCJ20170736] [PMID: 29170160]

[35]   Pohjanvirta R. AHR in energy balance regulation. Curr Opin Toxicol 2017; 2: 8-14.
[http://dx.doi.org/10.1016/j.cotox.2017.01.002]

[36]   Enriori PJ, Sinnayah P, Simonds SE, Garcia Rudaz C, Cowley MA. Leptin action in the dorsomedial hypothalamus increases sympathetic tone to brown adipose tissue in spite of systemic leptin resistance. J Neurosci 2011; 31(34): 12189-97.
[http://dx.doi.org/10.1523/JNEUROSCI.2336-11.2011] [PMID: 21865462]

[37] Côté I, Sakarya Y, Green SM, *et al.* iBAT sympathetic innervation is not required for body weight loss induced by central leptin delivery. Am J Physiol Endocrinol Metab 2018; 314(3): E224-31.
[http://dx.doi.org/10.1152/ajpendo.00219.2017] [PMID: 29089334]

[38] Bell BB, Harlan SM, Morgan DA, Guo DF, Rahmouni K, Rahmouni K. Differential contribution of POMC and AgRP neurons to the regulation of regional autonomic nerve activity by leptin. Mol Metab 2018; 8: 1-12.
[http://dx.doi.org/10.1016/j.molmet.2017.12.006] [PMID: 29289646]

[39] Martins FF, Bargut TCL, Aguila MB, Mandarim-de-Lacerda CA. Thermogenesis, fatty acid synthesis with oxidation, and inflammation in the brown adipose tissue of ob/ob (−/−) mice. Ann Anat 2017; 210: 44-51.
[http://dx.doi.org/10.1016/j.aanat.2016.11.013] [PMID: 27986616]

[40] Han J, Bae JH, Kim SY, *et al.* Taurine increases glucose sensitivity of UCP2-overexpressing β-cells by ameliorating mitochondrial metabolism. Am J Physiol Endocrinol Metab 2004; 287(5): E1008-18.
[http://dx.doi.org/10.1152/ajpendo.00008.2004] [PMID: 15265758]

[41] Kim KS, Oh DH, Kim JY, *et al.* Taurine ameliorates hyperglycemia and dyslipidemia by reducing insulin resistance and leptin level in Otsuka Long-Evans Tokushima fatty (OLETF) rats with long-term diabetes. Exp Mol Med 2012; 44(11): 665-73.
[http://dx.doi.org/10.3858/emm.2012.44.11.075] [PMID: 23114424]

[42] Camargo RL, Batista TM, Ribeiro RA, *et al.* Taurine supplementation preserves hypothalamic leptin action in normal and protein-restricted mice fed on a high-fat diet. Amino Acids 2015; 47(11): 2419-35.
[http://dx.doi.org/10.1007/s00726-015-2035-9] [PMID: 26133737]

[43] Weiner J, Kranz M, Klöting N, *et al.* Thyroid hormone status defines brown adipose tissue activity and browning of white adipose tissues in mice. Sci Rep 2016; 6(1): 38124.
[http://dx.doi.org/10.1038/srep38124] [PMID: 27941950]

[44] López M, Varela L, Vázquez MJ, *et al.* Hypothalamic AMPK and fatty acid metabolism mediate thyroid regulation of energy balance. Nat Med 2010; 16(9): 1001-8.
[http://dx.doi.org/10.1038/nm.2207] [PMID: 20802499]

[45] Martínez-Sánchez N, Moreno-Navarrete JM, Contreras C, *et al.* Thyroid hormones induce browning of white fat. J Endocrinol 2017; 232(2): 351-62.
[http://dx.doi.org/10.1530/JOE-16-0425] [PMID: 27913573]

[46] Martínez-Sánchez N, Seoane-Collazo P, Contreras C, *et al.* Hypothalamic AMPK-ER Stress-JNK1 axis mediates the central actions of thyroid hormones on energy balance. Cell Metab 2017; 26(1): 212-229.e12.
[http://dx.doi.org/10.1016/j.cmet.2017.06.014] [PMID: 28683288]

[47] Gavrila A, Hasselgren PO, Glasgow A, *et al.* Variable cold-induced brown adipose tissue response to thyroid hormone status. Thyroid 2017; 27(1): 1-10.
[http://dx.doi.org/10.1089/thy.2015.0646] [PMID: 27750020]

[48] Than A, Xu S, Li R, Leow MS, Sun L, Chen P. Angiotensin type 2 receptor activation promotes browning of white adipose tissue and brown adipogenesis. Signal Transduct Target Ther 2017; 2(1): 17022.
[http://dx.doi.org/10.1038/sigtrans.2017.22] [PMID: 29263921]

[49] Tsukuda K, Mogi M, Iwanami J, *et al.* Enhancement of Adipocyte Browning by Angiotensin II Type 1 Receptor Blockade. PLoS One 2016; 11(12): e0167704.
[http://dx.doi.org/10.1371/journal.pone.0167704] [PMID: 27992452]

[50] Watanabe M, Houten SM, Mataki C, *et al.* Bile acids induce energy expenditure by promoting intracellular thyroid hormone activation. Nature 2006; 439(7075): 484-9.
[http://dx.doi.org/10.1038/nature04330] [PMID: 16400329]

[51]   Taş S, Dirican M, Sarandöl E, Serdar Z. The effect of taurine supplementation on oxidative stress in experimental hypothyroidism. Cell Biochem Funct 2006; 24(2): 153-8.
[http://dx.doi.org/10.1002/cbf.1198] [PMID: 15617030]

[52]   Frank AP, Palmer BF, Clegg DJ. Do estrogens enhance activation of brown and beiging of adipose tissues? Physiol Behav 2018; 187: 24-31.
[http://dx.doi.org/10.1016/j.physbeh.2017.09.026] [PMID: 28988965]

[53]   López M, Tena-Sempere M. Estradiol and brown fat. Best Pract Res Clin Endocrinol Metab 2016; 30(4): 527-36.
[http://dx.doi.org/10.1016/j.beem.2016.08.004] [PMID: 27697213]

[54]   López M, Tena-Sempere M. Estradiol effects on hypothalamic AMPK and BAT thermogenesis: A gateway for obesity treatment? Pharmacol Ther 2017; 178: 109-22.
[http://dx.doi.org/10.1016/j.pharmthera.2017.03.014] [PMID: 28351720]

[55]   Ponnusamy S, Tran Q, Harvey I, Smallwood H, Thiyagarajan T, Banerjee S, *et al.* Pharmacologic activation of estrogen receptor increases mitochondrial function, energy expenditure, and brown adipose tissue. FASEB J 2016; 31.
[PMID: 27733447]

[56]   Roysommuti S, Suwanich A, Lerdweeraphon W, Thaeomor A, Jirakulsomchok D, Wyss JM. Sex dependent effects of perinatal taurine exposure on the arterial pressure control in adult offspring. Adv Exp Med Biol 2009; 643: 135-44.
[http://dx.doi.org/10.1007/978-0-387-75681-3_14] [PMID: 19239144]

[57]   McIlvride S, Mushtaq A, Papacleovoulou G, *et al.* A progesterone-brown fat axis is involved in regulating fetal growth. Sci Rep 2017; 7(1): 10671.
[http://dx.doi.org/10.1038/s41598-017-10979-7] [PMID: 28878263]

[58]   Liu P, Ji Y, Yuen T, *et al.* Blocking FSH induces thermogenic adipose tissue and reduces body fat. Nature 2017; 546(7656): 107-12.
[http://dx.doi.org/10.1038/nature22342] [PMID: 28538730]

[59]   Singh R, Braga M, Reddy ST, *et al.* Follistatin targets distinct pathways To promote brown adipocyte characteristics in brown and white adipose tissues. Endocrinology 2017; 158(5): 1217-30.
[http://dx.doi.org/10.1210/en.2016-1607] [PMID: 28324027]

[60]   Hashimoto O, Noda T, Morita A, *et al.* Castration induced browning in subcutaneous white adipose tissue in male mice. Biochem Biophys Res Commun 2016; 478(4): 1746-50.
[http://dx.doi.org/10.1016/j.bbrc.2016.09.017] [PMID: 27608598]

[61]   Alzubaidi NAK, Al Diwan MA. The effect of taurine on reproductive efficiency in male rats fed high cholesterol diet. Bas j vet Res. 2013;12(1):30-40.

[62]   Chondronikola M, Porter C, Malagaris I, Nella AA, Sidossis LS. Brown adipose tissue is associated with systemic concentrations of peptides secreted from the gastrointestinal system and involved in appetite regulation. Eur J Endocrinol 2017; 177(1): 33-40.
[http://dx.doi.org/10.1530/EJE-16-0958] [PMID: 28566533]

[63]   Kodo K, Sugimoto S, Nakajima H, *et al.* Erythropoietin (EPO) ameliorates obesity and glucose homeostasis by promoting thermogenesis and endocrine function of classical brown adipose tissue (BAT) in diet-induced obese mice. PLoS One 2017; 12(3): e0173661.
[http://dx.doi.org/10.1371/journal.pone.0173661] [PMID: 28288167]

[64]   Bookout AL, de Groot MHM, Owen BM, *et al.* FGF21 regulates metabolism and circadian behavior by acting on the nervous system. Nat Med 2013; 19(9): 1147-52.
[http://dx.doi.org/10.1038/nm.3249] [PMID: 23933984]

[65]   Owen BM, Ding X, Morgan DA, *et al.* FGF21 acts centrally to induce sympathetic nerve activity, energy expenditure, and weight loss. Cell Metab 2014; 20(4): 670-7.
[http://dx.doi.org/10.1016/j.cmet.2014.07.012] [PMID: 25130400]

[66]   Douris N, Stevanovic DM, Fisher M, *et al.* Central fibroblast growth factor 21 browns white fat *via* sympathetic action in male mice. Endocrinology 2015; 156(7): 2470-81.
[http://dx.doi.org/10.1210/en.2014-2001] [PMID: 25924103]

[67]   Haidari F, Asadi M, Mohammadi-asl J, Ahmadi-angali K. Evaluation of the effect of oral taurine supplementation on levels of fibroblast growth factors, β-Klotho co-receptor, some biochemical indices and body composition in obese women on a weight-loss diet: a study protocol for a double-blind randomized controlled trial. Research Square 2019.
[http://dx.doi.org/10.21203/rs.2.219/v2]

[68]   Zouhar P, Janovska P, Stanic S, *et al.* A pyrexic effect of FGF21 independent of energy expenditure and UCP1. Mol Metab 2021; 53: 101324.
[http://dx.doi.org/10.1016/j.molmet.2021.101324] [PMID: 34418595]

[69]   Moore TL, Podilakrishna R, Rao A, Alexis F. Systemic administration of polymer-coated nano-graphene to deliver drugs to glioblastoma. Part Part Syst Charact 2014; 31(8): 886-94.
[http://dx.doi.org/10.1002/ppsc.201300379]

[70]   Dutchak PA, Katafuchi T, Bookout AL, *et al.* Fibroblast growth factor-21 regulates PPARγ activity and the antidiabetic actions of thiazolidinediones. Cell 2012; 148(3): 556-67.
[http://dx.doi.org/10.1016/j.cell.2011.11.062] [PMID: 22304921]

[71]   Fisher M, Kleiner S, Douris N, *et al.* FGF21 regulates PGC-1α and browning of white adipose tissues in adaptive thermogenesis. Genes Dev 2012; 26(3): 271-81.
[http://dx.doi.org/10.1101/gad.177857.111] [PMID: 22302939]

[72]   Evans RM, Barish GD, Wang YX. PPARs and the complex journey to obesity. Nat Med 2004; 10(4): 355-61.
[http://dx.doi.org/10.1038/nm1025] [PMID: 15057233]

[73]   Tsuboyama-Kasaoka N, Shozawa C, Sano K, *et al.* Taurine (2-aminoethanesulfonic acid) deficiency creates a vicious circle promoting obesity. Endocrinology 2006; 147(7): 3276-84.
[http://dx.doi.org/10.1210/en.2005-1007] [PMID: 16627576]

[74]   Gaich G, Chien JY, Fu H, *et al.* The effects of LY2405319, an FGF21 analog, in obese human subjects with type 2 diabetes. Cell Metab 2013; 18(3): 333-40.
[http://dx.doi.org/10.1016/j.cmet.2013.08.005] [PMID: 24011069]

[75]   Villarroya F, Gavaldà-Navarro A, Peyrou M, Villarroya J, Giralt M. The Lives and Times of Brown Adipokines. Trends Endocrinol Metab 2017; 28(12): 855-67.
[http://dx.doi.org/10.1016/j.tem.2017.10.005] [PMID: 29113711]

[76]   Wills EJ. The powerhouse of the cell. Ultrastruct Pathol 1992; 16(3): iii-vi.
[http://dx.doi.org/10.3109/01913129209061353] [PMID: 1585494]

[77]   Pagliarini DJ, Rutter J. Hallmarks of a new era in mitochondrial biochemistry. Genes Dev 2013; 27(24): 2615-27.
[http://dx.doi.org/10.1101/gad.229724.113] [PMID: 24352419]

[78]   McBride HM, Neuspiel M, Wasiak S. Mitochondria: more than just a powerhouse. Curr Biol 2006; 16(14): R551-60.
[http://dx.doi.org/10.1016/j.cub.2006.06.054] [PMID: 16860735]

[79]   Wang X. The expanding role of mitochondria in apoptosis. Genes Dev 2001; 15(22): 2922-33.
[PMID: 11711427]

[80]   Ommati MM, Heidari R, Manthari RK, *et al.* Paternal exposure to arsenic resulted in oxidative stress, autophagy, and mitochondrial impairments in the HPG axis of pubertal male offspring. Chemosphere 2019; 236: 124325.
[http://dx.doi.org/10.1016/j.chemosphere.2019.07.056] [PMID: 31326754]

[81]   Ommati MM, Manthari RK, Tikka C, *et al.* Arsenic-induced autophagic alterations and mitochondrial

impairments in HPG-S axis of mature male mice offspring (F1-generation): A persistent toxicity study. Toxicol Lett 2020; 326: 83-98.
[http://dx.doi.org/10.1016/j.toxlet.2020.02.013] [PMID: 32112876]

[82]   Ommati MM, Shi X, Li H, *et al.* The mechanisms of arsenic-induced ovotoxicity, ultrastructural alterations, and autophagic related paths: An enduring developmental study in folliculogenesis of mice. Ecotoxicol Environ Saf 2020; 204: 110973.
[http://dx.doi.org/10.1016/j.ecoenv.2020.110973] [PMID: 32781346]

[83]   Green DR, Galluzzi L, Kroemer G. Mitochondria and the autophagy-inflammation-cell death axis in organismal aging. Science 2011; 333(6046): 1109-12.
[http://dx.doi.org/10.1126/science.1201940] [PMID: 21868666]

[84]   Granneman JG, Li P, Zhu Z, Lu Y. Metabolic and cellular plasticity in white adipose tissue I: effects of β_3-adrenergic receptor activation. Am J Physiol Endocrinol Metab 2005; 289(4): E608-16.
[http://dx.doi.org/10.1152/ajpendo.00009.2005] [PMID: 15941787]

[85]   Boudina S, Graham TE. Mitochondrial function/dysfunction in white adipose tissue. Exp Physiol 2014; 99(9): 1168-78.
[http://dx.doi.org/10.1113/expphysiol.2014.081414] [PMID: 25128326]

[86]   Gregoire FM, Smas CM, Sul HS. Understanding adipocyte differentiation. Physiol Rev 1998; 78(3): 783-809.
[http://dx.doi.org/10.1152/physrev.1998.78.3.783] [PMID: 9674695]

[87]   Vernochet C, Damilano F, Mourier A, *et al.* Adipose tissue mitochondrial dysfunction triggers a lipodystrophic syndrome with insulin resistance, hepatosteatosis, and cardiovascular complications. FASEB J 2014; 28(10): 4408-19.
[http://dx.doi.org/10.1096/fj.14-253971] [PMID: 25005176]

[88]   Keuper M, Jastroch M, Yi CX, *et al.* Spare mitochondrial respiratory capacity permits human adipocytes to maintain ATP homeostasis under hypoglycemic conditions. FASEB J 2014; 28(2): 761-70.
[http://dx.doi.org/10.1096/fj.13-238725] [PMID: 24200885]

[89]   Cinti S. Transdifferentiation properties of adipocytes in the adipose organ. Am J Physiol Endocrinol Metab 2009; 297(5): E977-86.
[http://dx.doi.org/10.1152/ajpendo.00183.2009] [PMID: 19458063]

[90]   Enerbäck S. The origins of brown adipose tissue. N Engl J Med 2009; 360(19): 2021-3.
[http://dx.doi.org/10.1056/NEJMcibr0809610] [PMID: 19420373]

[91]   Tormos KV, Anso E, Hamanaka RB, *et al.* Mitochondrial complex III ROS regulate adipocyte differentiation. Cell Metab 2011; 14(4): 537-44.
[http://dx.doi.org/10.1016/j.cmet.2011.08.007] [PMID: 21982713]

[92]   Orava J, Nuutila P, Lidell ME, *et al.* Different metabolic responses of human brown adipose tissue to activation by cold and insulin. Cell Metab 2011; 14(2): 272-9.
[http://dx.doi.org/10.1016/j.cmet.2011.06.012] [PMID: 21803297]

[93]   Cannon B, Nedergaard J. Brown adipose tissue: function and physiological significance. Physiol Rev 2004; 84(1): 277-359.
[http://dx.doi.org/10.1152/physrev.00015.2003] [PMID: 14715917]

[94]   Yehuda-Shnaidman E, Buehrer B, Pi J, Kumar N, Collins S. Acute stimulation of white adipocyte respiration by PKA-induced lipolysis. Diabetes 2010; 59(10): 2474-83.
[http://dx.doi.org/10.2337/db10-0245] [PMID: 20682684]

[95]   Rosell M, Kaforou M, Frontini A, *et al.* Brown and white adipose tissues: intrinsic differences in gene expression and response to cold exposure in mice. Am J Physiol Endocrinol Metab 2014; 306(8): E945-64.
[http://dx.doi.org/10.1152/ajpendo.00473.2013] [PMID: 24549398]

[96]   Forner F, Kumar C, Luber CA, Fromme T, Klingenspor M, Mann M. Proteome differences between brown and white fat mitochondria reveal specialized metabolic functions. Cell Metab 2009; 10(4): 324-35.
[http://dx.doi.org/10.1016/j.cmet.2009.08.014] [PMID: 19808025]

[97]   Nicholls DG, Locke RM. Thermogenic mechanisms in brown fat. Physiol Rev 1984; 64(1): 1-64.
[http://dx.doi.org/10.1152/physrev.1984.64.1.1] [PMID: 6320232]

[98]   Kajimura S, Saito M. A new era in brown adipose tissue biology: molecular control of brown fat development and energy homeostasis. Annu Rev Physiol 2014; 76(1): 225-49.
[http://dx.doi.org/10.1146/annurev-physiol-021113-170252] [PMID: 24188710]

[99]   Jamshidzadeh A, Niknahad H, Heidari R, Zarei M, Ommati MM, Khodaei F. Carnosine protects brain mitochondria under hyperammonemic conditions: Relevance to hepatic encephalopathy treatment. PharmaNutrition 2017; 5(2): 58-63.
[http://dx.doi.org/10.1016/j.phanu.2017.02.004]

[100]   Heidari R, Niknahad H, Sadeghi A, *et al.* Betaine treatment protects liver through regulating mitochondrial function and counteracting oxidative stress in acute and chronic animal models of hepatic injury. Biomed Pharmacother 2018; 103: 75-86.
[http://dx.doi.org/10.1016/j.biopha.2018.04.010] [PMID: 29635131]

[101]   Heidari R, Ghanbarinejad V, Ommati MM, Jamshidzadeh A, Niknahad H. Mitochondria protecting amino acids: Application against a wide range of mitochondria-linked complications. PharmaNutrition 2018; 6(4): 180-90.
[http://dx.doi.org/10.1016/j.phanu.2018.09.001]

[102]   Heidari R, Abdoli N, Ommati MM, Jamshidzadeh A, Niknahad H. Mitochondrial impairment induced by chenodeoxycholic acid: The protective effect of taurine and carnosine supplementation. Trends in Pharmaceutical Sciences. 2018;4(2).

[103]   Heidari R, Ghanbarinejad V, Ommati MM, Jamshidzadeh A, Niknahad H. 2018. Regulation of mitochondrial function and energy metabolism: A primary mechanism of cytoprotection provided by carnosine. Trends in Pharmaceutical Sciences. 2018;4(1).

[104]   Ahmadi N, Ghanbarinejad V, Ommati MM, Jamshidzadeh A, Heidari R. Taurine prevents mitochondrial membrane permeabilization and swelling upon interaction with manganese: Implication in the treatment of cirrhosis-associated central nervous system complications. J Biochem Mol Toxicol 2018; 32(11): e22216.
[http://dx.doi.org/10.1002/jbt.22216] [PMID: 30152904]

[105]   Ommati MM, Jamshidzadeh A, Heidari R, *et al.* Carnosine and histidine supplementation blunt lead-induced reproductive toxicity through antioxidative and mitochondria-dependent mechanisms. Biol Trace Elem Res 2019; 187(1): 151-62.
[http://dx.doi.org/10.1007/s12011-018-1358-2] [PMID: 29767280]

[106]   Mohammadi H, Ommati MM, Farshad O, Jamshidzadeh A, Niknahad H, Heidari R. Taurine and isolated mitochondria: A concentration-response study. Trends Pharmacol Sci 2019; 5(4): 5-6.

[107]   Heidari R, Arabnezhad MR, Ommati MM, Azarpira N, Ghodsimanesh E, Niknahad H. Boldine supplementation regulates mitochondrial function and oxidative stress in a rat model of hepatotoxicity. Ulum-i Daruyi 2019; 25(1): 1-10.
[http://dx.doi.org/10.15171/PS.2019.1]

[108]   Ommati MM, Farshad O, Jamshidzadeh A, Heidari R. Taurine enhances skeletal muscle mitochondrial function in a rat model of resistance training. PharmaNutrition 2019; 9: 100161.
[http://dx.doi.org/10.1016/j.phanu.2019.100161]

[109]   Ommati MM, Heidari R, Ghanbarinejad V, Abdoli N, Niknahad H. Taurine treatment provides neuroprotection in a mouse model of manganism. Biol Trace Elem Res 2019; 190(2): 384-95.
[http://dx.doi.org/10.1007/s12011-018-1552-2] [PMID: 30357569]

[110] Heidari R, Behnamrad S, Khodami Z, Ommati MM, Azarpira N, Vazin A. The nephroprotective properties of taurine in colistin-treated mice is mediated through the regulation of mitochondrial function and mitigation of oxidative stress. Biomed Pharmacother 2019; 109: 103-11.
[http://dx.doi.org/10.1016/j.biopha.2018.10.093] [PMID: 30396066]

[111] Ommati MM, Farshad O, Mousavi K, *et al.* Betaine supplementation mitigates intestinal damage and decreases serum bacterial endotoxin in cirrhotic rats. PharmaNutrition 2020; 12: 100179.
[http://dx.doi.org/10.1016/j.phanu.2020.100179]

[112] Ommati MM, Farshad O, Mousavi K, Khalili M, Jamshidzadeh A, Heidari R. Chlorogenic acid supplementation improves skeletal muscle mitochondrial function in a rat model of resistance training. Biologia (Bratisl) 2020; 75(8): 1221-30.
[http://dx.doi.org/10.2478/s11756-020-00429-7]

[113] Ommati MM, Farshad O, Ghanbarinejad V, *et al.* The nephroprotective role of carnosine against ifosfamide-induced renal injury and electrolytes imbalance is mediated *via* the regulation of mitochondrial function and alleviation of oxidative stress. Drug Res (Stuttg) 2020; 70(1): 49-56.
[http://dx.doi.org/10.1055/a-1017-5085] [PMID: 31671464]

[114] Ommati MM, Attari H, Siavashpour A, *et al.* Mitigation of cholestasis-associated hepatic and renal injury by edaravone treatment: Evaluation of its effects on oxidative stress and mitochondrial function. Liver Res 2021; 5(3): 181-93.
[http://dx.doi.org/10.1016/j.livres.2020.10.003]

[115] Ommati MM, Mohammadi H, Mousavi K, *et al.* Metformin alleviates cholestasis-associated nephropathy through regulating oxidative stress and mitochondrial function. Liver Res 2021; 5(3): 171-80.
[http://dx.doi.org/10.1016/j.livres.2020.12.001]

[116] Abdoli N, Sadeghian I, Mousavi K, Azarpira N, Ommati MM, Heidari R. Suppression of cirrhosis-related renal injury by N-acetyl cysteine. Current Research in Pharmacology and Drug Discovery 2020; 1: 30-8.
[http://dx.doi.org/10.1016/j.crphar.2020.100006] [PMID: 34909640]

[117] Ommati MM, Heidari R, Ghanbarinejad V, Aminian A, Abdoli N, Niknahad H. The neuroprotective properties of carnosine in a mouse model of manganism is mediated *via* mitochondria regulating and antioxidative mechanisms. Nutr Neurosci 2020; 23(9): 731-43.
[http://dx.doi.org/10.1080/1028415X.2018.1552399] [PMID: 30856059]

[118] Ommati MM, Azarpira N, Khodaei F, Niknahad H, Gozashtegan V, Heidari R. Methylene blue treatment enhances mitochondrial function and locomotor activity in a C57BL/6 mouse model of multiple sclerosis. Trends Pharmacol Sci 2020; 6(1): 29-42.

[119] Abdoli N, Sadeghian I, Azarpira N, Ommati MM, Heidari R. Taurine mitigates bile duct obstruction-associated cholemic nephropathy: Effect on oxidative stress and mitochondrial parameters. Clin Exp Hepatol 2020.
[PMID: 34027113]

[120] Ahmadi A, Ommati MM, Niknahad H, Heidari R. Methylene blue improves mitochondrial function in the liver of cholestatic rats. 2020.

[121] Ommati MM, Farshad O, Mousavi K, *et al.* Agmatine alleviates hepatic and renal injury in a rat model of obstructive jaundice. PharmaNutrition 2020; 13: 100212.
[http://dx.doi.org/10.1016/j.phanu.2020.100212]

[122] Ommati MM, Heidari R. Betaine, heavy metal protection, oxidative stress, and the liver.Toxicology. Academic Press 2021; pp. 387-95.
[http://dx.doi.org/10.1016/B978-0-12-819092-0.00038-8]

[123] Ommati MM, Farshad O, Azarpira N, Ghazanfari E, Niknahad H, Heidari R. Silymarin mitigates bile duct obstruction-induced cholemic nephropathy. Naunyn Schmiedebergs Arch Pharmacol 2021;

394(6): 1301-14.
[http://dx.doi.org/10.1007/s00210-020-02040-8] [PMID: 33538845]

[124] Ommati MM, Farshad O, Azarpira N, Shafaghat M, Niknahad H, Heidari R. Betaine alleviates cholestasis-associated renal injury by mitigating oxidative stress and enhancing mitochondrial function. Biologia (Bratisl) 2021; 76(1): 351-65.
[http://dx.doi.org/10.2478/s11756-020-00576-x]

[125] Ommati MM, Li H, Jamshidzadeh A, *et al.* The crucial role of oxidative stress in non-alcoholic fatty liver disease-induced male reproductive toxicity: the ameliorative effects of Iranian indigenous probiotics. Naunyn Schmiedebergs Arch Pharmacol 2022; 395(2): 247-65.
[http://dx.doi.org/10.1007/s00210-021-02177-0] [PMID: 34994824]

[126] Ito T, Yoshikawa N, Ito H, Schaffer SW. Impact of taurine depletion on glucose control and insulin secretion in mice. J Pharmacol Sci 2015; 129(1): 59-64.
[http://dx.doi.org/10.1016/j.jphs.2015.08.007] [PMID: 26382103]

[127] Cawthorn WP, Sethi JK. TNF-α and adipocyte biology. FEBS Lett 2008; 582(1): 117-31.
[http://dx.doi.org/10.1016/j.febslet.2007.11.051] [PMID: 18037376]

[128] Ito T, Yoshikawa N, Schaffer SW, Azuma J. Tissue taurine depletion alters metabolic response to exercise and reduces running capacity in mice. J Amino Acids 2014; 2014: 1-10.
[http://dx.doi.org/10.1155/2014/964680] [PMID: 25478210]

[129] Wen C, Li F, Zhang L, *et al.* Taurine is Involved in Energy Metabolism in Muscles, Adipose Tissue, and the Liver. Mol Nutr Food Res 2019; 63(2): 1800536.
[http://dx.doi.org/10.1002/mnfr.201800536] [PMID: 30251429]

[130] Murakami S. Role of taurine in the pathogenesis of obesity. Mol Nutr Food Res 2015; 59(7): 1353-63.
[http://dx.doi.org/10.1002/mnfr.201500067] [PMID: 25787113]

[131] Murakami S. The physiological and pathophysiological roles of taurine in adipose tissue in relation to obesity. Life Sci 2017; 186: 80-6.
[http://dx.doi.org/10.1016/j.lfs.2017.08.008] [PMID: 28801262]

[132] Li F, Li Y, Duan Y, Hu CAA, Tang Y, Yin Y. Myokines and adipokines: Involvement in the crosstalk between skeletal muscle and adipose tissue. Cytokine Growth Factor Rev 2017; 33: 73-82.
[http://dx.doi.org/10.1016/j.cytogfr.2016.10.003] [PMID: 27765498]

[133] Zieba DA, Biernat W, Barć J. Roles of leptin and resistin in metabolism, reproduction, and leptin resistance. Domest Anim Endocrinol 2020; 73: 106472.
[http://dx.doi.org/10.1016/j.domaniend.2020.106472] [PMID: 32265081]

[134] Dos Santos E, Duval F, Vialard F, Dieudonné MN. The roles of leptin and adiponectin at the fetal-maternal interface in humans. Horm Mol Biol Clin Investig 2015; 24(1): 47-63.
[http://dx.doi.org/10.1515/hmbci-2015-0031] [PMID: 26509784]

[135] Singh A, Choubey M, Bora P, Krishna A. Adiponectin and chemerin: Contrary adipokines in regulating reproduction and metabolic disorders. Reprod Sci 2018; 25(10): 1462-73.
[http://dx.doi.org/10.1177/1933719118770547] [PMID: 29669464]

[136] Juge-Aubry CE, Henrichot E, Meier CA. Adipose tissue: a regulator of inflammation. Best Pract Res Clin Endocrinol Metab 2005; 19(4): 547-66.
[http://dx.doi.org/10.1016/j.beem.2005.07.009] [PMID: 16311216]

[137] Coppack SW. Pro-inflammatory cytokines and adipose tissue. Proc Nutr Soc 2001; 60(3): 349-56.
[http://dx.doi.org/10.1079/PNS2001110] [PMID: 11681809]

[138] Trayhurn P, Wood IS. Signalling role of adipose tissue: adipokines and inflammation in obesity. Biochem Soc Trans 2005; 33(5): 1078-81.
[http://dx.doi.org/10.1042/BST0331078] [PMID: 16246049]

[139] Pond CM. Physiological specialisation of adipose tissue. Prog Lipid Res 1999; 38(3): 225-48.

[http://dx.doi.org/10.1016/S0163-7827(99)00003-X] [PMID: 10664794]

[140] Marcinkiewicz J, Grabowska A, Bereta J, Stelmaszynska T. Taurine chloramine, a product of activated neutrophils, inhibits in vitro the generation of nitric oxide and other macrophage inflammatory mediators. J Leukoc Biol 1995; 58(6): 667-74.
[http://dx.doi.org/10.1002/jlb.58.6.667] [PMID: 7499964]

[141] Marcinkiewicz J, Grabowska A, Bereta J, Bryniarski K, Nowak B. Taurine chloramine down-regulates the generation of murine neutrophil inflammatory mediators. Immunopharmacology 1998; 40(1): 27-38.
[http://dx.doi.org/10.1016/S0162-3109(98)00023-X] [PMID: 9776476]

[142] Park E, Jia J, Quinn MR, Schuller-Levis G. Taurine chloramine inhibits lymphocyte proliferation and decreases cytokine production in activated human leukocytes. Clin Immunol 2002; 102(2): 179-84.
[http://dx.doi.org/10.1006/clim.2001.5160] [PMID: 11846460]

[143] Rosa FT, Freitas EC, Deminice R, Jordão AA, Marchini JS. Oxidative stress and inflammation in obesity after taurine supplementation: a double-blind, placebo-controlled study. Eur J Nutr 2014; 53(3): 823-30.
[http://dx.doi.org/10.1007/s00394-013-0586-7] [PMID: 24065043]

[144] Zhang J, Wu H, Ma S, *et al.* Transcription regulators and hormones involved in the development of brown fat and white fat browning: transcriptional and hormonal control of brown/beige fat development. Physiol Res 2018; 67(3): 347-62.
[http://dx.doi.org/10.33549/physiolres.933650] [PMID: 29527907]

[145] Tiraby C, Tavernier G, Lefort C, *et al.* Acquirement of brown fat cell features by human white adipocytes. J Biol Chem 2003; 278(35): 33370-6.
[http://dx.doi.org/10.1074/jbc.M305235200] [PMID: 12807871]

[146] Batista TM, Ribeiro RA, da Silva PMR, *et al.* Taurine supplementation improves liver glucose control in normal protein and malnourished mice fed a high-fat diet. Mol Nutr Food Res 2013; 57(3): 423-34.
[http://dx.doi.org/10.1002/mnfr.201200345] [PMID: 23280999]

[147] Ghadge AA, Khaire AA, Kuvalekar AA. Adiponectin: A potential therapeutic target for metabolic syndrome. Cytokine Growth Factor Rev 2018; 39: 151-8.
[http://dx.doi.org/10.1016/j.cytogfr.2018.01.004] [PMID: 29395659]

[148] You JS, Zhao X, Kim SH, Chang KJ, Eds. Positive correlation between serum taurine and adiponectin levels in high-fat diet-induced obesity rats Taurine 8. New York, NY: Springer New York 2013.
[http://dx.doi.org/10.1007/978-1-4614-6093-0_11]

[149] Chen X, Sebastian BM, Tang H, *et al.* Taurine supplementation prevents ethanol-induced decrease in serum adiponectin and reduces hepatic steatosis in rats. Hepatology 2009; 49(5): 1554-62.
[http://dx.doi.org/10.1002/hep.22811] [PMID: 19296466]

[150] Kim H, Do CH, Lee D. Characterization of taurine as anti-obesity agent in C. elegans. J Biomed Sci 2010; 17(Suppl 1) (Suppl. 1): S33.
[http://dx.doi.org/10.1186/1423-0127-17-S1-S33] [PMID: 20804609]

[151] de Almeida Martiniano AC, De Carvalho FG, Marchini JS, *et al.* Effects of taurine supplementation on adipose tissue of obese trained rats. Adv Exp Med Biol 2015; 803: 707-14.
[http://dx.doi.org/10.1007/978-3-319-15126-7_56] [PMID: 25833538]

[152] Lin S, Hirai S, Yamaguchi Y, *et al.* Taurine improves obesity-induced inflammatory responses and modulates the unbalanced phenotype of adipose tissue macrophages. Mol Nutr Food Res 2013; 57(12): 2155-65.
[http://dx.doi.org/10.1002/mnfr.201300150] [PMID: 23939816]

[153] Chang YY, Chou CH, Chiu CH, *et al.* Preventive effects of taurine on development of hepatic steatosis induced by a high-fat/cholesterol dietary habit. J Agric Food Chem 2011; 59(1): 450-7.
[http://dx.doi.org/10.1021/jf103167u] [PMID: 21126079]

[154] Piña-Zentella G, de la Rosa-Cuevas G, Vázquez-Meza H, Piña E, de Piña MZ. Taurine in adipocytes prevents insulin-mediated H2o2 generation and activates Pka and lipolysis. Amino Acids 2012; 42(5): 1927-35.
[http://dx.doi.org/10.1007/s00726-011-0919-x] [PMID: 21537880]

[155] Kim KS, Choi HM, Ji HI, *et al.* Effect of taurine chloramine on differentiation of human preadipocytes into adipocytes. Adv Exp Med Biol 2013; 775: 247-57.
[http://dx.doi.org/10.1007/978-1-4614-6130-2_21] [PMID: 23392940]

[156] Kim KS, Ji HI, Chung H, *et al.* Taurine chloramine modulates the expression of adipokines through inhibition of the STAT-3 signaling pathway in differentiated human adipocytes. Amino Acids 2013; 45(6): 1415-22.
[http://dx.doi.org/10.1007/s00726-013-1612-z] [PMID: 24178768]

[157] Cao P, Jin Y, Li M, Zhou R, Yang M. PGC-1α may associated with the anti-obesity effect of taurine on rats induced by arcuate nucleus lesion. Nutr Neurosci 2016; 19(2): 86-93.
[http://dx.doi.org/10.1179/1476830514Y.0000000153] [PMID: 25211138]

[158] Mikami N, Hosokawa M, Miyashita K. Dietary combination of fish oil and taurine decreases fat accumulation and ameliorates blood glucose levels in type 2 diabetic/obese KK-A(y) mice. J Food Sci 2012; 77(6): H114-20.
[http://dx.doi.org/10.1111/j.1750-3841.2012.02687.x] [PMID: 22582992]

[159] Mitsue Rikimaru, Yutaka Ohsawa. Taurine ameliorates impaired mitochondrial function and prevents stroke-like episodes in patients with MELAS. Intern Med 2013.

[160] Jong CJ, Azuma J, Schaffer S. Mechanism underlying the antioxidant activity of taurine: prevention of mitochondrial oxidant production. Amino Acids 2012; 42(6): 2223-32.
[http://dx.doi.org/10.1007/s00726-011-0962-7] [PMID: 21691752]

[161] Hansen SH, Andersen ML, Cornett C, Gradinaru R, Grunnet N. A role for taurine in mitochondrial function. J Biomed Sci. 2010;17 Suppl 1(Suppl 1):S23.

[162] Cedikova M, Kripnerová M, Dvorakova J, *et al.* Mitochondria in white, brown, and beige adipocytes. Stem Cells Int 2016; 2016: 1-11.
[http://dx.doi.org/10.1155/2016/6067349] [PMID: 27073398]

[163] Guo YY, Li BY, Peng WQ, Guo L, Tang QQ. Taurine-mediated browning of white adipose tissue is involved in its anti-obesity effect in mice. J Biol Chem 2019; 294(41): 15014-24.
[http://dx.doi.org/10.1074/jbc.RA119.009936] [PMID: 31427436]

[164] Kim KS, Doss HM, Kim HJ, Yang HI. Taurine stimulates thermoregulatory genes in brown Fat tissue and muscle without an influence on inguinal white fat tissue in a high-fat diet-induced obese mouse model. Foods 2020; 9(6): 688.
[http://dx.doi.org/10.3390/foods9060688] [PMID: 32466447]

[165] Stenson BM, Rydén M, Steffensen KR, *et al.* Activation of liver X receptor regulates substrate oxidation in white adipocytes. Endocrinology 2009; 150(9): 4104-13.
[http://dx.doi.org/10.1210/en.2009-0676] [PMID: 19556420]

[166] Willy PJ, Umesono K, Ong ES, Evans RM, Heyman RA, Mangelsdorf DJ. LXR, a nuclear receptor that defines a distinct retinoid response pathway. Genes Dev 1995; 9(9): 1033-45.
[http://dx.doi.org/10.1101/gad.9.9.1033] [PMID: 7744246]

[167] Lehmann JM, Kliewer SA, Moore LB, *et al.* Activation of the nuclear receptor LXR by oxysterols defines a new hormone response pathway. J Biol Chem 1997; 272(6): 3137-40.
[http://dx.doi.org/10.1074/jbc.272.6.3137] [PMID: 9013544]

[168] Zelcer N, Tontonoz P. Liver X receptors as integrators of metabolic and inflammatory signaling. J Clin Invest 2006; 116(3): 607-14.
[http://dx.doi.org/10.1172/JCI27883] [PMID: 16511593]

[169] Dib L, Bugge A, Collins S. LXRα fuels fatty acid-stimulated oxygen consumption in white adipocytes. J Lipid Res 2014; 55(2): 247-57.
[http://dx.doi.org/10.1194/jlr.M043422] [PMID: 24259533]

[170] Laffitte BA, Chao LC, Li J, *et al.* Activation of liver X receptor improves glucose tolerance through coordinate regulation of glucose metabolism in liver and adipose tissue. Proc Natl Acad Sci USA 2003; 100(9): 5419-24.
[http://dx.doi.org/10.1073/pnas.0830671100] [PMID: 12697904]

[171] Qian SW, Tang Y, Li X, *et al.* BMP4-mediated brown fat-like changes in white adipose tissue alter glucose and energy homeostasis. Proc Natl Acad Sci USA 2013; 110(9): E798-807.
[http://dx.doi.org/10.1073/pnas.1215236110] [PMID: 23388637]

[172] Rosen ED, Spiegelman BM. What we talk about when we talk about fat. Cell 2014; 156(1-2): 20-44.
[http://dx.doi.org/10.1016/j.cell.2013.12.012] [PMID: 24439368]

[173] Suwa M, Kumagai S, Nakano H, Eds. Effects of chronic AICAR treatment on fiber composition, enzyme activity, UCP3, and PGC-1 in rat muscles. International Conference on Enterprise Interoperability Ii-new Challenges & Industrial Approaches.
[http://dx.doi.org/10.1152/japplphysiol.00349.2003]

[174] Jäger S, Handschin C, St-Pierre J, Spiegelman BM. AMP-activated protein kinase (AMPK) action in skeletal muscle *via* direct phosphorylation of PGC-1alpha. Proc Natl Acad Sci USA 2007; 104(29): 12017-22.
[http://dx.doi.org/10.1073/pnas.0705070104] [PMID: 17609368]

[175] Cantó C, Auwerx J. PGC-1α, SIRT1 and AMPK, an energy sensing network that controls energy expenditure. Curr Opin Lipidol 2009; 20(2): 98-105.
[http://dx.doi.org/10.1097/MOL.0b013e328328d0a4] [PMID: 19276888]

[176] Cantó C, Gerhart-Hines Z, Feige JN, *et al.* AMPK regulates energy expenditure by modulating NAD+ metabolism and SIRT1 activity. Nature 2009; 458(7241): 1056-60.
[http://dx.doi.org/10.1038/nature07813] [PMID: 19262508]

[177] Li Y, Wei H, Li F, Duan Y, Guo Q, Yin Y. Effects of low-protein diets supplemented with branched-chain amino acid on lipid metabolism in white adipose tissue of piglets. J Agric Food Chem 2017; 65(13): 2839-48.
[http://dx.doi.org/10.1021/acs.jafc.7b00488] [PMID: 28296401]

[178] Duan Y, Li F, Li Y, *et al.* The role of leucine and its metabolites in protein and energy metabolism. Amino Acids 2016; 48(1): 41-51.
[http://dx.doi.org/10.1007/s00726-015-2067-1] [PMID: 26255285]

CHAPTER 12

The Importance of Appropriate Taurine Formulations to Target Mitochondria

Abstract: As repeatedly mentioned in the current book, taurine (TAU) is a very hydrophilic molecule. Hence, the passage of this amino acid through the physiological barriers (*e.g.*, blood-brain barrier; BBB) is weak. In this context, experimental and clinical studies that mentioned the positive effects of TAU on CNS disorders administered a high dose of this amino acid (*e.g.*, 12 g/day). For example, in an animal model of hepatic encephalopathy, we administered 1 g/kg of TAU to hyperammonemic rats to preserve their brain energy status and normalize their locomotor activity. In some cases, where anticonvulsant effects of TAU were evaluated; also, and a high dose of this amino acid was used (150 mg/kg). In other circumstances, such as investigations on the reproductive system, the blood-testis barrier (BTB) could act as an obstacle to the bioavailability of TAU. On the other hand, recent studies mentioned the importance of targeted delivery of molecules to organelles such as mitochondria. These data mention the importance of appropriate formulations of this amino acid to target brain tissue as well as cellular mitochondria. Perhaps, TAU failed to show significant and optimum therapeutic effects against human disease (*e.g.*, neurological disorders) because of its inappropriate drug delivery system. Therefore, targeting tissues such as the brain with appropriate TAU-containing formulations is critical. The current chapter discusses possible formulations for bypassing physiological barriers (*e.g.*, blood-brain barrier; BBB or BTB) and effectively targeting subcellular compartments with TAU. These data could help develop effective formulations for managing human diseases (*e.g.*, CNS disorders or infertility issues in men).

Keywords: Amino acid, Drug delivery, Drug therapy, Mitochondria, Mitochondria-targeted antioxidants, Oxidative stress.

INTRODUCTION

As mentioned in several parts of this book, studies on the therapeutic potential of TAU against various human disorders usually administered very high doses (*e.g.*, 6-12 g/day) of this amino acid [1 - 4]. On the other hand, it is well known that TAU transporters such as TauT effectively facilitate the uptake of this amino acid by organs such as the skeletal muscle and the heart [5 - 11]. However, as TAU is a very hydrophilic compound, its transport to tissues with physiological barriers (*e.g.*, brain and testis) could be complex. Interestingly, the investigations that used very high doses of TAU were those conducted on CNS complications (*e.g.*, seizure) [12 - 14].

Another critical issue after increasing TAU's tissue (cellular) level is its appropriate mitochondria targeting. As mentioned in different chapters of this book, the acceleration of mitochondria-mediated ROS generation, decreased oxidative phosphorylation, and reduced ATP metabolism play a pivotal role in the pathogenesis of many human diseases [15 - 19]. These events could be related to a disturbed mitochondrial redox environment, indicating that endogenous mitochondrial antioxidants are insufficient to encounter excess ROS [15 - 19]. Many studies show that TAU effectively decreases mitochondria-mediated ROS formation and improves mitochondria antioxidant capacity [20 - 43]. Moreover, as noted in previous chapters, TAU acts as a buffering agent for the mitochondrial matrix [44, 45]. It is well-known that the activity of many mitochondria-embedded enzymes involved in energy metabolism is significantly increased by TAU [33, 45]. TAU also enhanced mitochondrial membrane potential ($\Delta\Psi_m$), a driving force for ATP metabolism [20 - 31, 42, 46 - 49]. It is also well-known that TAU robustly inhibits mitochondria-mediated cell death by preventing the induction of mitochondrial permeabilization [50]. All these data indicate that TAU should be effectively targeted to mitochondria; thus, the maximum benefit of this precious amino acid will be achieved in managing mitochondria-related disorders.

In the following parts, some novel strategies for targeting mitochondria are explained, and their relevance to the delivery of TAU to mitochondria is highlighted.

THE IMPORTANCE OF ENHANCING TAURINE BIOAVAILABILITY IN SPECIFIC ORGANS

As repeatedly mentioned in the current book, the passage of taurine (TAU) through physiological barriers such as BBB and BTB is challenging due to its hydrophilicity feature [51, 52]. BBB acts as a solid and selective interface between systemic blood flow and neuronal extracellular fluids (Fig. **1**). Therefore, this barrier regulates CNS homeostatic microenvironment [53 - 57]. Several cell types, including tight junctions between the endothelial cells and the interplay between astrocytes, podocytes, and vascular endothelial cells, form the basics of BBB (Fig. **1**). An intact and functional BBB guarantees the normal physiological function of the CNS [53 - 57] (Fig. **1**). BBB acts as a barrier for hydrophilic drugs in the drug delivery system that affects the brain function, and cellular gene expression, protecting many other organs and targeting mitochondria [58 - 77].

This issue highlights the necessity of designing therapeutic strategies for delivering drugs to the CNS to manage a wide range of CNS disorders.

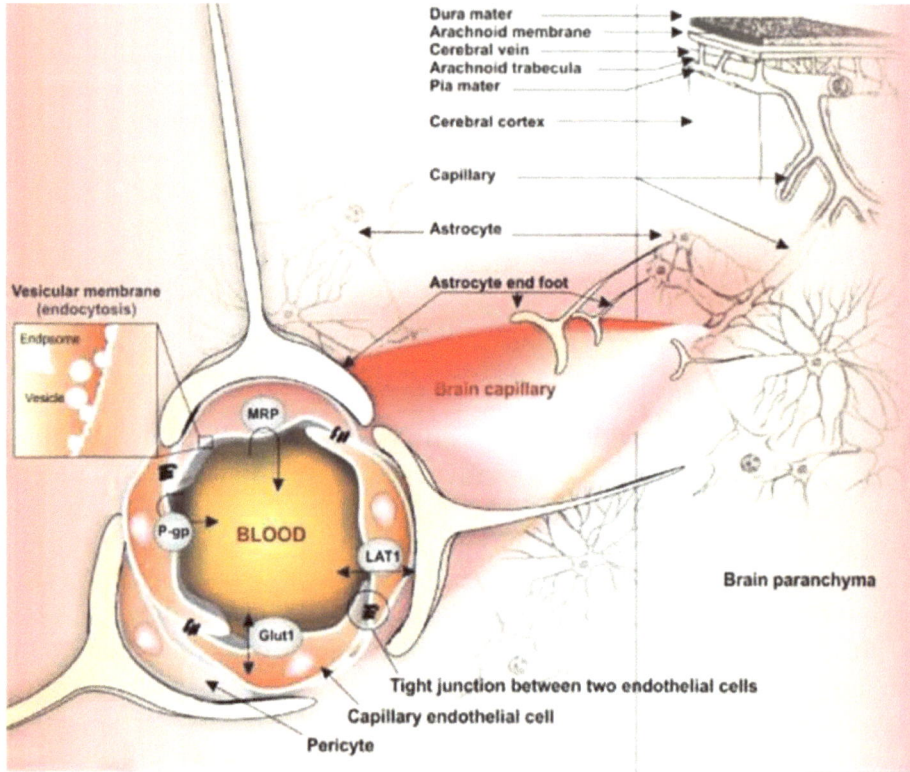

Fig. (1). Schematic representation of blood-brain barrier (BBB). Various cells are involved in BBB and prevent the entry of molecules (*e.g.*, very hydrophilic molecules) into the brain. Designing appropriate formulations of very hydrophilic drugs such as taurine could enhance its delivery to the CNS. MRP: multidrug resistance protein; LAT1: Large amino acid transporter; P-gp: P-glycoprotein; Glut1: Glucose transporter 1. Note: This figure is adapted from " [86]" (CC-BY license).

Several formulations have been designed in the context of bypassing BBB to deliver drugs to the CNS [55, 78 - 85] (Fig. **2**). Nanogels, liposomes, nano-capsules, neosomes, micelles, and nano-spheres are among the most-applied formulations for drug delivery to the CNS [55, 78 - 84] (Fig. **2**). It has been found that these formulations could effectively bypass the BBB and significantly increase the CNS level of drugs [55, 78 - 84]. Therefore, these drug delivery systems could be applied to effectively deliver a significant amount of TAU to the CNS by administrating lower doses of this amino acid (Fig. **2**). Further research on novel TAU formulations could help develop therapeutic strategies to manage a wide range of CNS disorders.

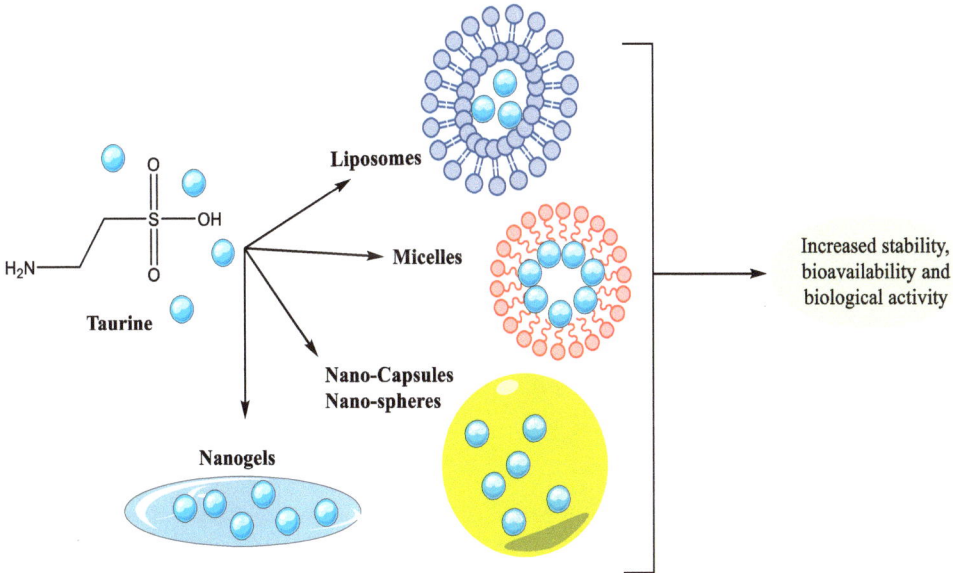

Fig. (2). Importance of target therapy and appropriate formulations of taurine (TAU). As mentioned in different parts of the current investigation, targeting cellular mitochondria with appropriate TAU formulations could serve as a promising strategy for treating many human diseases. TAU is a very hydrophilic compound. Hence, its distribution through lipid layers seems somewhat difficult.

In the BTB case, there is also tight junction and transporters (*e.g.*, multidrug resistance protein; MRP; and P-glycoprotein; P-gp) that significantly exclude drugs from Sertoli cells to the bloodstream and prevent their delivery to the apicolateral compartment of the Sertoli cells [87] (Fig. **3**). Actually, this could act as a physiological strategy to protect spermatozoa from xenobiotics damage (Fig. **3**). However, BTB could serve as a barrier to proper drug delivery to the testis (*e.g.*, for very hydrophilic drugs) [87 - 90] (Fig. **3**).

As mentioned in this book (Chapter 10), TAU has several positive effects on sperm parameters [36, 91 - 97]. TAU is able to enhance sperm motility and viability and significantly decrease oxidative stress parameters in testis [36, 91 - 97]. Hence, the effective delivery of TAU to sperm and other cells in the testis tissue is an important issue. For this purpose, some barriers, such as BTB, should be passed. This is important, especially when the drug is a very hydrophilic molecule (*e.g.*, TAU) (Fig. **2**). Further research on novel drug delivery systems (*e.g.*, nanocarriers, liposomes) for bypassing BTB could help appropriate TAU delivery to the testis tissue and its application against complications such as infertility (Fig. **3**).

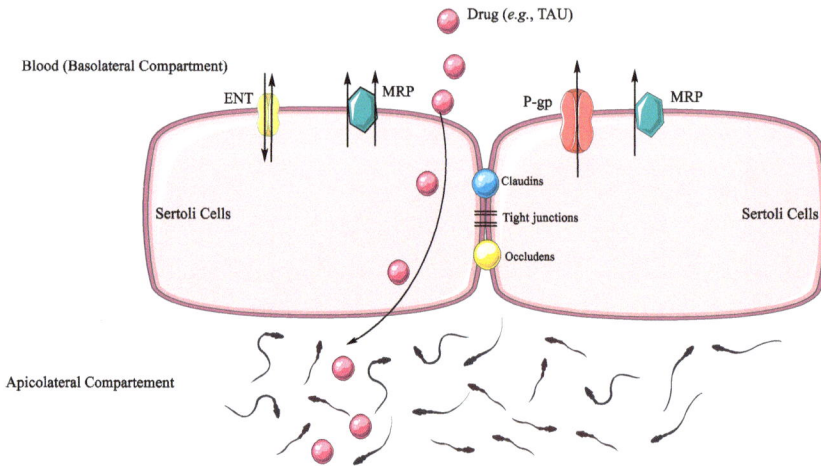

Fig. (3). Schematic representation of blood-testis barrier (BTB). Some drugs (*e.g.*, very hydrophilic agents) may not easily cross BTB. Designing appropriate formulations of taurine (TAU) could enhance its transport to tests for pharmaceutical purposes. MRP: Multidrug resistance protein; ENT: Equilibrative nucleoside transporters; P-gp: P-glycoprotein.

NOVEL STRATEGIES FOR TARGETING MITOCHONDRIA

Many studies revealed that when antioxidants such as vitamin C, E, and *β*-carotene are administered in traditional and not-targeted ways, surprisingly, they may not only have no antioxidant, or minimum antioxidant effects, but could also induce several side effects [98, 99]. Park *et al.* revealed that the risk of these adverse effects could be higher in cardiovascular diseases and cancer [98]. An important issue about the administration of antioxidants is that we should consider that redox signaling and the production of a basic level of ROS are essential for many physiological processes [100 - 103]. Therefore, a concern is that excessive or unsuitable administration of antioxidants (*e.g.*, at high doses and traditional non-targeted ways) could abolish all ROS levels and interrupt normal cellular physiology [99]. Antioxidants may also not absorb properly or metabolize at a high level when not targeted to a specific organ/organelle [99]. Finally, it should also be mentioned that we might waste antioxidants (some have a high price) by high doses and non-targeted administration of these molecules.

All the above data indicate that we should proceed with targeted antioxidant therapy. In the case of TAU, the main cellular target is mitochondria. Fortunately, several strategies have been developed for transporting molecules to mitochondria. Some techniques which could be applied for enhancing the delivery of TAU to mitochondria in future studies are mentioned in the forthcoming parts.

Several strategies have been developed for the accumulation of antioxidants in the mitochondria. Using lipophilic cations-conjugated compounds is an old and effective example of mitochondria-targeting drugs [99]. Since the identification of mitochondrial membrane potential ($\Delta\Psi_m$) in 1969, researchers have designed lipophilic cations that could easily penetrate the cell and mitochondrial membrane and accumulate in the mitochondrial matrix, which is negatively charged [99]. Therefore, drugs and antioxidant molecules could be conjugated with lipophilic cations to target mitochondria (Fig. 4). Triphenylphosphonium (TPP) is one of the well-known cations used for this purpose [99] (Fig. 4). MitoTEMPO, MitoQ, MitoE, and SkQ1 are TPP-linked agents used to alleviate mitochondria-linked disorders such as mitochondria-mediated ROS formation and oxidative stress in various human diseases [104 - 111] (Fig. 4). These molecules are extensively used in experimental models [104 - 111]. Interestingly, several clinical studies also revealed the positive effects of mitochondria-targeted antioxidants (TPP-conjugated) in clinical trials [99, 112 - 114].

The evolvement of mitochondrial toxicity is an important issue about applying cations such as TPP in drug delivery to mitochondria [99]. Several studies reported that higher doses of TPP could impair mitochondrial membrane potential, disrupt mitochondria respiratory chain activity, and decrease ATP metabolism [99, 111, 115]. These studies mention that the dose and treatment schedule of TPP-conjugated antioxidants should be strictly controlled.

Liposome encapsulation is another effective strategy for delivering antioxidants to various organs and subcellular compartments (*e.g.*, mitochondria) (Fig. 2). Liposomes are lipid bilayer vesicles widely used as a drug delivery strategy in pharmaceutical sciences [99, 116 - 118]. It has been well-documented that antioxidants such as vitamin E, N-Acetyl cysteine, and quercetin had a higher therapeutic effect in their liposomal formulations [119 - 125]. The advantages of liposomal formulations in comparison with methods such as conjugation with TPP are that the bioactive component remains intact, and there is no concern for the toxicity of molecules such as lipophilic cations [99]. On the other hand, a significant problem with liposomes is their degradation in the cytoplasm before delivering their cargo to subcellular compartments such as mitochondria [99]. Therefore, more sophisticated systems such as decorated liposomes have been developed to provide molecules to mitochondria better. For example, liposomes have been decorated with sphingomyelin, 1,2-dioleoyl-5n-glyce-o-3-phosphatidylethanolamine, and stearylated octaarginine peptide to decrease their cytoplasmic degradation and enhance their delivery to mitochondria [99, 126 - 130]. The delivery of TAU to specific organs (*e.g.*, the brain), as well as the enhancement of its concentration in the mitochondrial matrix, might be achieved by strategies such as liposomal drug delivery systems (Fig. 2). More research studies on this system are expected to be carried out in the future to enhance the delivery of TAU to its cellular targets and/or its transportation through physiological barriers (*e.g.*, BBB).

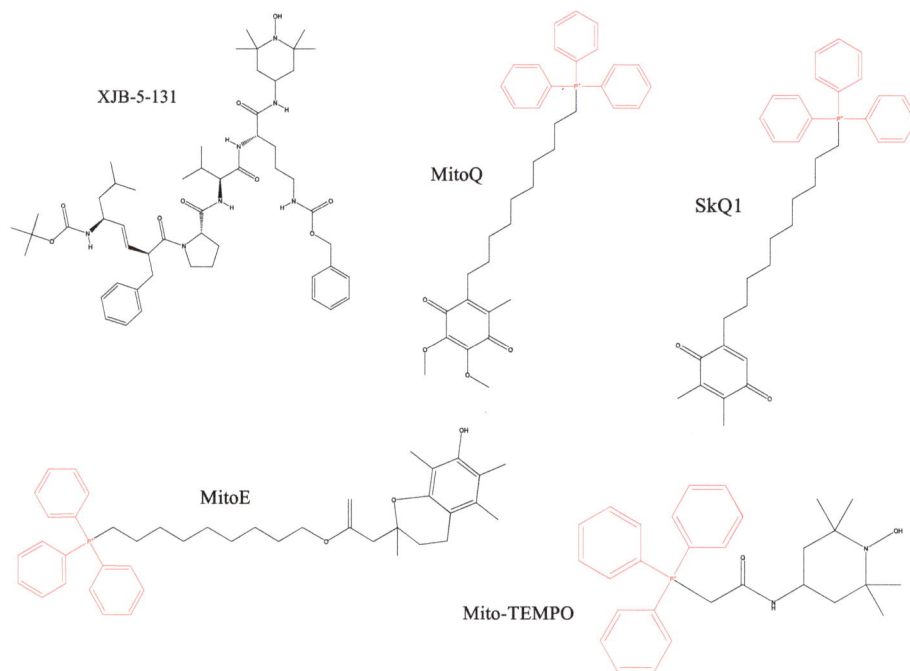

Fig. (4).   Mitochondria-targeted structures are designed for accumulation in the mitochondrial matrix. Conjugation of antioxidants with lipophilic cations such as triphenylphosphonium ion (TPP; the red part of the mentioned structures in this figure) is an efficient strategy for enhancing their delivery to the mitochondrial matrix. Other techniques, such as peptide-based mitochondrial antioxidants (*e.g.*, XJB-5-131 in this figure) have also been developed to target mitochondria with antioxidants. This field provides more information on comprehensive reviews (*e.g.*, Reference [99]).

Another antioxidant delivery system that has been widely studied is the peptide-based delivery of molecules to mitochondria [68, 99, 131 - 133]. Peptide-based drug delivery system is widely applied against various pathological conditions linked with oxidative stress and mitochondrial impairment [134 - 154]. XJB-5-131 is an example of mitochondria-penetrating peptides used for scavenging mitochondria-mediated ROS [99, 155 - 158] (Fig. **4**). Mitochondria-penetrating peptides such as XJB-5-131 are positively charged and hydrophobic molecules are widely used to deliver small molecules to mitochondria with the help of $\Delta\Psi_m$ [99, 159] (Fig. **4**). Several experimental studies revealed the positive effects of mitochondria-targeted antioxidants such as XJB-5-131 against oxidative stress and mitochondrial impairment [155 - 157, 160 - 164]. Peptide delivery systems have several advantages, such as unsaturated transport and uptake by cells, no degradation in the cytoplasm, efficient transportation to mitochondria, and an easy method of synthesis [99]. These properties made them favorite agents to deliver mitochondria antioxidants [99, 132, 133, 165 - 167]. Interestingly, it has been found that the speed of peptide-based antioxidant uptake by mitochondria is a $\Delta\Psi_m$ independent process [99, 168]. Moreover, these agents did not affect mitochondrial membrane polarization [99]. Finally, some peptide-based mitochondria-targeted antioxidants, such as BBB, readily penetrate the physiological barriers and could be used as neuroprotective agents [99, 169, 170].

Although peptide-based systems seem to be a safe method for delivering molecules to mitochondria, some studies mentioned that monitoring the effects of these peptides on parameters such as mitochondrial membrane potential could give a good estimate of any adverse effects of these molecules on mitochondria [131].

The data presented in this section indicate the importance of novel delivery systems for TAU as an effective mitochondrion protecting agent. More research on these delivery systems is warranted to reveal the potential therapeutic properties of TAU in a wide range of pathological conditions linked with mitochondrial impairment.

CONCLUSION

The data collected in this chapter highlights the importance of designing appropriate drug delivery systems for the optimum effectiveness of TAU in human disease. In this context, formulations that could help overcome physiological barriers (*e.g.*, BBB and BTB) and targeted drug delivery systems (*e.g.*, conjugation of TAU with mitochondria-targeted molecules) could enhance its pharmacological effects. Future studies in this field could significantly improve our understanding of the effects of TAU in various pathological conditions, especially those connected with oxidative stress and mitochondrial impairment.

REFERENCES

[1]   Hansen SH. The role of taurine in diabetes and the development of diabetic complications. Diabetes Metab Res Rev 2001; 17(5): 330-46.
        [http://dx.doi.org/10.1002/dmrr.229] [PMID: 11747139]

[2]   Kumar S, Goel R. Taurine supplementation to anti-seizure drugs as the promising approach to treat pharmacoresistant epilepsy: A pre-clinical study. Int J Epilepsy 2017; 4(2): 119-24.
        [http://dx.doi.org/10.1016/j.ijep.2017.07.001]

[3]   Nandhini TA, Anuradha CV. Inhibition of lipid peroxidation, protein glycation and elevation of membrane ion pump activity by taurine in RBC exposed to high glucose. Clin Chim Acta 2003; 336(1-2): 129-35.
        [http://dx.doi.org/10.1016/S0009-8981(03)00337-1] [PMID: 14500045]

[4]   Rikimaru M, Ohsawa Y, Wolf AM, *et al.* Taurine ameliorates impaired the mitochondrial function and prevents stroke-like episodes in patients with MELAS. Intern Med 2012; 51(24): 3351-7.
[http://dx.doi.org/10.2169/internalmedicine.51.7529] [PMID: 23257519]

[5]   Ito T, Hanahata Y, Kine K, Murakami S, Schaffer SW. Tissue taurine depletion induces profibrotic pattern of gene expression and causes aging-related cardiac fibrosis in heart in mice. Biol Pharm Bull 2018; 41(10): 1561-6.
[http://dx.doi.org/10.1248/bpb.b18-00217] [PMID: 30270325]

[6]   Ito T, Kimura Y, Uozumi Y, *et al.* Taurine depletion caused by knocking out the taurine transporter gene leads to cardiomyopathy with cardiac atrophy. J Mol Cell Cardiol 2008; 44(5): 927-37.
[http://dx.doi.org/10.1016/j.yjmcc.2008.03.001] [PMID: 18407290]

[7]   Jong C, Ito T, Prentice H, Wu JY, Schaffer S. Role of mitochondria and endoplasmic reticulum in taurine-deficiency-mediated apoptosis. Nutrients 2017; 9(8): 795.
[http://dx.doi.org/10.3390/nu9080795] [PMID: 28757580]

[8]   Warskulat U, Heller-Stilb B, Oermann E, *et al.* Phenotype of the taurine transporter knockout mouse. Methods Enzymol 2007; 428: 439-58.
[http://dx.doi.org/10.1016/S0076-6879(07)28025-5] [PMID: 17875433]

[9]   Horvath DM, Murphy RM, Mollica JP, Hayes A, Goodman CA. The effect of taurine and β-alanine supplementation on taurine transporter protein and fatigue resistance in skeletal muscle from mdx mice. Amino Acids 2016; 48(11): 2635-45.
[http://dx.doi.org/10.1007/s00726-016-2292-2] [PMID: 27444300]

[10]   Ito T, Yoshikawa N, Inui T, Miyazaki N, Schaffer SW, Azuma J. Tissue depletion of taurine accelerates skeletal muscle senescence and leads to early death in mice. PLoS One 2014; 9(9): e107409.
[http://dx.doi.org/10.1371/journal.pone.0107409] [PMID: 25229346]

[11]   Najibi A, Rezaei H, Kumar Manthari R, *et al.* Cellular and mitochondrial taurine depletion in bile duct ligated rats: a justification for taurine supplementation in cholestasis/cirrhosis. Clin Exp Hepatol 2022; 8(3): 195-210.
[http://dx.doi.org/10.5114/ceh.2022.119216] [PMID: 36685263]

[12]   Keränen T, Partanen VSJ, Koivisto K, Tokola O, Neuvonen PJ, Riekkinen PJ. Effects of taltrimide, an experimental taurine derivative, on photoconvulsive response in epileptic patients. Epilepsia 1987; 28(2): 133-7.
[http://dx.doi.org/10.1111/j.1528-1157.1987.tb03638.x] [PMID: 3816708]

[13]   Van Gelder NM, Sherwin AL, Sacks C, Andermann F. Biochemical observations following administration of taurine to patients with epilepsy. Brain Res 1975; 94(2): 297-306.
[http://dx.doi.org/10.1016/0006-8993(75)90063-3] [PMID: 807299]

[14]   Mantovani J, DeVivo DC. Effects of taurine on seizures and growth hormone release in epileptic patients. Arch Neurol 1979; 36(11): 672-4.
[http://dx.doi.org/10.1001/archneur.1979.00500470042006] [PMID: 508122]

[15]   Kaludercic N, Di Lisa F. Mitochondrial ROS formation in the pathogenesis of diabetic cardiomyopathy. Front Cardiovasc Med 2020; 7: 12.
[http://dx.doi.org/10.3389/fcvm.2020.00012] [PMID: 32133373]

[16]   Zorov DB, Juhaszova M, Sollott SJ. Mitochondrial reactive oxygen species (ROS) and ROS-induced ROS release. Physiol Rev 2014; 94(3): 909-50.
[http://dx.doi.org/10.1152/physrev.00026.2013] [PMID: 24987008]

[17]   Johannsen DL, Ravussin E. The role of mitochondria in health and disease. Curr Opin Pharmacol 2009; 9(6): 780-6.
[http://dx.doi.org/10.1016/j.coph.2009.09.002] [PMID: 19796990]

[18]   Picard M, Wallace DC, Burelle Y. The rise of mitochondria in medicine. Mitochondrion 2016; 30:

105-16.
[http://dx.doi.org/10.1016/j.mito.2016.07.003] [PMID: 27423788]

[19]   Larsson NG, Wedell A. Mitochondria in human disease. J Intern Med 2020; 287(6): 589-91.
[http://dx.doi.org/10.1111/joim.13088] [PMID: 32406555]

[20]   Schaffer S, Ito T, Azuma J, Jong C, Kramer J. Mechanisms underlying development of taurine-deficient cardiomyopathy. Hearts 2020; 1(2): 86-98.
[http://dx.doi.org/10.3390/hearts1020010]

[21]   Mohammadi H, Ommati MM, Farshad O, Jamshidzadeh A, Nikbakht MR, Niknahad H, *et al.* Taurine and isolated mitochondria: A concentration-response study. Trends Pharmacol Sci 2019; 5(4): 197-206.

[22]   Heidari R, Behnamrad S, Khodami Z, Ommati MM, Azarpira N, Vazin A. The nephroprotective properties of taurine in colistin-treated mice is mediated through the regulation of mitochondrial function and mitigation of oxidative stress. Biomed Pharmacother 2019; 109: 103-11.
[http://dx.doi.org/10.1016/j.biopha.2018.10.093] [PMID: 30396066]

[23]   Heidari R, Ghanbarinejad V, Ommati MM, Jamshidzadeh A, Niknahad H. Mitochondria protecting amino acids: Application against a wide range of mitochondria-linked complications. PharmaNutrition 2018; 6(4): 180-90.
[http://dx.doi.org/10.1016/j.phanu.2018.09.001]

[24]   Jamshidzadeh A, Heidari R, Abasvali M, *et al.* Taurine treatment preserves brain and liver mitochondrial function in a rat model of fulminant hepatic failure and hyperammonemia. Biomed Pharmacother 2017; 86: 514-20.
[http://dx.doi.org/10.1016/j.biopha.2016.11.095] [PMID: 28024286]

[25]   Schaffer SW, Shimada-Takaura K, Jong CJ, Ito T, Takahashi K. Impaired energy metabolism of the taurine-deficient heart. Amino Acids 2016; 48(2): 549-58.
[http://dx.doi.org/10.1007/s00726-015-2110-2] [PMID: 26475290]

[26]   Ahmadian E, Babaei H, Mohajjel Nayebi A, Eftekhari A, Eghbal MA. Venlafaxine-induced cytotoxicity towards isolated rat hepatocytes involves oxidative stress and mitochondrial/lysosomal dysfunction. Adv Pharm Bull 2016; 6(4): 521-30.
[http://dx.doi.org/10.15171/apb.2016.066] [PMID: 28101459]

[27]   Xu S, He M, Zhong M, *et al.* The neuroprotective effects of taurine against nickel by reducing oxidative stress and maintaining mitochondrial function in cortical neurons. Neurosci Lett 2015; 590 (Suppl. C): 52-7.
[http://dx.doi.org/10.1016/j.neulet.2015.01.065] [PMID: 25637701]

[28]   Hansen SH, Grunnet N. Taurine, glutathione and bioenergetics.Taurine 8 Advances in Experimental Medicine and Biology: Springer New York. 2013; pp. 3-12.

[29]   Sun M, Gu Y, Zhao Y, Xu C. Protective functions of taurine against experimental stroke through depressing mitochondria-mediated cell death in rats. Amino Acids 2011; 40(5): 1419-29.
[http://dx.doi.org/10.1007/s00726-010-0751-8] [PMID: 20862501]

[30]   Schaffer SW, Azuma J, Mozaffari M. Role of antioxidant activity of taurine in diabetesThis article is one of a selection of papers from the NATO Advanced Research Workshop on Translational Knowledge for Heart Health (published in part 1 of a 2-part Special Issue). Can J Physiol Pharmacol 2009; 87(2): 91-9.
[http://dx.doi.org/10.1139/Y08-110] [PMID: 19234572]

[31]   Chang L, Zhao J, Xu J, Jiang W, Tang CS, Qi YF. Effects of taurine and homocysteine on calcium homeostasis and hydrogen peroxide and superoxide anions in rat myocardial mitochondria. Clin Exp Pharmacol Physiol 2004; 31(4): 237-43.
[http://dx.doi.org/10.1111/j.1440-1681.2004.03983.x] [PMID: 15053820]

[32]   Jong CJ, Azuma J, Schaffer S. Mechanism underlying the antioxidant activity of taurine: prevention of

mitochondrial oxidant production. Amino Acids 2012; 42(6): 2223-32.
[http://dx.doi.org/10.1007/s00726-011-0962-7] [PMID: 21691752]

[33]   Seidel U, Huebbe P, Rimbach G. Taurine: A regulator of cellular redox homeostasis and skeletal muscle function. Mol Nutr Food Res 2019; 63(16): 1800569.
[http://dx.doi.org/10.1002/mnfr.201800569] [PMID: 30211983]

[34]   Shimada K, Jong CJ, Takahashi K, Schaffer SW, Eds. Role of ROS production and turnover in the antioxidant activity of taurine2015. Cham: Springer International Publishing 2015.

[35]   Hansen S, Andersen M, Cornett C, Gradinaru R, Grunnet N. A role for taurine in mitochondrial function. J Biomed Sci 2010; 17(Suppl 1) (Suppl. 1): S23.
[http://dx.doi.org/10.1186/1423-0127-17-S1-S23] [PMID: 20804598]

[36]   Das J, Ghosh J, Manna P, Sinha M, Sil PC. Taurine protects rat testes against NaAsO2-induced oxidative stress and apoptosis *via* mitochondrial dependent and independent pathways. Toxicol Lett 2009; 187(3): 201-10.
[http://dx.doi.org/10.1016/j.toxlet.2009.03.001] [PMID: 19429265]

[37]   Chang L, Xu J, Yu F, Zhao J, Tang X, Tang C. Taurine protected myocardial mitochondria injury induced by hyperhomocysteinemia in rats. Amino Acids 2004; 27(1): 37-48.
[http://dx.doi.org/10.1007/s00726-004-0096-2] [PMID: 15309570]

[38]   Schuller-Levis GB, Park E. Taurine: new implications for an old amino acid. FEMS Microbiol Lett 2003; 226(2): 195-202.
[http://dx.doi.org/10.1016/S0378-1097(03)00611-6] [PMID: 14553911]

[39]   Schaffer S, Azuma J, Takahashi K, Mozaffari M. Why is taurine cytoprotective?Taurine 5: Beginning the 21st Century Advances in Experimental Medicine and Biology. Boston, MA: Springer US 2003; pp. 307-21.
[http://dx.doi.org/10.1007/978-1-4615-0077-3_39]

[40]   Suzuki T, Suzuki T, Wada T, Saigo K, Watanabe K. Taurine as a constituent of mitochondrial tRNAs: new insights into the functions of taurine and human mitochondrial diseases. EMBO J 2002; 21(23): 6581-9.
[http://dx.doi.org/10.1093/emboj/cdf656] [PMID: 12456664]

[41]   Ahmadi N, Ghanbarinejad V, Ommati MM, Jamshidzadeh A, Heidari R. Taurine prevents mitochondrial membrane permeabilization and swelling upon interaction with manganese: Implication in the treatment of cirrhosis-associated central nervous system complications. J Biochem Mol Toxicol 2018; 32(11): e22216.
[http://dx.doi.org/10.1002/jbt.22216] [PMID: 30152904]

[42]   Abdoli N, Sadeghian I, Azarpira N, Ommati MM, Heidari R. Taurine mitigates bile duct obstruction-associated cholemic nephropathy: effect on oxidative stress and mitochondrial parameters. Clin Exp Hepatol 2021; 7(1): 30-40.
[http://dx.doi.org/10.5114/ceh.2021.104675] [PMID: 34027113]

[43]   Ommati MM, Mobasheri A, Ma Y, *et al.* Taurine mitigates the development of pulmonary inflammation, oxidative stress, and histopathological alterations in a rat model of bile duct ligation. Naunyn Schmiedebergs Arch Pharmacol 2022; 395(12): 1557-72.
[http://dx.doi.org/10.1007/s00210-022-02291-7] [PMID: 36097067]

[44]   Hansen SH, Andersen ML, Birkedal H, Cornett C, Wibrand F. The Important role of taurine in oxidative metabolism.Taurine 6 Advances in Experimental Medicine and Biology. Springer US 2006; pp. 129-35.
[http://dx.doi.org/10.1007/978-0-387-33504-9_13]

[45]   Hansen SH, Andersen ML, Birkedal H, Cornett C, Wibrand F. The important role of taurine in oxidative metabolism Taurine 6. Springer 2006; pp. 129-35.

[46]   Ommati MM, Farshad O, Jamshidzadeh A, Heidari R. Taurine enhances skeletal muscle mitochondrial

function in a rat model of resistance training. PharmaNutrition 2019; 9: 100161.
[http://dx.doi.org/10.1016/j.phanu.2019.100161]

[47] Heidari R, Abdoli N, Ommati MM, Jamshidzadeh A, Niknahad H. Mitochondrial impairment induced by chenodeoxycholic acid: The protective effect of taurine and carnosine supplementation. Trends Pharmacol Sci 2018; 4(2): 29-42.

[48] Mousavi K, Niknahad H, Ghalamfarsa A, *et al.* Taurine mitigates cirrhosis-associated heart injury through mitochondrial-dependent and antioxidative mechanisms. Clin Exp Hepatol 2020; 6(3): 207-19.
[http://dx.doi.org/10.5114/ceh.2020.99513] [PMID: 33145427]

[49] Heidari R, Babaei H, Eghbal MA. Cytoprotective effects of taurine against toxicity induced by isoniazid and hydrazine in isolated rat hepatocytes. Arh Hig Rada Toksikol 2013; 64(2): 201-10.
[http://dx.doi.org/10.2478/10004-1254-64-2013-2297] [PMID: 23819928]

[50] Palmi M, Youmbi GT, Sgaragli G, Meini A, Benocci A, Fusi F, *et al.* The mitochondrial permeability transition and taurine.Taurine 4: Taurine and Excitable Tissues Advances in Experimental Medicine and Biology. Boston, MA: Springer US 2002; pp. 87-96.
[http://dx.doi.org/10.1007/0-306-46838-7_8]

[51] Jakaria M, Azam S, Haque ME, *et al.* Taurine and its analogs in neurological disorders: Focus on therapeutic potential and molecular mechanisms. Redox Biol 2019; 24: 101223.
[http://dx.doi.org/10.1016/j.redox.2019.101223] [PMID: 31141786]

[52] Chung M, Malatesta P, Bosquesi P, Yamasaki P, Santos JL, Vizioli E. Advances in drug design based on the amino Acid approach: taurine analogues for the treatment of CNS diseases. Pharmaceuticals (Basel) 2012; 5(10): 1128-46.
[http://dx.doi.org/10.3390/ph5101128] [PMID: 24281261]

[53] Scherrmann JM. Drug delivery to brain *via* the blood-brain barrier. Vascul Pharmacol 2002; 38(6): 349-54.
[http://dx.doi.org/10.1016/S1537-1891(02)00202-1] [PMID: 12529929]

[54] Bellettato CM, Scarpa M. Possible strategies to cross the blood-brain barrier. Ital J Pediatr 2018; 44(S2) (Suppl. 2): 131.
[http://dx.doi.org/10.1186/s13052-018-0563-0] [PMID: 30442184]

[55] Ahlawat J, Guillama Barroso G, Masoudi Asil S, *et al.* Nanocarriers as potential drug delivery candidates for overcoming the blood-brain barrier: Challenges and possibilities. ACS Omega 2020; 5(22): 12583-95.
[http://dx.doi.org/10.1021/acsomega.0c01592] [PMID: 32548442]

[56] Pardridge WM. Blood-brain barrier and delivery of protein and gene therapeutics to brain. Front Aging Neurosci 2020; 11: 373.
[http://dx.doi.org/10.3389/fnagi.2019.00373] [PMID: 31998120]

[57] Mulvihill JJE, Cunnane EM, Ross AM, Duskey JT, Tosi G, Grabrucker AM. Drug delivery across the blood-brain barrier: recent advances in the use of nanocarriers. Nanomedicine (Lond) 2020; 15(2): 205-14.
[http://dx.doi.org/10.2217/nnm-2019-0367] [PMID: 31916480]

[58] Banks WA. From blood-brain barrier to blood-brain interface: new opportunities for CNS drug delivery. Nat Rev Drug Discov 2016; 15(4): 275-92.
[http://dx.doi.org/10.1038/nrd.2015.21] [PMID: 26794270]

[59] Abbott NJ. Blood-brain barrier structure and function and the challenges for CNS drug delivery. J Inherit Metab Dis 2013; 36(3): 437-49.
[http://dx.doi.org/10.1007/s10545-013-9608-0] [PMID: 23609350]

[60] Banks WA. Characteristics of compounds that cross the blood-brain barrier. BMC Neurol 2009; 9(Suppl 1) (Suppl. 1): S3.

[http://dx.doi.org/10.1186/1471-2377-9-S1-S3] [PMID: 19534732]

[61]   Masjedi M, Azadi A, Heidari R, Mohammadi-Samani S. Nose-to-brain delivery of sumatriptan-loaded nanostructured lipid carriers: preparation, optimization, characterization and pharmacokinetic evaluation. J Pharm Pharmacol 2020; 72(10): 1341-51.
[http://dx.doi.org/10.1111/jphp.13316] [PMID: 32579251]

[62]   Masjedi M, Azadi A, Heidari R, Mohammadi-Samani S. Brain targeted delivery of sumatriptan succinate loaded chitosan nanoparticles: Preparation, *In vitro* characterization, and (Neuro-)pharmacokinetic evaluations. J Drug Deliv Sci Technol 2021; 61: 102179.
[http://dx.doi.org/10.1016/j.jddst.2020.102179]

[63]   Jafari M, Abolmaali SS, Borandeh S, *et al.* Amphiphilic hyperbranched polyglycerol nanoarchitectures for Amphotericin B delivery in Candida infections. Biomaterials Advances 2022; 139: 212996.
[http://dx.doi.org/10.1016/j.bioadv.2022.212996] [PMID: 35891600]

[64]   Mozafari N, Dehshahri A, Ashrafi H, *et al.* Vesicles of yeast cell wall-sitagliptin to alleviate neuroinflammation in Alzheimer's disease. Nanomedicine 2022; 44: 102575.
[http://dx.doi.org/10.1016/j.nano.2022.102575] [PMID: 35714923]

[65]   Sadeghian I, Heidari R, Raee MJ, Negahdaripour M. Cell-penetrating peptide-mediated delivery of therapeutic peptides/proteins to manage the diseases involving oxidative stress, inflammatory response and apoptosis. J Pharm Pharmacol 2022; 74(8): 1085-116.
[http://dx.doi.org/10.1093/jpp/rgac038] [PMID: 35728949]

[66]   Heidari R, Taghizadeh SM, Karami-Darehnaranji M, Mirzaei E, Berenjian A, Ebrahiminezhad A. Application of FeOOH nano-ellipsoids as a novel nano-based iron supplement: an in vivo study. Biol Trace Elem Res 2022; 200(5): 2174-82.
[http://dx.doi.org/10.1007/s12011-021-02811-1] [PMID: 34392478]

[67]   Monajati M, Tamaddon AM, Abolmaali SS, *et al.* Novel self-assembled nanogels of PEG-grafted poly HPMA with bis(α-cyclodextrin) containing disulfide linkage: synthesis, bio-disintegration, and *in vivo* biocompatibility. New J Chem 2022; 46(20): 9931-43.
[http://dx.doi.org/10.1039/D1NJ05974B]

[68]   Sadeghian I, Heidari R, Sadeghian S, Raee MJ, Negahdaripour M. Potential of cell-penetrating peptides (CPPs) in delivery of antiviral therapeutics and vaccines. Eur J Pharm Sci 2022; 169: 106094.
[http://dx.doi.org/10.1016/j.ejps.2021.106094] [PMID: 34896590]

[69]   Entezar-Almahdi E, Heidari R, Ghasemi S, Mohammadi-Samani S, Farjadian F. Integrin receptor mediated pH-responsive nano-hydrogel based on histidine-modified poly(aminoethyl methacrylamide) as targeted cisplatin delivery system. J Drug Deliv Sci Technol 2021; 62: 102402.
[http://dx.doi.org/10.1016/j.jddst.2021.102402]

[70]   Ommati MM, Farshad O, Mousavi K, Khalili M, Jamshidzadeh A, Heidari R. Chlorogenic acid supplementation improves skeletal muscle mitochondrial function in a rat model of resistance training. Biologia (Bratisl) 2020; 75(8): 1221-30.
[http://dx.doi.org/10.2478/s11756-020-00429-7]

[71]   Heidari R, Mousavi K, Amin S, Ommati MM, Niknahad H. N-acetylcysteine Treatment Protects Intestinal Mitochondria in a Surgical Stress Model. Trends Pharmacol Sci 2020; 6(2): 87-96.

[72]   Heidari R, Ahmadi A, Ommati MM, Niknahad H. Methylene blue improves mitochondrial function in the liver of cholestatic rats. Trends Pharmacol Sci 2020; 6(2): 73-86.

[73]   Nouri F, Sadeghpour H, Heidari R, Dehshahri A. Preparation, characterization, and transfection efficiency of low molecular weight polyethylenimine-based nanoparticles for delivery of the plasmid encoding CD200 gene. Int J Nanomedicine 2017; 12: 5557-69.
[http://dx.doi.org/10.2147/IJN.S140734] [PMID: 28831252]

[74]   Abedi M, Abolmaali SS, Heidari R, Mohammadi Samani S, Tamaddon AM. Hierarchical mesoporous zinc-imidazole dicarboxylic acid MOFs: Surfactant-directed synthesis, pH-responsive degradation, and

drug delivery. Int J Pharm 2021; 602: 120685.
[http://dx.doi.org/10.1016/j.ijpharm.2021.120685] [PMID: 33964340]

[75]   Najafi H, Abolmaali SS, Heidari R, Valizadeh H, Tamaddon AM, Azarpira N. Integrin receptor-binding nanofibrous peptide hydrogel for combined mesenchymal stem cell therapy and nitric oxide delivery in renal ischemia/reperfusion injury. Stem Cell Res Ther 2022; 13(1): 344.
[http://dx.doi.org/10.1186/s13287-022-03045-1] [PMID: 35883125]

[76]   Ourani-Pourdashti S, Mirzaei E, Heidari R, Ashrafi H, Azadi A. Preparation and evaluation of niosomal chitosan-based in situ gel formulation for direct nose-to-brain methotrexate delivery. Int J Biol Macromol 2022; 213: 1115-26.
[http://dx.doi.org/10.1016/j.ijbiomac.2022.06.031] [PMID: 35691430]

[77]   Najafi H, Abolmaali SS, Heidari R, *et al*. Nitric oxide releasing nanofibrous Fmoc-dipeptide hydrogels for amelioration of renal ischemia/reperfusion injury. J Control Release 2021; 337: 1-13.
[http://dx.doi.org/10.1016/j.jconrel.2021.07.016] [PMID: 34271033]

[78]   Dong X. Current strategies for brain drug delivery. Theranostics 2018; 8(6): 1481-93.
[http://dx.doi.org/10.7150/thno.21254] [PMID: 29556336]

[79]   Vieira D, Gamarra L. Getting into the brain: liposome-based strategies for effective drug delivery across the blood-brain barrier. Int J Nanomedicine 2016; 11: 5381-414.
[http://dx.doi.org/10.2147/IJN.S117210] [PMID: 27799765]

[80]   Gharbavi M, Amani J, Kheiri-Manjili H, Danafar H, Sharafi A. Niosome: A promising nanocarrier for natural drug delivery through blood-brain barrier. Adv Pharmacol Sci 2018; 2018: 1-15.
[http://dx.doi.org/10.1155/2018/6847971] [PMID: 30651728]

[81]   Tsou YH, Zhang XQ, Zhu H, Syed S, Xu X. Drug delivery to the brain across the blood-brain barrier using nanomaterials. Small 2017; 13(43): 1701921.
[http://dx.doi.org/10.1002/smll.201701921] [PMID: 29045030]

[82]   Craparo EF, Bondì ML, Pitarresi G, Cavallaro G. Nanoparticulate systems for drug delivery and targeting to the central nervous system. CNS Neurosci Ther 2011; 17(6): 670-7.
[http://dx.doi.org/10.1111/j.1755-5949.2010.00199.x] [PMID: 20950327]

[83]   Zhou Y, Peng Z, Seven ES, Leblanc RM. Crossing the blood-brain barrier with nanoparticles. J Control Release 2018; 270: 290-303.
[http://dx.doi.org/10.1016/j.jconrel.2017.12.015] [PMID: 29269142]

[84]   Md S, Bhattmisra SK, Zeeshan F, *et al*. Nano-carrier enabled drug delivery systems for nose to brain targeting for the treatment of neurodegenerative disorders. J Drug Deliv Sci Technol 2018; 43: 295-310.
[http://dx.doi.org/10.1016/j.jddst.2017.09.022]

[85]   Mehdi-alamdarlou S, Ahmadi F, Azadi A, Shahbazi MA, Heidari R, Ashrafi H. A cell-mimicking platelet-based drug delivery system as a potential carrier of dimethyl fumarate for multiple sclerosis. Int J Pharm 2022; 625: 122084.
[http://dx.doi.org/10.1016/j.ijpharm.2022.122084] [PMID: 35944590]

[86]   Omidi Y, Barar J. Impacts of blood-brain barrier in drug delivery and targeting of brain tumors. Bioimpacts 2012; 2(1): 5-22.
[PMID: 23678437]

[87]   Mruk DD, Su L, Cheng CY. Emerging role for drug transporters at the blood-testis barrier. Trends Pharmacol Sci 2011; 32(2): 99-106.
[http://dx.doi.org/10.1016/j.tips.2010.11.007] [PMID: 21168226]

[88]   Mao B, Bu T, Mruk D, Li C, Sun F, Cheng CY. Modulating the blood-testis barrier towards increasing drug delivery. Trends Pharmacol Sci 2020; 41(10): 690-700.
[http://dx.doi.org/10.1016/j.tips.2020.07.002] [PMID: 32792159]

[89]   Su L, Mruk DD, Cheng CY. Drug transporters, the blood-testis barrier, and spermatogenesis. J

Endocrinol 2011; 208(3): 207-23.
[PMID: 21134990]

[90]   Naidu ECS, Olojede SO, Lawal SK, Rennie CO, Azu OO. Nanoparticle delivery system, highly active antiretroviral therapy, and testicular morphology: The role of stereology. Pharmacol Res Perspect 2021; 9(3): e00776.
[http://dx.doi.org/10.1002/prp2.776] [PMID: 34107163]

[91]   Schaffer S, Takahashi K, Azuma J. Role of osmoregulation in the actions of taurine. Amino Acids 2000; 19(3-4): 527-46.
[http://dx.doi.org/10.1007/s007260070004] [PMID: 11140357]

[92]   Bucak MN, Ateşşahin A, Varışlı Ö, Yüce A, Tekin N, Akçay A. The influence of trehalose, taurine, cysteamine and hyaluronan on ram semen. Theriogenology 2007; 67(5): 1060-7.
[http://dx.doi.org/10.1016/j.theriogenology.2006.12.004] [PMID: 17280711]

[93]   Motawi TK, Abd Elgawad HM, Shahin NN. Modulation of indomethacin-induced gastric injury by spermine and taurine in rats. J Biochem Mol Toxicol 2007; 21(5): 280-8.
[http://dx.doi.org/10.1002/jbt.20194] [PMID: 17912696]

[94]   Sarıözkan S, Bucak MN, Tuncer PB, Ulutaş PA, Bilgen A. The influence of cysteine and taurine on microscopic-oxidative stress parameters and fertilizing ability of bull semen following cryopreservation. Cryobiology 2009; 58(2): 134-8.
[http://dx.doi.org/10.1016/j.cryobiol.2008.11.006] [PMID: 19070613]

[95]   Yang J, Wu G, Feng Y, Lv Q, Lin S, Hu J. Effects of taurine on male reproduction in rats of different ages. J Biomed Sci 2010; 17(Suppl 1) (Suppl. 1): S9.
[http://dx.doi.org/10.1186/1423-0127-17-S1-S9] [PMID: 20804629]

[96]   Aly HAA, Khafagy RM. Taurine reverses endosulfan-induced oxidative stress and apoptosis in adult rat testis. Food Chem Toxicol 2014; 64: 1-9.
[http://dx.doi.org/10.1016/j.fct.2013.11.007] [PMID: 24262488]

[97]   Yang W, Huang J, Xiao B, *et al.* Taurine protects mouse spermatocytes from ionizing radiation-induced damage through activation of Nrf2/HO-1 signaling. Cell Physiol Biochem 2017; 44(4): 1629-39.
[http://dx.doi.org/10.1159/000485762] [PMID: 29216642]

[98]   Park Y, Spiegelman D, Hunter DJ, *et al.* Intakes of vitamins A, C, and E and use of multiple vitamin supplements and risk of colon cancer: a pooled analysis of prospective cohort studies. Cancer Causes Control 2010; 21(11): 1745-57.
[http://dx.doi.org/10.1007/s10552-010-9549-y] [PMID: 20820901]

[99]   Jiang Q, Yin J, Chen J, *et al.* Mitochondria-targeted antioxidants: A step towards disease treatment. Oxid Med Cell Longev 2020; 2020: 1-18.
[http://dx.doi.org/10.1155/2020/8837893] [PMID: 33354280]

[100] Burgoyne JR, Mongue-Din H, Eaton P, Shah AM. Redox signaling in cardiac physiology and pathology. Circ Res 2012; 111(8): 1091-106.
[http://dx.doi.org/10.1161/CIRCRESAHA.111.255216] [PMID: 23023511]

[101] Schieber M, Chandel NS. ROS function in redox signaling and oxidative stress. Curr Biol 2014; 24(10): R453-62.
[http://dx.doi.org/10.1016/j.cub.2014.03.034] [PMID: 24845678]

[102] Forman HJ, Torres M, Fukuto J. Redox signaling. Mol Cell Biochem 2002; 234/235(1): 49-62.
[http://dx.doi.org/10.1023/A:1015913229650] [PMID: 12162460]

[103] Olguín-Albuerne M, Morán J. Redox signaling mechanisms in nervous system development. Antioxid Redox Signal 2018; 28(18): 1603-25.
[http://dx.doi.org/10.1089/ars.2017.7284] [PMID: 28817955]

[104] Dong LF, Jameson VJA, Tilly D, *et al.* Mitochondrial targeting of vitamin E succinate enhances its

pro-apoptotic and anti-cancer activity *via* mitochondrial complex II. J Biol Chem 2011; 286(5): 3717-28.
[http://dx.doi.org/10.1074/jbc.M110.186643] [PMID: 21059645]

[105]   Jameson VJA, Cochemé HM, Logan A, Hanton LR, Smith RAJ, Murphy MP. Synthesis of triphenylphosphonium vitamin E derivatives as mitochondria-targeted antioxidants. Tetrahedron 2015; 71(44): 8444-53.
[http://dx.doi.org/10.1016/j.tet.2015.09.014] [PMID: 26549895]

[106]   Zielonka J, Joseph J, Sikora A, *et al.* Mitochondria-targeted triphenylphosphonium-based compounds: Syntheses, mechanisms of action, and therapeutic and diagnostic applications. Chem Rev 2017; 117(15): 10043-120.
[http://dx.doi.org/10.1021/acs.chemrev.7b00042] [PMID: 28654243]

[107]   Bakeeva LE, Barskov IV, Egorov MV, *et al.* Mitochondria-targeted plastoquinone derivatives as tools to interrupt execution of the aging program. 2. Treatment of some ROS- and Age-related diseases (heart arrhythmia, heart infarctions, kidney ischemia, and stroke). Biochemistry (Mosc) 2008; 73(12): 1288-99.
[http://dx.doi.org/10.1134/S000629790812002X] [PMID: 19120015]

[108]   Skulachev VP, Antonenko YN, Cherepanov DA, *et al.* Prevention of cardiolipin oxidation and fatty acid cycling as two antioxidant mechanisms of cationic derivatives of plastoquinone (SkQs). Biochim Biophys Acta Bioenerg 2010; 1797(6-7): 878-89.
[http://dx.doi.org/10.1016/j.bbabio.2010.03.015] [PMID: 20307489]

[109]   Tauskela JS. MitoQ-a mitochondria-targeted antioxidant. The investigational drugs journal. 2007;10(6):399-412.

[110]   Adlam VJ, Harrison JC, Porteous CM, *et al.* Targeting an antioxidant to mitochondria decreases cardiac ischemia-reperfusion injury. FASEB J 2005; 19(9): 1088-95.
[http://dx.doi.org/10.1096/fj.05-3718com] [PMID: 15985532]

[111]   Smith RAJ, Porteous CM, Gane AM, Murphy MP. Delivery of bioactive molecules to mitochondria *in vivo*. Proc Natl Acad Sci USA 2003; 100(9): 5407-12.
[http://dx.doi.org/10.1073/pnas.0931245100] [PMID: 12697897]

[112]   Rossman MJ, Santos-Parker JR, Steward CAC, *et al.* Chronic supplementation with a mitochondrial antioxidant (MitoQ) improves vascular function in healthy older adults. Hypertension 2018; 71(6): 1056-63.
[http://dx.doi.org/10.1161/HYPERTENSIONAHA.117.10787] [PMID: 29661838]

[113]   Gane EJ, Weilert F, Orr DW, *et al.* The mitochondria-targeted anti-oxidant mitoquinone decreases liver damage in a phase II study of hepatitis C patients. Liver Int 2010; 30(7): 1019-26.
[http://dx.doi.org/10.1111/j.1478-3231.2010.02250.x] [PMID: 20492507]

[114]   Petrov A, Perekhvatova N, Skulachev M, Stein L, Ousler G. SkQ1 ophthalmic solution for dry eye treatment: Results of a phase 2 safety and efficacy clinical study in the environment and during challenge in the controlled adverse environment model. Adv Ther 2016; 33(1): 96-115.
[http://dx.doi.org/10.1007/s12325-015-0274-5] [PMID: 26733410]

[115]   Ross MF, Kelso GF, Blaikie FH, *et al.* Lipophilic triphenylphosphonium cations as tools in mitochondrial bioenergetics and free radical biology. Biochemistry (Mosc) 2005; 70(2): 222-30.
[http://dx.doi.org/10.1007/s10541-005-0104-5] [PMID: 15807662]

[116]   Lian T, Ho RJY. Trends and developments in liposome drug delivery systems. J Pharm Sci 2001; 90(6): 667-80.
[http://dx.doi.org/10.1002/jps.1023] [PMID: 11357170]

[117]   Zylberberg C, Matosevic S. Pharmaceutical liposomal drug delivery: a review of new delivery systems and a look at the regulatory landscape. Drug Deliv 2016; 23(9): 3319-29.
[http://dx.doi.org/10.1080/10717544.2016.1177136] [PMID: 27145899]

[118] Sercombe L, Veerati T, Moheimani F, Wu SY, Sood AK, Hua S. Advances and challenges of liposome assisted drug delivery. Front Pharmacol 2015; 6: 286.
[http://dx.doi.org/10.3389/fphar.2015.00286] [PMID: 26648870]

[119] Alipour M, Omri A, Smith MG, Suntres ZE. Prophylactic effect of liposomal N-acetylcysteine against LPS-induced liver injuries. J Endotoxin Res 2007; 13(5): 297-304.
[http://dx.doi.org/10.1177/0968051907085062] [PMID: 17986488]

[120] Rezaei-Sadabady R, Eidi A, Zarghami N, Barzegar A. Intracellular ROS protection efficiency and free radical-scavenging activity of quercetin and quercetin-encapsulated liposomes. Artif Cells Nanomed Biotechnol 2016; 44(1): 128-34.
[http://dx.doi.org/10.3109/21691401.2014.926456] [PMID: 24959911]

[121] Fan J, Shek PN, Suntres ZE, Li YH, Oreopoulos GD, Rotstein OD. Liposomal antioxidants provide prolonged protection against acute respiratory distress syndrome. Surgery 2000; 128(2): 332-8.
[http://dx.doi.org/10.1067/msy.2000.108060] [PMID: 10923013]

[122] Koudelka S, Turanek Knotigova P, Masek J, *et al.* Liposomal delivery systems for anti-cancer analogues of vitamin E. J Control Release 2015; 207: 59-69.
[http://dx.doi.org/10.1016/j.jconrel.2015.04.003] [PMID: 25861728]

[123] Loguercio C, Federico A, Trappoliere M, *et al.* The effect of a silybin-vitamin e-phospholipid complex on nonalcoholic fatty liver disease: a pilot study. Dig Dis Sci 2007; 52(9): 2387-95.
[http://dx.doi.org/10.1007/s10620-006-9703-2] [PMID: 17410454]

[124] Takahashi M, Uechi S, Takara K, Asikin Y, Wada K. Evaluation of an oral carrier system in rats: bioavailability and antioxidant properties of liposome-encapsulated curcumin. J Agric Food Chem 2009; 57(19): 9141-6.
[http://dx.doi.org/10.1021/jf9013923] [PMID: 19757811]

[125] Chiu CH, Chang CC, Lin ST, Chyau CC, Peng R. Improved hepatoprotective effect of liposome-encapsulated astaxanthin in lipopolysaccharide-induced acute hepatotoxicity. Int J Mol Sci 2016; 17(7): 1128.
[http://dx.doi.org/10.3390/ijms17071128] [PMID: 27428953]

[126] Yamada Y, Harashima H. MITO-Porter for mitochondrial delivery and mitochondrial functional analysis. Handb Exp Pharmacol 2016; 240: 457-72.
[http://dx.doi.org/10.1007/164_2016_4] [PMID: 27830347]

[127] Yamada Y, Akita H, Kamiya H, *et al.* MITO-Porter: A liposome-based carrier system for delivery of macromolecules into mitochondria *via* membrane fusion. Biochim Biophys Acta Biomembr 2008; 1778(2): 423-32.
[http://dx.doi.org/10.1016/j.bbamem.2007.11.002] [PMID: 18054323]

[128] Yamada Y, Nakamura K, Abe J, *et al.* Mitochondrial delivery of Coenzyme Q10 *via* systemic administration using a MITO-Porter prevents ischemia/reperfusion injury in the mouse liver. J Control Release 2015; 213: 86-95.
[http://dx.doi.org/10.1016/j.jconrel.2015.06.037] [PMID: 26160304]

[129] Yamada Y, Daikuhara S, Tamura A, Nishida K, Yui N, Harashima H. Enhanced autophagy induction *via* the mitochondrial delivery of methylated β-cyclodextrin-threaded polyrotaxanes using a MITO-Porter. Chem Commun (Camb) 2019; 55(50): 7203-6.
[http://dx.doi.org/10.1039/C9CC03272J] [PMID: 31165120]

[130] Yamada Y, Furukawa R, Yasuzaki Y, Harashima H. Dual function MITO-Porter, a nano carrier integrating both efficient cytoplasmic delivery and mitochondrial macromolecule delivery. Mol Ther 2011; 19(8): 1449-56.
[http://dx.doi.org/10.1038/mt.2011.99] [PMID: 21694702]

[131] Cerrato CP, Pirisinu M, Vlachos EN, Langel Ü. Novel cell-penetrating peptide targeting mitochondria. FASEB J 2015; 29(11): 4589-99.

[http://dx.doi.org/10.1096/fj.14-269225] [PMID: 26195590]

[132]   Toyama S, Shimoyama N, Szeto HH, Schiller PW, Shimoyama M. Protective effect of a mitochondria-targeted peptide against the development of chemotherapy-induced peripheral neuropathy in mice. ACS Chem Neurosci 2018; 9(7): 1566-71.
[http://dx.doi.org/10.1021/acschemneuro.8b00013] [PMID: 29660270]

[133]   Qvit N, Rubin SJS, Urban TJ, Mochly-Rosen D, Gross ER. Peptidomimetic therapeutics: scientific approaches and opportunities. Drug Discov Today 2017; 22(2): 454-62.
[http://dx.doi.org/10.1016/j.drudis.2016.11.003] [PMID: 27856346]

[134]   Imai T, Mishiro K, Takagi T, *et al.* Protective effect of bendavia (SS-31) against oxygen/glucose-deprivation stress-induced mitochondrial damage in human brain microvascular endothelial cells. Curr Neurovasc Res 2017; 14(1): 53-9.
[http://dx.doi.org/10.2174/1567202614666161117110609] [PMID: 27855593]

[135]   Kuang X, Zhou S, Guo W, Wang Z, Sun Y, Liu H. SS-31 peptide enables mitochondrial targeting drug delivery: a promising therapeutic alteration to prevent hair cell damage from aminoglycosides. Drug Deliv 2017; 24(1): 1750-61.
[http://dx.doi.org/10.1080/10717544.2017.1402220] [PMID: 29214897]

[136]   Wu J, Hao S, Sun XR, *et al.* Elamipretide (SS-31) ameliorates isoflurane-induced long-term impairments of mitochondrial morphogenesis and cognition in developing rats. Front Cell Neurosci 2017; 11: 119.
[http://dx.doi.org/10.3389/fncel.2017.00119] [PMID: 28487636]

[137]   Zhang M, Zhao H, Cai J, *et al.* Chronic administration of mitochondrion-targeted peptide SS-31 prevents atherosclerotic development in ApoE knockout mice fed Western diet. PLoS One 2017; 12(9): e0185688.
[http://dx.doi.org/10.1371/journal.pone.0185688] [PMID: 28961281]

[138]   Zhao H, Liu Y, Liu Z, *et al.* Role of mitochondrial dysfunction in renal fibrosis promoted by hypochlorite-modified albumin in a remnant kidney model and protective effects of antioxidant peptide SS-31. Eur J Pharmacol 2017; 804: 57-67.
[http://dx.doi.org/10.1016/j.ejphar.2017.03.037] [PMID: 28322835]

[139]   Cai J, Jiang Y, Zhang M, *et al.* Protective effects of mitochondrion-targeted peptide SS-31 against hind limb ischemia-reperfusion injury. J Physiol Biochem 2018; 74(2): 335-43.
[http://dx.doi.org/10.1007/s13105-018-0617-1] [PMID: 29589186]

[140]   Campbell MD, Duan J, Samuelson AT, *et al.* Improving mitochondrial function with SS-31 reverses age-related redox stress and improves exercise tolerance in aged mice. Free Radic Biol Med 2019; 134: 268-81.
[http://dx.doi.org/10.1016/j.freeradbiomed.2018.12.031] [PMID: 30597195]

[141]   Escribano-Lopez I, Diaz-Morales N, Iannantuoni F, *et al.* The mitochondrial antioxidant SS-31 increases SIRT1 levels and ameliorates inflammation, oxidative stress and leukocyte-endothelium interactions in type 2 diabetes. Sci Rep 2018; 8(1): 15862.
[http://dx.doi.org/10.1038/s41598-018-34251-8] [PMID: 30367115]

[142]   Hou S, Yang Y, Zhou S, *et al.* Novel SS-31 modified liposomes for improved protective efficacy of minocycline against drug-induced hearing loss. Biomater Sci 2018; 6(6): 1627-35.
[http://dx.doi.org/10.1039/C7BM01181D] [PMID: 29740652]

[143]   Tarantini S, Valcarcel-Ares NM, Yabluchanskiy A, *et al.* Treatment with the mitochondrial-targeted antioxidant peptide SS-31 rescues neurovascular coupling responses and cerebrovascular endothelial function and improves cognition in aged mice. Aging Cell 2018; 17(2): e12731.
[http://dx.doi.org/10.1111/acel.12731] [PMID: 29405550]

[144]   Zhang W, Tam J, Shinozaki K, *et al.* Increased survival time with SS-31 after prolonged cardiac arrest in rats. Heart Lung Circ 2019; 28(3): 505-8.
[http://dx.doi.org/10.1016/j.hlc.2018.01.008] [PMID: 29503242]

[145] Czigler A, Toth L, Szarka N, *et al.* Hypertension exacerbates cerebrovascular oxidative stress induced by mild traumatic brain injury: Protective effects of the mitochondria-targeted antioxidative peptide SS-31. J Neurotrauma 2019; 36(23): 3309-15.
[http://dx.doi.org/10.1089/neu.2019.6439] [PMID: 31266393]

[146] Zhu Y, Wang H, Fang J, *et al.* SS-31 provides neuroprotection by reversing mitochondrial dysfunction after traumatic brain injury. Oxid Med Cell Longev 2018; 2018: 1-12.
[http://dx.doi.org/10.1155/2018/4783602] [PMID: 30224944]

[147] Chatfield KC, Sparagna GC, Chau S, *et al.* Elamipretide improves mitochondrial function in the failing human heart. JACC Basic Transl Sci 2019; 4(2): 147-57.
[http://dx.doi.org/10.1016/j.jacbts.2018.12.005] [PMID: 31061916]

[148] Daubert MA, Yow E, Dunn G, *et al.* Novel mitochondria-targeting peptide in heart failure treatment. Circ Heart Fail 2017; 10(12): e004389.
[http://dx.doi.org/10.1161/CIRCHEARTFAILURE.117.004389] [PMID: 29217757]

[149] Sabbah HN, Gupta RC, Singh-Gupta V, Zhang K. Effects of elamipretide on skeletal muscle in dogs with experimentally induced heart failure. ESC Heart Fail 2019; 6(2): 328-35.
[http://dx.doi.org/10.1002/ehf2.12408] [PMID: 30688415]

[150] Sabbah HN, Gupta RC, Singh-Gupta V, Zhang K, Lanfear DE. Abnormalities of mitochondrial dynamics in the failing heart: Normalization following long-term therapy with elamipretide. Cardiovasc Drugs Ther 2018; 32(4): 319-28.
[http://dx.doi.org/10.1007/s10557-018-6805-y] [PMID: 29951944]

[151] Forini F, Canale P, Nicolini G, Iervasi G. Mitochondria-targeted drug delivery in cardiovascular disease: A long road to nano-cardio medicine. Pharmaceutics 2020; 12(11): 1122.
[http://dx.doi.org/10.3390/pharmaceutics12111122] [PMID: 33233847]

[152] Liu D, Jin F, Shu G, *et al.* Enhanced efficiency of mitochondria-targeted peptide SS-31 for acute kidney injury by pH-responsive and AKI-kidney targeted nanopolyplexes. Biomaterials 2019; 211: 57-67.
[http://dx.doi.org/10.1016/j.biomaterials.2019.04.034] [PMID: 31085359]

[153] Saad A, Herrmann SMS, Eirin A, *et al.* Phase 2a clinical trial of mitochondrial protection (Elamipretide) during stent revascularization in patients with atherosclerotic renal artery stenosis. Circ Cardiovasc Interv 2017; 10(9): e005487.
[http://dx.doi.org/10.1161/CIRCINTERVENTIONS.117.005487] [PMID: 28916603]

[154] Sweetwyne MT, Pippin JW, Eng DG, *et al.* The mitochondrial-targeted peptide, SS-31, improves glomerular architecture in mice of advanced age. Kidney Int 2017; 91(5): 1126-45.
[http://dx.doi.org/10.1016/j.kint.2016.10.036] [PMID: 28063595]

[155] Polyzos A, Holt A, Brown C, *et al.* Mitochondrial targeting of XJB-5-131 attenuates or improves pathophysiology in HdhQ150 animals with well-developed disease phenotypes. Hum Mol Genet 2016; 25(9): 1792-802.
[http://dx.doi.org/10.1093/hmg/ddw051] [PMID: 26908614]

[156] Polyzos AA, Wood NI, Williams P, Wipf P, Morton AJ, McMurray CT. XJB-5-131-mediated improvement in physiology and behaviour of the R6/2 mouse model of Huntington's disease is age- and sex- dependent. PLoS One 2018; 13(4): e0194580.
[http://dx.doi.org/10.1371/journal.pone.0194580] [PMID: 29630611]

[157] Xun Z, Rivera-Sánchez S, Ayala-Peña S, *et al.* Targeting of XJB-5-131 to mitochondria suppresses oxidative DNA damage and motor decline in a mouse model of Huntington's disease. Cell Rep 2012; 2(5): 1137-42.
[http://dx.doi.org/10.1016/j.celrep.2012.10.001] [PMID: 23122961]

[158] Krainz T, Gaschler MM, Lim C, Sacher JR, Stockwell BR, Wipf P. A mitochondrial-targeted nitroxide is a potent inhibitor of ferroptosis. ACS Cent Sci 2016; 2(9): 653-9.

[http://dx.doi.org/10.1021/acscentsci.6b00199] [PMID: 27725964]

[159] Yousif LF, Stewart KM, Horton KL, Kelley SO. Mitochondria-penetrating peptides: sequence effects and model cargo transport. ChemBioChem 2009; 10(12): 2081-8.
[http://dx.doi.org/10.1002/cbic.200900017] [PMID: 19670199]

[160] Zhao Z, Wu J, Xu H, *et al.* XJB-5-131 inhibited ferroptosis in tubular epithelial cells after ischemia–reperfusion injury. Cell Death Dis 2020; 11(8): 629.
[http://dx.doi.org/10.1038/s41419-020-02871-6] [PMID: 32796819]

[161] Rao VR, Lautz JD, Kaja S, Foecking EM, Lukács E, Stubbs EB Jr. Mitochondrial-targeted antioxidants attenuate TGF-β2 signaling in human trabecular meshwork cells. Invest Ophthalmol Vis Sci 2019; 60(10): 3613-24.
[http://dx.doi.org/10.1167/iovs.19-27542] [PMID: 31433458]

[162] Saberi M, Zhang X, Mobasheri A. Targeting mitochondrial dysfunction with small molecules in intervertebral disc aging and degeneration. Geroscience 2021; 43(2): 517-37.
[http://dx.doi.org/10.1007/s11357-021-00341-1] [PMID: 33634362]

[163] Fink MP, Macias CA, Xiao J, *et al.* Hemigramicidin-TEMPO conjugates: Novel mitochondria-targeted anti-oxidants. Biochem Pharmacol 2007; 74(6): 801-9.
[http://dx.doi.org/10.1016/j.bcp.2007.05.019] [PMID: 17601494]

[164] Stelmashook EV, Isaev NK, Genrikhs EE, Novikova SV. Mitochondria-targeted antioxidants as potential therapy for the treatment of traumatic brain injury. Antioxidants 2019; 8(5): 124.
[http://dx.doi.org/10.3390/antiox8050124] [PMID: 31071926]

[165] Oliver DMA, Reddy PH. Small molecules as therapeutic drugs for Alzheimer's disease. Mol Cell Neurosci 2019; 96: 47-62.
[http://dx.doi.org/10.1016/j.mcn.2019.03.001] [PMID: 30877034]

[166] Kezic A, Spasojevic I, Lezaic V, Bajcetic M. Mitochondria-targeted antioxidants: Future perspectives in kidney ischemia reperfusion injury. Oxid Med Cell Longev 2016; 2016: 1-12.
[http://dx.doi.org/10.1155/2016/2950503] [PMID: 27313826]

[167] Böhmová E, Machová D, Pechar M, *et al.* Cell-penetrating peptides: a useful tool for the delivery of various cargoes into cells. Physiol Res 2018; 67 (Suppl. 2): S267-79.
[http://dx.doi.org/10.33549/physiolres.933975] [PMID: 30379549]

[168] Alder NN, Mitchell W, Ng E, *et al.* Biophysical approaches toward understanding the molecular mechanism of action of the mitochondrial therapeutic SS-31 (Elamipretide). Biophys J 2019; 116(3) (Suppl. 1): 511a-2a.
[http://dx.doi.org/10.1016/j.bpj.2018.11.2759]

[169] Galdiero S, Gomes P. Peptide-based drugs and drug delivery systems. Molecules 2017; 22(12): 2185.
[http://dx.doi.org/10.3390/molecules22122185] [PMID: 29292757]

[170] Szeto HH. Stealth peptides target cellular powerhouses to fight rare and common age-related diseases. Protein Pept Lett 2019; 25(12): 1108-23.
[http://dx.doi.org/10.2174/0929866525666181101105209] [PMID: 30381054]

SUBJECT INDEX

www.ingramcontent.com/pod-product-compliance
Lightning Source LLC
Chambersburg PA
CBHW050807220326
41598CB00006B/144